BRAIN AND BEHAVIOR

CORE BOOKS IN PSYCHOLOGY SERIES

Edward L. Walker, Editor

BRAIN AND BEHAVIOR

Thomas L. Bennett

Colorado State University

Brooks/Cole Publishing Company
Monterey, California

A Division of Wadsworth Publishing Company, Inc.

For my parents, Tom and Trudy,
my wife, Jackie,
and our children, Dean, Shannon, Brian,
and Laurie.

Printed in the United States of America

10 9 8 7 6 5 4 3 2 1

Library of Congress Cataloging in Publication Data

Bennett, Thomas L
    Brain and behavior.

    Bibliography: p. 299.
    Includes index.
    1. Psychology, Physiological.   I. Title.
[DNLM:1. Behavior. 2. Neurophysiology. WL102 B474b]
QP360.B47   612'.82   76-26091
ISBN 0-8185-0201-0

Production Editor: *Valerie Daigen*
Interior and Cover Design: *John Edeen*

Preface

The brain is the least-known area of our universe, and, although it has been extensively studied for many years, many of its functions in regulating behavior remain a mystery. Interest in brain research and in the light it sheds on human behavior is at an all-time high. This book is intended for an introductory course in physiological psychology or brain and behavior, and in it I deliberately emphasize those topics that I've found in my teaching to be of greatest interest to students. Therefore, although most of the studies involve nonhuman species, human research is discussed whenever possible.

The aim of this book is to provide a description of current knowledge about how the brain regulates behavior—a description that requires of the reader no special background in either psychology or the biological sciences. All concepts from these disciplines are defined when they are introduced in the text; I've also provided a glossary at the end of the book. It is my belief that brain research can be comprehensively discussed in an intelligible manner. Therefore, I have tried to write a book that is readable for all college students, regardless of their major field of study. I hope that my presentation of suggestions for future research and of unanswered major questions in the brain-and-behavior literature will stimulate the students to propose their own unique solutions to controversial problems.

Since this text is intended for the first course in physiological psychology, it begins, after an introductory chapter, with basic neurophysiology and neuroanatomy (Chapters 2 and 3). This information is the framework on which principles of brain functioning are constructed in the later chapters. Research methods are discussed next (Chapter 4), to acquaint the reader with the "tools of the trade." Chapters 5 and 6 complete the framework by describing input and output of behavior—in other words, sensory processes and brain control of movement. The chapters up to this point in the text, because of their nature, are not as heavily referenced as are the seven chapters that represent the real message of this book: how the brain controls behavior. In order, the topics considered in the second half of the book are arousal, sleep, and dreaming (Chapter 7), emotion and attempts at emotional control through psychosurgery (Chapter 8), motivation (Chapter 9), and learning and memory (Chapters 10 through 13). Each of these chapters provides both historic and recent findings regarding how the brain regulates behavior.

Many people contributed to the final development of this book. My greatest debt of gratitude is to my wife, Jackie, who critically read the entire manuscript and made many suggestions to improve the quality of my presentation. Several individuals reviewed parts of or the entire manuscript, and their suggestions improved the quality of the final product. For this help, I would like to thank Judith P. Goggin, University of Texas, El Paso, Kenneth F. Green, California State University, Long Beach, Laverne C. Johnson, Naval Regional Medical Center, San Diego, James

McGaugh, University of California, Irvine, James B. Ranck, Jr., State University of New York, Downstate Medical Center, and Charles Weiss, College of the Holy Cross.

Finally, I would like to thank the staff of Brooks/Cole Publishing Company for their help on this project; I would particularly like to acknowledge Claire Verduin, Project Development Editor, and Valerie Daigen, Production Editor, for their assistance at all stages of the manuscript's preparation.

Thomas L. Bennett

Contents

1
Introduction

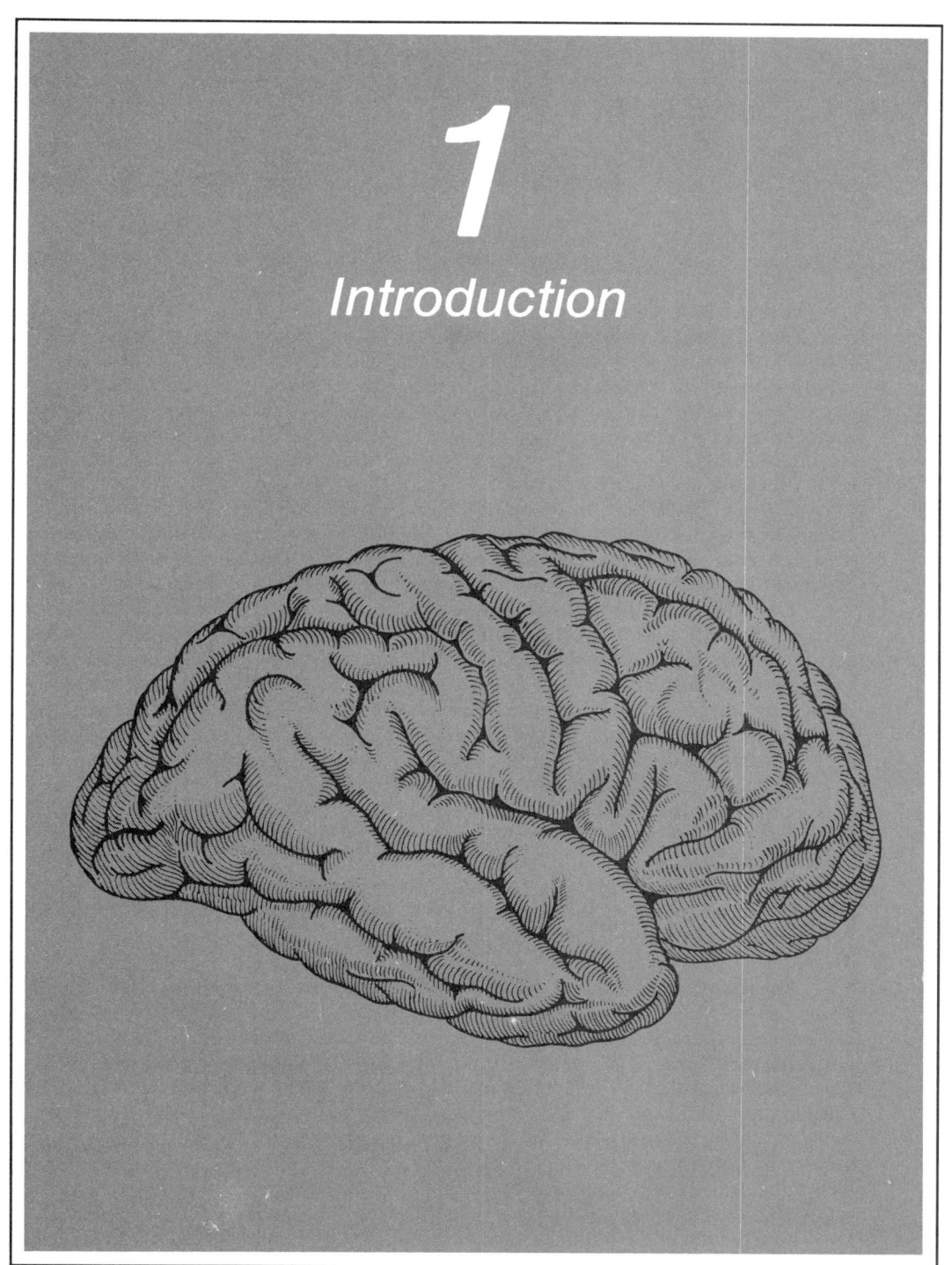

Just beneath the human skull is an exceedingly complex labyrinth of approximately 10–12 billion cells, called the **brain.** The brain is not very impressive to look at. It is pinkish gray in color and has the consistency of cooked oatmeal or soft cheese; it weighs only about 1.5 kg (3.5 lb.). However, this lump of living tissue is the most marvelous and intricate structure existing in nature; it is many times more complex than the most sophisticated of computers. Thousands of scientists throughout the world are dedicated to the task of unveiling the brain's secrets, but many, if not most of its functions are still mysterious.

Galen (129–199A.D.) was one of the first writers to recognize the importance of this master control organ. Galen localized the mind in the brain; Aristotle had placed it in the heart. It is not overstating the case to suggest that everything the human organism has ever been, is now, or will be is the product of its brain.

The purpose of this book is to describe the functions of the brain in regulating behavior. Scientists who investigate these functions call themselves by various names, including physiological psychologist, neuropsychologist, psychobiologist, and neuroscientist. They have a common goal, however—to clarify the role of the brain in regulating and controlling behavior. They strive to attain this goal with the belief that, by increasing our knowledge of the physiological mechanisms that underlie behavior, we will increase our understanding of behavior itself.

The answers to the questions that the neuropsychologist poses may someday shed light on the nature of the human species. For example, a neuropsychologist may ask "What happens when an object passes in front of us? What brain mechanisms allow us to detect the object, analyze it, and react to it?"

We spend a third of each day in a state of suspended animation called sleep. Why do we go to sleep? What is happening to our brains and bodies during this period? What events in the brain trigger the unique state of existence we call dreaming?

Aggression and violence are pressing problems in our society. How does the brain control these behaviors? In 1966, Charles Whitman killed his wife and his mother and then climbed to the top of the administration-building tower at the University of Texas and started firing a rifle at random at people walking below. Before he was killed by police, he shot 44 people, 14 of whom died. Postmortem examination indicated that Whitman had a cancerous tumor in his brain near a structure called the **amygdala.** Brain research has shown that the amygdala performs important functions in emotion. Did the tumor cause the man's aberrant behavior? Could this tragedy have been prevented if the diseased tissue had been detected and removed?

Satisfaction of the biological drives, including the drives for food, water, and sex, is an important determinant of behavior. How does the brain signal to an individual

2

to engage in behaviors that will diminish these drive states? How does the brain determine when these drive states have been satisfied?

The most fascinating thing about the brain is its capacity for storing millions of bits of information. Although an event may not have been recalled in years, the brain can bring that information into consciousness. We have all had the experience of suddenly remembering an experience we had years ago. Perhaps our memory was jogged by something a friend said. A most striking experience occurs during dream sleep; we may find ourselves visiting with a friend whom we have not seen or perhaps even thought about in years. What is memory? Are there particular brain regions required for information storage? How does memory get stored? How do memories remain intact and unmolested for years, able to suddenly reappear in our conscious minds?

The ultimate objective of brain-and-behavior research is to understand how the brain mediates human behavior. However, most of the research that I will discuss in this book has used nonhuman animals as the experimental subjects because the research often involves damaging or stimulating parts of the brain. I want to emphasize that, whenever researchers use animals in their experiments, they are very careful to conduct their work in a humane fashion and to make the animals as comfortable as possible. In my discussions, I will bring in human data where possible. The human data will be mostly of a clinical nature, which means that the investigators have studied the effects of brain disease or injury on behavior. I will also describe the available information regarding the effects of surgically induced brain lesions in human patients. This radical surgical procedure is sometimes used to alleviate intractable seizures accompanying severe epilepsy or to treat psychopathology, but it is done only after more conservative treatments have failed.

The topics of this book are organized as follows. The book begins, in the next chapter, with a description of the anatomy and physiology of the basic functional unit of the brain, the nerve cell or **neuron.** Chapter 3, on neuroanatomy, describes how neurons are organized into brain structures; both the phylogenetic (evolutionary) and ontogenetic (maturational) development of the brain will be discussed. With these basic concepts of neural or brain function in mind, you will then learn about the types of research methods used by neuroscientists to study brain-behavior relations. This chapter on techniques is followed by two chapters that describe the basic input and output of behavior: sensory processes and neural control of movement. The first six chapters thus give you the framework for considering the operations of the brain in the control of complex behavior processes.

Chapters 7–13 attempt to comprehensively discuss current evidence regarding brain-behavior relations. The topics that will be considered are arousal, sleep, and dreaming (Chapter 7), emotion (Chapter 8), motivation (Chapter 9), and learning and memory (Chapters 10–13). As you read this book, you will rapidly realize that often as many questions as answers arise from brain-and-behavior experiments. I have tried to suggest resolutions to apparent conflicts and possible directions for future research whenever possible. I'm sure that you will discover novel answers of your own to some of these questions as you read through these pages. When you have had that experience, you will know the excitement felt by researchers in this field.

2

The Neuron

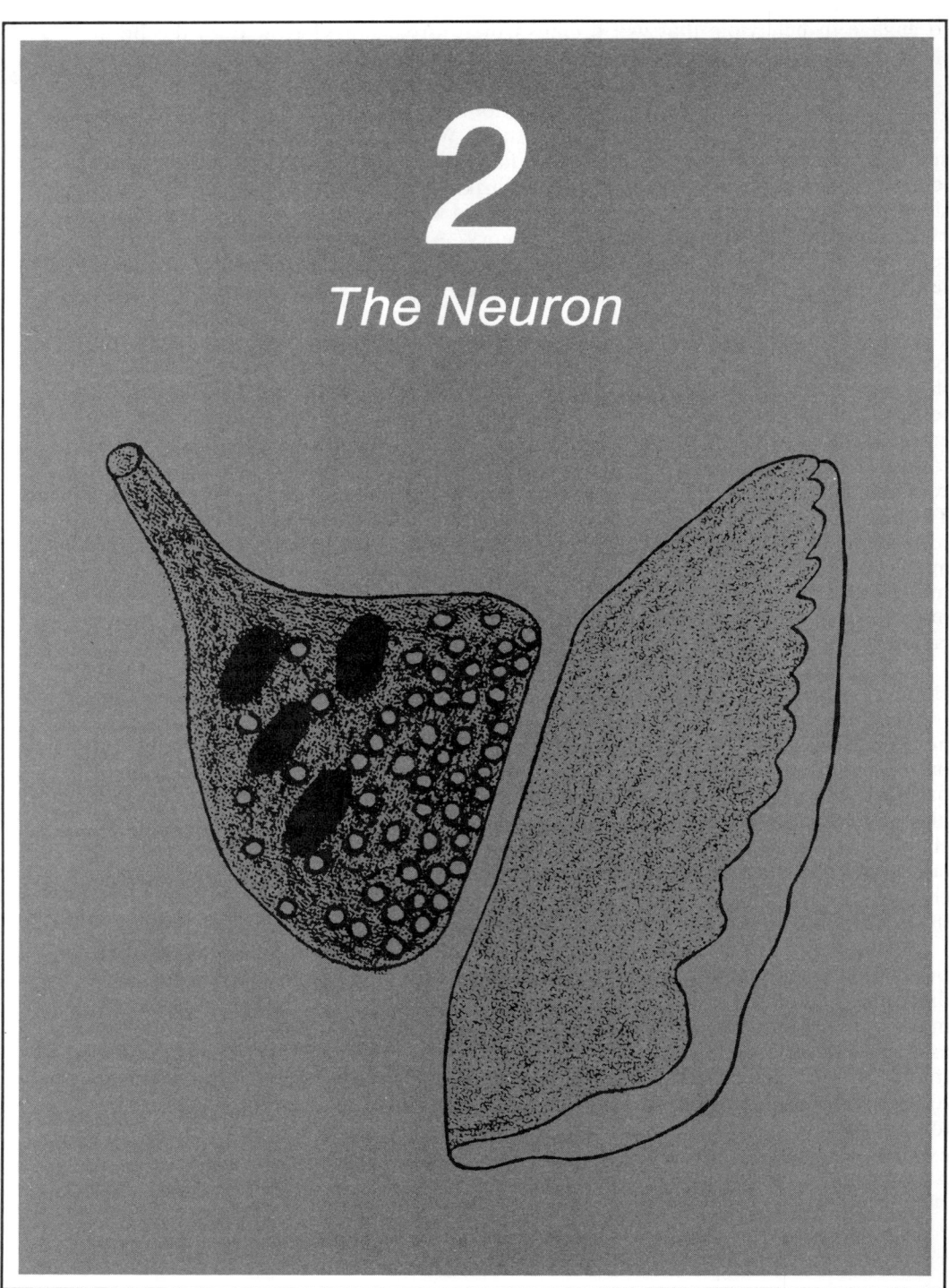

The cell is the building block of the body, and different types of cells are organized to perform different functions. For example, the gastrointestinal system functions to digest and absorb food, the respiratory system is specialized to take up oxygen and to eliminate carbon dioxide, and the reproductive system allows for preservation of the species. Our primary interest in this book is in the nervous system—a system that is specialized to mediate the activities of all other systems in the body and that is responsible for the behavior repertoire that makes us unique as individuals.

Around the beginning of the 20th century, it became well established that the nerve cell or **neuron** is the basic functional unit of the nervous system. Neurons are specialized for the transmission of information. In this chapter, an overview of how neurons transmit and process information will be presented. Before examining these functions of nervous tissue, it is important that you become familiar with some basic notions of cell biology. For a more detailed description than will be possible in this book, see Ganong (1975) or Guyton (1971).

Some Basic Principles of Cell Biology

At the risk of oversimplifying, it can be stated that the living cell consists of a **nucleus** surrounded by a liquid **cytoplasm.** The **cellular membrane** forms the outer boundary of the cell, which separates the **intracellular fluid** (interior of the cell) from the **extracellular fluid** in the spaces outside the cells. From the extracellular fluid, the cells take up oxygen, various nutrients, and ions essential for maintaining life; waste products from the cells are discharged into this fluid compartment.

There are differences between the extracellular and intracellular fluids in terms of the concentrations of certain ions. An **ion** is an electrically charged particle. It is an atom or molecule that has gained or lost electrons to complete its outer electron shell and that, as a result, has acquired a net electrical charge. Since ions have a complete outer electron shell, they are relatively inert chemically; that is, one cannot join another to form a new chemical compound. However, because of their electrical charge—either positive or negative—ions will attract other ions having opposite charges and repel other ions having like charges. Positively charged ions are called *cations,* while negatively charged ions are referred to as *anions.* As you will see later in this chapter, the movement of ions through the cell membrane of neurons provides the basis for the transfer of information in nervous tissue.

As I indicated, there are differences in the concentrations of certain ions in the extracellular and intracellular fluids. The extracellular fluid contains large amounts of sodium (Na^+), chloride (Cl^-), calcium (Ca^+), and bicarbonate (HCO_3^-) ions and has a

5

relatively low content of protein anions. The intracellular fluid, on the other hand, has a high concentration of protein anions, potassium (K^+), magnesium (Mg^{++}), and phosphate (PO_4^{---}) ions. The differences in ion distribution across the cell membrane are at least partially mediated by special transport mechanisms, which will be discussed later in this chapter. At this point, just remember that these observed differences in the distribution of ions across the cell membrane are very important.

Associated with these differing ionic concentrations is a *potential difference*— that is, a *difference in voltage*— across the membrane of the cell. The magnitude of this **resting membrane potential** varies greatly from tissue to tissue but ranges from 10 to 100 millivolts (mv; 1 mv = 1/1000 volt), with the inside of the cell negatively charged with respect to the exterior. In nervous tissue, changes in the membrane potential due to the movements of ions across the cell membrane reflect and form the basis for information transfer. The processes by which these events occur will be elaborated on later in this chapter. Before we examine those processes, let's review the anatomy of a nerve cell.

The Anatomy of the Neuron

A spinal motor neuron is shown in Figure 2-1. The main body of the nerve cell is called the **soma**; typically, a soma is approximately 5–100 microns (μ) in diameter. A micron is equal to one-millionth of a meter. Extending out from the soma are a number of **dendrites,** which branch extensively, and a long **axon,** which originates from a thickened area of the soma called the **axon hillock.** The dendrites and the axon, which are sometimes called *processes,* serve to transmit information in the nervous system. The dendrites conduct information or **excitation** toward the body of the cell. This is referred to as the **afferent** direction with respect to the cell body. In contrast, axons carry information in an **efferent** direction—that is, away from the soma.

Figure 2-1
A motor neuron with a myelinated axon. From Review of Medical Physiology *(7th ed.), by W. F. Ganong. Copyright 1975 by Lange Medical Publications. Reprinted by permission.*

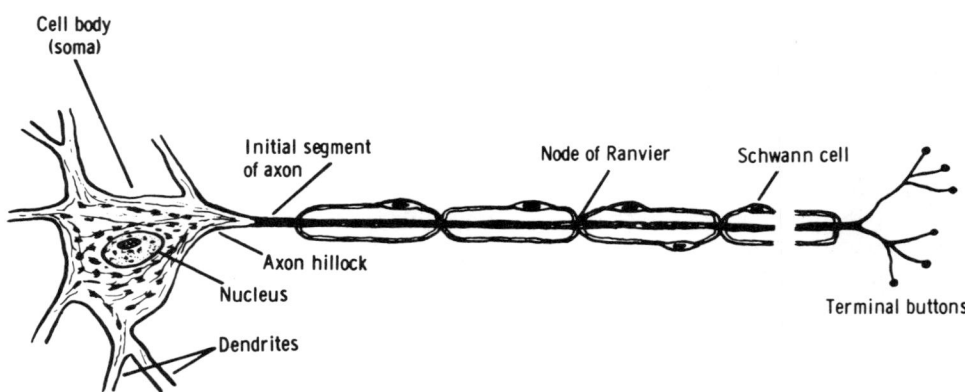

The size of a neuron's processes compared with the size of its soma is really amazing in some cases. Ganong (1975) gives as an example the spinal motor neurons that supply the muscles of the foot. Their axons can be up to several meters long. Ganong indicates that, if the cell body of one of these neurons were the size of a tennis ball, the dendrites of this cell would fill an average-sized living room; the axon would be up to 1.6 km (almost a mile) in length, although only about 13 mm in diameter.

If we follow the axon pictured in Figure 2-1 away from the cell body, toward its extremity, we find that it branches into a number of **terminal arborizations**; at the tip of each of these branches is a **terminal button.** An axon conducts information to adjacent nerve cells or to muscle fibers via these terminal buttons. It is important to note that an axon is not physically connected to the cells to which it relates. Rather, there is a discriminable space separating them. We call this functional junction between the terminal buttons of one neuron and the next cell a **synapse.** Approximately 100–500 angstroms (Å) separate the cell membranes at synaptic junctions. An angstrom is equal to one ten-billionth of a meter. The structure of a synapse is shown in Figure 2-2.

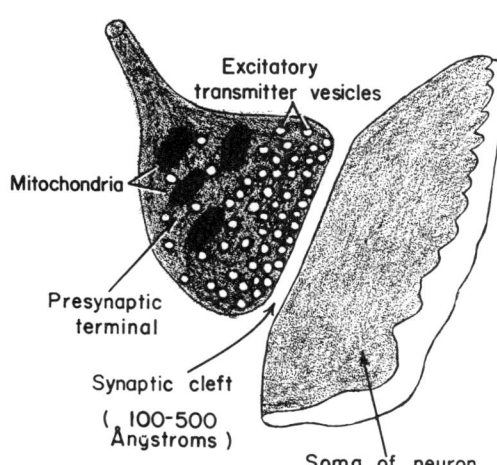

*Figure 2-2
The synapse. From* Textbook of Medical Physiology *(4th ed.), by A. C. Guyton. Copyright 1971 by W. B. Saunders Company. Reprinted by permission.*

A short distance from its origin on the axon hillock, the axon acquires a coating called the **myelin sheath.** The myelin sheath is made up of many layers of *Schwann cells* in the peripheral nervous system and *neuroglia* in the central nervous system. The Schwann cells and neuroglia actually coil around the axon, thereby forming the multiple layers that make up myelin. The myelin sheath is a characteristic of axons only. Neither the dendrites nor the cell body is covered with myelin.

Axons vary greatly with respect to their degree of myelinization. Large-diameter axons are typically heavily myelinated and appear white. In contrast, smaller axons are often poorly myelinated or essentially unmyelinated and appear gray. All axons are enveloped with Schwann cells or neuroglia, but in some cases these cells are not coiled around the fiber to produce the multiple layers characteristic of the myelin sheath. The degree of myelinization is a measure of the number of layers of cells that form the myelin sheath. Later in this chapter, you will see that the degree of myelinization is one of the factors determining the rate of information conduction by nerve cells.

Looking at Figure 2-1 again, you will note that the myelin sheath covers the axon except at its endings or terminal arborizations and except at regular interruptions or constrictions, which occur approximately 1 mm apart. These discontinuities in the myelin sheath, at which the axon comes into direct contact with the extracellular fluid, are called the **nodes of Ranvier.**

Nerve cells conduct information. This process is an electrical event and can be recorded. The conduction of information by a neuron is called the *nerve impulse.* To understand the nature of the nerve impulse, one must understand the electrical characteristics of the resting or inactive nerve cell. These characteristics make up the **resting membrane potential.**

Resting Membrane Potential

Earlier in this chapter, I indicated that there is an unequal distribution of certain ions on the two sides of the cellular membrane of living cells—that is, in the extracellular versus the intracellular fluid. I also indicated that a resting membrane potential of 10–100 mv was associated with this ionic distribution. This potential difference or voltage is determined by using two recording electrodes attached to an amplifier device. One of the electrodes is inserted into the cell, while the second electrode is placed on the cell's surface. The magnitude of the resting membrane potential has been found to be approximately 70 mv for most nerve cells. The resting membrane potential is conventionally expressed as a negative potential, $^-70$ mv, because *the inside of the neuron is negatively charged relative to the exterior.*

Of all the ions present in the intracellular and extracellular compartments, the distributions of four seem to be especially important in determining the resting membrane potential. These are Na^+, Cl^-, K^+, and intracellular proteins and other organic anions, which will be represented by the symbol A^-. The cell membrane varies greatly with respect to its permeability to these ions. **Permeability** refers to how easily a substance can pass through the cell membrane. The cell membrane is essentially impermeable to A^-, moderately permeable to Na^+, and highly permeable to K^+ and Cl^- ions. The basis for the observed differences in membrane permeability to various small ions is not clear. However, it has been proposed that the membrane contains small pores or holes and that differences in permeability can be explained on the basis of ion size. For example, the diameter of an Na^+ ion is about 50% greater than that of either K^+ or Cl^- ions. These latter two ions (K^+ and Cl^-) are about the same size (Eccles, 1957).

There appear to be two major factors accounting for the unequal distribution of ions and the resulting resting membrane potential in cells. The first of these is the synthesis within the cell of A^-; again, these are large protein molecules and other organic anions, to which the cell membrane is impermeable. The second factor is the operation of the sodium-potassium pump.

Factors Influencing the Transmembrane Ionic Distribution

As indicated earlier, there are more Cl^- ions in the extracellular fluid compartment than in the cell, and, for this reason, the ions tend to diffuse into the cell along this **concentration gradient.** However, they cannot reach an equal distribution across the membrane, because the interior of the cell is negatively charged, due to the presence of A^- ions. Thus, the Cl^- ions flow into the cell along the concentration gradient, but they are pushed out along an **electrical gradient.** An equilibrium is reached in this system when the Cl^- influx and Cl^- efflux become equal and the net exchange is zero. When this point is reached, we find that Cl⁻ ions are approximately 14 times more concentrated on the outside than on the inside of the cell.

The membrane potential that should exist when this observed equilibrium distribution of Cl⁻ ions has been attained can be calculated, and it is called the **equilibrium potential.** The calculated value is almost identical to the observed resting membrane potential. For this reason, it can be concluded that no forces affect the movement of Cl⁻ ions across the membrane other than the electrical and the concentration gradients.

In the case of potassium ions (K^+), the concentration gradient tends to move them outward, while the electrical gradient tends to move them inward. We find that K^+ ions are approximately 30 times more concentrated on the inside of the cell than on the outside. We can again calculate the electrical gradient that would be required to account for this relative distribution. In the case of K^+ ions, it turns out that the calculated equilibrium potential (-100 mv) is actually larger than what naturally occurs across the membrane of nerve cells. Thus, something in addition to the chemical and electrical gradients must be affecting the movement of K^+ ions. Specifically, this additional factor is the active transport of K^+ ions into the cell. The mechanism involved in this active transport process will be described below.

The forces acting on the distribution of sodium ions (Na^+) across the cell membrane result in a different situation from that seen with the K^+ and Cl⁻ ions. For Na^+ ions, the concentration and the electrical gradients are working in the same direction. Both influence the flow of Na^+ ions in an inward direction. Although the membrane is permeable to the flow of Na^+ ions, the intracellular level of Na^+ remains low. In fact, Na^+ is approximately ten times as concentrated on the outside of the cell membrane as it is on the inside. The electrical gradient that would be required to produce this concentration gradient would have to be approximately 50 mv *positive inside* with respect to the exterior. However, as indicated, it is known that the interior is approximately 70 mv negative with respect to the exterior. Hence, to obtain the observed concentrations of Na^+ across the cell membrane, there must be an active transport system that moves Na^+ ions out of the cell against a steep inward diffusion gradient composed of the combined forces of the electrical and concentration gradients.

The Sodium-Potassium Pump. The mechanism responsible for this active transport process is the **sodium-potassium pump;** it is often referred to simply as the *sodium pump.* The pump is responsible for both the active transport of Na^+ out of the cell and the active inward transport of K^+. The details of the operation of the sodium-potassium pump are gradually being filled in by researchers but still require a great deal of further clarification.

The postulated operation of the sodium-potassium pump is diagramed in Figure 2-3. The pump is located in the cell membrane and derives its energy from metabolic processes in the interior of the cell. According to this model (see Guyton, 1971, for details), Na^+ inside the cell combines with a carrier Y at the inner surface of the membrane to form large quantities of the combination NaY. NaY is transported to the exterior, where Na^+ is released and the carrier Y changes its chemical composition slightly to become carrier X. Carrier X next combines with K^+ to form KX. KX then moves to the interior of the membrane. On the inner surface of the membrane, energy is provided to split K from X via the influence of the enzyme ATPase. The energy is derived from the compound MgATP (magnesium adenosine triphosphate). The omnipresent ATP molecule is the principal source of energy for cellular processes.

The sodium-potassium pump is believed to be more effective in transporting Na^+ than in transporting K^+ ions. Usually, approximately three Na^+ ions are transported for every two K^+ ions. Presumably, the operation of this pump is regulated by the internal Na^+ concentration, so that the 10:1 external-to-internal concentration ratio of Na^+ ions is maintained despite the combined electrical and concentration gradients, which tend to force Na^+ ions inward.

Figure 2-3
The postulated mechanism for active transport of sodium and potassium through the cell membrane. From Textbook of Medical Physiology *(4th ed.), by A. C. Guyton. Copyright 1971 by W. B. Saunders Company. Reprinted by permission.*

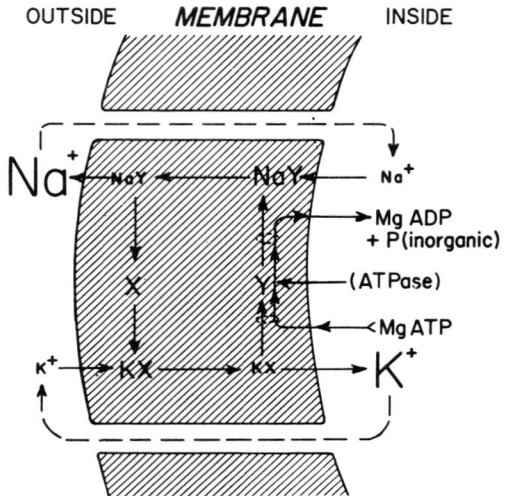

The factors described above are the basis for the observed ionic distribution across the membrane of a resting neuron. This distribution results in the resting membrane potential. It should be emphasized that the number of ions accounting for the resting membrane potential represents only a minute fraction of the total number of ions present. As I've said, changes in the membrane potential due to changes in the distribution of ions relative to the resting state form the basis for information transmission in nervous tissue. We next turn to an examination of this process.

The Action Potential

As long as the cell membrane remains undisturbed, the resting membrane potential remains at a level of approximately -70 mv. However, if an adequate stimulus is applied to this membrane, a *nerve impulse* or **action potential** will occur. The action potential is the physiological basis of information transfer in the nervous system. Information is conducted as the frequency of impulses per second. The action potential is a sequence of rapid changes in membrane potential lasting a fraction of a millisecond (1 millisecond = 1/1000 second). During this sequence, the resting membrane potential is reversed and then immediately returns to its resting level. This means that, during the fraction of a millisecond in which the nerve impulse occurs, the membrane potential becomes internally positive with respect to the exterior. The ionic movements that form the basis for these electrical events will be detailed next.

We normally think of the action potential as occurring in two successive stages—namely, **depolarization** and **repolarization.** These stages are illustrated in Figure 2-4. Part A of the illustration depicts the resting membrane potential, the interior being negatively charged and the exterior being positively charged. *Depolarization occurs when a stimulus suddenly increases the permeability of the membrane to Na^+ ions.* The Na^+ ions rush into the cell. This inward movement of these positively charged particles yields a reversal of the transmembrane potential, so that the inside is now positive and the outside negative. This process is illustrated by section B in Figure 2-4 and is called *depolarization.*

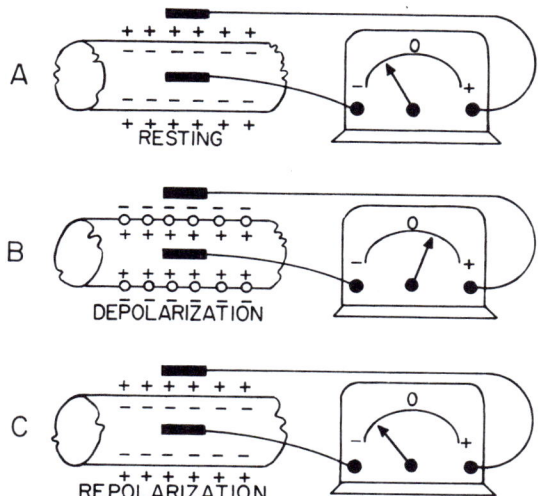

Figure 2-4
The sequence of events during the action potential. From Textbook of Medical Physiology *(4th ed.), by A. C. Guyton. Copyright 1971 by W. B. Saunders Company. Reprinted by permission.*

Almost immediately after depolarization takes place, the membrane pores again become impermeable to Na^+ ions. The reversed potential then disappears, followed by a return of the resting membrane potential. This latter process, *repolarization,* is depicted in section C. To give you further understanding of the processes underlying the nerve impulse, I'll describe how this sequence of events occurs. For my discussion, I'll use the model detailed by Guyton (1971).

Changes in Sodium Conductance during Depolarization

As indicated, a nerve impulse is initiated when there is a sudden, dramatic increase in the permeability of the membrane to Na^+. It is postulated that this alteration in the membrane permeability is mediated by calcium (Ca^+) ions in the following way. Experimental evidence has suggested the existence of sodium channels of some type, through which Na^+ ions can flow to bring about a reversal of the membrane potential during depolarization. It has been further postulated that, during the resting state, an influx of Na^+ ions is prevented by the presence of calcium

(Ca^+) ions, which are attached to the sides of these channels. Because of their positive charge, the Ca^+ ions repel Na^+ and other positively charged ions and thereby prevent their movement through these channels.

It is further thought that the effect of an action-potential-inducing stimulus is to displace some of these Ca^+ ions. This allows an initial inflow of Na^+ ions. As the Na^+ ions rush into the cell, they displace more of the Ca^+ ions from their sites, and this process accelerates until most of the Ca^+ ions have been displaced. The resistance to a Na^+ influx is thereby abolished. This change in Na^+ conductance is plotted in Figure 2-5. This figure demonstrates that the permeability of the membrane to the inward flow of Na^+ ions increases several thousandfold in only a fraction of a millisecond.

Figure 2-5
Changes in sodium and potassium conductance during the action potential in a giant-squid axon. The dotted line represents the action potential superimposed on the same time coordinate. The unit of conductance—the mmho—is the reciprocal of the unit of resistance—the mohm (milliohm). From "Ionic Movements and Electrical Activity in Giant Nerve Fibers," by A. L. Hodgkin, Proceedings of the Royal Society of London, 1958, B.148, 1–37. Copyright 1958 by the Royal Society. (Adapted by Ganong, 1975.) Reprinted by permission.

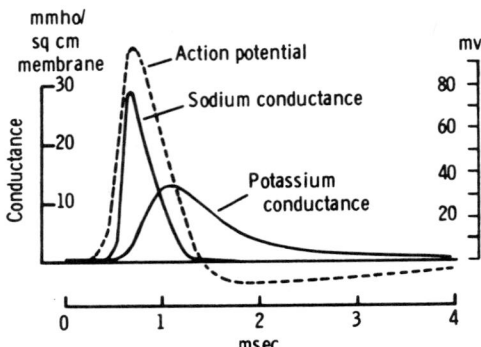

The effect of the movement of the positively charged Na^+ ions is to bring about a reversal of the membrane potential in a fraction of a millisecond. With the inside of the membrane now positive, further inflow of Na^+ ions is blocked. According to the theory, the cessation of the Na^+ influx permits the Ca^+ ions to rebind to the sodium channels until the channels again become almost totally impermeable to Na^+ ions. Thus, at the onset of an action potential, the flow of Na^+ into the cell dramatically increases in a fraction of a millisecond; the flow then decreases to its original resting level in another fraction of a millisecond. It is the inward movement of Na^+ ions that accounts for the depolarization of the cell membrane.

The Ionic Basis of Repolarization

Before a neuron can fire again, the resting membrane potential must be reestablished; that is, repolarization must occur. On first thought, a likely explanation for repolarization would be the ejection of Na^+ ions via the activity of the sodium pump, but it has been demonstrated that the sodium pump plays almost no role in this process. The sodium pump operates much too slowly to recharge the membrane in the fraction of a millisecond that has been shown to elapse before the neuron can be excited again. Instead, the immediate recovery of the resting membrane potential is accomplished by an outflow of potassium (K^+) ions.

Referring back to Figure 2-5, we can see that K^+ conductance does not change significantly during the first half of the action potential. However, it increases approximately 30 to 40 times toward the end of the action potential. The mechanism for the observed K$^+$ conductance alterations is hypothetical, as is the mechanism that governs the influx of Na$^+$. It is thought that the reversal of the membrane potential initiates the outward flow of K$^+$ ions, which in turn opens potassium channels in much the same way as was outlined for the sodium channels. Researchers believe that these potassium channels are separate from the sodium channels, but this fact remains to be established.

The important point to be made here is that the outflow of K$^+$ ions brings about the repolarization of the cell membrane. Figure 2-5 illustrates that, as Na$^+$ conductance returns to its resting level, the outward flow of K$^+$ ions increases greatly. It has been experimentally verified that the observed rapid outward movement of K$^+$ ions is capable of returning the membrane potential to its resting level of approximately -70 mv.

Only a tiny fraction of the available Na$^+$ and K$^+$ ions are exchanged during a single action potential. For this reason, the occurrence of many thousands of successive nerve impulses will not seriously alter the relative external and internal concentrations of these ions. Moreover, although the sodium-potassium pump is not rapid enough to eject Na$^+$ ions for recovery of excitability during a millisecond, the pump still operates continuously and replaces the external K$^+$ ions with Na$^+$ ions during those periods when the neuron is inactive.

In summary, the excitation of a neuron is signaled by the occurrence of an action potential. The observed changes in the membrane potential result from the movements of Na$^+$ and K$^+$ ions. Na$^+$ inflow occurs first and causes depolarization—that is, a reversal of the polarity of the membrane. K$^+$ outflow promptly follows and brings about a restoration of the resting membrane potential. With an overall view of the ionic basis of the nerve impulse in mind, let's next examine the characteristics of the nerve impulse.

Characteristics of the Action Potential

The All-or-None Law. One of the most notable features of a nerve impulse is that, in order for one to occur, the intensity of stimulation must be above a certain level, which is called the **threshold** for firing the neuron. This threshold will vary according to the experimental conditions and the characteristics of the nerve fiber, but, once the firing threshold is surpassed, a full-blown action potential will be produced. Another feature of interest is that, if the intensity of stimulation is increased beyond the firing threshold, no changes in the action potential will occur. Thus, subthreshold stimuli will fail to produce an action potential, but, once the threshold for firing a given neuron is surpassed, the resultant action potentials are always of the same form and amplitude. For this reason, it is said that the action potential follows the **all-or-none law.** According to the all-or-none law, a nerve impulse either takes place at a certain amplitude or not at all. Furthermore, once a nerve impulse is initiated on a nerve fiber or axon, it is conducted to the end of the axon without a decrease in magnitude. The mechanisms underlying the propagation of a nerve impulse down an axon will be described later in this chapter.

Changes in Excitability Correlated with Phases of the Action Potential. There are changes in the excitability of a neuron—that is, in the ease of initiation of subsequent nerve impulses—that are correlated with different phases of the action potential. The changes in excitability are illustrated in Figure 2-6, which depicts a typical action potential. The initial, very large change in membrane potential, which corresponds to membrane depolarization, is called the *spike potential.* The term *spike potential* may be used interchangeably with *action potential* or *nerve impulse.* As indicated, the spike potential is of constant magnitude for any given neuron, and, once initiated, it passes unaltered along the length of the axon. The **absolute refractory period** corresponds to the interval during which the spike appears, and no additional activity can be induced by a stimulus of any strength until the spike has been completed and the membrane potential has begun to return to its resting level.

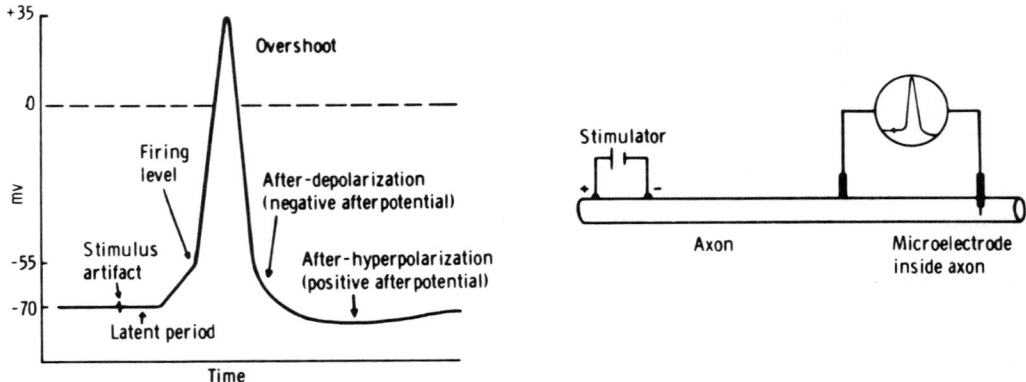

Figure 2-6
An action potential ("spike potential") recorded with one electrode inside the cell. From Review of Medical Physiology *(7th ed.), by W. F. Ganong. Copyright 1975 by Lange Medical Publications. Reprinted by permission.*

The **relative refractory period** corresponds to the short period during the tail of the spike. During this interval, only a stimulus much stronger than is normally required can initiate an action potential. The relative refractory period is followed by the **negative afterpotential,** which is seen in Figure 2-6 as the broad base at the end of the tail of the spike. When the negative afterpotential occurs, the neuron is partially depolarized. This is a period of increased excitability; a stimulus of less strength than is normally required is capable of producing an action potential.

The negative afterpotential is in turn followed by the **positive afterpotential,** which is seen below the level of the resting membrane potential. The positive afterpotential corresponds to a period of decreased excitability or hyperpolarization during which a stimulus of greater than normal strength is required for production of a nerve impulse. Presumably, this period of hyperpolarization results from a K^+ overshoot; that is, more than enough K^+ ions rush to the outside of the cell membrane than are required for recovery of the resting membrane potential. Finally, although this change is not depicted on the graph, the neuron regains its normal sensitivity. The spike potential is the message carrier of the nervous system, while the afterpotentials determine the readiness with which subsequent messages will be accepted.

Conduction of the Nerve Impulse

The Rate of Conduction

Once a nerve impulse is initiated in an axon, it is conducted to the end of the fiber without a decrease in magnitude. This process is referred to as **propagation of the action potential.** The rate of conduction of the nerve impulse varies as a direct

function of the diameter of the nerve fiber and the thickness of the myelin sheath.
Specifically, the rate at which the action potential is propagated increases with increases in the cross-sectional diameter of the axon and with increases in the thickness of the surrounding myelin sheath. The velocity of conduction varies from as little as 0.5 meter per second in very small, unmyelinated fibers to as fast as 130 meters (the length of a football field) per second in some very-large-diameter, heavily myelinated fibers (Guyton, 1971).

The Ionic Basis of Conduction

Unmyelinated Fibers. On the basis of the information already presented about ionic transfer during the nerve impulse, a simple model to account for conduction can be constructed. If a stimulus is applied to an axon and if this stimulus is above the threshold for firing the axon, then an action potential will occur. When the membrane potential is reversed, during the action potential, because of the Na^+ influx, the excited area becomes a "sink" into which Na^+ ions from adjacent, nonexcited regions flow. By drawing off positive charges, this flow partially depolarizes these adjacent regions. The resultant decrease in polarity in the adjoining sections of the axon leads to a local action potential, which then partially depolarizes the region that is in turn next to it, and the wave of depolarization is thereby propagated down the axon. The depolarization appears to travel like a wave on the ocean.

If a stimulus is applied at the center of a long fiber, the excitation wave proceeds toward both ends until the entire membrane has become depolarized. Fibers conduct equally in all directions. Repolarization of the fiber will first occur at the initial point of stimulation and then spread progressively along the membrane, following the depolarization process by a few ten-thousandths of a second.

Myelinated Fibers. In a heavily myelinated fiber, the process of propagation is slightly different from that in unmyelinated fibers. In the case of myelinated axons, the fiber is, in effect, insulated by the myelin sheath. However, as indicated earlier in this chapter, the myelin sheath is interrupted at approximately 1-mm intervals by the nodes of Ranvier. The axon comes into direct contact with the extracellular fluid at these discontinuities in the myelin sheath. Although ions cannot flow through the sheath, they can easily flow through the membrane at the nodes of Ranvier. It has been estimated that the membrane at these points is 500 times more permeable to the flow of ions than is the membrane of some unmyelinated fibers (Guyton, 1971). At the nodes, depolarization and the action potential occur as described previously. The result is that the wave of depolarization appears to jump from node to node. This phenomenon has given rise to the use of the term **saltatory conduction** to describe propagation of nerve impulses in myelinated fibers. Between the nodes, the electrical current flows passively through the axoplasm (the protoplasm of an axon), exciting successive nodes one after another. Saltatory conduction along a myelinated axon is depicted in Figure 2-7.

Synaptic Transmission

Earlier in this chapter, I indicated that the exceedingly narrow (100–500 Å) junction between the terminal buttons of an axon and an adjacent cell is called a synapse. Propagation or transmission across this protoplasmic discontinuity is a

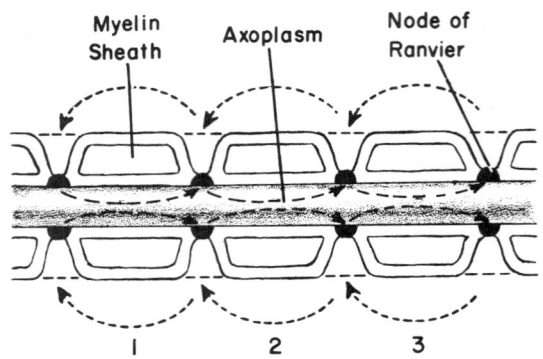

Figure 2-7
*Saltatory
conduction along a
myelinated axon.
From* Textbook of
Medical Physiology
*(4th ed.), by A. C.
Guyton. Copyright
1971 by W. B.
Saunders Company.
Reprinted by
permission.*

Myelin
Sheath   Axoplasm   Node of
Ranvier

1   2   3

different process from transmission in the axon. One very important distinction is that transmission can move in only one direction.

The number of terminal buttons varies from as few as one per postsynaptic cell for some midbrain synapses to as many as approximately 5500 on a single postsynaptic spinal neuron (see Figure 2-8). There are three types of synapses. Axons may end on a dendrite (*axo-dendritic*), the cell body (*axo-somatic*), or the axon (*axo-axonic*) of another cell. According to Ganong (1975), there are approximately 10^{14} synapses in the human brain. On the average, each of the 10 billion neurons in the brain has 100 inputs converging on it. In turn, each neuron diverges to 100 other neurons. Thus, the number of possible pathways that can be taken by a nerve impulse is incredibly large.

Figure 2-8
*A typical
motor neuron,
showing synapses
with presynaptic
terminals that
originate from other
neurons. From*
Textbook of
Medical Physiology
*(4th ed.), by A. C.
Guyton. Copyright
1971 by W. B.
Saunders Company.
Reprinted by
permission.*

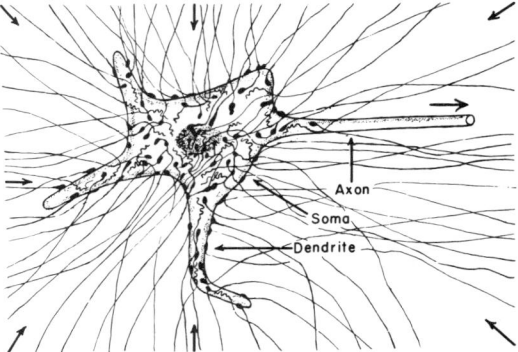

Axon

Soma

Dendrite

Propagation of impulses across the synaptic junction is usually called transmission rather than conduction, to reflect the fact that the processes that mediate the transmission of information at the synapse are different from those that operate within the neuron. With the exception of some excitatory and inhibitory electrical synapses in certain invertebrates and fish (for example, the abdominal ganglia of the crayfish and the Mauthner cells of fish), synaptic transmission is a chemical process. Since most synaptic transmission is chemical, I will confine my discussion in this chapter to chemical transmission.

The fine structure of a synapse is depicted in Figure 2-9. The presynaptic terminals excite the postsynaptic neuron by means of a secreted **excitatory transmitter** substance. Two structures crucial for the transmission of impulses across the synaptic cleft are shown in Figure 2-9. These are the **synaptic vesicles** and the **mitochondria.** The synaptic vesicles contain the excitatory transmitter, which excites the postsynaptic membrane when it is released into the synaptic cleft. The ATP required for synthesis of the transmitter substance is provided by the mitochondria, and it has been suggested that the mitochondria may even synthesize the transmitter substance. This synthesizing process must be extremely rapid because the total amount of the transmitter substance in the terminal button is enough for only a few minutes of synaptic activity at normal operating rates (Guyton, 1971).

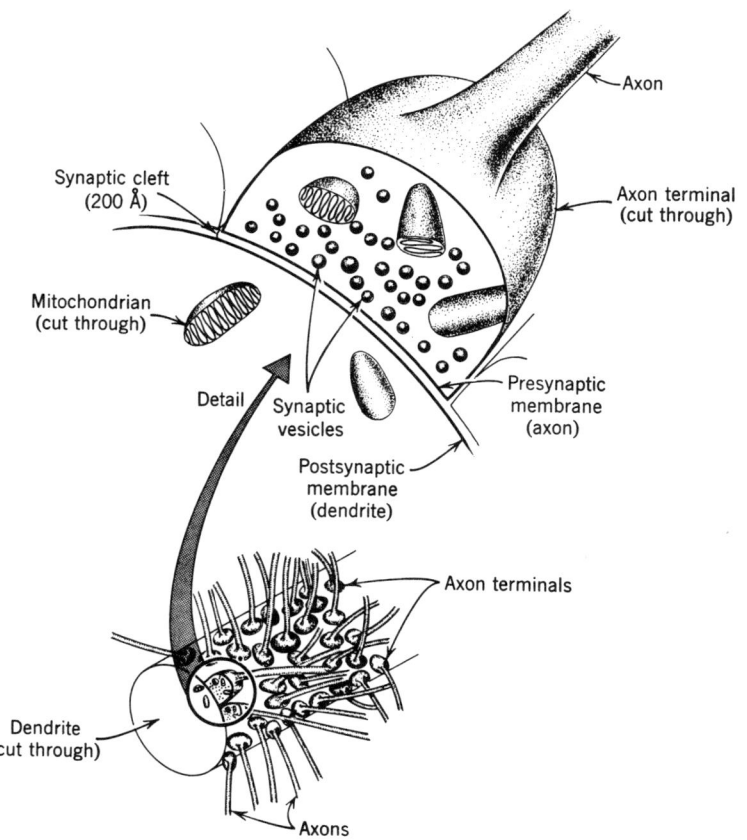

Figure 2-9
The fine structure of the synapse (schematic). From Neurophysiology: A Primer, *by C. F. Stevens. Copyright 1966 by John Wiley & Sons, Inc. Reprinted by permission.*

The Mechanism of Transmitter Release

The mechanisms responsible for the release of transmitter substance are not entirely understood, but the following account is suggested by most of the available data (Guyton, 1971). As I indicated, the transmitter is released from the terminal buttons in response to action potentials arriving at these axonal endings. It appears likely that the wave of depolarization causes electrical attraction of the transmitter vesicles to the presynaptic membrane. Simultaneously, the porosity or permeability of this membrane dramatically increases, allowing calcium ions (Ca^+) to enter, and these ions in turn stimulate the rupture of the vesicles. The contents of the vesicles then pour into the synaptic cleft and diffuse across to the postsynaptic membrane, where they increase the permeability of the postsynaptic membrane to Na^+.

The Chemical Nature of Excitatory Transmitters

It is now generally agreed that, at the neuromuscular junction (the junction between a muscle and the nerve fiber that activates it) and at certain autonomic nervous system synapses, a chemical substance called **acetylcholine (ACh)** is the transmitter. Further, in the central nervous system, injected acetylcholine will excite some neurons. For this reason, it is believed that at least some of the presynaptic terminals of the central nervous system secrete ACh. Neurons that release ACh are referred to as **cholinergic** neurons. It has been determined that each cholinergic vesicle contains about 3000 molecules of ACh and that each terminal button contains enough vesicles to transmit approximately 10,000 impulses (Guyton, 1971). Following its release from the vesicles, ACh diffuses across the synaptic cleft and causes an increase in the Na^+ permeability of the postsynaptic membrane.

The action of ACh on the postjunctional membrane is short-lived because of the presence of an acetylcholine-destroying enzyme, **acetylcholinesterase (AChE),** in the junctional region. The destruction of ACh by AChE reduces the permeability of the postsynaptic membrane to Na^+ and allows the postsynaptic membrane potential to return to its resting level.

Norepinephrine is another proposed excitatory transmitter for central nervous system neurons, and it has been shown to mediate activity in the autonomic nervous system. Neurons that secrete norepinephrine are called **adrenergic** neurons. *Dopamine* and *5-hydroxytryptamine (serotonin)* are also thought to be excitatory transmitters, as are *histamine* and the polypeptide *"substance P."*

The Excitatory Postsynaptic Potential

Approximately 0.5 millisecond (msec) after an excitatory nerve impulse reaches the presynaptic membrane, an electrical response can be recorded from the postsynaptic membrane. This response is called the **excitatory postsynaptic potential (EPSP),** and it lasts for as long as 15 msec, decreasing in strength as a function of time. An EPSP represents a period of partial depolarization during which the excitability of the neuron to other stimuli is increased—hence the name *excitatory postsynaptic potential.* If the potential rises above the threshold for firing the neuron, an action potential will be generated in the neuron. For example, the average threshold for an anterior motorneuron in the spinal cord is 11 mv above the resting level. Therefore, if the resting potential of −70 mv gives way to an EPSP of −59 mv, an action potential will be produced (Guyton, 1971).

What conditions will result in an EPSP being above the threshold for firing the neuron? Basically, a nerve impulse will occur when there is sufficient transmitter operating on the postsynaptic membrane. This is because the degree of postsynaptic depolarization depends directly upon local transmitter concentration. Although the EPSP due to the activity of a single synaptic knob may be small, the depolarizations produced by adjacent synaptic knobs may summate. There are two types of synaptic summation: **spatial** and **temporal.**

Spatial Summation. Spatial summation is illustrated in Figure 2-10. Spatial summation occurs when activity is simultaneously present in more than one synaptic knob. As shown in the figure, simultaneous excitation of progressively greater numbers of excitatory presynaptic terminals yields increases in the size of the EPSP. If the threshold level is surpassed, an action potential will be generated at the axon hillock. The axon hillock discharges first because its threshold for excitation is lower than that of the soma. For example, in the case of the anterior motorneuron, the threshold for firing at the axon hillock is only 11 mv from the resting level, while it is 25 mv from the resting level on the soma (Guyton, 1971). After the axon hillock discharges, the impulse travels forward over the axon and backward over the soma.

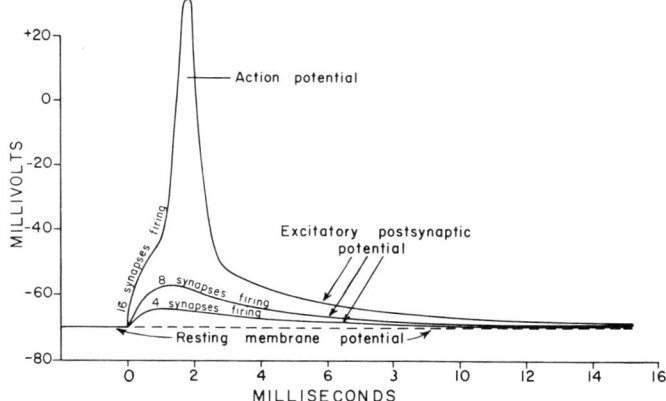

Figure 2-10
Excitatory postsynaptic potentials. Note that the simultaneous firing of only a few synapses will not cause sufficient summated potential to elicit an action potential but that the simultaneous firing of many synapses will raise the summated potential to the threshold for excitation and cause an action potential. (The exact number of synapses firing is hypothetical.) From Textbook of Medical Physiology *(4th ed.), by A. C. Guyton. Copyright 1971 by W. B. Saunders Company. Reprinted by permission.*

Temporal Summation. Temporal summation occurs when a new EPSP occurs before the previous EPSPs have completely decayed. As indicated, each EPSP lasts up to 15 msec. If the postsynaptic membrane is again depolarized before the existing EPSP has disappeared, then the new EPSP will simply add to what remains of the first EPSP. The phenomenon of temporal summation is depicted in Figure 2-11. In the initial section of this graph, two EPSPs are separated by 15 msec, and no summation occurs. In the middle section, it is shown that potentials separated by 3 msec do summate, at least moderately. Finally, potentials separated by only 1 msec yield a large summated potential and result in the generation of an action potential.

Figure 2-11 additionally portrays one of the most notable characteristics of the postsynaptic potential. This is the fact that the size of an EPSP is directly proportional to the strength of the stimulus producing it. This property contrasts with the all-or-none response of the axon. If the EPSP is large enough to surpass the threshold for firing the cell, then a full-blown action potential will occur.

Figure 2-11
*Temporal
summation of
excitatory
postsynaptic
potentials. From*
Textbook of
Medical Physiology
*(4th ed.), by A. C.
Guyton. Copyright
1971 by W. B.
Saunders Company.
Reprinted by
permission.*

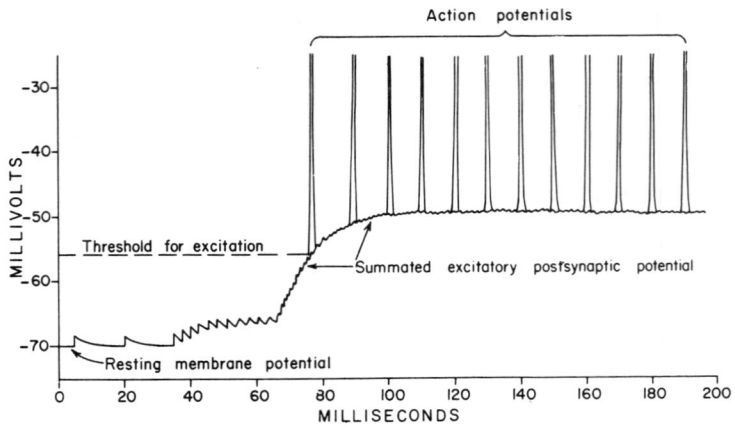

The Inhibitory Postsynaptic Potential

In contrast to the EPSP, which involves a partial depolarization of the postsynaptic membrane, other potentials may involve the opposite effect—namely, hyperpolarization. During this second type of postsynaptic potential, the excitability of the nerve cell to subsequent stimuli is decreased. For this reason, it is referred to as an **inhibitory postsynaptic potential (IPSP).** As was the case for EPSPs, both spatial and temporal summation can occur. This type of inhibition is called *direct* or *postsynaptic inhibition* (Ganong, 1975).

Figure 2-12
*A mechanism of
postsynaptic
inhibition, showing:
(A) a single inhibitory
postsynaptic
potential and (B)
decreased summated
postsynaptic
potential caused by
superimposition of
an inhibitory
postsynaptic
potential on an
excitatory
postsynaptic
potential. From*
Textbook of
Medical Physiology
*(4th ed.), by A. C.
Guyton. Copyright
1971 by W. B.
Saunders Company.
Reprinted by
permission.*

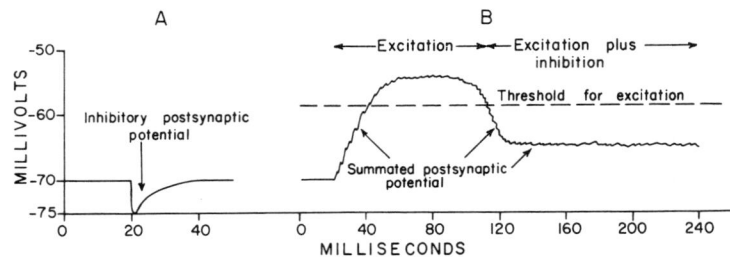

An IPSP is shown in the A section of Figure 2-12; it is the mirror image of an EPSP. Again, an IPSP has an effect opposite to that of an EPSP. An IPSP results in the inside of the cell becoming more negative, with respect to the exterior, than during the normal resting state. This voltage change is in a direction opposite to that required for generating a nerve impulse. This hyperpolarizing effect is shown in the B section of Figure 2-12. As was also the case with the EPSP, an IPSP persists for about 15 msec.

The hyperpolarizing effect of an IPSP is actually to drive the membrane potential toward a value of −80 mv. This can be demonstrated experimentally. If the membrane potential is artifically held at −80 mv, the application of a new inhibitory impulse will have absolutely no effect on the membrane potential. A further interesting observation is that, if the membrane potential is artificially hyperpolarized beyond this −80 mv level (for example, to −90 mv by the passage of current), the

20

next inhibitory impulse that arrives will cause a depolarizing effect, driving the potential toward the −80 mv level (Eccles, 1964).

The mechanism of postsynaptic inhibition is not known for sure, but researchers believe that an inhibitory transmitter substance increases the permeability of the neuronal membrane to potassium and chloride ions but not to sodium ions. As indicated earlier, sodium ions are about 50% bigger than potassium and chloride ions. Presumably the inhibitory substance opens only those pores that will allow the passage of the smaller ions. Since Cl⁻ ions are already in an exact distribution in accordance with their electrochemical gradient, few of these ions move across the membrane. In contrast, the K⁺ ions do move across the membrane to the exterior in response to the existing electrical and chemical gradients. Movement of K⁺ ions out of the neuron results in a greater degree of negativity inside the cell and thus in the observed hyperpolarization.

A second type of inhibition occurring in the nervous system is **presynaptic inhibition** (Ganong, 1975), and it involves a process by which the amount of excitatory transmitter released by action potentials arriving at terminal buttons is reduced. This in turn results in a decrease in the magnitude of the following EPSP. Neurons that produce presynaptic inhibition terminate on the surfaces of excitatory presynaptic nerve terminals. These are *axo-axonic* synapses. When inhibitory presynaptic neurons release their transmitter, they produce a partial depolarization of the excitatory endings. This results in the arriving nerve impulse being attenuated in size. The net result is that less excitatory transmitter is released and consequently less postsynaptic excitation ensues (Ganong, 1975). Neurons that produce presynaptic inhibition often fire repetitively. As a result, the partial depolarization that yields the presynaptic inhibition may last for 100 msec or longer. The physical arrangement of neurons that produce presynaptic and postsynaptic inhibition is depicted in Figure 2-13.

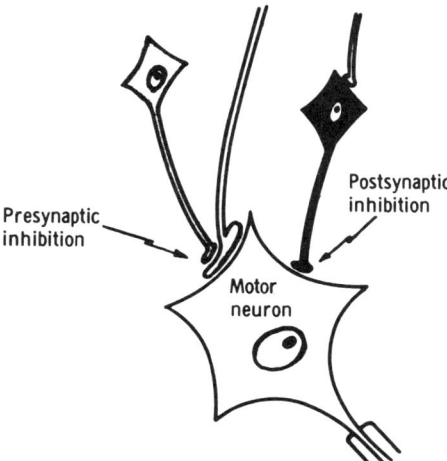

Presynaptic inhibition

Postsynaptic inhibition

Motor neuron

*Figure 2-13
The arrangement of neurons producing presynaptic and postsynaptic inhibition. The neuron producing presynaptic inhibition is shown ending on an excitatory synaptic knob. Many of these neurons actually end higher up along the axon of the excitatory cell. From* Review of Medical Physiology *(7th ed.), by W. F. Ganong. Copyright 1975 by Lange Medical Publications. Reprinted by permission.*

The Chemical Nature of Inhibitory Transmitters

The chemical nature of the inhibitory transmitter or transmitters has not been definitely determined. One favored candidate is the amino acid *glycine*, which may mediate inhibitory impulses arising from inhibitory interneurons in the spinal cord.

(An *interneuron* is a neuron that lies between, and synapses with, two other neurons.) Another candidate is *gamma aminobutyric acid* (GABA), which has been implicated in presynaptic inhibition. Other possibilities include *Factor I* and *5-hydroxytryptamine* (*serotonin*). Serotonin was also mentioned as a possible candidate for an excitatory transmitter agent. This brings up an important point; there is some evidence suggesting that a given transmitter may have excitatory or inhibitory effects, depending upon the characteristics of the postsynaptic membrane to which it attaches (Eccles, 1964). More specifically, Gardner and Kandel (1972) have demonstrated that a specific neurotransmitter, such as acetylcholine, can have either an excitatory or an inhibitory effect, depending on the part of the neuron (dendrites, soma, or axon) it acts upon.

The Origin of the Action Potential in the Postsynaptic Neuron

From the picture that has been drawn of the various excitatory and inhibitory influences impinging on the postsynaptic membrane, one can envision the constant interplay of excitatory and inhibitory activity that occurs on any given postsynaptic membrane. In order for a postsynaptic neuron in the central nervous system to fire, there must be a virtually simultaneous arrival of a number of impulses at different excitatory terminal buttons that synapse with the to-be-excited neuron's soma and dendrites. If their summated depolarization is greater than the 10–15 mv of depolarization that is required, an action potential will be generated at the axon hillock.

Another requisite for the firing of the postsynaptic neuron is that not too many impulses arrive at inhibitory terminals at the same time. If too many arrive, the depolarizing excitatory effects will be nullified. Therefore, within the central nervous system, whether or not a neuron fires is determined by the algebraic sum of the effects of impulses arriving at excitatory and inhibitory terminals that synapse with the neuron. This process of algebraic summation of EPSPs and IPSPs is called **central summation.** When an action potential is generated, the wave of excitation is carried in both directions: down the axon toward the next neuron and backward over the soma. The net effect is that the slate is wiped clean after each nerve impulse, allowing for a renewed interplay of excitatory and inhibitory influences.

Chapter Summary and Conclusions

In this chapter, the anatomy and physiology of the basic functional unit of the nervous system —the neuron—were presented. It was shown that, like all living cells, the neuron has a membrane potential that arises from an unequal distribution of ions across the membrane. In nervous tissue, the resting membrane potential is −70 mv. Changes in this membrane potential associated with shifts in the distribution of certain ions are the physiological processes underlying the transfer of information in nervous tissue.

The anatomy of the neuron was discussed. A neuron has a cell body or soma, from which a number of processes or arms extend. These processes—the axon and the dendrites—serve to transmit information in the nervous system. Dendrites conduct information toward the cell body, and the axon conducts information away from it.

Nerve impulses or action potentials, which reflect the coding and transmission of information, are generated in the initial segment of the axon, which is called the axon hillock. Axons are covered with a myelin sheath that varies in thickness according to the type of cell. At its end, an axon branches. At the end of each branch is a terminal button, through which the neuron relates to other neurons. A neuron is not anatomically connected to adjacent neurons; rather, it is functionally related via the synapse. Transmission across synapses is usually a chemical process.

The ionic distribution across the cell membrane during the resting membrane potential was reviewed. It was shown that four ions are primarily responsible for the resting potential. These are sodium and chloride ions, which are predominantly located in the extracellular space, and potassium and large organic anions, which are concentrated inside the cell. Factors that influence the distribution of the ions were described. The nerve impulse was related to shifts in the distribution of these ions. It was indicated that the nerve impulse or depolarization results from the influx of sodium ions. Electrical recovery in preparation for another firing of the neuron is accomplished by the outflow of potassium ions. The entire process—depolarization and recovery—requires only a fraction of a millisecond. Similar ionic movements account for propagation of the nerve impulse down the axon. Some details of the nerve impulse, including changes in the excitability of the neuron correlated with phases of the action potential, were reviewed. Conduction of a nerve impulse down the axon and transmission across the synaptic junction were detailed next.

Two kinds of influences can act across the synapse and influence the postsynaptic neuron: excitatory and inhibitory. These influences algebraically summate at the axon hillock. Whether an action potential is generated by the postsynaptic neuron depends upon whether the sum of excitatory and inhibitory influences exceeds the threshold for firing the neuron. If it does, an action potential will be generated. Several potential candidates for the role of excitatory and inhibitory transmitter agents were suggested, but much work is needed in order to verify their role in synaptic transmission.

It is almost overwhelming to realize that the basis for information processing and transfer by nervous tissue is the movement of certain ions. Think about it for a moment. All that we do and feel is the product of the movement of ions. Our loves, our feelings of distaste, and all of our other emotional reactions reflect the movements of ions and the interplay of excitatory and inhibitory impulses on postsynaptic membranes in that complex labyrinth we call the brain.

3
The Anatomy of the Brain

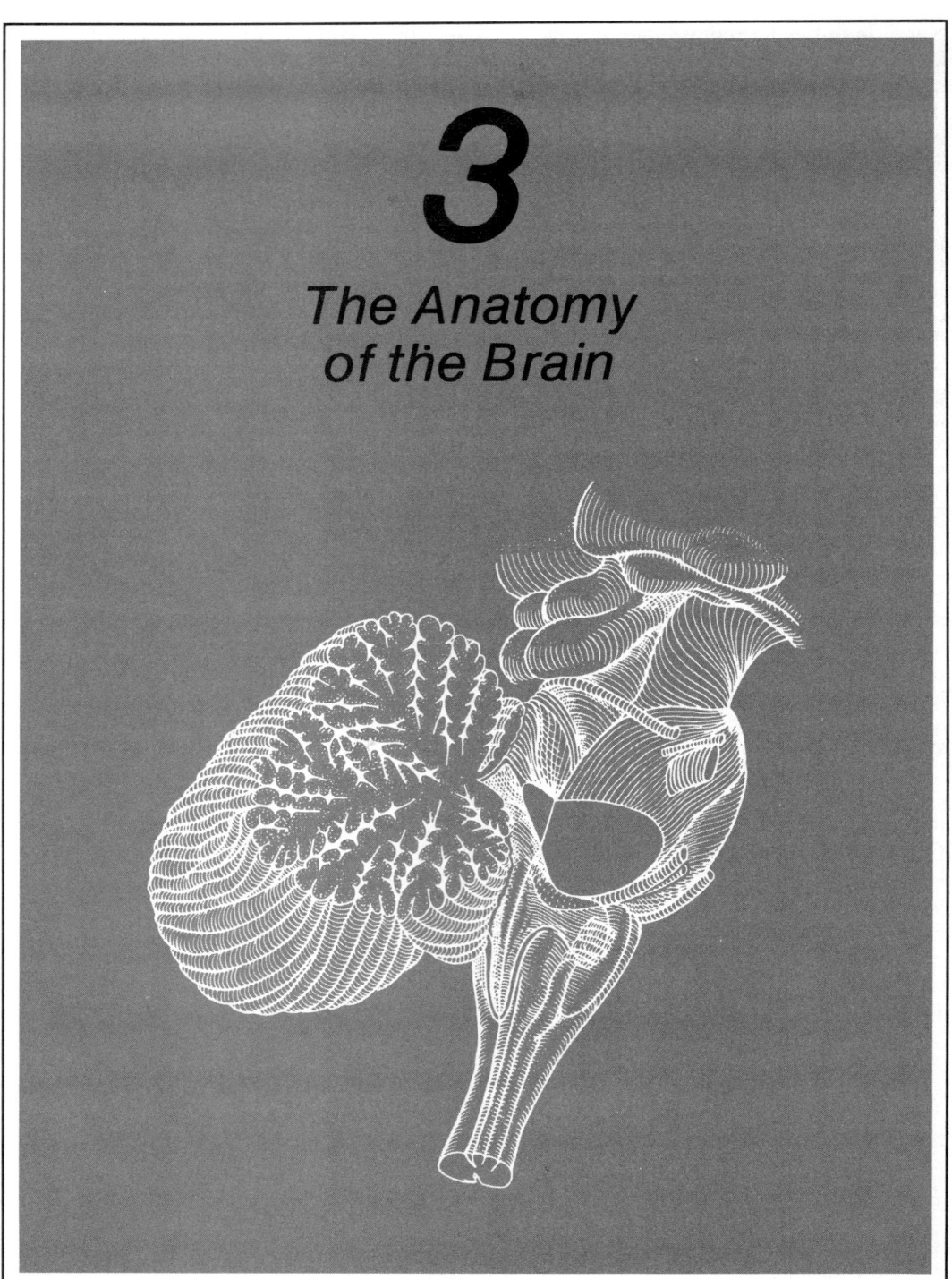

The nervous system of vertebrates is usually considered to be divisible into three major sectors: (1) the **central nervous system,** which consists of the brain and spinal cord, (2) the **peripheral nervous system,** which includes the cranial and spinal nerves, and (3) the **autonomic nervous system,** which includes the autonomic nerves and ganglia. Since this text emphasizes the role of the brain in mediating behavior, the anatomy chapter will do likewise. The anatomy of the spinal cord, the spinal nerves, and the autonomic nervous system will be elaborated on in later chapters whenever such elaboration is appropriate. In this chapter, I'll first present general directional terms used by neuroanatomists. Next, some basic features of the central nervous system will be outlined. The general anatomy of the human brain will then be presented, and, finally, the development of the vertebrate brain will be considered.

Directional Terms in Neuroanatomy

Anatomically speaking, the brain is the most complex of all biological structures. Nevertheless, a number of simple principles have been developed that allow us to conceptualize clearly the anatomical relationships within this structure. One aid has been the development of a number of simple directional terms that indicate the relative locations of structures. The purpose of these directional terms is simply to indicate whether a brain structure or substructure is at the top or bottom, in the front or back, or toward the middle or side of the brain. Other terms indicate from which direction the piece of brain is being viewed. Most of these directional terms are shown in Figure 3-1.

The term **dorsal** denotes the back, **ventral** the front or belly surface, **medial** toward the middle, and **lateral** to either side. The head end is called **anterior,** *cephalic,* or *rostral,* while the tail end is termed **posterior** or *caudal.* Quite often these directional terms are employed to name *nuclei*—groupings of nerve-cell bodies—within various structures. The nuclei are named according to their location in the particular brain structure. For example, the ventroanterior nucleus of the thalamus is located in the anterior region of the thalamus and toward the ventral surface of this structure. The ventromedial nucleus of the hypothalamus is located in the ventral region and toward the midline of the hypothalamus. The terms **ipsilateral** and **contralateral** are also often used in describing anatomical regions. Ipsilateral means on the same side, and contralateral means on the opposite side.

The terms *dorsal* and *ventral* can sometimes lead to confusion. In the case of four-legged animals, *dorsal* refers to the back of the animal and the top of the head, while *ventral* refers to both the belly surface and the underside of the head. In contrast, for primates, including humans, the top of the head is at a right angle to the

Figure 3-1
The anatomical
terminology used to
describe position
and location in
reference to the axes
of the body.

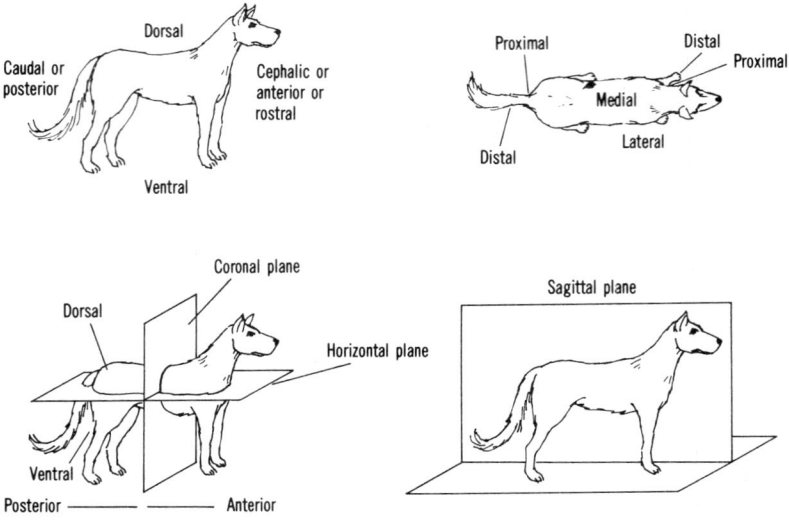

back of the body. Instead of changing terms when talking about the brains of rats and humans, anatomists have placed a right-angle bend in their directional terms. Hence, for primates, just as for quadrupeds, the top of the brain is referred to as *dorsal,* the bottom *ventral,* the front *anterior,* and the back *posterior.*

A set of terms has also been developed to denote from what direction a particular structure or slice of brain tissue is being viewed. For example, during **histology** after an experiment, when brains are sliced very thin, mounted on slides, and stained so that the exact site of a lesion or electrode placement can be verified, brain sections are usually cut perpendicular to the anterior/posterior axis. In this case, they are referred to as *frontal* or **coronal** sections. (Look at Figure 3-1 for an illustration of the various planes.) Vertical sections that extend from the front to the back of the head are called *longitudinal* or *sagittal* sections. The brain is divided into its two hemispheres by the medial sagittal section. Finally, *horizontal* sections are perpendicular to the sagittal plane. The horizontal plane divides the brain into dorsal and ventral portions.

Basic Features of the
Central Nervous System

The central nervous system consists of the brain and the spinal cord. The term *brain* refers to the large collection of nerve cells and fibers at the head end of all vertebrates. The functional anatomy of the brain will be detailed below. As the central nervous system leaves the skull, it becomes the spinal cord. I will elaborate on the anatomy and functions of the spinal cord in later chapters whenever I feel that it will help you. A simplified overview of the structure and function of the spinal cord follows.

26

The Spinal Cord

The spinal cord has two primary functions. First, it mediates reflex actions. Second, it conducts nerve impulses to and from the brain. The spinal cord is organized into segments corresponding to the different vertebrae of the spine. Sensory nerves feed into the dorsal side of each segment of the cord, and motor nerves emerge from the ventral side. A cross-sectional view of the spinal cord is shown in Figure 3-2. The cord consists of two major portions: the central **gray matter** and a surrounding **white matter.**

The central core of gray matter is shaped roughly like a butterfly and contains primarily cell bodies of neurons. The protrusions of gray matter at the top are called the **dorsal horns,** while the ones at the bottom are called the **ventral horns.** The dorsal horns contain the cell bodies of neurons involved in transmitting sensory information. In contrast, the ventral horns contain cells whose axons travel out of the spinal cord to influence movement.

The peripheral white matter consists primarily of ascending and descending sensory and motor tracts that are heavily myelinated. These tracts are shown in Figure 3-2. Their functional significance will be discussed in Chapter 5 ("Sensory Processes") and Chapter 6 ("Movement").

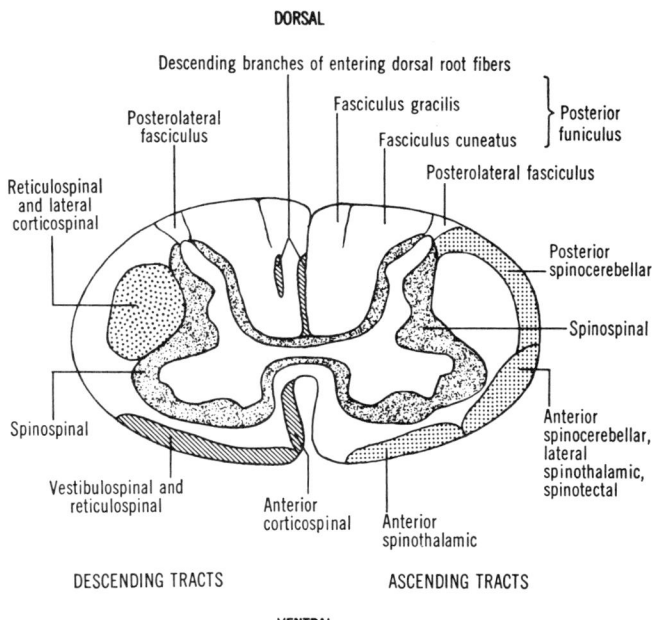

DORSAL

Descending branches of entering dorsal root fibers

Posterolateral fasciculus

Fasciculus gracilis

Fasciculus cuneatus

Posterolateral fasciculus

} Posterior funiculus

Reticulospinal and lateral corticospinal

Posterior spinocerebellar

Spinospinal

Spinospinal

Anterior spinocerebellar, lateral spinothalamic, spinotectal

Vestibulospinal and reticulospinal

Anterior corticospinal

Anterior spinothalamic

DESCENDING TRACTS

ASCENDING TRACTS

VENTRAL

Figure 3-2
The main tracts of the spinal cord. Afferent (ascending) tracts are on the right side; efferent (descending) tracts are on the left. It must be remembered, however, that both ascending and descending fibers are present on each side. From Fundamentals of Neurology *(5th ed.), by E. Gardner. Copyright 1968 by W. B. Saunders Company. Reprinted by permission.*

The Meninges and Cerebrospinal Fluid

The brain and spinal cord are wrapped in a continuous covering of three layers of nonnervous supportive tissue called the **meninges,** which are in turn enclosed in bone—the skull and vertebrae. The meninges are important in physically supporting the central nervous system, which, as was indicated earlier, is actually quite soft. The meninges also enclose the cerebrospinal fluid, which bathes the entire central nervous system.

The outermost layer of the meninges is called the *dura mater.* It is a tough, fibrous membrane. The innermost of the three layers, and the one that actually comes into contact with the nervous tissue, is the *pia mater.* Sandwiched between the dura and the pia is a fibrous mass referred to as the *arachnoid.* The outer part of the pia contains the blood vessels that supply the brain and spinal cord. **Cerebrospinal fluid,** which is similar to blood plasma in composition, circulates in the **subarachnoid space**—between the arachnoid and the pia mater. The fluid interacts both with the cerebrospinal fluid contained in four interconnected spaces or **ventricles** within the brain and with the cerebrospinal fluid that circulates down the length of the spinal cord in the **central canal.**

Cerebrospinal fluid performs a role in the nutrition of the brain and the spinal cord. If an interference with absorption or circulation of cerebrospinal fluid occurs in the developing infant, excess cerebrospinal fluid will accumulate in the brain, producing a condition called **hydrocephalus.** Since the skull bones do not unite until many years after birth, the excess fluid in the hydrocephalic infant forces the bones apart until the head reaches an enormous size. The brain is usually severely compressed, and extreme mental retardation results. If diagnosed early, hydrocephalus can be relieved by the implantation of a pressure-sensitive valve that opens and drains the fluid into the bladder via a tube whenever too much fluid accumulates.

The Brain

Sir Charles Sherrington once called the brain "the great ravelled knot"—an appropriate name, considering that the neurons are interwoven into such an incredibly intricate meshwork that a neuron is probably never active without influencing some of its neighbors. In this chapter, I'll present an overview of the anatomy of the brain and describe some of the functions of the major brain structures. Analyses of some of the finer aspects of the anatomy of selected structures will appear in later chapters.

In presenting a functional overview of anatomically distinct structures, I don't want to convey the idea that each structure has an independent function that it performs in mediating behavior. Rather, the brain must be conceived of as a dynamic organization of distinct but highly interrelated structures. Neural structures are organized into a hierarchy or "chain of command," with the activity at certain levels profoundly affecting the activity of other levels. The lowest levels—those that evolved initially—are responsible for the basic expression of behavior. That is, they are involved in controlling behaviors, such as eating, fighting, fleeing, and sexual behavior, that are necessary for survival of the individual and the species. Higher levels in the brain are responsible for making these behaviors more goal oriented or stimulus directed. I will elaborate this view in later chapters, but, for the present, consider the brain a group of differentiated parts whose activity is continually modified by the influence of higher and lower-level parts. The activity that occurs in any single part of the brain can influence the activity in any other region. With this view of neural function in mind, let's examine the overall functional anatomy of the brain.

All vertebrate brains can be subdivided into five regions, each containing specific structures. Not all vertebrate brains have all of the structures that will be discussed, but they all have these five regions; comparisons of the brains of reptiles, birds, rats, and humans are thus possible. The regions are the *myelencephalon,* the *metencephalon,* the *mesencephalon,* the *diencephalon,* and the *telencephalon.* The term **hindbrain** collectively refers to the myelencephalon and metencephalon, **midbrain** denotes the mesencephalon, and the diencephalon and telencephalon together compose the **forebrain.** The divisions and the major brain structures that they include are summarized in Table 3-1.

Table 3-1.   Subdivisions of the Brain and Their Major Structures

Subdivisions	*Structures*
hindbrain:	
myelencephalon	medulla
metencephalon	pons
	cerebellum
midbrain:	
mesencephalon	superior colliculi
	inferior colliculi
forebrain:	
diencephalon	hypothalamus
	pituitary
	optic tracts
	subthalamus
	thalamus
telencephalon	cerebral hemispheres
	basal ganglia
	rhinencephalon

Another division of the brain that is commonly referred to is the **brain stem.** Diagrams of the human brain stem are shown in Figures 3-3 and 3-4. Anatomists generally use the term *brain stem* to refer to the combined hindbrain and midbrain. Sometimes the diencephalon and even the basal ganglia are included in the term, in which case *brain stem* is being used to refer to everything between the spinal cord and the cerebral hemispheres.

Myelencephalon

Medulla. The **medulla oblongata** is the major structure of the myelencephalon, and it is essentially a continuation of the spinal cord into the brain. The medulla contains ascending sensory-fiber tracts and descending motor tracts that connect the brain with the spinal cord. A number of important nerve-cell nuclei are located in this

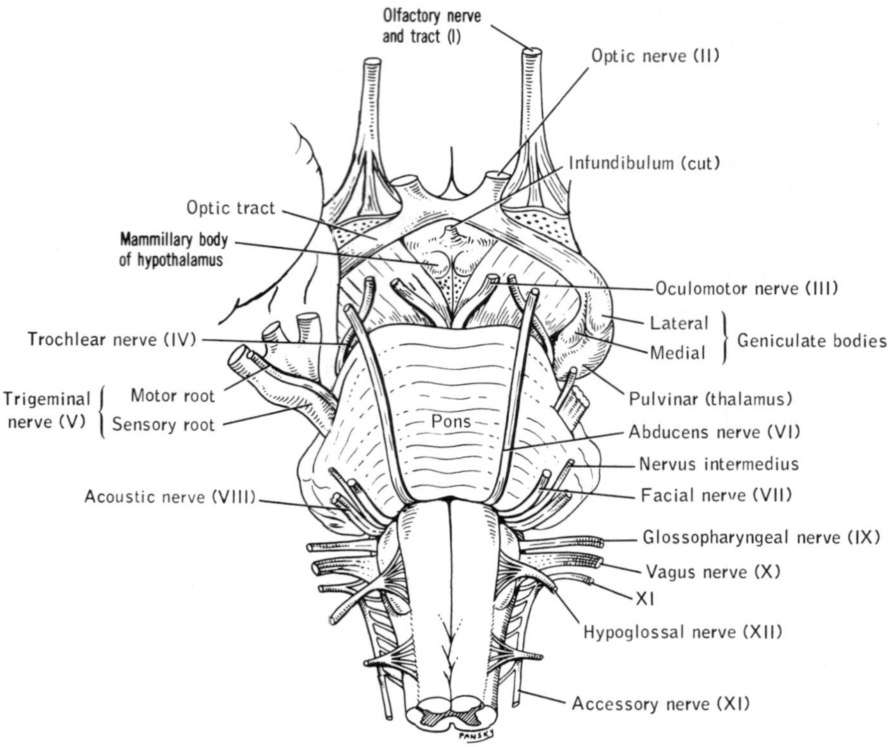

Figure 3-3
The central portion of the basal aspect of the human brain stem. Adapted from A Functional Approach to Neuroanatomy, *by E. L. House and B. Pansky. Copyright 1967 by McGraw-Hill, Inc. Reprinted by permission.*

structure. Several nuclei of the cranial nerves, which control sensory and motor functions of the head, are located here. And several so-called "vital nuclei" are located in the medulla. These nuclei of the autonomic nervous system are concerned with such critical functions as respiration, heart action, and gastrointestinal function. Because these vital nuclei are concerned with the primary control of these functions, damage to the medulla due to trauma is usually fatal. Such was the case when Robert F. Kennedy was felled by an assassin's bullet during the United States Presidential primary elections of 1968.

At the level of the medulla, the **cranial nerves** are first encountered. The brain is connected to the receptors and effectors of the head by the 12 pairs of cranial nerves that emerge from the brain stem. The cranial nerves are numbered according to the order in which they emerge from the brain stem, from anterior to posterior. The cranial nerves, along with their places of origin in the brain stem and their most important functions, are shown in Table 3-2. In this table, *afferent* (sensory) indicates that the nerve carries information to the brain. *Efferent* (motor) indicates that the nerve conducts impulses from the brain to the part of the body being activated. The origins of each of the cranial nerves can be seen in Figure 3-3 (see also Figure 3-8). For the student who has to memorize the names of the cranial nerves, a bit of verse has been devised. Each word in this phrase starts with the first letter of one of the cranial nerves, taken in order from the first through the twelfth: **O**n **o**ld **O**lympus' **t**owering **t**op, **a** French-speaking German viewed some hops.

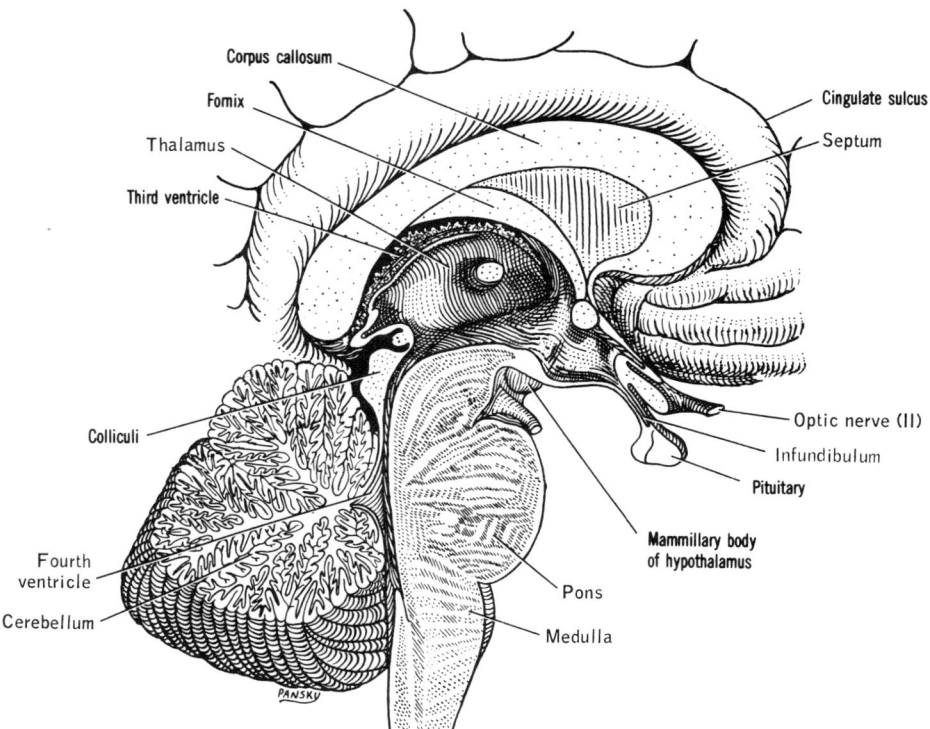

Corpus callosum
Fornix
Thalamus
Third ventricle
Cingulate sulcus
Septum
Colliculi
Fourth ventricle
Cerebellum
Optic nerve (II)
Infundibulum
Pituitary
Mammillary body of hypothalamus
Pons
Medulla
PANSKY

*Figure 3-4
A median sagittal
section through the
human brain stem.
Adapted from* A
Functional
Approach to
Neuroanatomy, *by
E. L. House and B.
Pansky. Copyright
1967 by
McGraw-Hill, Inc.
Reprinted by
permission.*

Reticular Formation. The **reticular formation** is located, in part, in the myelencephalon. It is an anatomically complex meshwork of cell bodies, nuclei, and fibers that extends from the spinal cord into the hypothalamus and central portion of the thalamus of the diencephalon. The location of the reticular formation in the human brain is diagramed in Figure 3-5. It occupies a ventral location in the brain stem.

There are two major influences exerted by the reticular formation on behavior; one operates through descending and the other through ascending fibers. **Descending** fibers of the reticular formation affect the activity of spinal and cranial motor neurons. This part of the reticular formation is part of a large system that mediates movement, called the **extrapyramidal motor system** (see Chapter 6). Stimulation that activates the descending reticular formation may produce either inhibition or facilitation of the activity of motor neurons that control the skeletal muscles.

The ascending reticular formation plays a crucial role in behavior arousal. As a result, it is often referred to as the *ascending reticular activating system* (ARAS). The importance of the ARAS in behavioral arousal was first demonstrated by Moruzzi and Magoun (1949). These researchers reported that stimulation of these pathways resulted in a pattern of low-voltage, fast, cortical brain-wave activity. This type of brain-wave activity is normal in alert animals. In a complementary inquiry, Lindsley, Bowden, and Magoun (1949) found that midbrain lesions that interrupted these ascending influences produced a constantly stuporous or sleeping animal. These results supported the theory that the ARAS is a critical component of the neural

Table 3-2. *The Cranial Nerves*

Number	Name	Origin in Brain Stem	Functions (afferent = sensory; efferent = motor)
I	olfactory	olfactory bulb	afferent for smell
II	optic	thalamus	afferent for vision
III	oculomotor	midbrain	afferent and efferent for eye movement
IV	trochlear	midbrain	afferent and efferent for eye movement
V	trigeminal	pons and midbrain	afferent from skin and mucous membranes of head; afferent and efferent for chewing
VI	abducens	medulla	afferent and efferent for eye movement
VII	facial	medulla	afferent from taste buds of anterior 2/3 of tongue; efferent for facial movements
VIII	statoacoustic	medulla	afferent from inner ear for hearing and balance
IX	glossopharyngeal	medulla	afferent from throat, rear of tongue, and taste buds of posterior 1/3 of tongue; efferent to throat
X	vagus	medulla	afferent and efferent for heart, blood vessels, and viscera
XI	spinal accessory	medulla	efferent to viscera (via vagus); efferent to throat, larynx, and neck and shoulder muscles
XII	hypoglossal	medulla	afferent and efferent for tongue muscles

system mediating sleeping and waking. The functions of the reticular formation in arousal will be considered in greater detail in Chapter 7, where I'll discuss the physiological determinants of arousal, sleep, and dreaming.

Metencephalon

Cerebellum. The metencephalon consists of two major structures: the **cerebellum** and the **pons.** Located just above and behind the medulla are the two lobes of the cerebellum, a phylogenetically old structure that was the first brain region to be specialized for sensory-motor coordination. Even slight damage to this structure can seriously disrupt motor responses, such as walking, that require a good deal of coordination. The cerebellum as viewed from the dorsal surface is pictured in Figure 3-6. Figure 3-7 depicts a midsagittal section through this structure.

Pons. The **pons** lies above the medulla and in front of the cerebellum. In fact, the dorsal surface of the pons is completely obscured by the cerebellum. The position of the pons is clearly depicted in the diagrams of the brain stem, Figures 3-3 and 3-4.

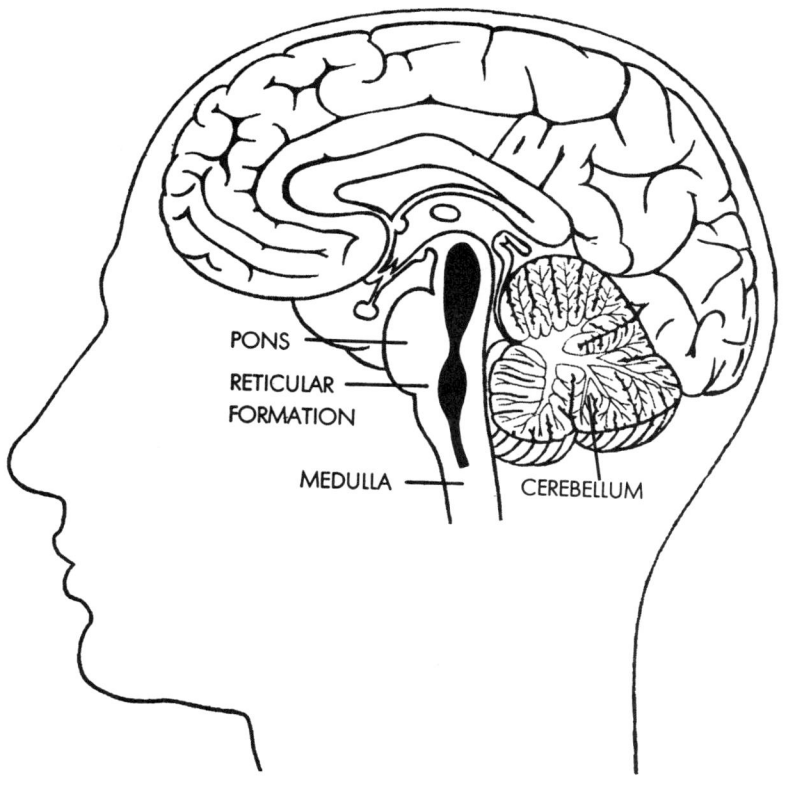

PONS

RETICULAR
FORMATION

MEDULLA

CEREBELLUM

Figure 3-5
*The relationship of
the reticular
formation (black
area) to various
parts of the brain.
From "The
Reticular
Formation," by J.
D. French,* Scientific
American, *1957,
196, 54–60.
Copyright © 1957
by Scientific
American, Inc.
Reprinted by
permission.*

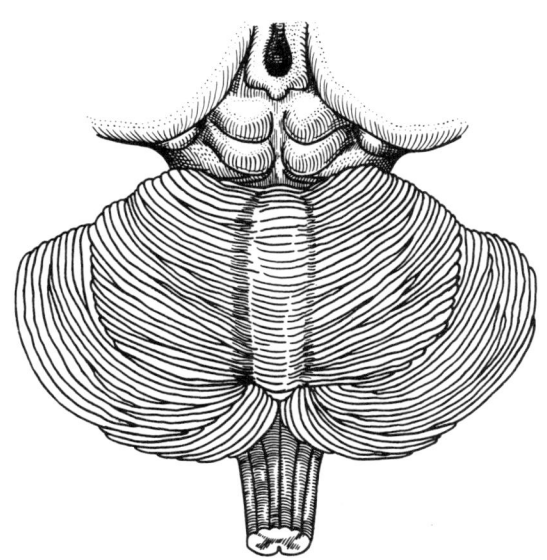

Figure 3-6
*The cerebellum as
seen from the dorsal
side. Adapted from*
A Functional
Approach to
Neuroanatomy, *by
E. L. House and B.
Pansky. Copyright
1967 by
McGraw-Hill, Inc.
Reprinted by
permission.*

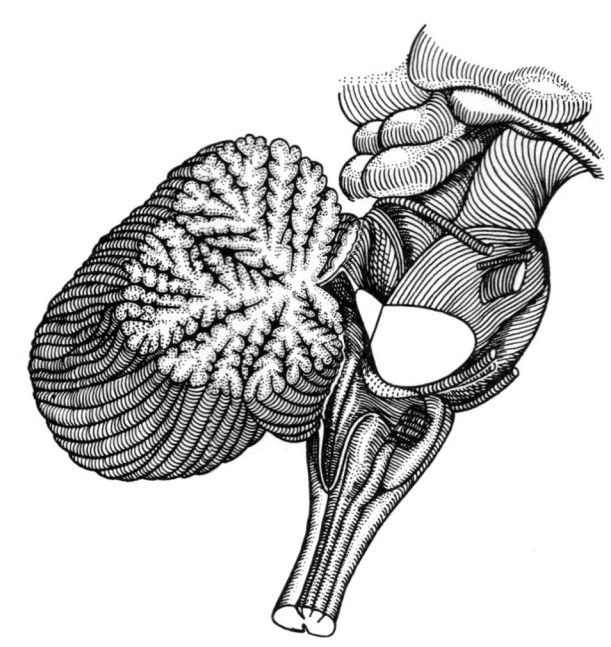

Figure 3-7
A midsagittal
section through the
cerebellum. Adapted
from A Functional
Approach to
Neuroanatomy, *by*
E. L. House and B.
Pansky. Copyright
1967 by
McGraw-Hill, Inc.
Reprinted by
permission.

The pons contains fibers that connect the two hemispheres of the cerebellum and also fibers that carry ascending and descending information within the central nervous system. Relays for the auditory system, as well as nuclei influencing respiration, feeding, movement, and facial expression, are situated in this structure.

Mesencephalon

Tectum. The most recently evolved portion of the central nervous system that still maintains the basic tubular structure of the spinal cord is the mesencephalon or midbrain. The midbrain forms a bridge between the hindbrain and the forebrain by merging anteriorly into the hypothalamus and thalamus. When the cerebral hemispheres and the cerebellum have been removed, as in Figure 3-8, it can easily be seen that the dorsal surface or **tectum** of the mesencephalon consists of four rounded swellings called the *quadrigeminal bodies* or *colliculi.* Two furrows, forming a cross, divide the four into paired **inferior** and **superior colliculi.** The inferior colliculi are primitive centers for audition, and the superior colliculi are lower centers for vision.

Fiber bands associated with each colliculus can be seen as elevations along the lateral surface of the midbrain. One of these bands, the **brachium of the inferior colliculus,** joins the inferior colliculus to the *medial geniculate body of the thalamus*—a center for processing auditory information. The other band, the **brachium of the superior colliculus,** connects the superior colliculus with the *lateral geniculate body of the thalamus*—a center for vision.

Tegmentum. The ventral portion of the mesencephalon is called the **tegmentum.** Ascending and descending fiber tracts connecting higher and lower regions of the brain pass through this region. Certain cell groups are located in the tegmentum.

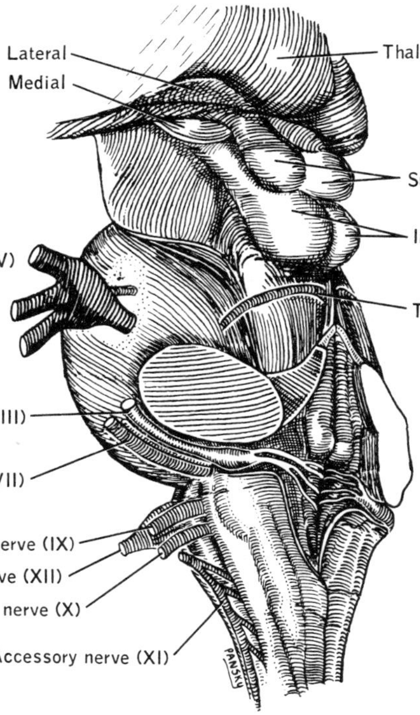

Geniculate bodies { Lateral — / / / —— Thalamus
                  { Medial —

— Superior colliculi

— Inferior colliculi

Trigeminal nerve (V)

— Trochlear nerve (IV)

Acoustic nerve (VIII)

Facial nerve (VII)

Glossopharyngeal nerve (IX)
Hypoglossal nerve (XII)
Vagus nerve (X)

Accessory nerve (XI)

Figure 3-8
*The human brain
stem viewed from
the side. Adapted
from* A Functional
Approach to
Neuroanatomy, *by
E. L. House and B.
Pansky. Copyright
1967 by
McGraw-Hill, Inc.
Reprinted by
permission.*

For example, the nuclei of cranial nerves III and IV, which mediate eye movements, are located here. In addition, some nuclear groups in this area apparently mediate the expression of aggressive behavior. Flynn and his associates have reported that attack by a cat on a rat can be elicited by stimulation of the tegmentum (Flynn, Vanegas, Foote, and Edwards, 1970). The neural substrates of emotion will be considered in Chapter 8.

Diencephalon

Thalamus. When the cerebral hemispheres are in place, the diencephalon is almost completely hidden from view. The largest portion of the diencephalon is the **thalamus,** which is bounded ventrally by the **hypothalamus.** These two areas are separated by the *hypothalamic sulcus.* (A sulcus is a groove, or fissure.) The thalamus looks somewhat like two footballs lying side by side, one in each hemisphere. The two halves of the thalamus are joined across the midline by a bridge known as the **massa intermedia.** Overlying the thalamus are the **basal ganglia** of the telencephalon. The major nuclear divisions of the thalamus and the relation of the thalamus to the midbrain and the basal ganglia are shown in Figures 3-9 and 3-10.

The thalamus is a large mass of gray matter that is divided into a number of nuclear groups. Although some information processing occurs at thalamic levels, the thalamus may still be conceived of as primarily a relay station for sensory and motor information. Fibers coursing through this region conduct information between the

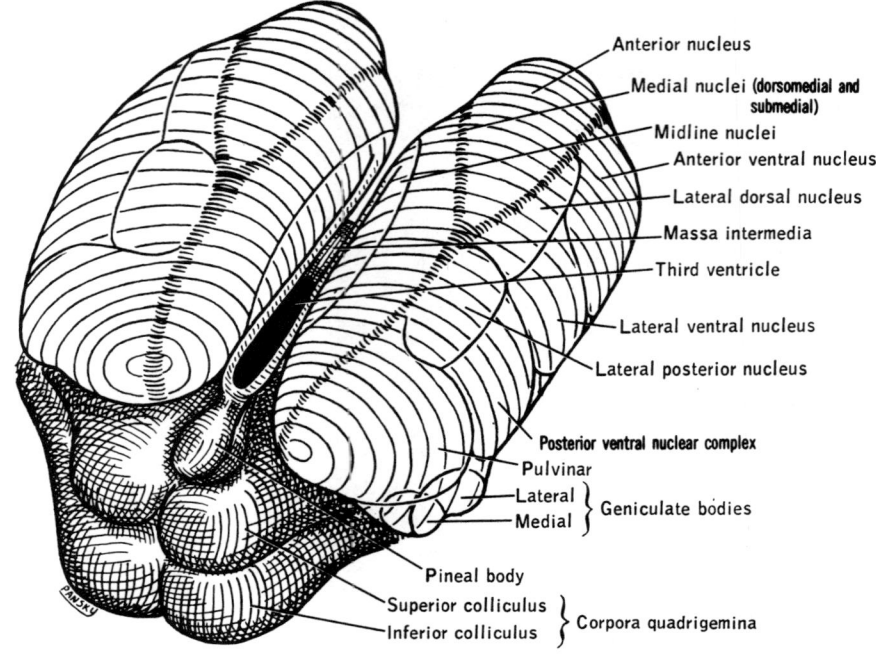

Anterior nucleus
Medial nuclei (dorsomedial and submedial)
Midline nuclei
Anterior ventral nucleus
Lateral dorsal nucleus
Massa intermedia
Third ventricle
Lateral ventral nucleus
Lateral posterior nucleus
Posterior ventral nuclear complex
Pulvinar
Lateral ⎱ Geniculate bodies
Medial ⎰
Pineal body
Superior colliculus ⎱ Corpora quadrigemina
Inferior colliculus ⎰

cerebral hemispheres and lower, subcortical regions and additionally interconnect various subcortical areas. Several classification schemes are used to group the thalamic nuclei, but probably the simplest of these, and the one that I will use, is classification in terms of connections. When this is done, three classes of nuclei may be distinguished: **cortical relay nuclei, association nuclei,** and **intrinsic** or *subcortical* **nuclei.**

Cortical relay nuclei. The cortical relay nuclei receive information from specific ascending sensory pathways and in turn send efferents to specific sensory areas of the neocortex on the surface of the brain. The major cortical relay nuclei are the *lateral geniculate body,* the *medial geniculate body,* the *posterior ventral nuclear complex,* which includes the posteromedial ventral and posterolateral ventral nuclei, the *accessory arcuate nucleus,* and the *lateral ventral nucleus.* With the exception of the accessory arcuate, which lies medial to the posterior ventral nuclear complex, these nuclei may be found in Figures 3-9 and 3-10. As indicated, these nuclei project to specific receiving areas of the neocortex; these areas are shown in Figure 3-11. The numbers of the different cortical areas refer to the commonly used classification system devised by Brodmann more than 50 years ago to map the cortex according to variations in structural characteristics.

The lateral geniculate body is a specific relay nucleus for vision. It receives afferents from the optic tract and also from the superior colliculi via the brachium of the superior colliculus. The lateral geniculate body relays information on to the visual cortex (area 17). The medial geniculate body receives auditory projections from the inferior colliculi via the brachium of the inferior colliculus and sends efferent projections to the auditory cortex (areas 41 and 42). The posterior ventral nuclear complex receives projections from the somesthetic and proprioception systems.

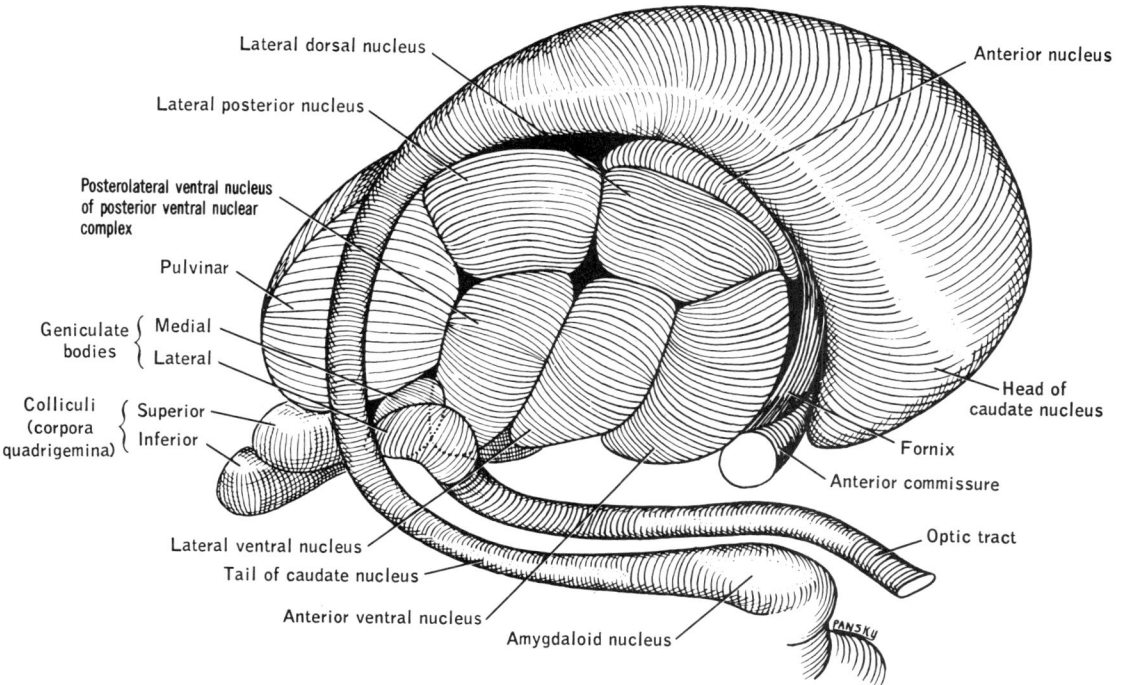

Lateral dorsal nucleus

Lateral posterior nucleus

Posterolateral ventral nucleus
of posterior ventral nuclear
complex

Pulvinar

Geniculate { Medial
bodies { Lateral

Colliculi { Superior
(corpora
quadrigemina) { Inferior

Lateral ventral nucleus

Tail of caudate nucleus

Anterior ventral nucleus

Amygdaloid nucleus

Anterior nucleus

Head of
caudate nucleus

Fornix

Anterior commissure

Optic tract

PANSKY

Figure 3-10
*The thalamic nuclei
as seen from the
lateral aspect. Some
of the related
structures are also
shown. Adapted
from* A Functional
Approach to
Neuroanatomy, *by
E. L. House and B.
Pansky. Copyright
1967 by
McGraw-Hill, Inc.
Reprinted by
permission.*

Somesthesis refers to the senses of the skin, including the perception of heat, pressure, and pain. *Proprioception* refers to the sensation of movement. Efferents from this nuclear complex are projected to the somatosensory cortex (areas 3, 2, and 1). The accessory arcuate nucleus is a relay for taste. The afferents are derived from the taste system, and the efferents project to area 43. Finally, the lateral ventral nucleus receives fibers from the cerebellum and relays information on to the motor (area 4) and premotor (areas 6 and 8) cortical areas. **Ablation** (surgical removal) of the lateral ventral nucleus of the thalamus has been used quite successfully over the years to relieve the rigidity and tremor associated with Parkinson's disease.

Association nuclei. The association nuclei, the second major class of thalamic nuclei, also project to the cerebral cortex. However, they receive few, if any, direct projections from ascending sensory fibers. The afferents of the association nuclei come from other parts of the brain, and their efferents project mainly to association areas of the cortex. **Association cortex** is cortex that is neither sensory nor motor and has generally been assumed to be involved in higher or complex behavior functions. The major thalamic association nuclei are the *anterior nucleus,* the *dorsomedial nucleus* (medial nuclear group), the *submedial nucleus* (medial nuclear group), the *lateral dorsal nucleus,* the *lateral posterior nucleus,* and the *pulvinar.* These nuclei can be located on Figures 3-9 and 3-10. The cortical areas to which they project are indicated in Figure 3-12.

The afferents to the anterior nucleus are chiefly derived from the mammilothalamic tract, which originates in the mammillary region of the hypothalamus. Most of the efferents from this nucleus go to the cingulate gyrus (areas 23, 24, 29, and

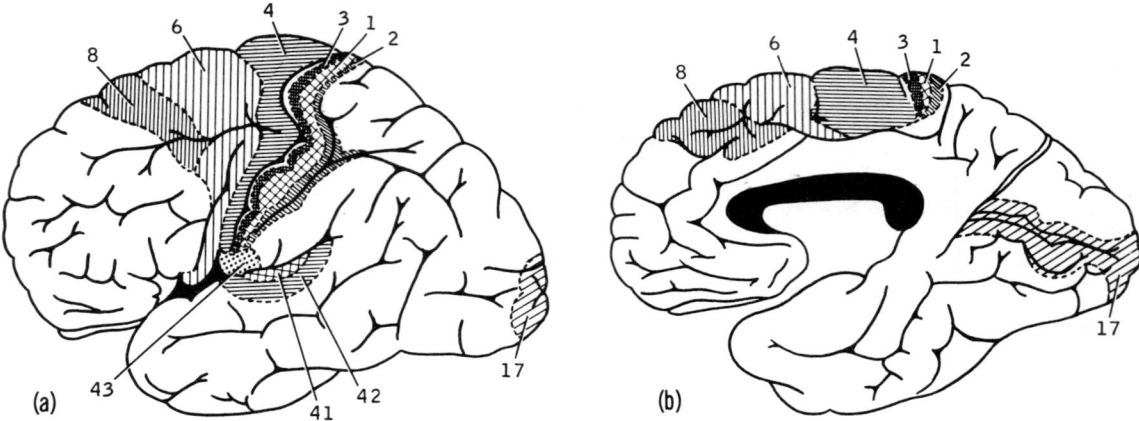

Figure 3-11
The primary sensory
areas of the cortex.
Diagram (a) is a
lateral view and (b)
a medial view of the
areas related to the
thalamic relay
nuclei. The
posterolateral and
posteromedial
ventral nuclei relate
to areas 1, 2, and 3,
the medial
geniculate body to
areas 41 and 42, the
lateral geniculate
body to area 17, the
accessory arcuate
body to area 43, and
the lateral ventral
nucleus to areas 4,
6, and 8. Adapted
from The
Neuroanatomical
Basis for Clinical
Neurology, by T. L.
Peele. Copyright
1954 by
McGraw-Hill,Inc.
Reprinted by
permission.

32). Afferents to the dorsomedial nucleus come from a variety of sources, including portions of the thalamus, hypothalamus, and prefrontal cortex. Its efferents are also widespread, but most of them make their way to frontal association areas (areas 8, 9, 10, 11, 12, 45, 46, and 47). The afferents to the submedial nucleus are similar to those to the dorsomedial nucleus. And, like the dorsomedial nucleus, the submedial nucleus sends most of its efferents to the frontal cortex—to areas 8 and 46 in particular. The lateral dorsal and the lateral posterior nuclei receive their afferents from other thalamic nuclei and send efferents primarily to the parietal lobe (areas 5, 7, 39, and 40), although they send some efferents to the postcentral gyrus (area 19). The dorsomedial nucleus also sends some efferents to area 19. The pulvinar is a large association nucleus on the most posterior part of the lateral thalamus. It receives most of its afferents from other parts of the thalamus, but afferents are also contributed to it by the amygdala and by the inferior portion of the temporal lobe. Its efferents project to posterior association areas of the cortex (areas 5, 7, 19, 39, and 40).

Intrinsic or subcortical nuclei. Also called the *midline* or *intralaminar nuclei,* the intrinsic or subcortical nuclei have no projections to the neocortex. The intrinsic nuclei have connections with other thalamic nuclei, the reticular formation, and various structures of the limbic system. These nuclei have been functionally related to attention shifts and to the mediation of impulses arising from the viscera.

Hypothalamus. The *hypothalamus* is a grouping of small nuclei lying ventral to the thalamus, and it forms a junction between the midbrain and the thalamus. The major nuclei of this structure are shown in Figure 3-13. The function of the hypothalamus is to regulate the expression of basic drive states and related behaviors that are necessary for the survival of the individual and the species. It does this in two ways. First, it mediates overt, observable behavior. Second, through its action as the highest integration region for the autonomic nervous system, it physiologically prepares the organism to engage in a particular behavior pattern. The **autonomic nervous system** is the part of the nervous system that controls visceral functions of the body. To understand the second action, it might help to think of the hypothalamus as translating instructions from structures higher in the chain of command into the physiological correlates of an overt behavior. This function will be elaborated on in Chapter 8 when the physiological substrates of emotion are discussed.

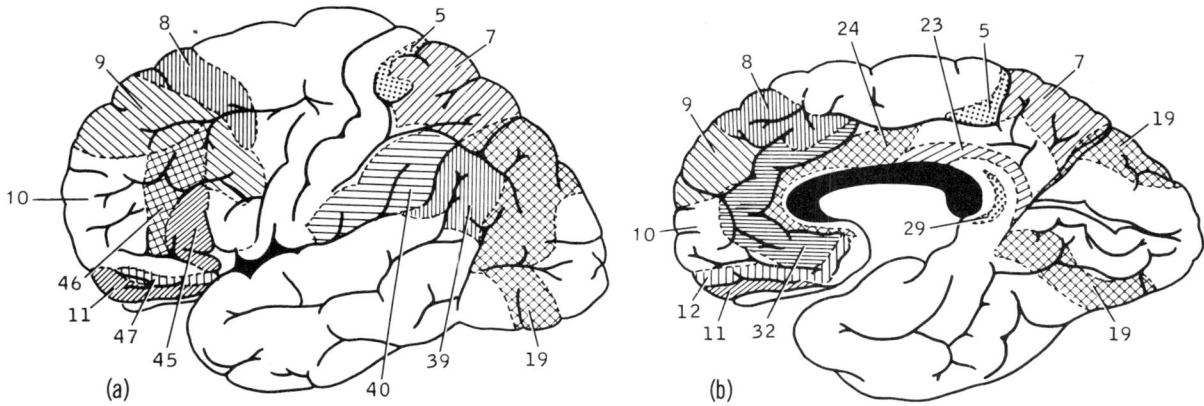

Figure 3-12
*The areas of the
cortex related to the
associative thalamic
nuclei. Diagram (a)
is a lateral view, and
diagram (b) is a
medial view. The
anterior nucleus
relates to areas, 23,
24, 29, and 32, the
dorsal medial
nucleus to areas 8,
9, 10, 11, 12, 19, 45,
46, and 47, the
submedial nucleus
to areas 8 and 46,
the lateral dorsal
and lateral posterior
nuclei to areas 5, 7,
19, 39, and 40, and
the pulvinar to areas
5, 7, 19, 39, and 40.
Adapted from* The
Neuroanatomical
Basis for Clinical
Neurology, *by T. L.
Peele. Copyright
1954 by
McGraw-Hill, Inc.
Reprinted by
permission.*

The hypothalamic control of behavior is a gross control and yields poorly directed and integrated behavior. This point can be verified by the removal of all brain tissue that lies on top of this structure. If this is done, the behavior patterns of the animal will be very primitively organized and poorly directed. Higher brain regions elaborate and refine the crude patterns of behavior that the hypothalamus is capable of initiating. As was indicated, the hypothalamus has been implicated in the mediation of a number of survival behaviors. Among these are sleep and waking, emotion, reproductive behavior, and hunger and thirst. Its functions in governing these processes will be described in later chapters.

The most prominent afferent input to the hypothalamus is the **fornix.** This pathway begins in the hippocampus, which is a structure in the phylogenetically older "rhinencephalic" portion of the cerebral hemispheres. The fornix projects primarily to the posterior hypothalamus. The **medial forebrain bundle** joins the anterior and lateral hypothalamic regions with other rhinencephalic areas. The anterior hypothalamus also receives afferents from the amygdala, via the **stria terminalis.**

The major efferent connections of the hypothalamus are as follows. As mentioned before, the **mammilothalamic tract** sends efferents to one of the major association nuclei of the thalamus—the anterior nucleus. The anterior nucleus in turn projects primarily to the cingulate gyrus of the cerebral hemispheres. The **mammilo-tegmental tract** relates many regions of the hypothalamus to the brain stem reticular formation. The **periventricular fibers** carry impulses upward to the dorsomedial and midline nuclei of the thalamus. Most periventricular fibers are descending and terminate in the brain stem reticular formation or in the "vital centers" of the medulla. **Hypothalamicohypophyseal fibers** arise primarily in the supraoptic and periventricular nuclei of the hypothalamus and project into the subjacent **pituitary** (hypophysis) via a stalk known as the **infundibulum** (see Figure 3-3). Most of these fibers terminate in the posterior pituitary lobe (neurohypophysis). These hypothalamicohypophyseal relations, as depicted in Figure 3-14, are crucial in the neural regulation of endocrine-gland functions.

Subthalamus. The **subthalamus** is a transitional zone between the dorsal thalamus and the tegmental portion of the mesencephalon. It contains a number of distinct nuclei that form part of the extrapyramidal motor system. The hypothalamus lies medial and rostral to the subthalamus.

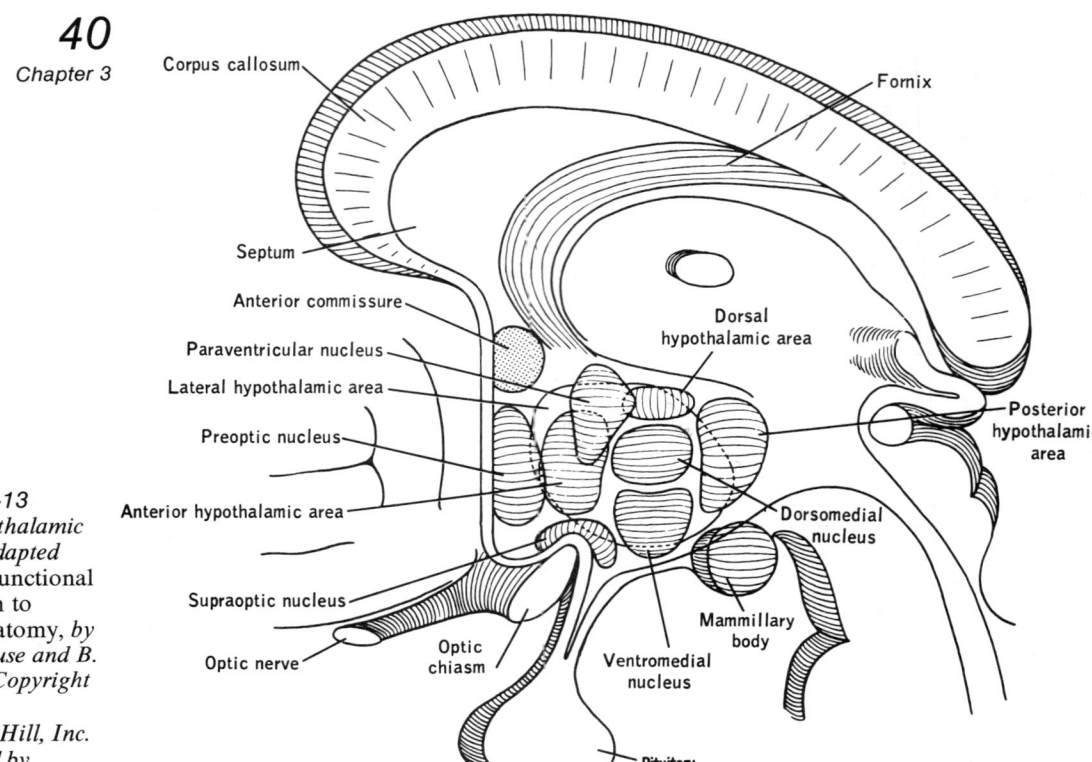

Figure 3-13
The hypothalamic nuclei. Adapted from A Functional Approach to Neuroanatomy, *by E. L. House and B. Pansky. Copyright 1967 by McGraw-Hill, Inc. Reprinted by permission.*

Telencephalon

Basal Ganglia. The telencephalic division of the brain has three parts: the **basal ganglia,** the **rhinencephalon,** and the **neocortex.** The basal ganglia form a large group of nuclei lying in the central regions of the cerebral hemispheres. The basal ganglia partially surround the thalamus, as shown in Figure 3-10, and they are in turn enclosed by the neocortex. The nuclei most often included under the heading *basal ganglia* are the *caudate nucleus,* the *putamen,* and the *globus pallidus.* The putamen and globus pallidus together make up the *lenticular nucleus.* When the caudate and lenticular nuclear complexes are taken together, they are referred to as the *corpus striatum.* Figure 3-15 shows various views of the basal ganglia.

The basal ganglia appear to control movement and have at least indirect connections with motor neurons. They apparently mediate gross movements that we normally perform unconsciously (for example, walking). In contrast, the motor cortex controls more highly discrete movements—that is, delicate movements that require great concentration. Another function of the basal ganglia seems to be to inhibit muscle tone. Damage to the basal ganglia may produce **hypertonia**—a significantly increased level of muscle tone that tends to restrict body movement and facial expression. It is thought that loss of basal-ganglia influences through disease results in the tremor associated with Parkinson's disease.

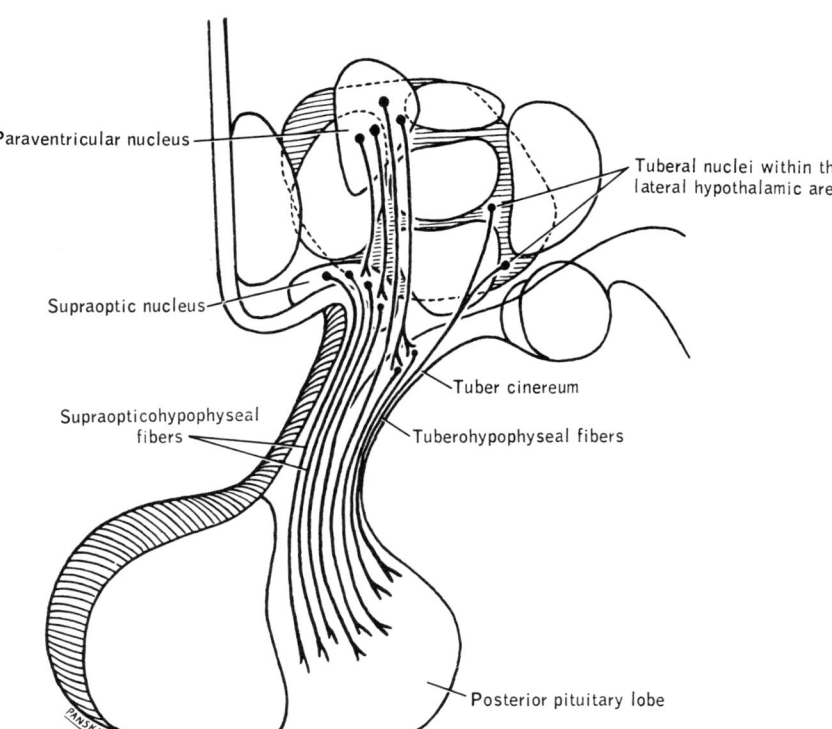

Paraventricular nucleus

Tuberal nuclei within the
lateral hypothalamic area

Supraoptic nucleus

Tuber cinereum

Supraopticohypophyseal
fibers

Tuberohypophyseal fibers

Posterior pituitary lobe

Figure 3-14
*The
hypothalamicohypophyseal
paths. From* A
Functional
Approach to
Neuroanatomy, *by
E. L. House and B.
Pansky. Copyright
1967 by
McGraw-Hill, Inc.
Reprinted by
permission.*

Rhinencephalon. In the past, the term *rhinencephalon* was used as a designation for those regions of the brain thought to process olfactory information, but it is now generally accepted that certain rhinencephalic structures probably have no olfactory function. In addition to the olfactory bulb and tracts, the major structures or regions in the rhinencephalon are (as shown in Figure 3-16) the *septal area,* the *hippocampal formation,* and the *amygdala.* The amygdala is also often classified as belonging to the basal ganglia because the tail of the caudate nucleus merges posteriorly with the amygdala. However, since the amygdala does not directly function to control movement, it is more logically grouped with the rhinencephalic structures, which perform functions related to those of the amygdala in mediating behavior. The *cingulate gyrus* is also at times classified as a rhinencephalic structure.

If one adds the hypothalamus and certain portions of the thalamus to all of the rhinencephalic structures enumerated above, then the *limbic system* is defined. The limbic system is a subneocortex-level network of structures. As will be seen in later chapters, these structures are involved in the control of behaviors related to emotion, motivation, and learning.

Neocortex

The neocortex of the telencephalon was the last region of the brain to evolve, and it is greatly enlarged in primates, particularly humans. The entire dorsal and

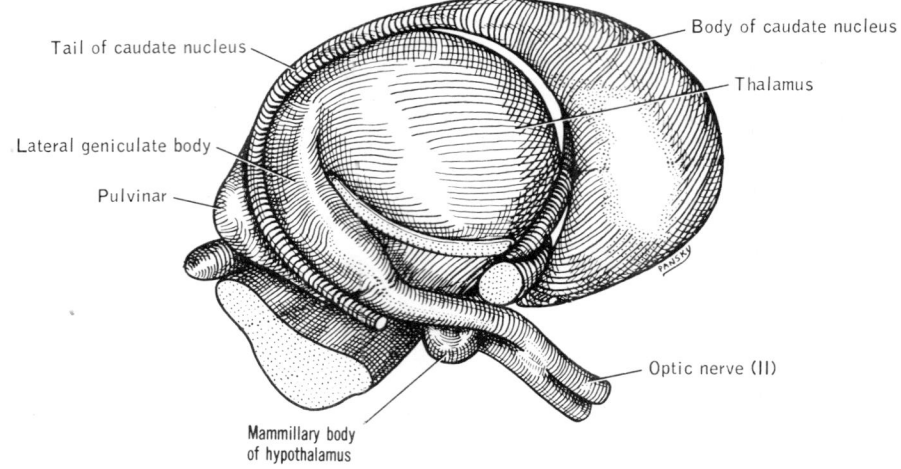

Tail of caudate nucleus

Body of caudate nucleus

Thalamus

Lateral geniculate body

Pulvinar

Optic nerve (II)

Mammillary body
of hypothalamus

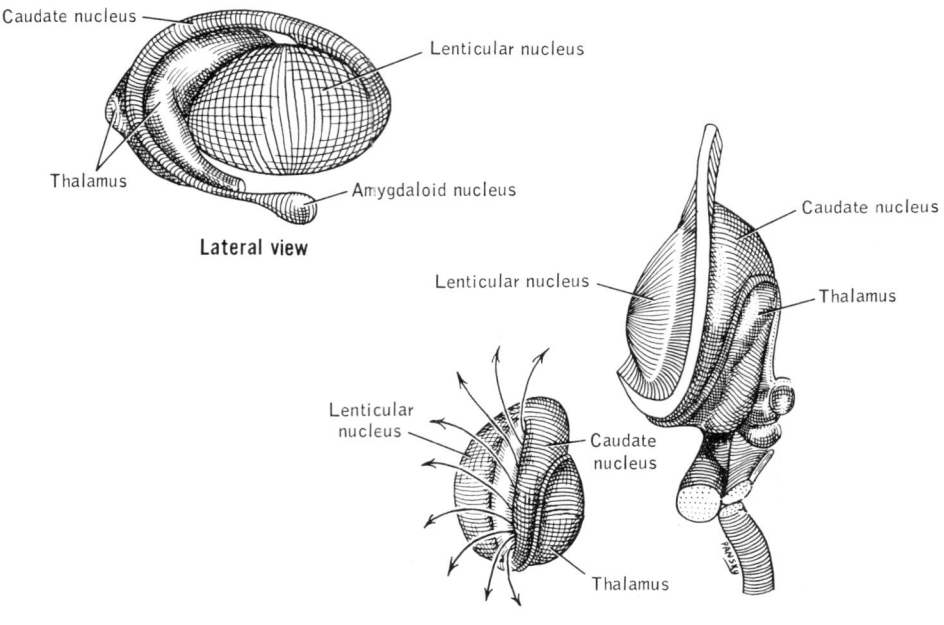

Caudate nucleus

Lenticular nucleus

Thalamus

Amygdaloid nucleus

Lateral view

Lenticular nucleus

Caudate nucleus

Thalamus

Lenticular
nucleus

Caudate
nucleus

Thalamus

Dorsal view

Caudate nucleus

Putamen

Tail of
caudate
nucleus

Amygdaloid
nucleus

Anterior view

Posterior view

Figure 3-15
Various views of the
basal ganglia.
Adapted from A
Functional
Approach to
Neuroanatomy, *by*
E. L. House and B.
Pansky. Copyright
1967 by
McGraw-Hill, Inc.
Reprinted by
permission.

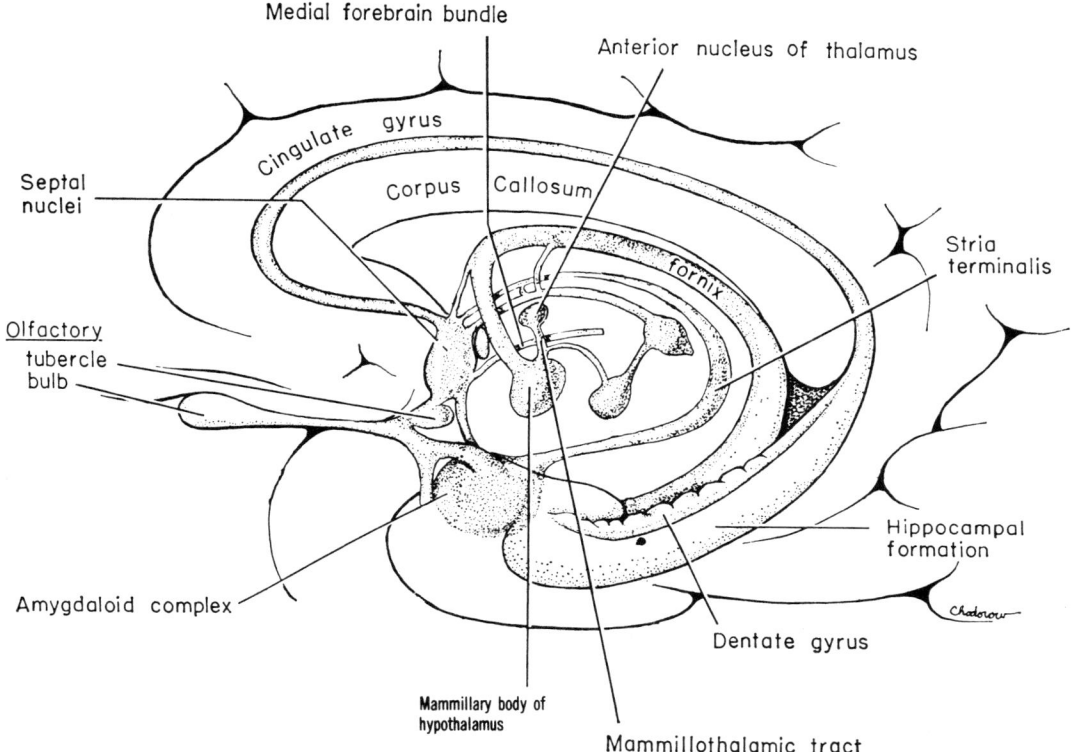

Medial forebrain bundle

Anterior nucleus of thalamus

Cingulate gyrus

Corpus Callosum

Septal nuclei

fornix

Stria terminalis

Olfactory
tubercle
bulb

Amygdaloid complex

Hippocampal formation

Dentate gyrus

Mammillary body of hypothalamus

Mammillothalamic tract

Figure 3-16
The rhinencephalic structural relationships as seen in a medial view of the right hemisphere. Adapted from Strong and Elwyn's Human Neuroanatomy (5th ed.), by R. C. Truex and M. B. Carpenter. Copyright © 1964 by the Williams & Wilkins Co., Baltimore. Reprinted by permission.

lateral surfaces and much of the ventral surface of the cerebral hemispheres consist of neocortex.

The neocortex is the most complex tissue in the brain and consists of six distinct layers of cells. In contrast, the phylogenetically old areas of the rhinencephalon (such as the hippocampus) consist of only three layers of cells. The cingulate gyrus is a transitional zone of cortex and is composed of four cell layers.

Communication between the hemispheres is conveyed via several commissures or pathways, the most prominent of which is the **corpus callosum** (Figure 3-16).

The surface of the cerebral hemispheres of humans is convoluted. The ridges are called *gyri* (the singular is *gyrus*). The grooves are called *fissures* or *sulci* (the singular is *sulcus*). These have all been named, as shown in Figure 3-17, and may be used as landmarks. Each hemisphere can be divided into four lobes: *frontal, parietal, occipital,* and *temporal.*

Frontal Lobe. The *frontal lobes* include all the cortex lying anterior to the *central sulcus.* Immediately anterior to the central sulcus is the *precentral gyrus,* which makes up the **primary motor area** (area 4; see Figure 3-11). This region controls discrete movements, particularly of the fingers. Areas 6 and 8, lying anterior to area 4, are referred to as the **premotor areas** (see Figure 3-11). Stimulation of area 6 will produce gross movements of the limbs, and stimulation of area 8 will produce discrete

43

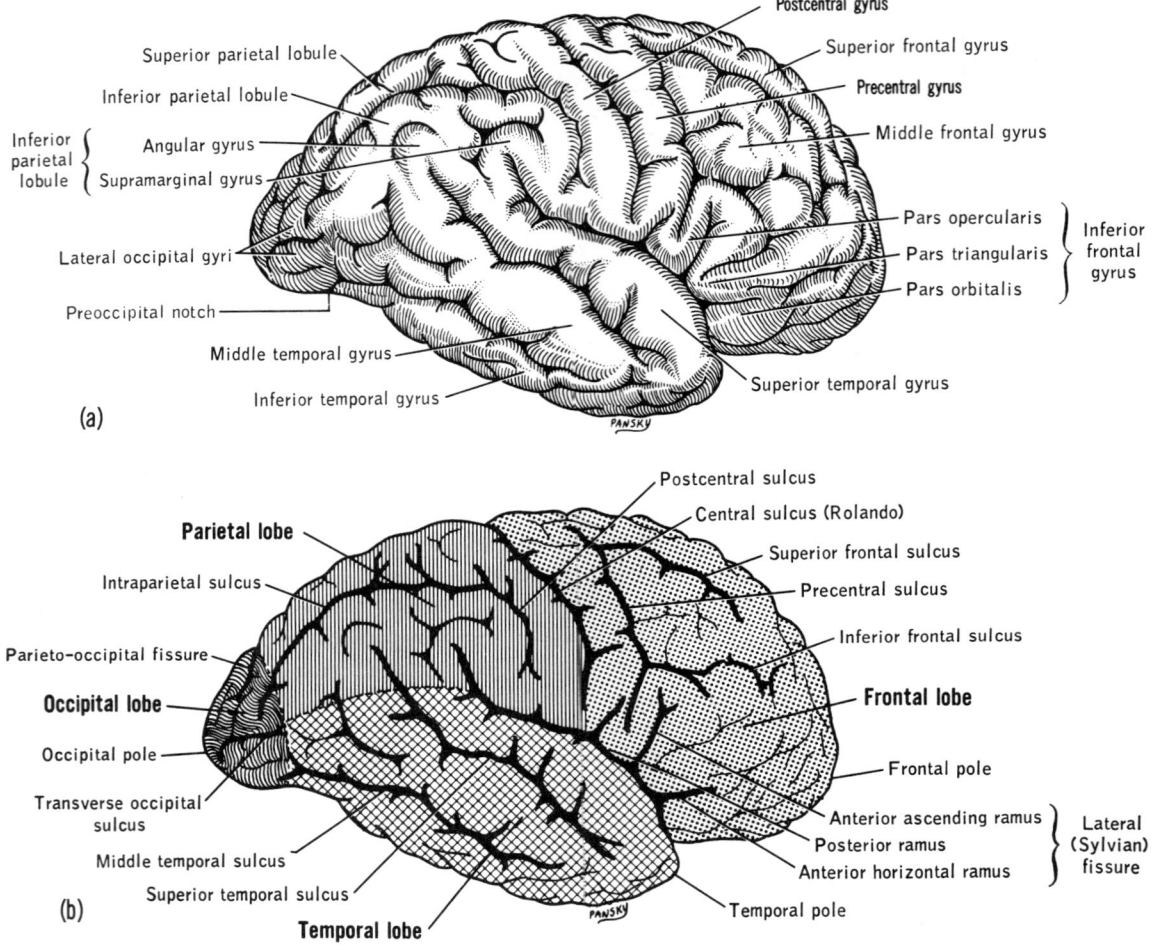

Figure 3-17
(a) *A lateral view of the human cerebral hemispheres, illustrating the principal gyri.* (b) *A lateral view of the human cerebral hemispheres, illustrating the principal sulci and lobes. From* A Functional Approach to Neuroanatomy, *by E. L. House and B. Pansky. Copyright 1967 by McGraw-Hill, Inc. Reprinted by permission.*

head and/or eye movements. I pointed out earlier that areas 4, 6, and 8 receive projections from the lateral ventral nucleus, one of the cortical relay nuclei of the thalamus.

The remainder of the frontal lobe, which is anterior to the motor and premotor areas, is the **prefrontal association cortex** (areas 9, 10, 11, 12, 45, 46, and 47); it receives afferents primarily from the dorsomedial nucleus of the thalamus—an association nucleus. As I've indicated, association cortex is cortex that is neither sensory nor motor and that is assumed to be involved in higher or more complex behavior processes, such as emotion and memory.

Parietal Lobe. The *parietal lobe* lies posterior to the central sulcus, which serves as a dividing line between it and the frontal lobe (see Figure 3-17). The parietal lobe is separated from the subjacent *temporal lobe* by the **lateral fissure** and by an imaginary line extending from the angle of the posterior ramus of the lateral fissure to the occipital pole (see Figure 3-17). The portion of the parietal lobe directly posterior to the central sulcus contains the somatosensory projection areas (areas 3, 2, and 1; see Figure 3-11), which receive fibers from the posteroventral nuclear complex of the thalamus. The specific projection region for taste is located at the ventral end of the postcentral gyrus of this lobe (area 43; see Figure 3-11). The parietal lobe contains association cortex areas 5, 7, 39, and 40 (see Figure 3-12), which receive thalamic projections from the pulvinar, lateral dorsal, and lateral posterior association nuclei.

Occipital Lobe. As shown in Figure 3-17, the *occipital lobes* are not clearly demarcated by any major fissures. The occipital lobe contains the **primary visual projection area** (area 17; see Figure 3-11), which receives projections from the lateral geniculate body of the thalamus. Fibers from area 17 project to the adjacent visual association area (area 18) and through it to area 19 (see Figure 3-12). Both areas 18 and 19 send fibers back to area 17, thus establishing potential **reverberatory circuits.** (A reverberatory circuit is a circular nervous pathway that, once activated, can reactivate itself over and over again.) Area 19 also receives projections from a majority of the thalamic association nuclei.

Hebb (1949) and others have suggested that memories in humans are stored in sensory association areas that border specific sensory projection regions of the cortex. It has been further suggested that short-term memory of an event that has just transpired is mediated by activity in reverberatory circuits such as could potentially exist in areas 17, 18, and 19. Evidence bearing on this possibility will be discussed in Chapter 10.

Temporal Lobe. The *temporal lobes* are situated lateral and ventral to the lateral fissure (see Figure 3-17). The **primary auditory projection areas** (areas 41 and 42; see Figure 3-11) are located in this lobe. Much of the auditory projection area and most of the adjacent auditory association areas are hidden in the folds of the lateral fissure. The auditory projection area receives afferents from the medial geniculate body of the thalamus. Stimulation of this specific sensory area yields auditory sensations.

Most of the remaining temporal lobe is classified as association cortex. Many researchers have suggested that the temporal lobe association areas serve as repositories for long-term memory. In support of this hypothesis, Penfield (1965) has reported that stimulation of the human temporal lobe can sometimes elicit complex memories.

The Development of the Vertebrate Brain

Phylogenetic Considerations

As indicated earlier in this chapter, all vertebrate brains can be divided into five regions: myelencephalon, metencephalon, mesencephalon, diencephalon, and telencephalon. However, when you examine a series of successively more highly evolved vertebrate brains, such as that shown in Figure 3-18, you might think that everything has changed. There certainly have been changes in the vertebrate brain as it evolved from fish to human over time, but most of these changes have involved only the addition of something new or the modification or enlargement of some existing region. Some of the changes that the brain has experienced during its evolution from fish to human are as follows.

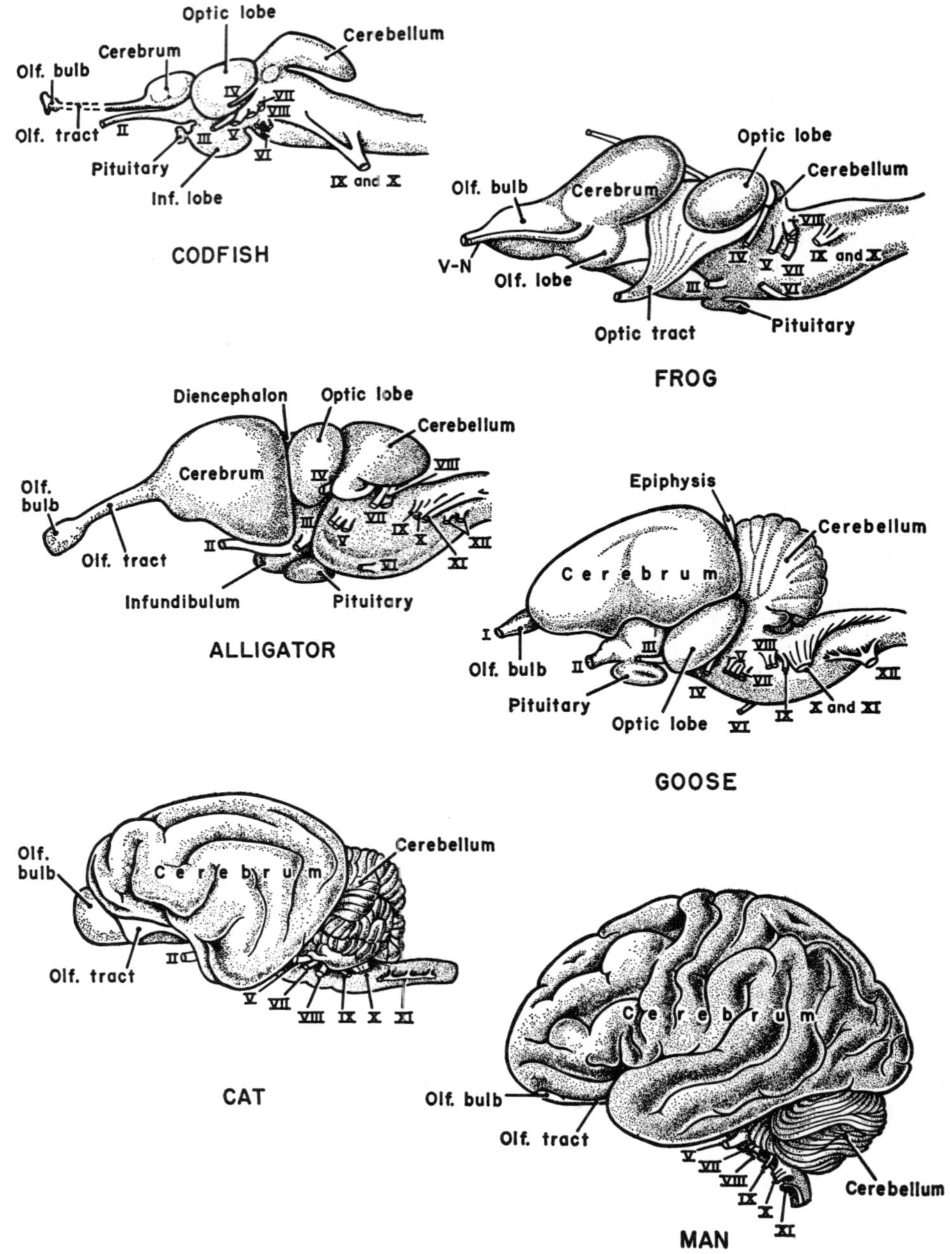

CODFISH

FROG

ALLIGATOR

GOOSE

*Figure 3-18
A representative
series of vertebrate
brains. From Strong
and Elwyn's
Human
Neuroanatomy (5th
ed.), by R. C. Truex
and M. B.
Carpenter.
Copyright © 1964
by the Williams &
Wilkins Co.,
Baltimore.
Reprinted by
permission.*

CAT

MAN

One notable characteristic of the human brain is the largeness of the cerebellum. This has probably resulted from two factors: the assumption of an upright posture and the discrete movements made possible by the evolution of the hands, particularly the development of the opposable thumb. The ventral surface of the midbrain became larger to accommodate the masses of descending motor fibers that developed with the increase in motor control.

The most striking evolutionary change that occurred was the tremendous growth of the cerebral hemispheres, which are markedly enlarged in primates and especially in humans. Fish have no cerebral cortex. The forebrain of fish is made up of only the olfactory bulbs and a primitive thalamus and corpus striatum. The first cortex appears in amphibia and reptiles, in the form of a nucleus of cell bodies located between the olfactory bulbs and the remainder of the forebrain.

The first cortex having nonolfactory functions appears in birds, but it is small and poorly developed. Only in mammals does the cerebral cortex become a true cortex with a definite cortical structure devoted to higher behavioral processes. As the cerebrum increased in size, the necessity arose to increase the area of the hemispheres without enlarging the total brain size too much. This increase in surface area was accomplished by the formation of folds or convolutions. The rat has a very simple cortex, with no convolutions. However, in carnivora such as dogs and cats, the principal fissures used to demarcate the human brain are beginning to develop. As you saw in Figure 3-17, the number of convolutions in the human brain is indeed large.

It is important to note that the basic organization of the cortical sensory and motor areas does not vary greatly among mammals. However, as the mammalian scale of evolution is ascended, the amount of cortex that is association cortex increases greatly. As you can see in Figure 3-19, most of the rabbit cortex is concerned with sensory and motor functions, while most of the primate cortex is association cortex. This difference is further accentuated in the human brain. Hence, as the phylogenetic scale is ascended, not only does the size of the cerebrum increase; the relative amount of the cortex that is association cortex also increases.

Figure 3-19
Maps of the sensory, motor, and association (unlabeled) areas of the cerebral cortex of the rabbit, the cat, and the monkey. Adapted from "Patterns of Sensory Representation in the Cerebral Cortex," by C. N. Woolsey, Federation Proceedings, 1947, 6, 437–441. Copyright 1947 by Federation of American Societies for Experimental Biology. Reprinted by permission.

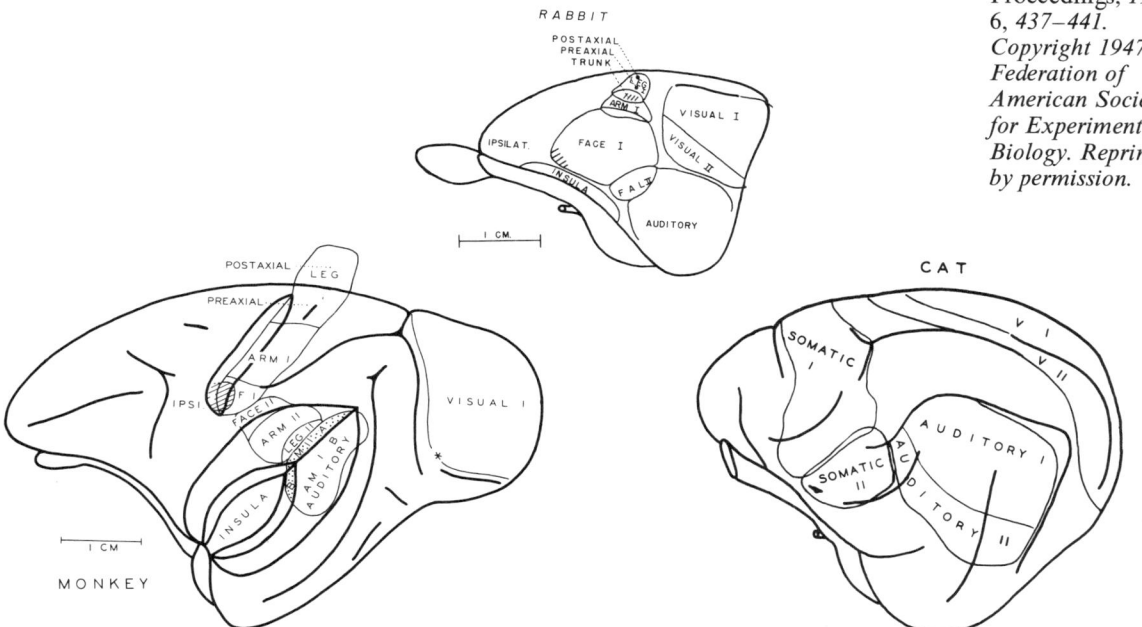

In its embryonic development, the human brain reenacts its phyletic history. The earliest stages of development of the human brain are shown in Figures 3-20 and 3-21. The brain begins as a relatively straight **neural tube** (Figures 3-20A and 3-21A). From the beginning, when the neural tube is formed, three primary brain regions may be distinguished. These early subdivisions include a cephalic **prosencephalon** (forebrain), a middle **mesencephalon** (midbrain) and a caudal **rhombencephalon** (hindbrain).

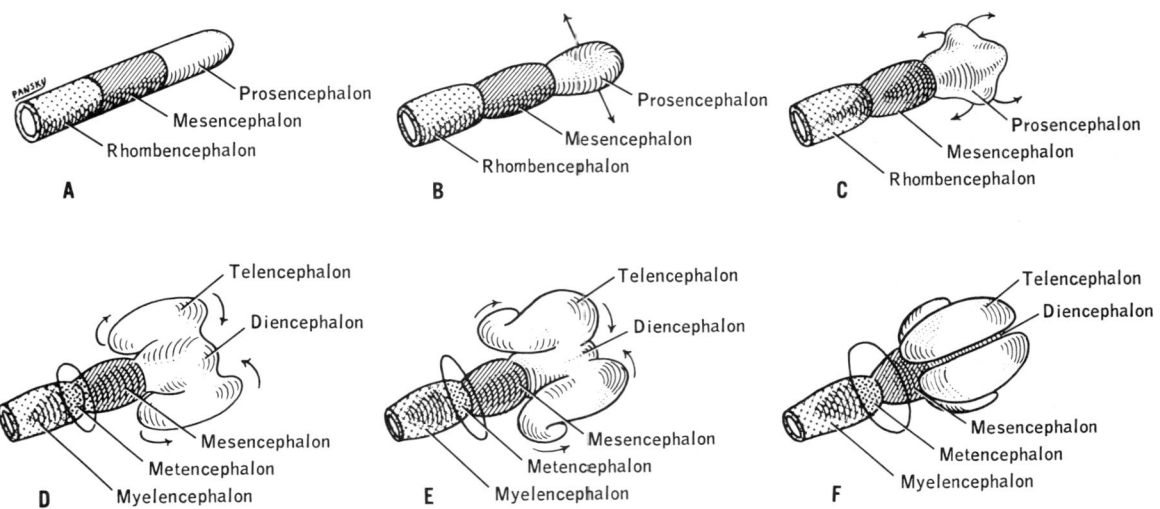

Figure 3-20
The embryonic development of the brain, as seen from the dorsal aspect. From A Functional Approach to Neuroanatomy *by E. L. House and B. Pansky. Copyright 1967 by McGraw-Hill, Inc. Reprinted by permission.*

Rapid changes occur in the developing brain during the fourth and fifth weeks of embryonic life (Figures 3-20B and C and 3-21B and C). By early in the sixth week, five brain components can be identified (Figures 3-20D and 3-21D). The forebrain now has a cephalic telencephalon and a more caudal part, the diencephalon. The mesencephalon has remained small, but the rhombencephalon has divided into two segments—the metencephalon and the myelencephalon. The more cephalic metencephalon will later form the pons and cerebellum, and the caudal myelencephalon will become the medulla.

As the brain develops further (Figures 3-20E and F and 3-21D), the telencephalon grows out and overlays the diencephalon, and the cerebellum develops. During the first four months of development, the surfaces of the cerebral hemispheres are smooth. Then the surfaces of the hemispheres begin to grow rapidly and develop convolutions (gyri) separated by furrows (sulci, fissures). As a result of this folding process, two-thirds of the cerebral cortex is buried in the walls and floors of the sulci by the time the brain reaches adult size.

It is interesting to note that sulci appear in the fetal brain in an orderly sequence. The phylogenetically older sulci appear first in the developing cerebrum, and the more recently evolved sulci appear later. By the time the fetus reaches full term, the principal sulci and gyri that mark the human cerebral cortex can all be identified.

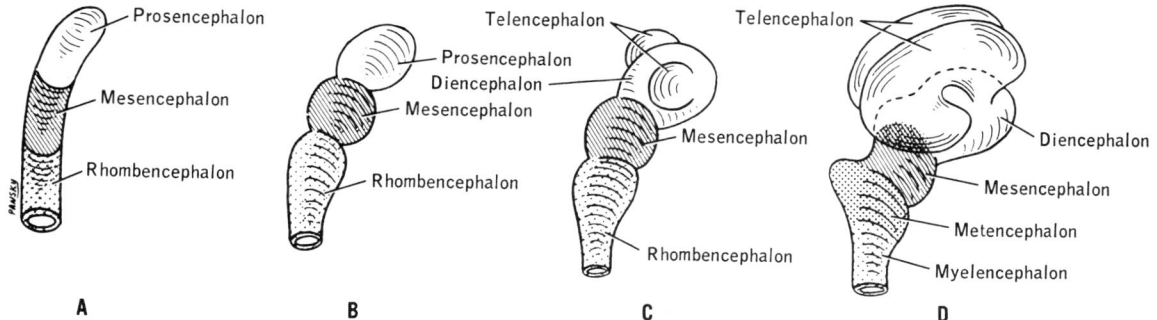

A   B   C   D

Figure 3-21
Approximately the same stages of embryonic development as shown in Figure 3-20, seen from the side. From A Functional Approach to Neuroanatomy *by E. L. House and B. Pansky. Copyright 1967 by McGraw-Hill, Inc. Reprinted by permission.*

Chapter Summary and Conclusions

The purpose of this chapter was to provide an overview of the functional anatomy of the brain.

The nervous system becomes the brain upon entering the skull, and the spinal cord thereupon merges with the most posterior region of the brain—the medulla. The medulla is the major structure of the myelencephalon, and, together with the metencephalic structures (the pons and the cerebellum), it forms the hindbrain. The next division of the brain is the mesencephalon or midbrain. It includes the tegmentum and the superior and inferior colliculi. The forebrain, composed of the diencephalon and telencephalon, is the most recently evolved portion of the brain.

The diencephalon contains the hypothalamus, pituitary, subthalamus, and thalamus. The diencephalon also contains the anterior portion of the reticular formation, which originates in the medulla. The remaining forebrain structures constitute the telencephalon.

The telencephalon includes the basal ganglia, rhinencephalon, and cerebral hemispheres. Major regions or structures in the rhinencephalon include the septal area, hippocampal formation, and amygdala. The cingulate gyrus is also at times classified as part of the rhinencephalon, while the amygdala is often considered to be part of the basal ganglia.

The neocortex of the cerebral hemispheres was the last region of the brain to evolve, and it is greatly enlarged in primates, particularly humans. For convenience, scientists divide each hemisphere into four lobes: frontal, parietal, occipital, and temporal. There are three functionally distinct types of neocortex making up the hemispheres: sensory, motor, and association cortex. It is the third type of cortex—association cortex—that places humans apart from the remainder of the animal kingdom.

If one examines the phylogenetic development of the brain, the most striking fact that one finds is the tremendous growth of the neocortical mantle. Fish have no cerebral cortex, reptiles and amphibia have a very rudimentary cortex, and in birds the neocortex is small and poorly developed. Only in mammals does the cortex become a true cortex. Among mammals, there is a tremendous difference in the proportion of neocortex that is association cortex. (Association cortex is cortex that is neither sensory nor motor in function but rather seems to be related to higher behavioral processes.) In lower mammals, such as rats and rabbits, there is very little association cortex; almost all of their cortex is devoted to specific sensory or motor

49

functions. However, in the human brain, the majority of the cortex is association cortex.

The final topic of this chapter was the ontogenetic development of the human brain. It was indicated that, during its embryonic development, the human brain goes through a series of stages that reenact its phylogenetic history. Even the sulci appear in an orderly sequence that recapitulates their phyletic emergence. With an overview of the brain's anatomy and of how the functional unit of the brain—the neuron—processes information, we are now almost ready to investigate neural functions in behavior processes. Before we can do this, an understanding of some of the research methods used by neuroscientists is needed. These methods are discussed in the next chapter.

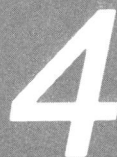

Research Methods
in the Neurosciences

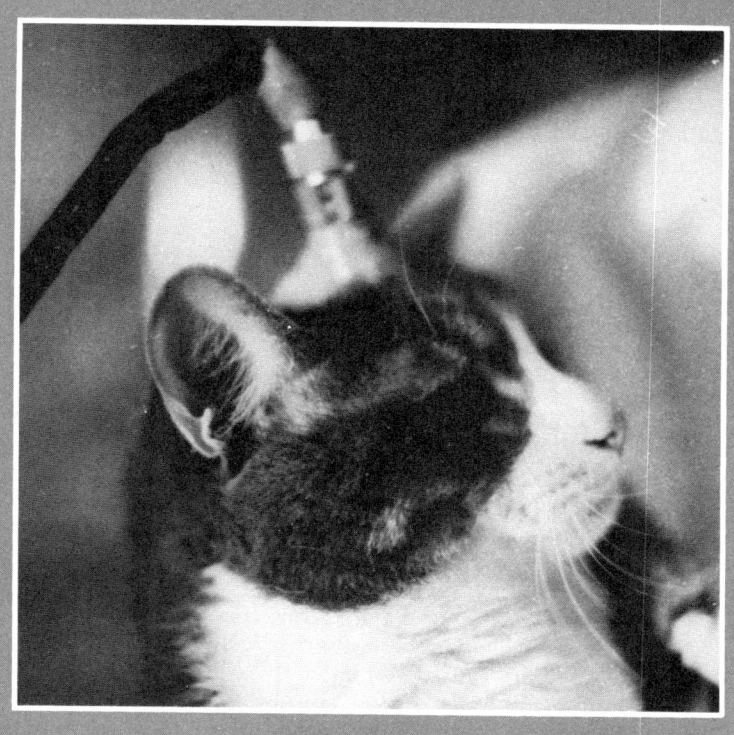

The goal of the physiological psychologist is to define the physiological substrates of behavior. In order to accomplish this, researchers have developed some new research methods and borrowed others from other branches of science. To get a clear understanding of the findings produced by neuroscience research, you'll need to be familiar with these techniques.

A detailed description of these research technologies is beyond the scope of this book. The reader who would like detailed information regarding how these techniques are used should refer to one of the excellent physiological psychology techniques books that are available (for example, Hart, 1969; Myers, 1971; Singh & Avery, 1975; Skinner, 1971). Basically, four techniques are currently used by investigators in this field: lesions, electrical stimulation, chemical stimulation, and electrical recording. These methods may be employed either separately or in combination. All surgical procedures are conducted under anesthesia.

Lesions

Ablation

The oldest and still most widely used technique for studying neural functions is the **ablation** (also called *lesion or extirpation*) method, in which all of the cells in a region of the brain are removed or destroyed and the effects on behavior evaluated. Since the brain is bilaterally symmetrical, the lesions must bilaterally destroy the structure or region being studied in order to produce an alteration in behavior.

Lesion studies have produced a great deal of our current knowledge about the functions performed by various brain areas in mediating behavior. However, one must always be aware of the fact that a change in behavior following a neural ablation does not necessarily imply that the structure is a "center" regulating the behavior under consideration. The neural area is more likely only a portion of a system that is intimately concerned with the behavior. Further, it is often hard to determine the basis for the observed changes in behavior. Did they result from a change in motivation, in level of arousal, in general activity level, or from something else?

The ablation technique was pioneered by Pierre Flourens (1794–1867) in the early 19th century, when, using infrahuman subjects, he examined the effects on behavior of removing different parts of the brain. This technique was almost the only method available to neuroscientists until the 1930s. Victor Horsley (1857–1916) must be credited with laying the foundations for modern neurosurgical techniques, for both clinical and research applications. Horsley performed his first brain operation in 1886, and during his career he contributed many innovative operative techniques to the field. His development of the **stereotaxic method,** with R. H. Clarke in 1908, was a milestone.

The stereotaxic method made it possible to destroy structures buried in the depths of the brain without causing significant damage to overlying tissues. A modern stereotaxic device is shown in Figure 4-1. This apparatus consists of a frame that holds the animal's head firmly in a standard or reference-zero position. Attached micro-manipulators or electrode carriers allow a lesioning **electrode** to be moved into an exact position with respect to the reference zero. In this way, an electrode can be directed to any preselected point in the brain.

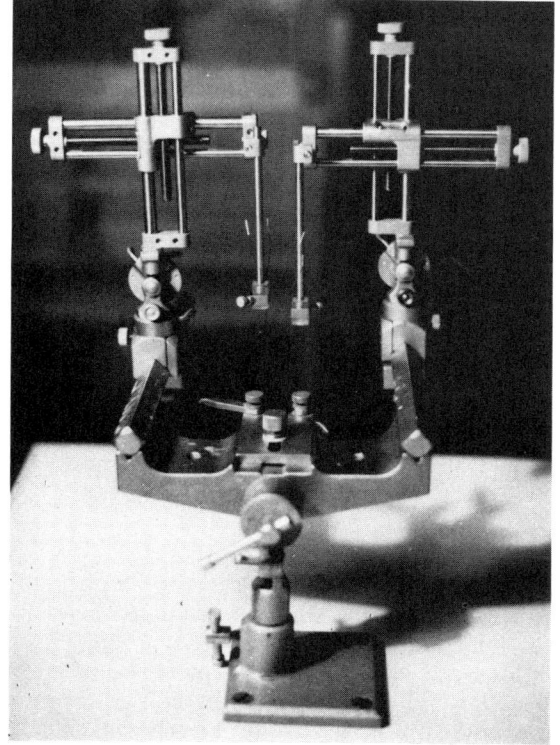

Figure 4-1
*A modern
stereotaxic device.*

To properly use the stereotaxic device, it is necessary to know the exact location of the structure being studied with respect to the reference zero. To make this task relatively easy, *brain atlases* have been published for the species most commonly used in brain research. A sample page from the Pellegrino and Cushman (1967) atlas of the rat brain is shown in Figure 4-2. The atlas indicates where an electrode should be placed in the three principal axes (anterior/posterior, lateral, and vertical) to reach a given brain locus.

A number of different procedures are utilized to produce an ablation of neural tissue. Ablation of the neocortex surface is probably best accomplished via aspiration using weak suction and small pipettes. This procedure results in a small piece of the brain being removed. Depth lesions are usually made electrically, by Horsley and

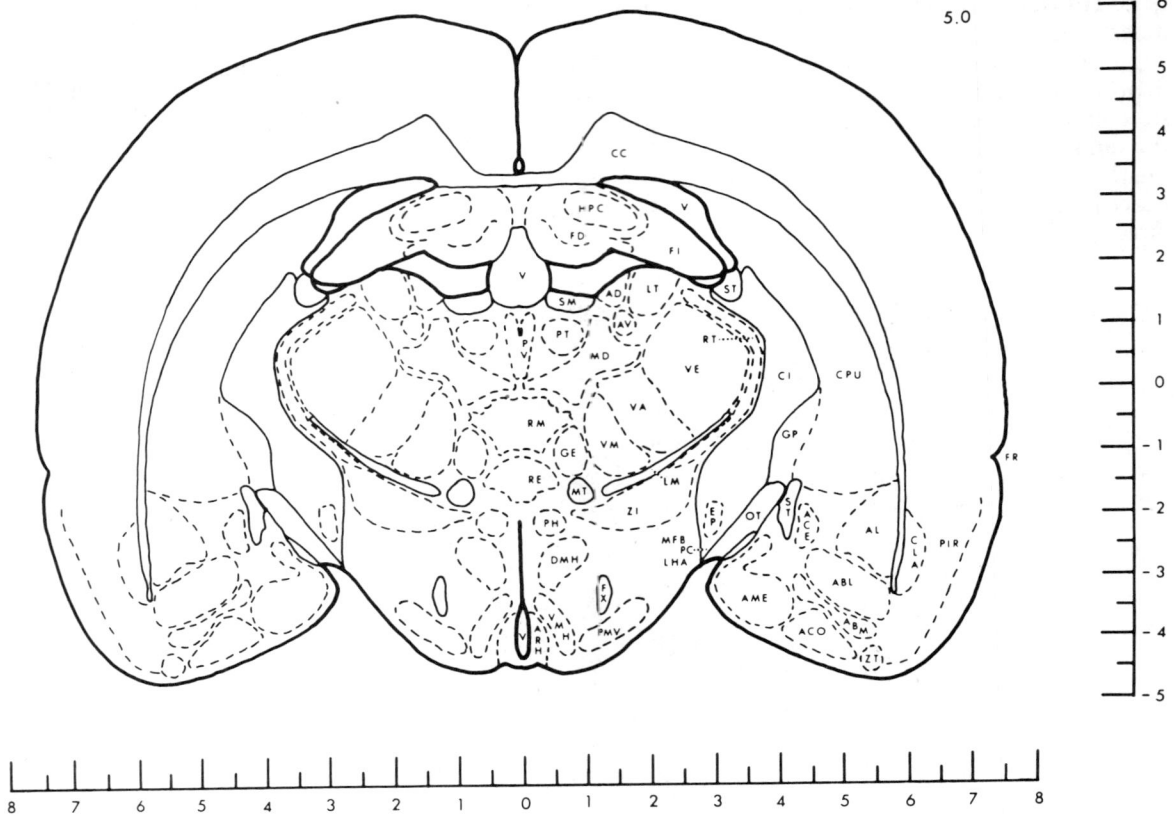

5.0

Figure 4-2
A plate from the Pellegrino and Cushman stereotaxic atlas of the rat brain, showing an anterior plane. The dorsal/ventral and medial/lateral coordinates are given in millimeters. From A Stereotaxic Atlas of the Rat Brain, *by L. J. Pellegrino and A. J. Cushman. Copyright 1967 by Plenum Publishing Corporation. Reprinted by permission.*

Clarke's stereotaxic method. Although this latter technique is fairly accurate, the exact placement and extent of the lesions must later be verified histologically. Histological methods will be discussed later in this chapter.

Electrolytic lesions are easily made by passing direct current through an electrode that has been lowered to the desired place. Most commonly, stainless steel wires, insulated except at the tip, are used for this purpose. When a continuous flow of fairly intense (1–4 milliamperes) direct current is passed through the electrode, tissue is destroyed in the region of the uninsulated tip, thereby yielding a discrete and localized lesion.

Although the electrode-produced-lesion technique is widely utilized, it does have several disadvantages. The most obvious problem is controlling the exact position and size of the ablation. Another problem is that the shape of the destruction is roughly spherical, which is not always the shape desired. Finally, the lesion does not have distinct borders. Hence, it is often difficult to determine whether the observed changes following the lesion were due to the destruction of a distinct structure or to the interruption of fiber pathways located next to the destroyed structure.

The effect of a brain lesion on the behavior of adult nonhuman animals can be critically affected by the age of the subjects when the ablation is made. Lesions made in young animals may not yield any behavior effects when these same subjects are later tested as adults. Even animals that have undergone ablation as adults will sometimes show recovery of function. Therefore, the interval elapsing between surgery and assessment can significantly influence the outcome and interpretation of an experiment. Although the rationale for doing brain-lesion studies is that a lesion will tell something about what the destroyed area normally does, it is certainly possible that the results will instead indicate what the remaining brain tissue does once the influences of the lesioned area have been removed. When brain researchers conduct an experiment, their most challenging and perplexing problem is often that of determining the basis for their obtained results.

Reversible Lesions

Another disadvantage of the ablation technique is its irreversibility. Once the ablation is completed, it is thereafter impossible to obtain samples of "normal" behavior. This problem can be circumvented by the use of reversible or temporary lesions, and several methods for making reversible lesions have been reported.

A reversible lesion of cortical and subcortical regions can sometimes be made by either topical or intracerebral administrations of potassium-chloride solution. This procedure is called **spreading depression,** and it causes a temporary inactivation of brain cells. Bureš and his associates (for example, Bureš & Burešová, 1963) have used this technique in a number of studies examining the memory-consolidation process. Microinjections of drugs, such as procaine, that temporarily interfere with neural functions have also been used to cause temporary lesions to subcortical regions. Agents that selectively block the transmission of information across certain categories of synapses (for example, cholinergic or adrenergic) are also commonly used.

Another interesting method for creating a reversible lesion is to cool a selected area of the brain below a temperature of about 25° C. Many brain cells cease to operate at this temperature. When the affected region is allowed to return to normal body temperature, the cells recover their normal functioning. Special probes have been devised to produce discrete lesions of this sort. These cryoprobes can also be used to yield permanent ablations of the target region by reducing the temperature below freezing. In this case, the affected cells are destroyed by the formation of ice crystals.

Electrical Stimulation

The converse of the lesion technique, in terms of its usual effect on neural tissue, is electrical stimulation. It produces excitation or activation of an area. The historical highlights of the use of this technique in brain research are summarized below. More detailed historical accounts of this method, as well as more general historical reviews of research in the neural sciences, are provided by Sheer (1961) and Valenstein (1973).

In 1870, Fritsch and Hitzig excited the scientific world when they published the results of their systematic experiments on the electrical stimulation of the cortex of dogs. The stage for their inquiries was set when Hitzig observed that electrical stimulation of the human cortex produced eye movements. In their monumental inquiry, Fritsch and Hitzig used bipolar (two wires side by side) platinum electrodes stuck through a cork to apply their electrical stimulation, and they carefully explored the entire surface of the cortex.

Using weak current, Fritsch and Hitzig were able to map regions of the motor cortex by showing that stimulation of discrete areas produced specific movements of the neck, face, and limbs. Their findings were confirmed by other researchers, and, within a few years, a more detailed map of the motor areas had been developed by Ferrier (1876) and others.

Other researchers studied the effects of stimulation of the human neocortex and successfully elaborated on Hitzig's initial observations. In 1909, for example, Harvey Cushing demonstrated that electrical stimulation of the postcentral gyrus of the cerebral cortex in conscious human patients would produce gross sensations in the contralateral limbs. Principles developed by these early investigators have formed the basis for present-day usage of electrical stimulation as a tool in clinical neurosurgery and brain research.

The procedures used when applying electrical stimulation to the brain have some features in common with the electrical lesioning method. Stainless steel electrodes, insulated except at their tips, are normally used. Depth placements are accomplished by the stereotaxic technique. The animal surgical preparation can be either acute or chronic. In the **acute preparation,** the animal is stimulated during surgery and then sacrificed at the end of the session. **Chronic preparations** are stimulated following recovery from surgery. In the case of chronic preparations, the stimulating electrodes are permanently anchored in their proper location, and stimulation is applied through wires connecting the electrodes with a plug permanently attached to the skull. A chronically implanted cat is shown in Figure 4-3. A second plug attaches to the one permanently mounted on the skull, and a cable attached to this second plug connects the implant with the stimulating device. Similar preparations are used to record the electrical activity of the brain; in this case, the cable connects the animal to a recording device.

The electrodes used to electrically stimulate the brain may be either *monopolar* or *bipolar* in construction. A monopolar electrode is a single wire inserted into the brain. Since current must flow in a closed circuit, an *indifferent* or *reference* electrode attached to the skull or imbedded in the skin must be used to complete the circuit. Bipolar electrodes consist of two leads placed close together. The most commonly used bipolar electrode consists of two wires either lying side by side or twisted together. Another type of bipolar electrode is the bipolar concentric electrode, which is made by placing a central insulated wire inside a surrounding tube. In all of these cases, the leads are insulated except for the tip. An advantage of the bipolar electrode is that the area of the brain being stimulated is more discrete than the area stimulated by a monopolar electrode.

Although there has been controversy regarding what parameters of electrical stimulation are preferred, the generally accepted procedure is to apply a train of short-duration pulses (0.1–10.0 milliseconds) of approximately 10–100 microvolts between the electrodes. The experimenter will usually start with a stimulus strength at the lower end of this microvolt range and then gradually increase it until a behavioral response to the stimulation occurs (Avery, 1975).

A crucial problem in electrical-stimulation studies is localization of the effective site of stimulation. The tip of the electrode can be localized via histology following completion of the experiment. However, the location of the tip of the stimulating electrode is not necessarily the effective site of stimulation. In some cases, the structure or pathway that is activated by electrical stimulation is several millimeters from the electrode tip but has a much lower threshold for electrical activation than closer structures or pathways.

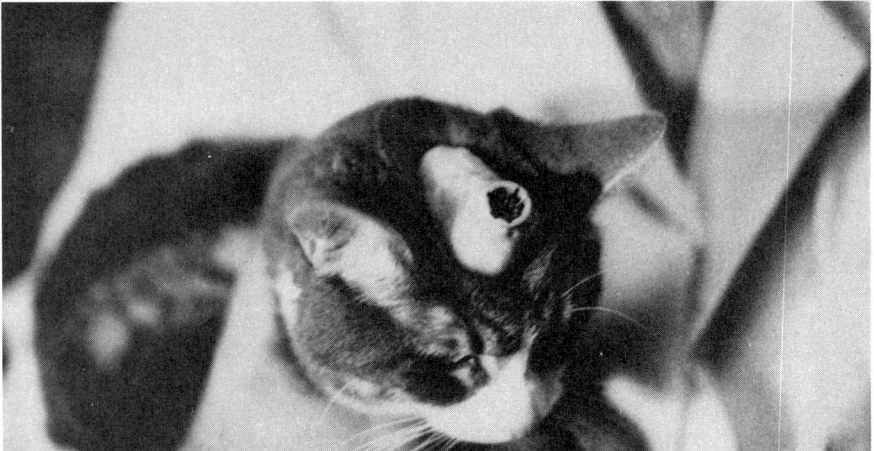

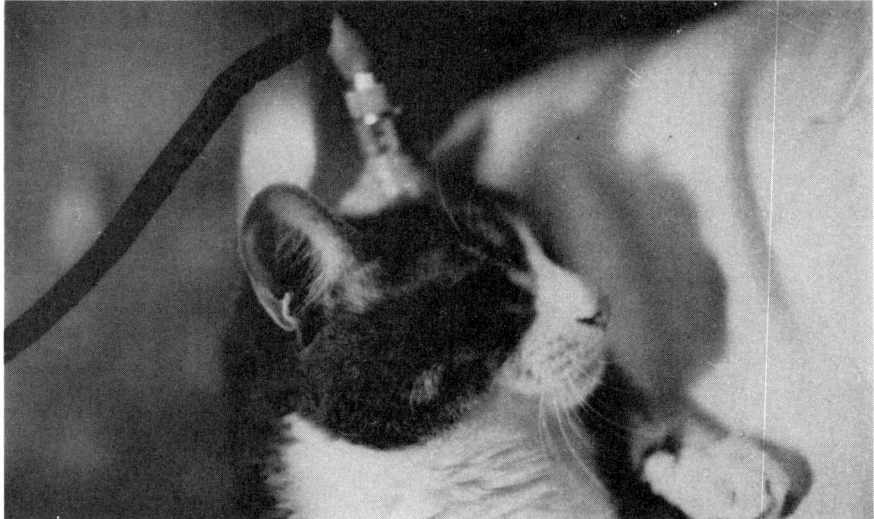

*Figure 4-3
A chronically
implanted cat.*

Intracranial Chemical Stimulation

A technique that has been developed relatively recently to study brain processes is the injection of chemicals directly into the brain. This method is called **intracranial chemical injection** or **stimulation.** Earlier in this chapter, I indicated that intracranial injections have been used by a number of researchers to cause reversible brain lesions, and these types of studies fall into the general category of intracranial chemical stimulation. In this section of the chapter, an historical overview of the development of this method and a description of how it is currently employed will be presented.

The first major studies using this technique were conducted by Andersson in the early 1950s. His findings have greatly increased our understanding of the mechanisms regulating water intake. Andersson originally was examining the hormonal regulation of lactation by electrically stimulating the hypothalamus of the goat. During his research, he noted that stimulation of the anterior region of the hypothalamus produced rumination and licking (Andersson, 1951).

A great researcher takes advantage of accidents, and Andersson was a great researcher. He was struck by the similarity between the electrical-stimulation-elicited behavior that he was observing and normal responses that occur during eating and drinking. If the area being stimulated did indeed contribute to the regulation of water intake, Andersson reasoned, then Verney's (1947) postulated thirst-regulating **osmoreceptor** cells might be situated in this region. (Osmoreceptor cells change their firing rate in response to changes in the concentration of solutes in the extracellular fluid.) He reasoned that if this were true, direct contact of hypertonic (higher concentration than normally found in the body) saline solutions with these cells would produce cellular dehydration, which in turn would elicit drinking. To test his hypothesis, Andersson (1952) injected 0.1 cc hypertonic saline solution directly into the hypothalamus of nonanesthetized goats via modified hypodermic needles (cannulas), which were cemented to their skulls. Within 30–90 seconds after the injections, the water-satiated goats began drinking water, and they consumed up to a gallon of water before the effects of the chemical stimulation disappeared.

Andersson's very intriguing report set the stage for later uses of the intracranial chemical-stimulation technique. A few years after Andersson's observations were made public, Feldberg and his associates published a report on their initial inquiries into the effects on body temperature of injecting various drugs into the cerebral ventricles (Feldberg & Sherwood, 1954), and Fisher (1956) reported his provocative observations of the effects on reproductive behavior of injecting sex hormones directly into the hypothalamus of rats.

The great importance of and research potential for intracranial chemical stimulation was not firmly established until Grossman (1960, 1962a, 1962b) published his exhaustive inquiries into hypothalamic neurochemical control of eating and drinking. In these experiments, crystalline chemicals were repeatedly applied to the lateral hypothalamic area—a region that by this time had been clearly implicated in the control of these behaviors. His research differed from the other studies I've described in that substances thought to act as synaptic transmitters were injected.

Grossman found that applications of adrenergic transmitter substances (epinephrine or norepinephrine) produced eating in fully satiated animals. Injections of cholinergic transmitters (acetylcholine or carbachol) through the identical cannulas produced vigorous and prolonged drinking. Further, Grossman found that injections of either adrenergic or cholinergic blocking agents selectively inhibited these behaviors. Applications of atropine sulfate—an anticholinergic agent—inhibited drinking in a water-deprived rat, and injections of the adrenergic blocking agent ethomoxane blocked eating in hungry animals.

Grossman's results showed that chemical stimulation could be used to selectively activate anatomically overlapping but functionally distinct neural systems mediating behavior. This cannot be accomplished using electrical stimulation. Encouraged by these results, many investigators began to employ intracranial chemical stimulation in a wide variety of experimental inquiries. Presently, this technique is enjoying great popularity among brain researchers.

The basic methodology developed in the early intracranial chemical stimulation studies is still used. It is often called the **double-cannula system.** An excellent critical review of the use of this method in the study of behavior processes is provided by

Routtenberg (1972). To accomplish intracranial chemical stimulation, an *outer cannula,* which serves as a guide through which the *injection cannula* can be introduced, is stereotaxically implanted and attached to the skull, and the animal is allowed to recover from surgery. This guide cannula can also be combined with an electrode, for electrical stimulation or recording.

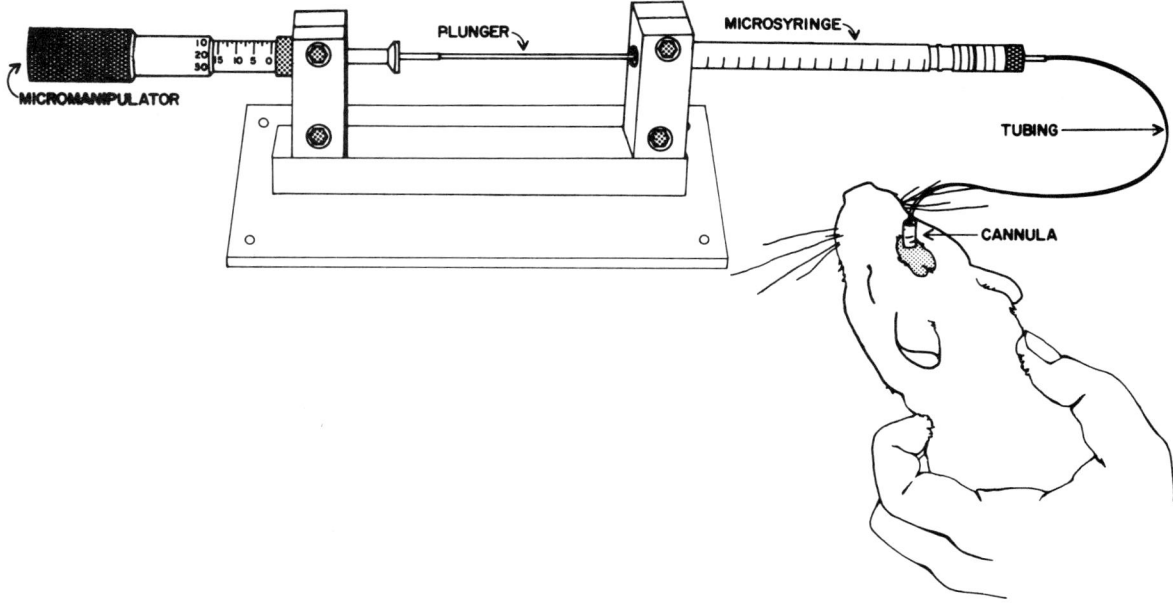

To administer chemicals into the brain, a smaller-diameter injection cannula is inserted through the outer guide. A polyethylene tube connects the injection cannula to a microsyringe or other infusion device, which contains the solution to be injected (see Figure 4-4). To avoid damage to the tissues near the tip of the cannula, only a few microliters of fluid are injected at a time, and the injection is performed slowly over a period of at least a minute. The injection cannula is subsequently left in place for another minute to prevent the injected substance from backing up through the system. A dummy cannula, consisting of a length of stainless steel wire, is then placed into the guide, where it remains until the next injection.

The chemical-stimulation technique has some of the same drawbacks that electrical stimulation has. Most important is the difficulty of localizing the effective site of stimulation. The tip of the cannula can be located histologically, but the observed effects of the chemical injection may be due to the effect of the chemical on neurons located up to several millimeters from the tip. This problem has been lessened by recently developed techniques that allow the researcher to determine the extent of the area reached by the injected chemical. These control procedures involve the use of either dyes or radioactively labeled substances. It is imperative that these control methods be used by researchers employing intracranial stimulation in attempts to determine localization of function.

A second problem confronted by investigators using the chemical-stimulation technique to study brain functions is the difficulty of controlling the duration of the stimulus being applied. Using electrical stimulation, one can end the stimulus by

Figure 4-4
Apparatus for intracranial chemical stimulation. From Physiological Techniques in Behavioral Research, *by D. Singh and D. D. Avery. Copyright © 1975 by Wadsworth Publishing Company, Inc. Reprinted by permission of the publisher, Brooks/Cole Publishing Company, Monterey, California.*

simply turning off the electric current. In contrast, the duration of a chemical stimulus will depend on such factors as the rate of dissolution of the injected chemical into the tissue, the rate of metabolic degradation of the chemical, and how widely the chemical is distributed in the tissue surrounding the tip of the cannula (Myers, 1974).

Technological advances have lessened the problems of localizing the effective site of a chemical stimulus and controlling the duration of the chemical's stimulation (see Myers, 1974). These modern techniques involve localized perfusion of neural tissue by means of a **push-pull cannula system.** A push-pull cannula consists of two cannulas, located either side by side or one inside the other. A precision infusion-withdrawal pump, attached to the cannula, is used to inject the chemical through one of the tubes and withdraw it through the other. Using this method, the researcher can use smaller concentrations of the injected chemical than was possible with traditional chemical-stimulation methods. In fact, the actual concentrations bathing the neural tissue are close to levels that normally occur in the brain. This aspect of the method, which restricts the spread of the chemical to the area of the cannula tip, makes it possible to localize the effective site of the chemical stimulation more precisely than was previously possible. Since the injected chemical is withdrawn soon after it is infused, the investigator can quickly terminate the chemical stimulation.

Electrical Recording

The same electrodes that are used for electrical stimulation can be employed to record bioelectric potentials in the brain. Three types of electrical recording are popular among brain researchers. These include the recording of large populations of neurons (electroencephalography), the recording of the firing pattern of single brain cells, and the recording of the DC or steady potentials.

Electroencephalography

Modern electroencephalography began in 1929, when Hans Berger, a German psychiatrist, reported a method for recording the electrical activity of the brain from the intact skull. Berger had been recording electroencephalograph (EEG) patterns from the brains of lower animals since 1902 and from humans since 1924. However, it was a number of years earlier, in 1875, that Richard Caton of England had made the original discovery that the brain continuously exhibits very-low-voltage electrical fluctuations or waves, which are rarely over several hundred microvolts in amplitude.

In the 1930s, Berger's findings were developed into a clinical tool for the study of brain pathology. In 1935, Gibbs, Davis, and Lennox discovered the brain-wave pattern typical of petit mal epilepsy, and, in 1936, Grey Walter demonstrated that tumors could be located through the unopened skull because tissue adjoining a tumor shows abnormally slow potential shifts. Other scientists, such as Jung and Kornmüller (1938), set the stage for later experimental inquiries regarding the physiological significance of specific EEG patterns recorded from discrete areas of the brain. Their inquiries served as a basis for much of the current interest in determining the EEG correlates of behavior.

A major breakthrough for the physiological study of the sleep/waking continuum also occurred in the 1930s. Loomis, Harvey, and Hobart (1935, 1937) demonstrated that brain waves of cortical origin exhibited distinct change with the onset of sleep and continued to change throughout the sleep period. Loomis and his colleagues devised a system for classifying these EEG patterns into five stages considered representative of increasing sleep depth.

Many different methodologies have been used over the years to record the electrical activity of the brain. The electrical activity of the cortex directly under the skull can be recorded through small plate or disc electrodes lying on the surface of the scalp or through needles inserted under the scalp. In nonhuman animals, records are additionally obtained via silver-ball electrodes applied directly to the exposed cortex. For recording the local activity of subcortical regions, stereotaxically implanted electrodes with tip diameters of several hundred microns are generally employed. Monopolar or bipolar electrodes can be used, but bipolar are preferred because they allow the recording area to be more clearly delineated. A cat chronically implanted with depth electrodes was shown in Figure 4-3.

Electrodes serve as pickups for bioelectric potentials. Since the electrical activity of the brain is in the microvolt range, the signal must be greatly amplified before it can be recorded as an **electroencephalogram.** Therefore, between the electrode and the device used to make a record of the brain's electrical activity are high-gain amplifiers. A permanent record of the electrical activity, which allows for later analysis, is usually obtained either on a polygraph or on magnetic tape via an FM tape recorder. A modern polygraph is shown in Figure 4-5.

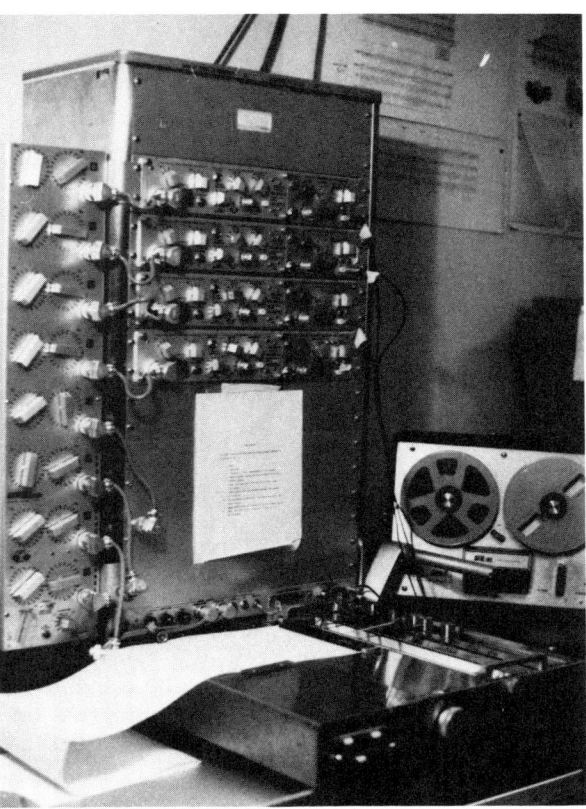

Figure 4-5
A modern polygraph.

Brain waves are rarely over several hundred microvolts in amplitude; their frequencies range from one wave approximately every half second to 50 or more per second. A **brain wave** is an undulation in the electrical activity of the brain, and an electroencephalogram (EEG) is a record of these waves. The basis for the EEG is most likely the waxing and waning of summed postsynaptic potentials from a large population of neurons adjacent to the tip of the recording electrode.

Much of the time, the EEG records a pattern of electrical activity that can best be described as irregular, low-amplitude, **desynchronized activity** having no general pattern. An example of desynchronized activity recorded from the dorsal hippocampus of an awake cat is shown in the top tracing of Figure 11-1 (page 213). At other times, distinct patterns can be detected in the EEG. Sometimes these patterns are indicative of brain pathology such as a tumor or epilepsy. Other patterns occur even in normal individuals, and these are called **synchronous activity.** Synchronous activity involves a very regular pattern of EEG waves, in which the waves are all approximately of the same height or amplitude and occur with regular frequency. An example of synchronous activity recorded from the dorsal hippocampus of an awake cat is shown in the bottom tracing of Figure 11-1. Different patterns of synchronous activity have been given Greek-letter names according to their frequency—that is, according to the number of waves or cycles per second. The abbreviation *Hz* is used to denote cycles per second. The Greek-letter classification system differentiates four types of synchronous activity: *alpha, beta, theta,* and *delta* waves. Examples of these patterns of synchronous EEG patterns are shown in Figure 4-6.

Figure 4-6
Different types of
normal
electroencephalographic
waves. From
Textbook of
Medical Physiology
(4th ed.), by A. C.
Guyton. Copyright
1971 by W. B.
Saunders Company.
Reprinted by
permission.

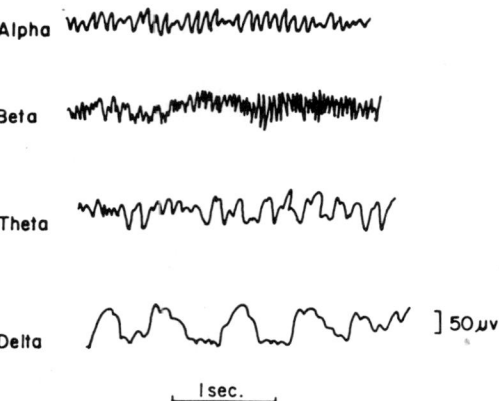

Alpha waves are synchronous brain waves in the frequency range of 8–12 Hz. They are most easily observed from electrodes situated over the occipital cortex. They occur in the EEGs of normal persons when they are awake but in a quiet, resting state with their eyes shut. If an individual is demonstrating alpha activity and if we have the subject try to solve a mental problem or if the subject's eyes are opened, a phenomenon called *alpha blocking* occurs. In alpha blocking, the 8–12 Hz synchronous wave train is blocked and replaced by desynchronized activity, which is a correlate of behavioral arousal. When the eyes are again closed or the individual again enters a resting state, the alpha activity reappears in the occipital leads. This phenomenon is depicted in Figure 4-7.

Beta waves occur at frequencies of 18 Hz and above and are most commonly recorded from the frontal and parietal regions. Sheer and his associates have studied patterns of synchronous activity in the beta range that occur in the neocortex during learning and performance of a visual-discrimination problem by cats. Sheer has suggested that 40-Hz activity may be related to memory processes and has called this pattern the **consolidation rhythm.** His very intriguing work on this subject will be described in Chapter 11.

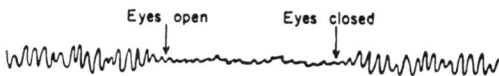

*Figure 4-7
Replacement of
alpha waves by
desynchronized
activity on opening
the eyes. From
Textbook of
Medical Physiology
(4th ed.), by A. C.
Guyton. Copyright
1971 by W. B.
Saunders Company.
Reprinted by
permission.*

Theta waves have frequencies in the range of 4–7 Hz. Theta waves of cortical origin are mainly observed in the temporal and parietal regions of children, but they can sometimes be observed during emotional stress in adults, particularly if the stress is produced by disappointment or frustration. Theta waves of hippocampal origin have intrigued neuroscientists since the mid-1950s because of what they may tell about the functions of the hippocampus in regulating behavior. As we will see in later chapters, the hippocampus has been implicated in many behavior processes, including arousal, attention, voluntary movement, and learning and memory. We will examine research on the significance of hippocampal electrical activity in Chapter 11.

Delta waves include all electrical activity of 0.5–3 Hz in frequency. Delta waves occur in serious organic brain diseases and, as will be discussed in Chapter 7, during deep sleep.

EEG records can be analyzed by gross visual inspection or by computer. Visual analysis allows an investigator to determine the presence or absence of a particular EEG pattern and to consider the relationship of the pattern to behavior that was observed during the recording. Computer analysis allows for a more detailed analysis of the frequency characteristics of an EEG signal and can also be used to determine the similarity between EEG patterns recorded successively or simultaneously from different regions in the brain. With **spectral analysis**—a type of computer analysis— the investigator can determine the most common frequency from a sample of EEG activity. **Cross correlation** allows the researcher to determine the extent of the relationship between brain potentials simultaneously recorded from different brain regions. This computer analysis plots a correlation coefficient that indicates how similar the two signals are. The time relationship between two signals is also plotted. With this analysis, if two signals are correlated, then it is possible to determine whether the activity of one region temporally leads that of another. Thus one can determine whether electrical activity arising in one region carried a signal to some other structure.

As our methods for analysis of the electroencephalogram become more sophisticated, it is important for us to remember that the relationship between the EEG and behavior is only a correlation. As is true for all correlations, it does not necessarily indicate a causal relationship. Thus, we cannot say for certain that a change in the EEG causes a behavioral alteration or that a behavior change causes a shift in the EEG.

Unit recording is the procedure of recording the electrical activity of single cells. Some researchers have argued that, since macroelectrodes (such as the electrodes discussed in the previous section) record regional EEG patterns and since neurons that are located near each other are not necessarily functionally related, it is hard, if not impossible, to obtain meaningful correlations between EEG patterns obtained from macroelectrodes and brain functions. Such an argument is considerably weakened by a number of reports (for example, Ranck 1973a) demonstrating a close correspondence between single-cell activity and EEG potentials obtained from macroelectrodes. Ranck has reported that the pattern of firing of specific cells in the hippocampus is correlated with the same behavior repertoire that accompanies one of the major EEG patterns of this structure. These findings will be discussed in Chapter 11, where I'll review what is known about the electrophysiological correlates of learning and performance.

Microelectrodes are used to record the electrical activity of individual brain cells. Until the 1960s, microelectrode studies were almost exclusively confined to acute surgical preparations. With subsequent technological advancements, it has become possible to record the firing pattern of a single cell for several hours in an unrestrained, vigorously moving animal with almost no distortion of the record due to movement (see Ranck, 1973b).

Microelectrodes are usually not more than ten microns in diameter at the tip, as compared with macroelectrodes used to record EEG potentials, which are several hundred microns in diameter at the tip. There are two basic types of microelectrodes: metal microelectrodes insulated except at the tip and glass pipettes filled with a conducting electrolyte such as potassium-chloride solution. A detailed description of the construction and uses of various types of microelectrodes is provided by Bureš, Petráň, and Zachar (1962).

Microelectrode investigations of the electrical activity of single cells are accomplished by recording either intracellularly or extracellularly. Intracellular recording involves penetrating the cell membrane and allows the researcher to record the potential difference across the membrane from the inside to the outside of the cell. The extracellular method involves placing the electrode outside the cell and makes possible the recording of nerve impulses from the cell.

Extracellular unit recording is technically much easier than intracellular recording and has other advantages over the intracellular method. First, extracellular recording allows the investigator to monitor simultaneously the electrical activity of several neurons. Second, the possibility of damaging the nerve cell under study is much less when using the extracellular recording technique.

DC, or Steady Potentials

While the EEG measures changes in bioelectric potentials in terms of milliseconds, there are brain voltages that change more slowly—over a period of seconds or minutes. These latter changes are called *DC* or **steady potentials.** They can be recorded only with a type of amplifier different from that normally used to record EEG responses. Special electrodes must also be used (see Rowland, 1968, for details of construction). The study of steady potentials in neural tissues has an interesting history.

Earlier in this chapter, I indicated that Richard Caton discovered the EEG in 1875. In his research, he was actually interested in finding out the effects of using various stimuli to induce shifts in the steady cortical potential of awake animals. During his experiments, Caton noted small, continuous fluctuations that were driving his recorder in the absence of any experimental stimuli. The discovery of these fluctuations was the discovery of the EEG. Caton was really interested, however, in the DC or steady potentials (SP) of the brain. Brazier (1961) has suggested that Caton's emphasis on the SP phenomena actually obstructed the early investigation of the EEG waves. As Rowland (1968) has justly noted, the vast literature of the EEG now obscures what little has been learned regarding stimulus-induced changes in SP since Caton's pioneering investigations.

It is interesting to note that Caton considered the EEG to be "noise." Investigators of EEG phenomena now consider SP and shifts that occur in this electrophysiological response to be a nuisance or "noise." Modern EEG amplifiers are constructed in such a way that they lose this DC information, but EEG researchers, fascinated with fluctuating EEG rhythms, have not seemed to mind that the SP is not preserved. As I pointed out earlier, special amplifiers and electrodes have been developed to study SP phenomena in modern laboratories.

The term *steady potential,* as it pertains to the cortex, denotes ". . . the maintained or nonrhythmic difference of potential between the surface of the cortex and the immediately subjacent white matter" (Rowland, 1968, p. 5). It ranges in amplitude from 0.5 to 5 mv and exhibits a slow shift as a function of time but rarely changes by more than about 0.5 mv over several hours under normal conditions. If a stimulus is presented to the subject, an SP shift will be elicited. If the stimulus is neutral, the shift will rapidly diminish in size, but SP shifts having significance for survival (for example, in response to the presentation of food) do not diminish simply as a function of repeated presentations. In this latter case, diminution of the SP shift is apparently related to a decrease in the stimulus-relevant drive state.

Current interest in SP phenomena has followed Caton's lead and centered around investigating the relationship between SP shifts and behavior. Excellent reviews of the SP phenomena are provided by Rowland (1968) and by Rowland and Anderson (1971). I will discuss some of these findings when we consider the electrophysiological correlates of behavior processes related to learning and performance.

Histological Procedures

Regardless of the method used by the neuroscientist, it is essential that the researcher verify the exact site at which an electrode or cannula was implanted or determine the exact locus and extent of a lesion. Certain histological procedures have been developed for this purpose. In some cases, histology can be accomplished through gross dissection of the brain after its structural features have been preserved by fixation with formalin or alcohol. More often, the location of the brain probe or lesion must be verified through microscopic procedures. The techniques used are as follows.

Prior to microscopic examination of brain tissue, the brain must be fixed and hardened. It is fixed by perfusion with either formalin or alcohol. This procedure preserves the structural features of the brain. The neural tissue is then hardened by being frozen or by being impregnated with either paraffin or celloidin. After the brain has been fixed and hardened, it is cut into very thin slices.

A *microtome* is used to slice the hardened tissue. The microtome is a specially mounted knife that can be set to cut tissues of a predetermined thickness—usually approximately 5 to 100 microns. In slicing a brain, the researcher attempts to cut the tissue in such a way that the slices duplicate the pattern of the stereotaxic atlas being used as a reference. After sectioning, the slices are stained by immersion in stains that selectively dye certain features of the tissue. Some stains will accentuate only the cell bodies, others only nerve fibers, while still other staining techniques bring out only degenerating fibers and cell bodies. This last technique has been especially valuable in determining the connections or pathways that exist among various brain regions. Knowledge of these pathways is crucial to interpreting the effects observed in lesion and stimulation experiments. Either during or after staining, the tissues are mounted on glass slides and dried. They are then ready for microscopic examination. The location of the lesion or brain probe can be verified by comparison of the prepared tissue with corresponding sections in the stereotaxic atlas.

Chapter Summary and Conclusions

This chapter presented an overview of research methods used by brain researchers. It was indicated that the four most commonly used techniques are lesioning, electrical stimulation, chemical stimulation, and electrical recording. These methods are used either singly or together. Some of the advantages and disadvantages of each of these methods were discussed.

The lesion technique is the oldest and still most widely used method for studying brain functions. Ablation of the neocortex is probably best accomplished by weak suction, while subcortical structures in the depths of the brain are best destroyed by using stereotaxic surgery and electrolytic lesions. It is also possible to perform reversible or temporary lesions either on the surface of the brain or in subcortical regions.

Stimulation techniques have been very popular in recent years. Electrical stimulation involves the application of trains of short-duration pulses through electrodes, while chemical stimulation involves the administration of various chemicals directly to brain tissue. Both methods attempt to replicate what are thought to be normal brain processes.

Electrical recording methods do not interfere with the ongoing processes in the brain. Rather, they attempt to record electrical activity that is thought to reflect these processes. Three types of electrophysiological approaches are popular. These are the recording of large populations of neurons (electroencephalography), the recording of single units, and the recording of steady potentials.

The final topic reviewed in this chapter was histology. Histology allows the researcher to verify the exact location of a brain probe or the anatomical boundaries of a brain lesion. All experiments in the neurosciences must end in the histology lab. Careful histological analysis can often lead to the integration of many apparently contradictory findings in the experimental-brain-research literature. Histological techniques are also used to define the pathways that connect various brain regions. Knowledge of these pathways is crucial for interpretation of the effects observed in lesion and stimulation experiments.

Every method used by the brain researcher has certain advantages and drawbacks, and every method has enhanced our knowledge of how the brain processes information and mediates behavior. I believe that it would be naïve to state that there is a best or preferred method. Neural functions will be completely clarified only through the use of a variety of research methods.

5
Sensory Processes

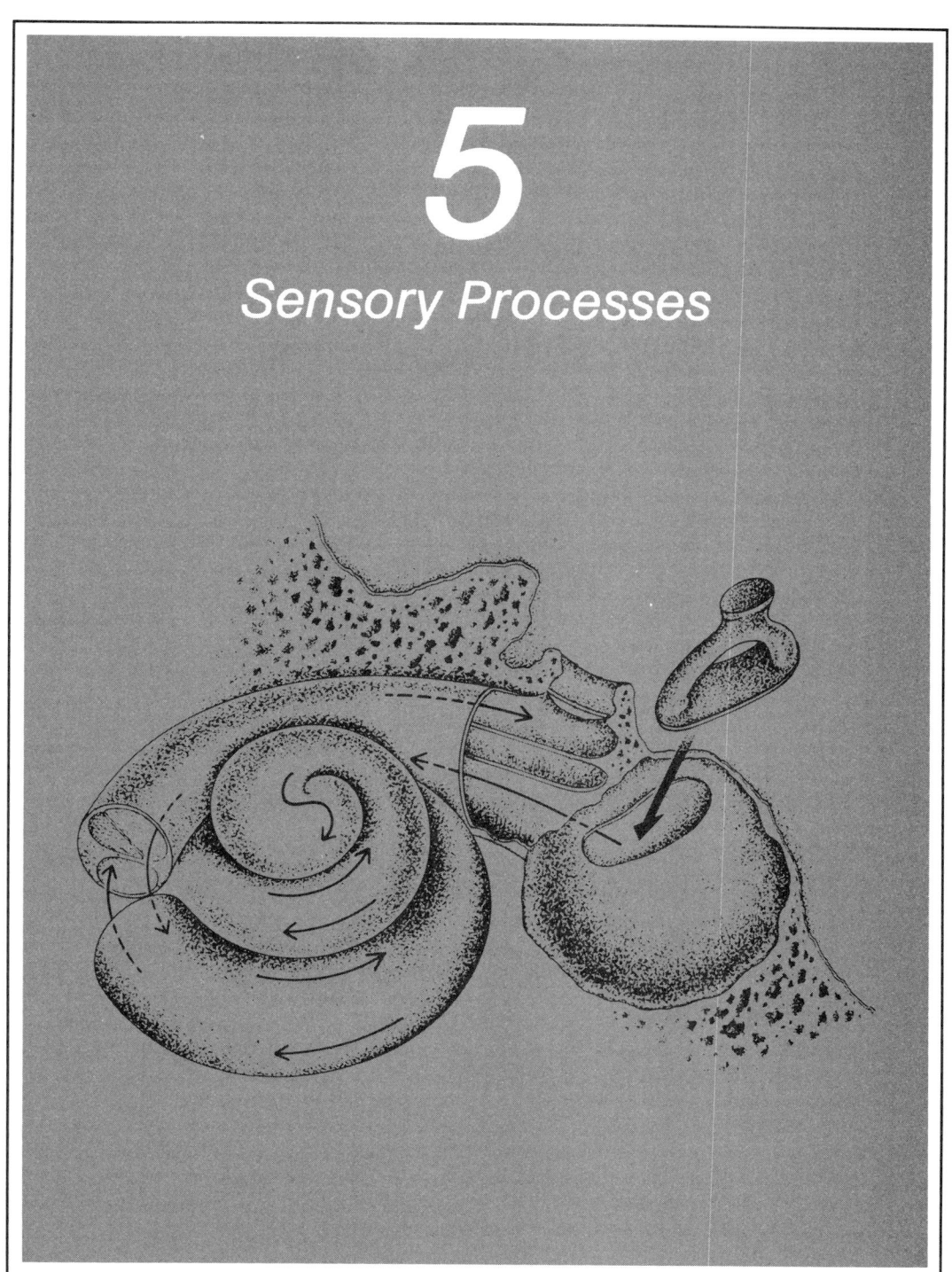

Behavior is adaptive in that it allows an organism to survive in its environment. However, for adaptive responding to occur, the organism must receive and process information from the tremendous amount of stimulation with which it is continuously being bombarded. The reception of stimulus information from the environment and the transmission of this information to the central nervous system, where the information is processed, are the roles performed by our sensory systems in mediating behavior. In this chapter, we will examine the performance of these roles by the visual, auditory, olfactory, taste, and somatosensory systems. The study of sensory processes has a long and distinguished history in experimental psychology. The first psychological laboratory was devoted to the study of sensation and perception and was established in Germany in 1879 by the founder of experimental psychology, Wilhelm Wundt.

Principles of Receptor-Cell Function

A receptor cell is unique among the cells in our body in that it is specialized to react to environmental changes. There are basically four kinds of receptors. **Mechanoreceptors** detect bending or displacement of either the receptor or cells adjacent to it. Mechanoreceptors are involved in the detection of stimulus changes associated with our tactile sensitivities and hearing. **Thermoreceptors** are sensitive to changes in temperature. Some receptors of this type detect cold, while others detect warmth. **Electromagnetic receptors** detect light on the receptive surface of the eye (the retina). Finally, **chemoreceptors** are involved in the sensations of taste and smell.

All receptors actually are responsive to a wide variety of stimuli, but they are maximally sensitive to only one type of stimulus. This stimulus, called the **adequate stimulus** for exciting the receptor, is the basis for the classification of receptors given above. It should be pointed out, however, that, no matter what type of stimulus initiates a receptor response, activation of that receptor will always yield the same sensory experience. For example, the receptors in the eye are mainly sensitive to light. However, if we apply gentle pressure to the eyeball with the eyelid closed, the sensation that is experienced is one of light. This phenomenon is a demonstration of the **doctrine of specific nerve energies,** formulated by Johannes Müller in 1838. This doctrine states that, regardless of the nature of the initiating stimulus, a given receptor always gives rise to the same psychological experience.

The sensory process begins when a receptor is stimulated. Examples of receptors are the rods and cones of the retina in the eye and the hair cells of the cochlea in the ear. Regardless of the type of stimulus that activates the receptor, the stimulus produces an electrical potential. It is similar to the postsynaptic potential you studied in Chapter 2 in that it is a **graded potential**; that is, the size of the **receptor potential** is directly proportional to the intensity of the sensory stimulus producing it.

A sensory neuron is located in close proximity to the receptor cell. The two are separated by a synapse. The receptor potential is transmitted across this synapse to produce on the dendrite a graded potential that spreads through the sensory neuron. If this graded potential reaches sufficient size and the threshold for firing the sensory neuron is surpassed, then an action potential will be generated. Just as was the case for the excitatory postsynaptic potential, two successive graded potentials will summate if they occur close together (temporal summation) and thus yield an action potential in the sensory neuron. Regardless of the intensity and mechanism of stimulation, the sensory-nerve impulses are always the same; that is, the action potentials are of the same magnitude and travel at the same rate.

How is information about the intensity of stimulation conducted? This is accomplished by variation in the number of impulses per unit of time and in the duration of the impulses. A stimulus that is just above threshold will send only a few impulses for a short period of time. In contrast, an intense stimulus will result in a burst of nerve impulses for a sustained duration. Thus, stimulus intensity is coded by the number of nerve impulses that reach the cortex.

An important characteristic of all sensory receptors is that they show **adaptation** to stimuli after a period of time. If an adequate stimulus is applied to a receptor, a burst of impulses will occur. However, if the stimulus is maintained at a constant level for a period of time, the frequency of impulses will become lower and lower. The rate of impulses will become very low or will end completely, even though the stimulus is still present. Again, this phenomenon is referred to as *adaptation.* Adaptation is not due to fatigue, because, if the stimulus is begun again, after being only momentarily stopped, a burst of impulses will once more occur, and the adaptation process will be repeated. The rate of adaptation varies for the different receptors.

With these principles of receptor-cell function in mind, we can now proceed to an examination of how the various sensory systems process information. We will first examine the visual system. Vision is the most studied and best understood of all our sensory systems.

The Visual System

The Anatomy of the Visual System

The Structure of the Eye. The eye is designed to focus rays of light bouncing off objects in the environment onto the receptive surface of the eye—the **retina.** In terms of its method of operation, the eye has been compared to a camera. It has a **lens** that focuses light waves on a photosensitive area, the retina. An aperture, the **pupil,** regulates the amount of light falling on the receptive surface. The gross structure of the eye is shown in Figure 5-1.

The outer shell of the eyeball consists of three layers. The outermost layer is called the **sclera** or **sclerotic coat.** It is the "white" of our eyes. The frontal portion of the sclerotic coat is transparent and is called the **cornea.** The middle layer is the darkly pigmented **choroid coat.** This layer, which serves to darken the interior of

Figure 5-1
A cross section of
the human eye.
From Color in
Business, Science
and Industry (2nd
ed.), by D. B. Judd
and G. Wyszecki.
Copyright 1963 by
John Wiley & Sons,
Inc. Reprinted by
permission.

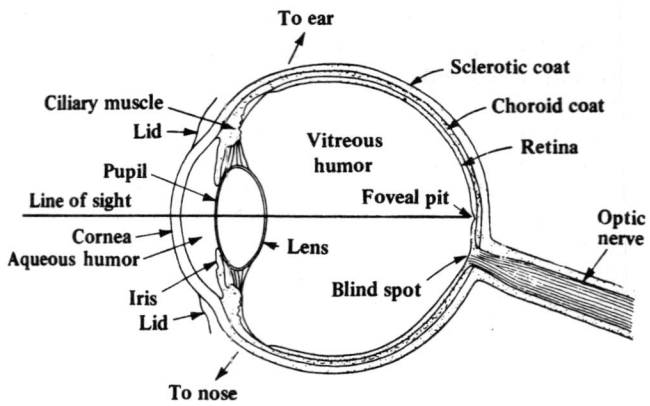

the eye, forms the **iris** or colored part of the eye at the front of the eye. The opening in the center of the iris is the pupil. The size of the pupil is reflexively controlled by muscles in the iris so that it becomes smaller in bright light and larger in dim light. An elastic crystalline lens is stretched across the anterior portion of the eyeball. Surrounding the outer margin of the lens and attached to it by fine strands are bundles of smooth muscle fibers, which form the **ciliary muscles.** Contraction of the ciliary muscles changes the thickness of the lens. This allows near objects to be brought into sharp focus. Relaxation of these muscles brings distant objects into focus. The process of self-adjustment of the lenses of the eyes to bring objects into focus is called **visual accommodation.** Finally, the innermost layer is the retina, and it contains the photosensitive receptor cells. The space between the cornea and the lens is filled with a thin, watery fluid called the **aqueous humor.** Behind the lens is a clear, viscous, gelatinous substance called the **vitreous humor.**

The Retina. The retina is part of the brain. In fact, it is the only part of the nervous system that can be directly observed in an intact organism. The retina, as you can see in Figure 5-2, is an exceptionally complex, multilayered tissue (Polyak, 1957). It contains two types of visual receptor cells: **rods** and **cones.** In addition to these photoreceptors, there are **horizontal, amacrine, bipolar,** and **ganglion cells** in the retina. The horizontal and amacrine cells collect and relay information within the retina, while the bipolar and ganglion cells relay information from the retina to the brain (Brown, 1975). As you can see in Figure 5-2, light has to pass through all of the other layers of the retina before reaching the photoreceptive cells. This may not seem to you to be a very efficient design. However, in the central regions of the retina, as will be discussed below, the layers in front of the rods and cones are pulled aside to prevent the loss of acuity that might result from the light waves passing through the retinal layers (Guyton, 1971). The image is projected on this central retinal region by the lens.

Again, the basic photoreceptor cells of the eye are the rods and the cones. There are approximately four times as many rods as cones in the retina. However, in a region in the center of the retina called the **macula,** the cones predominate, and, in the center of the macula, an area called the **fovea** is occupied exclusively by cones. The fovea is only about a millimeter square in area, but it is the point of clearest vision

70

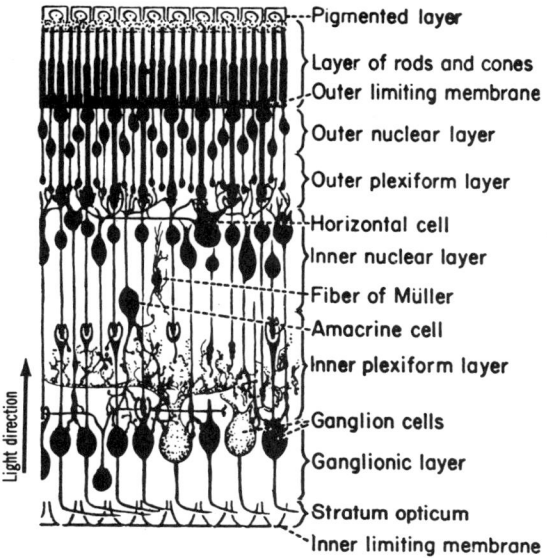

Pigmented layer

Layer of rods and cones
Outer limiting membrane

Outer nuclear layer

Outer plexiform layer

Horizontal cell
Inner nuclear layer

Fiber of Müller
Amacrine cell
Inner plexiform layer

Ganglion cells
Ganglionic layer

Stratum opticum
Inner limiting membrane

Light direction

Figure 5-2
The plan of the retinal neurons. From The Vertebrate Visual System, *by S. Polyak (H. Klüver, Ed.). Copyright ©* 1957 by the University of Chicago. © 1955 under the International Copyright Convention. Reprinted by permission of The University of Chicago Press.

because the lens focuses the image onto it. Further, to aid in detail vision, the blood vessels and cellular layers in front of the cones on the fovea are all displaced to the side so that light does not have to pass through them to reach the photosensitive cones. The cone density falls rapidly as one proceeds toward the periphery of the retina. The number of rods per square millimeter concurrently increases, until, at the extreme edge of the retina, the rods predominate (Brown, 1975).

The rods and cones, which you can see at the top of Figure 5-3, synapse with bipolar cells, which then synapse with ganglion cells. The ganglion cells send fibers toward the back of the eye, where they collect at the **optic disc** or "blind spot" to form the **optic nerve.** The region of the optic disc is completely devoid of rods and cones. Since light striking this area does not fall on any receptor cells, visual function is precluded. This is why this area is called the *blind spot.*

There are approximately 115 to 130 million rods and cones but only about one million optic nerve fibers (Abramov & Gordon, 1973). As a result, there is a good deal of convergence in the retina. In other words, a number of rods and cones will converge on a single bipolar cell, as shown in Figure 5-3a, or several bipolar cells may converge on a single ganglion cell, as shown in Figure 5-3c. Most ganglion cells receive inputs from thousands of photoreceptors. In contrast, in the foveal region, there is a one-to-one connection; a single cone cell synapses with a single bipolar cell, which in turn synapses with a single ganglion cell, as shown in Figure 5-3b. This is another property that provides for finer detail vision in the foveal region.

The Visual Pathway. Rods and cones synapse with bipolar cells, which in turn synapse with ganglion cells. Fibers from the ganglion cells course to the rear of the eye, where they collect on the optic disc to form the optic nerve. As shown in Figure 5-4, the optic nerves from the two eyes proceed in a posterior direction and converge to form the **optic chiasm.** At the optic chiasm, half of the nerve fibers cross over to the other side of the brain. Specifically, fibers that have arisen from the medial or nasal

71

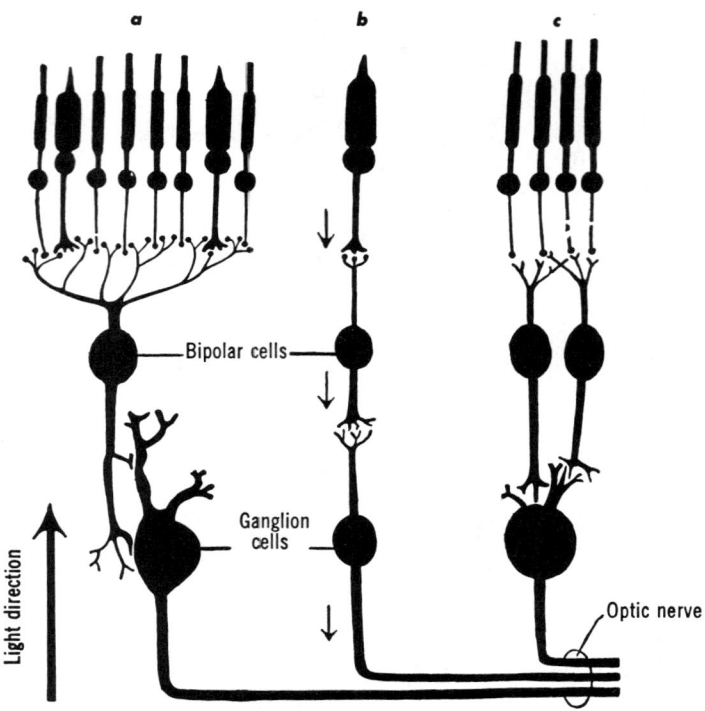

half of each retina cross over to the other side, while fibers that have arisen from the lateral or temporal half of each retina remain uncrossed. This crossing occurs immediately in front of the infundibulum, which connects the pituitary to the hypothalamus.

Posterior to the optic chiasm, the pathways now have fibers from both retinas, and they are called the **optic tracts.** The right optic tract is composed of axons from ganglion cells in the right half of each retina—that is, in the temporal half of the right retina and the nasal half of the left retina. Similarly, the left optic tract is composed of axons from ganglion cells in the left half of each retina.

Some of the axons terminate in the colliculi—the midbrain centers for vision—and then send fibers to the lateral geniculate bodies of the thalamus. However, most of the fibers of the optic tract travel directly to the lateral geniculate bodies of the thalamus, which thus serve as the primary visual relay station. Neurons that originate in the lateral geniculate bodies send their axons in turn to the visual cortex or occipital lobes via fiber bundles called the **optic radiations.** In humans, the retina/lateral geniculate/visual cortex pathway is the more important pathway for visual functioning (Brown, 1975). The retina/colliculi/lateral geniculate/visual cortex pathway, on the other hand, appears to be involved in relatively simple visual processes, such as reflex pupillary reactions and body movements in response to light. The functions of the retina, lateral geniculate body, and visual cortex in visual processes will be considered below.

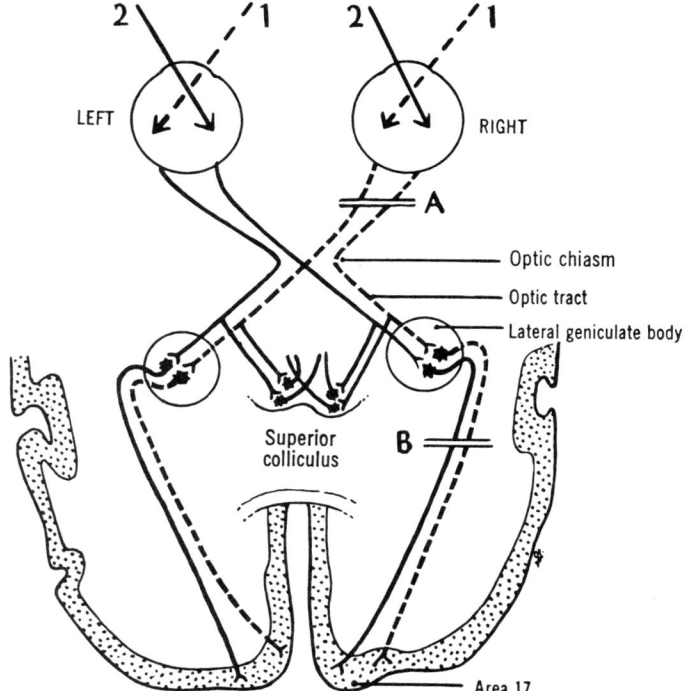

LEFT

RIGHT

A

Optic chiasm

Optic tract

Lateral geniculate body

Superior
colliculus

B

Area 17

*Figure 5-4
The visual
pathways. The
arrows numbered 1
represent light from
objects in the right
visual field, and the
arrows numbered 2
represent light from
the left visual field.
Cutting the optic
nerve at A causes
complete blindness
in that eye. A lesion
at B, however,
causes blindness in
the left half of each
field of vision
(arrows numbered 2).
From* Fundamentals
of Neurology *(5th
ed.), by E. Gardner.
Copyright 1968 by
W. B. Saunders
Company.
Reprinted by
permission.*

The Functions of the Retina

Light striking the photoreceptor cells on the retina touches off a series of processes that result in nerve impulses leaving the eye by way of the optic nerve fibers. These receptors—the rods and cones—contain visual pigments that decompose upon absorbing light. This chemical process results in an electrical charge, which activates the succeeding elements in the neural chain mediating vision.

Both rods and cones are found in the retinas of most mammals. However, nocturnal animals seem to have a marked preponderance of rods, while diurnal animals have cone-rich retinas. This finding helped to generate the **duplicity theory of vision.** According to the duplicity theory, the rods and the cones comprise two functional systems. The rod system functions at low levels of illumination. This would explain the fact that the retinas of nocturnal animals are often almost devoid of cones. Another characteristic of rods is that they are insensitive to color. In contrast, the cone system is sensitive to color and provides for more visual acuity than the rod system does. However, the cones need greater levels of illumination for their functioning than do the rods. Thus, each system has certain advantages and certain limitations.

The Physiology of the Rods. A visual pigment that accounts for the low-illumination sensitivity of the rods has been isolated. It is called **rhodopsin** or *visual purple.* Rhodopsin is a combination of an *opsin,* or protein material, called *scotopsin* and the yellow pigment *retinene.* When light energy is absorbed by rhodopsin, the rhodopsin immediately begins to decompose. It is thought that, during normal daylight vision, the rhodopsin of the rods remains decomposed and that the rods are therefore relatively unresponsive to light. However, this chemical reaction is reversible. When the eye is returned to a dark environment and is **dark-adapted,** rhodopsin is resynthesized. This allows the rods to regain their sensitivity and begin to function. The amount of light required to stimulate a dark-adapted eye is only about a thousandth of that required in daylight.

Vitamin A is involved in the metabolism of rhodopsin, and it is stored for later use in the pigment layer of the retina. Vitamin-A deficiency may result in a condition called **night blindness.** The vitamin-A deficiency results in a decreased level of rhodopsin in the rods, which in turn decreases the sensitivity of the rods to light. The result is that normal rod-mediated vision in dim light is precluded. Because so much vitamin A is stored in the liver for use in various parts of the body, night blindness usually won't develop unless an individual is on a vitamin-A-deficiency diet for several weeks or months. If it does occur, it can often be reversed after only half an hour or so of intravenous injection of vitamin A. However, if the vitamin-A deficiency is allowed to persist, permanent retinal damage can result (Guyton, 1971).

The Cones and Color Vision. A number of theories of color vision have been proposed over the years, but the two views that have received the widest support are the **Young-Helmholtz trichromatic theory** and **Hering's opponent-process theory.** Both of these theories have their roots in the 19th century, and both contend that the cones of the retina are the basic receptors for color vision. However, from that point on, they diverge.

According to the trichromatic theory of color vision, three different types of photosensitive pigments are present in different cones. These different pigments make each cone selectively sensitive to one of the three primary colors—that is, to red, green, or blue. Combinations of output from these receptors would determine the colors or hues that we see. If the influence of all of these outputs were approximately equal, the resulting sensation would be white. The existence of the three types of cones that are required by the trichromatic theory has now been shown for the retinas of fish, monkeys, and humans (MacNichol, 1964).

In some ingenious experiments, Brown and Wald (1964) and Marks, Dobelle, and MacNichol (1964) demonstrated the presence of these three types of cones in the human retina. They passed a narrow beam of light into *single* cones and then analyzed the characteristics of the light reflected off the retina. As shown in Figure 5-5, one group of cones absorbs light maximally at wavelengths of approximately 440 mμ (blue), another at approximately 540 mμ (green), and the third group at approximately 575 mμ (red). These data constitute experimental evidence for the idea that combinations of outputs from three color-receptor populations mediate our experience of color vision. The fact that there is convergence of several receptors onto a single bipolar cell also supports the theory. Thus, there is strong evidence to support the trichromatic theory of color vision—at least at the retinal level of the visual system. We will presently see, however, that behavioral studies, as well as electrophysiological studies of the lateral geniculate body of the thalamus, have supported the alternate theory of color vision—the opponent-process theory.

The basic assumption of Hering's opponent-process theory is that there are three visual pigments. One of these mediates black/white vision—that is, white, black, or gray sensations. A second pigment mediates red/green vision, while a third

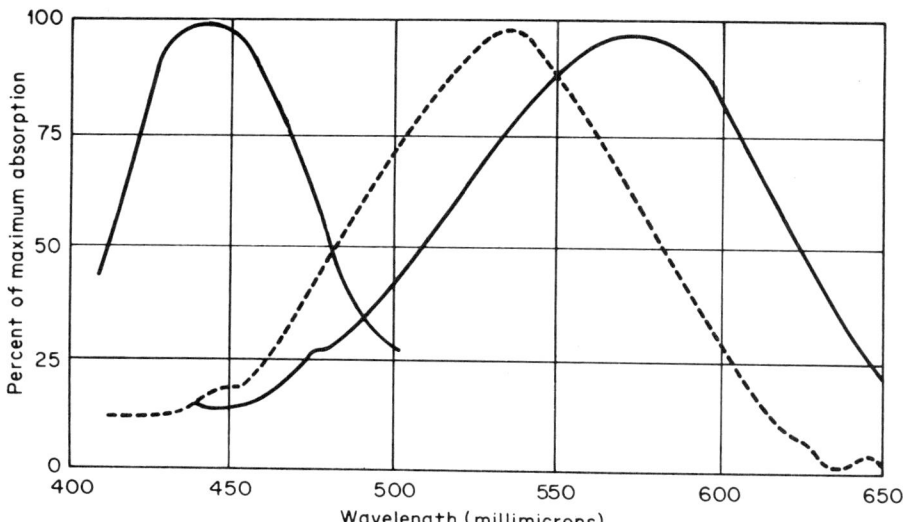

Figure 5-5
Color vision in primates may be mediated by three cone pigments responsible for sensing light in the blue, green, and red portions of the spectrum. These curves show the spectral sensitivity of the three types of cones (from the left, blue-, green-, and red-sensitive cones). The absorption spectrum of the blue pigment peaks at 447 millimicrons, of the green pigment at 540, and of the red-sensitive pigment at 577. The peak of the absorption of the red-sensitive pigment is actually in the yellow range, but it extends far enough into the red range to detect red wavelengths. From "Three Pigment Color Vision," by E. F. MacNichol, Scientific American, 1964, 211, 48–56. *Copyright © 1964 by Scientific American, Inc. All rights reserved. Reprinted by permission.*

pigment is involved in yellow/blue vision. An important difference between this theory and the trichromatic theory is that this theory holds that black/white sensations arise from stimulation of specific black/white, or luminosity, receptors. Luminosity sensations are not dependent on the mixing of colors, as the trichromatic theory would contend.

There are behavioral data to support Hering's theory. For example, if you stare at a blue light for a long period of time and then look at a yellow light, it will seem more yellow than it would normally seem. According to the opponent-process theory, this color-contrast phenomenon occurs because the prolonged exposure to the blue light causes the blue component of the yellow/blue system to be depleted. When the yellow light is subsequently observed, the yellow component is allowed to function free from the normally opposing blue component. Thus, the sensation of yellow is enhanced. In contrast, if the eye is extensively exposed to yellow light before observing a yellow stimulus, the second stimulus will appear less yellow than it normally would. Additional support for the opponent-process theory of color vision has come from electrophysiological studies of the lateral geniculate nucleus. These findings will be discussed below.

The Lateral Geniculate Body

As I said earlier, most of the fibers of the optic tract terminate in the lateral geniculate bodies of the thalamus. Neurons originating in the lateral geniculate nuclei in turn send projections to the visual cortex via the optic radiations. Each lateral geniculate body is composed of 6 nuclear layers. The layers are numbered 1 through 6, from the ventral to the dorsal surface of this nucleus. Layers 2, 3, and 5 receive fibers from the ipsilateral eye, while layers 1, 4, and 6 receive projections from the ganglion cells of the contralateral eye (Brown, 1975).

The firing patterns of single cells in the lateral geniculate of the monkey have been extensively studied by DeValois and his associates (DeValois, 1965; DeValois, Abramov, & Mead, 1967; DeValois & Jacobs, 1968; DeValois, Jacobs, & Jones, 1963). Using light of various wavelengths, they were able to distinguish two types of neurons. One type, called a **broad-band cell** was always either excited or inhibited by visual stimuli. They thought that this type of cell probably mediates information about light intensity. A second group of neurons, the **spectrally opponent cells,** fired in a manner consistent with the opponent-process theory of color vision. Spectrally opponent cells increased their rate of firing to one wavelength of light and decreased their rate of firing to another. For example, some of these single cells were excited by red and inhibited by green. Others reacted in the opposite way. Still other cells showed an increase in their rate of firing to blue light while decreasing their rate of firing to yellow light and vice versa. These observations suggest that the firing patterns of cells in the lateral geniculate nucleus conform to Hering's opponent-process theory of color vision.

When the color-vision data are taken together, it is not possible to decide whether the trichromatic or opponent-process theory explains how color vision is coded by the central nervous system. Retinal data tend to support the trichromatic theory, while electrophysiological studies of the lateral geniculate nucleus and some whether the trichromatic or the opponent-process theory explains how color vision is certainly possible that elements of both theories are correct. That is, it may be that a three-process system operates at the receptor level while a two-process system mediates color vision at higher levels.

The Visual Cortex

The ability of the mammalian nervous system to detect the shape of visual stimuli is dependent upon the visual cortex, the highest level of the visual system. Important inroads toward our understanding of how the visual cortex accomplishes this have been made by D. H. Hubel and T. N. Wiesel. They have examined the firing patterns of single neurons in the visual cortex of the cat (Hubel, 1963; Hubel & Wiesel, 1962, 1963, 1965) and of the monkey (Hubel & Wiesel, 1968). They have differentiated four types of visual-cortex neurons on the basis of their firing patterns. These are the **simple, complex, hypercomplex,** and **higher-order hypercomplex cells.**

Simple cells respond to line stimuli—bars of light, bars of darkness surrounded by light, and edges, such as a straight-line border between a light and a dark region. The stimulus must be of a specific orientation and in a fixed part of the receptive field to fire a simple cell. For example, a bar of light in a certain part of the **retinal receptive field** will fire a particular cortical cell if the bar of light is in a horizontal position. (The retinal receptive field is the region of the retina that activates the cell being studied.) However, the bar of light will fail to fire the cell if its orientation is moved slightly from the horizontal.

The criterion of specific orientation is also always true for complex cells; that is, a certain complex cell will fire only for a line stimulus of a specific orientation. However, a given complex cell will fire for a line stimulus of the required orientation regardless of its position in the field of vision. Further, and also in contrast with simple cells, a complex cell will fire continuously if the line stimulus is moved across the visual field. Simple cells will cease firing if the position of the line stimulus is changed, even if its orientation is maintained. In light of the observation that complex cells will fire continuously to a moving-line stimulus, it is thought that complex cells probably receive their inputs from a large number of simple cells that have identical orientations of their receptive fields but differ regarding the position in the visual field to which they are sensitive.

It is thought that hypercomplex cells receive both excitatory and inhibitory inputs from several complex cells. They also respond to line stimuli of a specific orientation, but they will not fire if the line stimulus exceeds a certain length. Finally, Hubel and Wiesel have described a small number of higher-order hypercomplex cells. These respond to an edge that moves across the visual field as long as the edge is of a specific width. Some of these higher-order hypercomplex neurons respond specifically to two edges that form a 90° angle. For this reason, they are called *corner detectors.*

Hubel and Wiesel have also shown that the visual cortex is functionally organized in columns of cells. Each column has a diameter of 0.5 mm or less and extends from the surface of the visual cortex down through its six layers. Each column of cells is excited by a line stimulus of a particular orientation. Immediately adjacent columns respond to line stimuli of slightly different orientations. The firing of these cells must be the basis for our ability to detect the features of stimuli, but the processes by which the various categories of visual-cortex neurons interact to allow us to perceive the incredibly complex visual world in which we live are far from understood.

You have seen that spatial coding of visual stimuli is accomplished at the cortical level of mammals. You might ask how animals lacking a highly developed cortex do it. In the frog—a species with only the beginnings of a cortex—it appears that much of the spatial coding takes place in the retina. This was demonstrated in research by Lettvin, Maturana, McCulloch, and Pitts (1959) and Maturana, Lettvin, McCulloch, and Pitts (1960). They moved a variety of stimuli, including lines, edges, dots, and checkered patterns, across the frog's visual field by means of a simple magnetic device, as shown in Figure 5-6. They then recorded the responses elicited by these stimuli in single optic fibers.

Figure 5-6
(A) The relationship between the frog and the hemisphere that constituted the experimental visual field. (B) Scale drawings of some of the objects used as stimuli. The degrees indicate their diameter when placed inside a hemisphere of the same radius as that represented in (A). The actual hemisphere used was larger—14 inches in diameter. From "*Anatomy and Physiology of Vision in the Frog* (Rana pipiens)," *by H. R. Maturana, J. Y. Lettvin, W. S. McCulloch, and W. H. Pitts,* Journal of General Physiology, *1960, 43, 129–175. Copyright 1960 by the Rockefeller University Press. Reprinted by permission.*

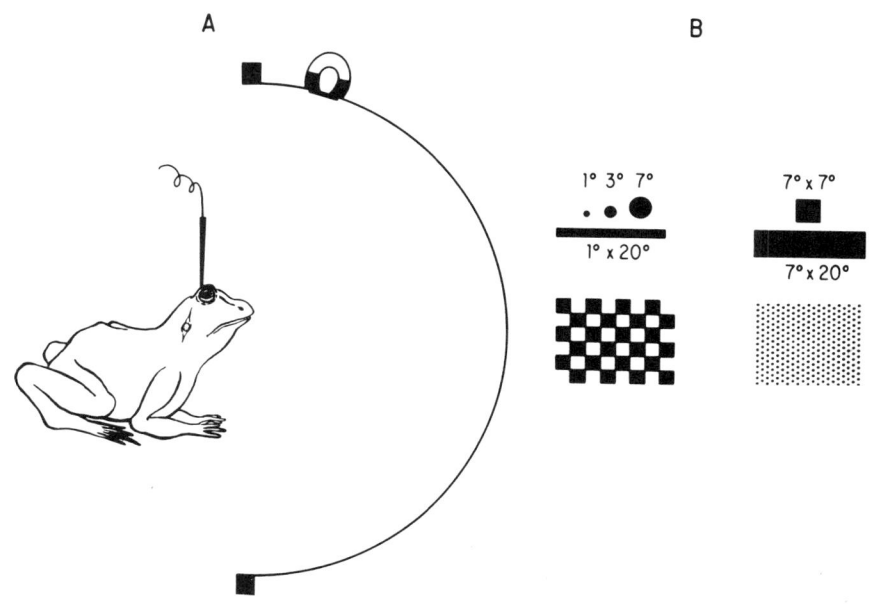

Maturana and his associates were able to delineate five categories of retinal detectors on the basis of the stimuli that elicited an optic-nerve response. Some of the fibers responded only to an edge that moved within the receptive field. Others responded most to an edge that was moved in a particular direction across the retinal receptive field. Some nerve fibers fired only when the receptive field was dimmed, and others fired continuously in inverse proportion to light intensity. The most interesting category of fibers described by these authors was one that they called "bug detectors." These fibers responded selectively to a small dark object that was moved irregularly across the visual field. The presence of these detectors is certainly helpful to the frog, but I imagine that flies and other insects do not universally applaud their existence!

The Auditory System

The physical bases for auditory stimuli are vibrations of the air that are produced by the vibration of a physical object. The vibrations or sound waves may be described in terms of their amplitude and frequency. *Amplitude* refers to the perceived loudness of a sound, while *frequency,* which is measured in cycles per second (Hz), is the physical correlate of perceived pitch. The greater the frequency of a sound, the higher the perceived pitch. We cannot hear all sound frequencies. In fact, the human ear only responds to sounds that fall in the frequency range of approximately 20–20,000 Hz. Furthermore, the human ear is most sensitive to sounds within the frequency range of approximately 1000–4000 Hz. The upper range of our auditory capabilities is exceeded by at least 23 other mammalian species. For example, bats can respond to sounds with a frequency of up to 120,000 Hz, while porpoises and the common seal react to sounds of frequencies up to 150,000 and 180,000 Hz, respectively.

The Structure of the Human Ear

The ear is composed of three major divisions: the **outer ear,** the **middle ear,** and the **inner ear.** The outer ear gathers sound stimuli, the middle ear transmits the sound to the inner ear, where the receptor cells are located, and the receptor cells in the inner ear transduce the mechanical sound energy into neural energy.

The Outer Ear. The outer ear consists of the *pinna*—the cartilaginous flappy structure that we normally call the ear—and the *external auditory meatus* (the ear canal). Although most humans have lost the ability, many animals can move their pinnae and thereby orient their outer ear so that more auditory information will be gathered.

The external auditory meatus is approximately 2.6 cm long in humans, and at the proximal end of the meatus is attached a rather taut, paper-thin *tympanic membrane* (eardrum). The tympanic membrane, which is the inner boundary of the outer ear, has an area of 69 square millimeters and is shaped like a cone with its apex pointed inward (Brown, 1975). Sound waves traveling down the meatus set the tympanic membrane into vibratory motion. The membrane vibrates freely between the outer and middle ear and faithfully reproduces the fluctuations of the sound waves.

The Middle Ear. The middle ear is a small, air-filled cavity adjacent to the tympanic membrane. The total volume of the middle ear is about 2 cc (Gulick, 1971). Figure 5-7 illustrates the basic anatomy of the middle ear. Air enters the middle ear from the mouth via the **eustachian tube,** which opens during swallowing. This passageway allows air pressure to be equalized on the two sides of the tympanic membrane. A difference in air pressure between the two sides would hamper the vibratory motion of this membrane and thus cause impaired hearing.

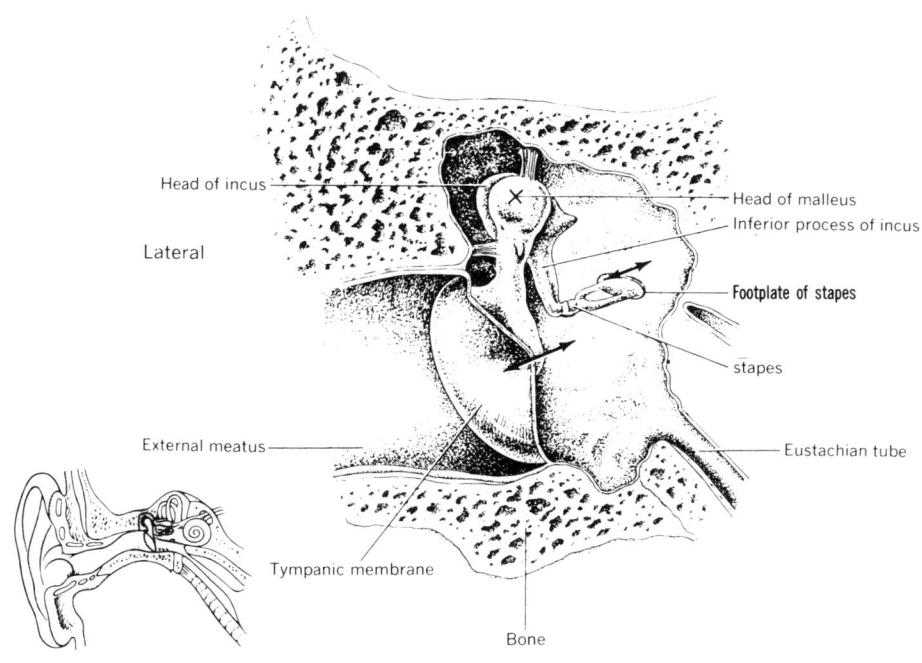

Head of incus

Lateral

Head of malleus

Inferior process of incus

Footplate of stapes

stapes

External meatus

Eustachian tube

Tympanic membrane

Bone

Figure 5-7
The anatomy of the middle ear. Adapted from Hearing: Physiology and Psychophysics, *by W. L. Gulick. Copyright © 1971 by Oxford University Press, Inc. Reprinted by permission.*

Suspended in the middle-ear space are three small bones, or **ossicles,** which transmit sound from the tympanic membrane to the inner ear (see Figure 5-8). The *malleus,* or hammer, is attached to the tympanic membrane. The *incus,* or anvil, is interposed between the malleus and the *stapes,* or stirrup. The *footplate* of the stapes fits up against the **oval window** (also see Figure 5-9). The oval window is a membrane-covered opening in the bony external wall of the inner ear. All three small ossicles are set in motion by vibrations of the tympanic membrane. As they in turn vibrate, the footplate is pushed in and out against the oval window.

The Inner Ear. The inner ear is filled with fluid and consists of the **cochlea.** Within the cochlea are the auditory receptor cells. As shown in Figure 5-9A, the cochlea is shaped like a coiled tube of decreasing diameter. The human cochlea has two and three-quarters turns and looks much like a snail's shell. A cross section of the cochlear canal is shown in Figure 5-9B. This cross section shows the three canals of the

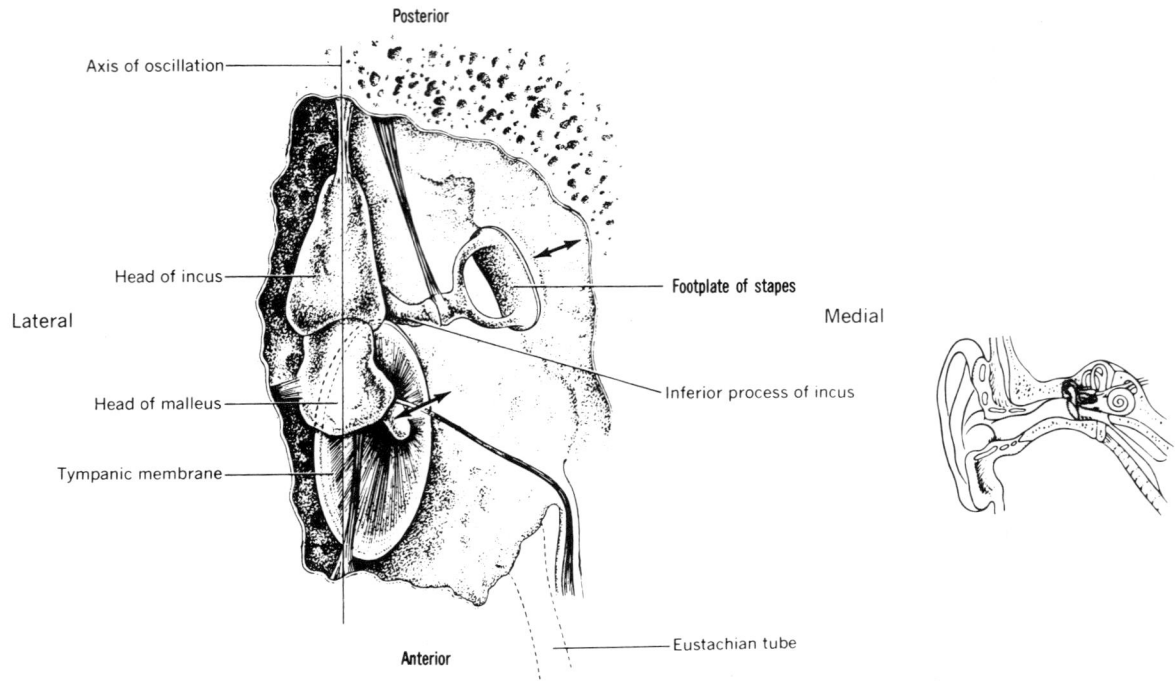

Axis of oscillation

Posterior

Lateral

Head of incus

Head of malleus

Tympanic membrane

Anterior

Footplate of stapes

Medial

Inferior process of incus

Eustachian tube

Figure 5-8
The anatomy of the
middle ear. Adapted
from Hearing:
Physiology and
Psychophysics, *by*
W. L. Gulick.
Copyright © 1971
by Oxford
University Press,
Inc. Reprinted by
permission.

cochlea: the *scala vestibuli,* the *scala media,* and the *scala tympani.* The scala vestibuli is separated from the scala media by *Reissner's membrane,* and the *basilar membrane* separates the scala media from the scala tympani. The scala media, which contains the auditory receptor cells, is completely enclosed and separated from the other two canals. It contains a viscous fluid called *endolymph* or *cochlear fluid,* which is set into motion by movements of the footplate of the stapes against the oval window.

Resting upon and running the length of the basilar membrane and projecting into the scala media is a group of structures collectively referred to as the **organ of Corti.** A cross section of this structure is shown in Figure 5-10. **Hair cells,** which are the receptor cells for hearing, are located in the organ of Corti. Pressure waves caused by movement of the stapes against the oval window are set up in the endolymph of the inner ear and cause the basilar membrane to move up and down. Suspended immediately above the basilar membrane is the **tectorial membrane.** It also moves up and down in response to the pressure waves but not in quite the same way as the basilar membrane. The difference in their movements causes the tectorial membrane to slide across the basilar membrane. This brushing, which is called *shearing,* somehow produces a generator potential or partial depolarization in the hair cells. If the generator potential exceeds threshold, an action potential is generated in the fibers of the auditory branch of the VIIIth cranial nerve and propagated toward the brain.

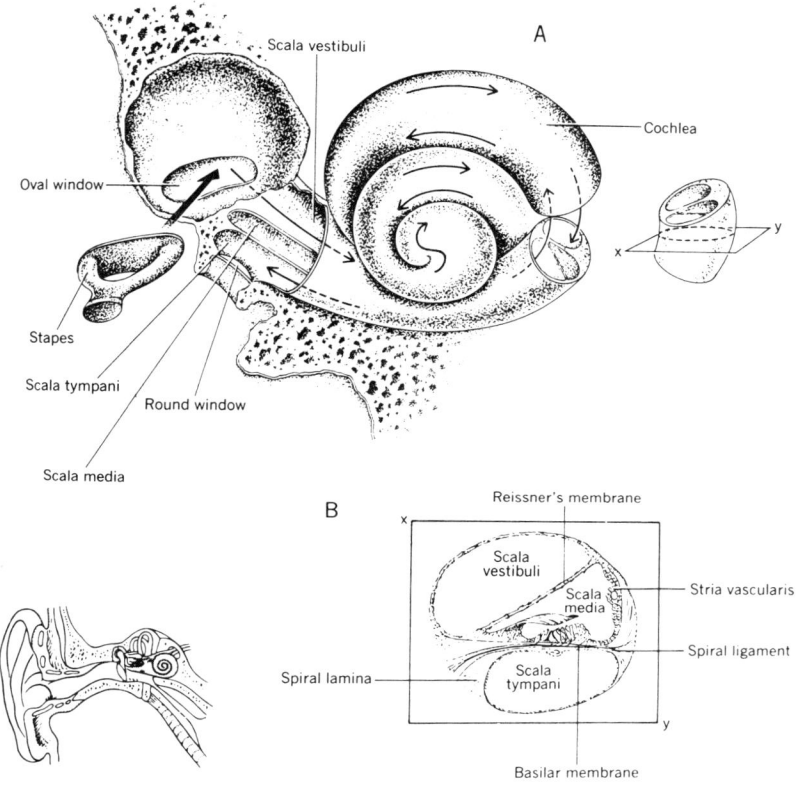

Figure 5-9
(A) The anatomy of
the inner ear. (B) A
cross section of the
cochlear canal.
From Hearing:
Physiology and
Psychophysics, by
W. L. Gulick.
Copyright © 1971
by Oxford
University Press,
Inc. Reprinted by
permission.

The Auditory Pathway

The pathways from the cochlea to the auditory cortex are probably the most complex of all sensory pathways. Figure 5-11 is a diagram of the main auditory pathways. As can be seen, there is extensive crossing of fibers from one side of the brain to the other. Fibers from the auditory branch of the VIIIth cranial nerve terminate in the *dorsal* and *ventral cochlear nuclei.* Separate fiber systems proceed from the two cochlear nuclei. Fibers from the dorsal cochlear nuclei cross the midline and then ascend toward the cortex via the **lateral lemniscus,** which terminates in the inferior colliculi of the midbrain. On the other hand, fibers from the ventral cochlear nucleus first synapse in both the ipsilateral and contralateral **superior olivary complex.** The superior olive is the first place in the auditory pathway where binaural (involving both ears) interactions occur. From the superior olivary complex, fibers ascend to the inferior colliculi via the lateral lemniscus.

Impulses are carried from the inferior colliculi to the medial geniculate body of the thalamus. The fiber tract interconnecting these two regions is the brachium of the inferior colliculus. From the medial geniculate body, fibers of the **auditory radiations**

81

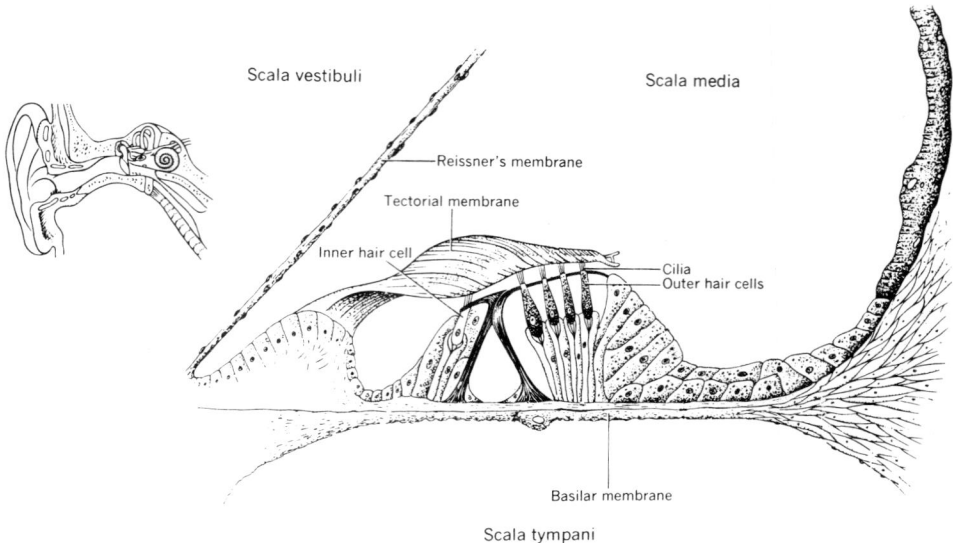

Figure 5-10
Cross section of the scala media, showing the organ of Corti. Adapted from Hearing: Physiology and Psychophysics, *by W. L. Gulick. Copyright © 1971 by Oxford University Press, Inc. Reprinted by permission.*

conduct impulses to the **superior gyrus of the temporal lobes** (areas 41 and 42)—the auditory cortex.

Auditory Abilities

Perception of Pitch. As was indicated earlier in this chapter, auditory stimuli vary along two dimensions: loudness (amplitude) and pitch (frequency). The greater the frequency of a sound, in cycles per second, the higher the perceived pitch. Over the years, a large research literature has been generated documenting attempts to determine how the auditory nervous system is able to decipher or code pitch. Two major theories have emerged to account for this ability: the **frequency theory** and the **place theory.** For a detailed description and assessment of these theories of hearing, consult Gulick (1971).

The frequency and place theories have their roots in the writings of Rutherford (1886) and Helmholtz (1863), respectively. According to the frequency theory, pitch is coded by the rate of firing of the axons in the auditory nerves. For example, if a tone with a frequency of 2000 Hz were presented, the first-order neurons of the auditory branch of the VIIIth cranial nerve would show 2000 nerve impulses per second. There is a problem with this simple frequency theory, however, because electrophysiological evidence indicates that axons of the size found in the auditory nerve cannot fire at a rate faster than 1000 Hz. Wever's (1949) frequency-place theory accounts for this problem—at least for tones of frequencies of up to 5000 Hz. Before his view is examined, the basic features of the place theory must be outlined.

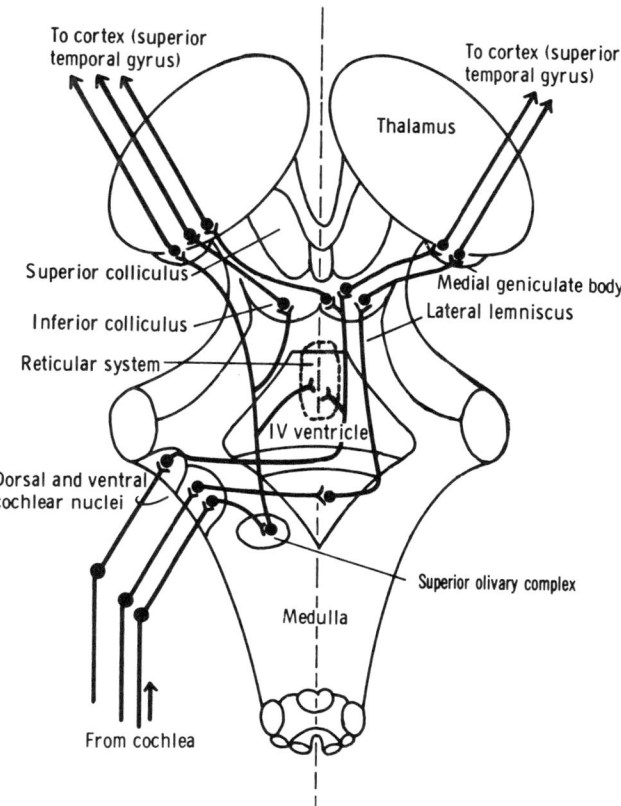

To cortex (superior
temporal gyrus)

To cortex (superior
temporal gyrus)

Thalamus

Superior colliculus

Medial geniculate body

Inferior colliculus

Lateral lemniscus

Reticular system

IV ventricle

Dorsal and ventral
cochlear nuclei

Superior olivary complex

Medulla

From cochlea

Figure 5-11
*A simplified
diagram of the main
auditory pathways
superimposed on a
dorsal view of the
brain stem. The
cerebellum and
cerebral cortex are
not shown. Adapted
from* Review of
Medical Physiology
*(7th ed.), by W. F.
Ganong. Copyright
1975 by Lange
Medical
Publications.
Reprinted by
permission.*

The place theory of hearing contends that the essential cues for pitch perception are provided first by the place of stimulation of the basilar membrane and later by the locus of activation in the auditory pathways. In 1928, Békésy published the first in a series of elegant studies of the physiological basis of pitch perception—studies that were to win him the Nobel Prize in medicine in 1961. Much of his research is summarized in a book titled *Experiments in Hearing,* published in 1960, and his findings provide strong support for the place theory.

Békésy took advantage of the fact that the peripheral auditory apparatus continues to function for some time after death to observe the functioning of the basilar membrane in a number of animal species, including humans. His observations indicated that, up to frequencies of 60 Hz, the entire basilar membrane vibrated—at a frequency corresponding to the frequency of the tone being presented. It appeared that, at frequencies of up to 60 Hz, the frequency theory was valid.

At frequencies above 60 Hz, a new phenomenon was observed. The surface of the basilar membrane now began to vibrate unevenly, and the place of maximum vibration varied as a function of the frequency of the auditory stimulus. Why would this occur? It occurred because of the physical characteristics of the basilar membrane. The basilar membrane is not of uniform thickness. Its thickness increases from its base, or stapes, end to its apex (the end at the top of the two and three-quarters turns of the cochlea). Correlated with this change in thickness is a difference in the ease with which the basilar membrane will vibrate. The stapes end is stiff and resistant to movement, while the wide apical end is very flexible. Békésy found that high-pitched or high-frequency sounds cause maximal activation of the basilar membrane at the stapes end, while low-pitched sounds have their maximum effect at the apical end. Middle tones activate the membrane maximally at intermediate distances along the basilar membrane.

Electrophysiological studies that have recorded action potentials in the auditory pathway have placed some restrictions on Békésy's observations regarding the actual frequency at which processing or encoding moves from frequency to place coding. Wever (1949, 1962) was able to demonstrate that fibers in the auditory tracts fire at the same frequency as tones ranging up to 5000 Hz. These data might seem in conflict with the observation made above that neurons in the auditory pathways cannot fire more rapidly than 1000 Hz. To circumvent this problem, Wever proposed that firing at higher rates is due to neural volleying.

Wever suggests that, at tone frequencies of up to 400 Hz, individual fibers follow the frequency by firing at the same frequency as the sound. However, at higher frequencies, neural volleying takes over. In neural volleying, the auditory pathway as a whole continues to follow the stimulus, but the individual fibers stagger their responses to fire in platoons. As the frequency gradually increases, individual fibers begin firing at a rate of only once every two, three, four, five, and so on cycles of the tone. Thus, no single fiber must fire more rapidly than is possible according to its physiological capacity, but frequency coding of pitch information can still occur. For the audible range of tones above 5000 Hz, Wever postulated that the place principle takes over. Place operates to some extent, along with volleying, at frequencies of up to 5000 Hz, according to Wever, but, beyond this upper limit, volleying fails, and place becomes the only basis for pitch coding. In summary, for tones of lower frequency (up to 5000 Hz), frequency theory appears to explain coding of pitch. At higher frequencies, the place of maximal activity along the basilar membrane is the critical factor in the transmission of pitch information.

An interesting finding with regard to place theory is that the auditory pathways, as they course upward to the cortex, are organized in a **tonotopic** manner. This means that neurons originating in adjacent parts of the basilar membrane are maximally sensitive to specific different tones and remain arranged in a systematic order throughout the different levels of the auditory system. Electrophysiological studies of single auditory neurons have shown that the cochlear nuclei (Rose, 1960), the lateral olivary nucleus (Tsuchitani & Boudreau, 1966), the nucleus of the lateral lemniscus (Aitkin, Anderson, & Brugge, 1970), and the inferior colliculus (Rose, Greenwood, Goldberg, & Hind, 1963) are organized in a tonotopic fashion. However, studies have thus far failed to uncover tonotopic organization at the thalamic level of the auditory system—namely, in the medial geniculate body (Brown, 1975).

The auditory cortex is probably not tonotopically organized (Evans, Ross, & Whitfield, 1965). Even if tonotopic organization does exist at the cortical level of the auditory system, it is probably not functional. It has been shown that ablation of the auditory cortex does not disrupt the ability of animals to make a frequency discrimination (Brown, Gedvilas, & Marco, 1967; Goldberg & Neff, 1961).

Perception of Loudness. As you know, sounds vary not only in pitch but also in loudness. Wever's theory of hearing also accounts for the perception of loudness, or stimulus intensity. He has proposed that increases in the intensity of a tone have two effects. First, the increase results in more fibers in the auditory pathway being fired. Second, those fibers that are already firing will respond earlier in their relative refractory periods. For example, a fiber that was firing only on every fourth cycle might now fire on every third peak. It also appears that certain hair cells do not become stimulated until a stimulus reaches a relatively high intensity. Activity in these hair cells and their efferent pathways may specifically code information regarding the intensity of a tone.

The processing of information about the intensity of tones takes place at subcortical levels. Cortical cells do not differentially react, in terms of their firing patterns, to changes in stimulus intensity. Animals with their auditory cortex removed show no loss in their ability to discriminate intensity (Raab & Ades, 1946). In fact, Raab and Ades found that this ability remained when the inferior colliculi were also destroyed, although there was a slight loss of sensitivity. Thus, the ability to discriminate between the intensity of two sounds is apparently for the most part mediated by levels of the auditory system below the inferior colliculi of the midbrain.

Detection of Auditory Patterns. Although complete bilateral removal of the auditory cortex does not disrupt an animal's ability to make either pitch or intensity discriminations, it does impair its ability to discriminate different patterns of tones. Suppose an animal is confronted with the following discrimination problem: There are two sound patterns, consisting of three tones each. In the first, the sequence of tones, according to pitch, is high-low-high. In the second, it is low-high-low.

To distinguish between these two tone patterns, the animal must make a frequency discrimination, but, in addition, the subject must learn the order in which the changes in frequency occur. This second process appears to be critically dependent upon the integrity of the auditory cortex, because, if the auditory cortex is bilaterally ablated, this ability is lost in cats (Diamond, Goldberg, & Neff, 1962; Diamond & Neff, 1957) and monkeys (Dewson, Cowey, & Weiskrantz, 1970).

Sound Localization. Determining the direction from which a sound arises in our environment depends on perception of the *temporal delay* between the arrival of the sound at one ear and its arrival at the other and perception of *differences between the intensities* of the sounds reaching the two ears. The temporal-delay mechanism appears to be more important for localizing tones with a pitch of less than 3000 Hz, and the intensity mechanism is more important for tones of higher frequencies. The bilateral interaction required for sound localization begins in the superior olivary nuclei, but the sound-localization process requires the integrity of the neural pathways all the way from these nuclei to the cortex. Interpretation of the temporal-delay and intensity-difference information takes place in the auditory cortex. If the auditory cortex is bilaterally destroyed, the ability to localize sound in space is severely impaired (Neff, 1961; Neff & Diamond, 1958; Strominger, 1969).

The Chemical Senses: Taste and Olfaction

The chemical sensations of taste and olfaction are usually considered together in discussions of sensory processes. For one thing, their transduction processes are similar. Both taste and olfactory receptors respond only to molecules of substances that are in a dissolved state. Both senses are intimately involved with eating. Flavor—that quality that determines our preferences in food and drink—is in large part a combination of taste and smell. We have all had the experience of "losing" our taste during a bad cold that depressed our sense of smell. Did you know that, if the nose is blocked, it is impossible to tell whether a slice of apple or of onion has been placed in the mouth? These examples illustrate the interdependence of taste and smell. However, as will be shown below, the two senses are anatomically distinct.

Taste

Taste Receptors. The sensory receptors for taste are contained in the **taste buds.** There are about 9000 taste buds on the human adult tongue and soft palate, and a few are found on the hard palate, pharynx, larynx, and other areas of the oral cavity. The majority of the taste buds are located in the areas shown in Figure 5-12. It is interesting to note that certain regions of the top of the tongue tend to be most sensitive to certain tastes. Sweet, sour, bitter, and salt are the primary taste qualities. The tip of the tongue is most sensitive to sweets, the sides to sour, the back of the tongue to bitter, and the sides toward the tip to salty tastes.

Taste buds are usually located on **papillae,** which are small elevations or ridges of tissue on the top and sides of the tongue. A papilla is shown in the middle drawing of Figure 5-12; each papilla contains many individual taste buds. A single taste bud with its efferent fiber is shown in the bottom drawing of Figure 5-12. Each taste bud contains several taste receptor cells, which have very fine, finger-like extensions called **microvilli.** The microvilli serve to increase the receptive surface of the taste cells. Chemical materials in solution in the fluids of the mouth reach the microvilli via pores in the papillae. In some way not yet completely understood, the chemicals produce a neural response in the taste receptor cells. The life span of a taste cell is only about three to five days in the cat and rabbit, and the same is probably true for human taste cells (Beidler, 1963). Investigators who once thought that they had discovered different types of sensory cells for the different taste qualities were probably simply observing receptors in different stages of development (Christman, 1971).

The Central Pathways for Taste. Fibers from three of the cranial nerves enter the taste buds and carry nervous signals from the taste receptor cells to the brain. Cells in the anterior two-thirds of the tongue transmit impulses via the *chorda tympani* branch of the facial nerve (VIIth cranial nerve). Fibers from the posterior third of the tongue reach the brain stem by way of the *glossopharyngeal nerve* (IXth cranial nerve). Finally, taste sensations arising from taste buds in areas other than the tongue are carried by the *vagus nerve* (Xth cranial nerve). The taste fibers in these three cranial nerves unite in the **solitary tract** or *tractus solitarius* in the medulla and end in the **nucleus solitarius** (see Figure 5-13). Fibers from this nucleus are thought to then cross the midline to join the medial lemniscus, which relays impulses to the accessory arcuate nucleus of the thalamus. From this thalamic relay for taste, efferent fibers project to the extreme ventral end of the postcentral gyrus—area 43.

Primary Tastes. For color vision, certain primary colors have been postulated, mixtures of which account for all possible hues. Similarly, **primary tastes** have been proposed, under the assumption that their mixtures can account for the broad spectrum of taste sensations that we encounter. These primary taste qualities are

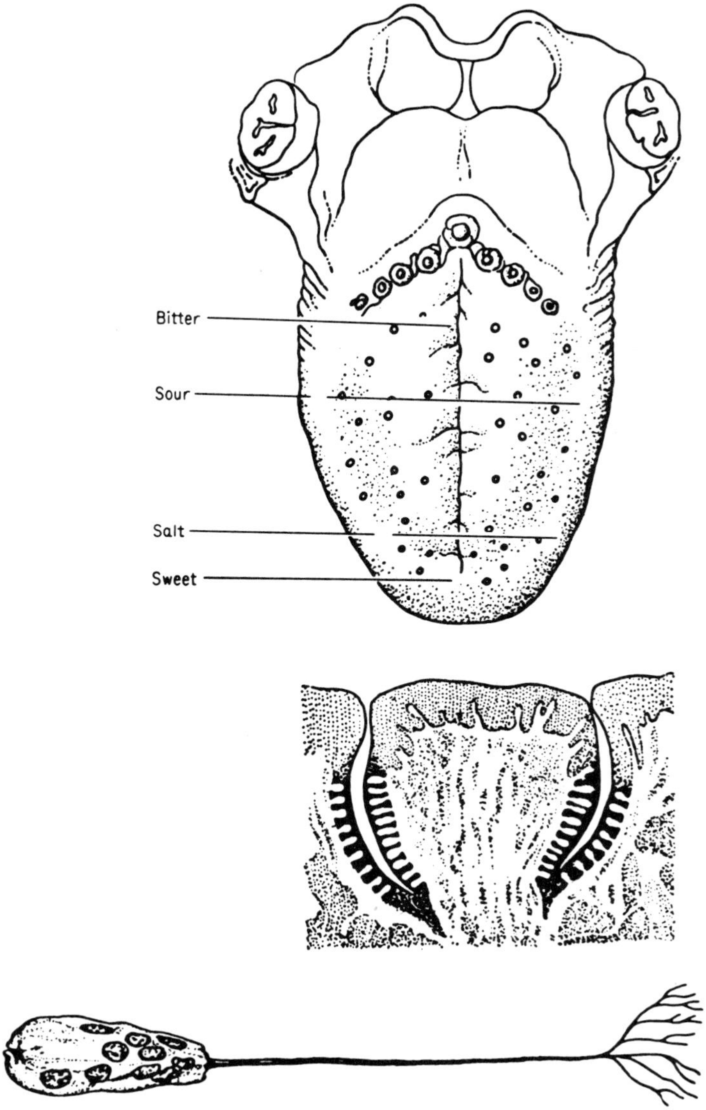

Bitter

Sour

Salt

Sweet

*Figure 5-12
The drawing at the
top shows the
surface of the
tongue; the small
circles indicate large
papillae. The middle
drawing shows a
cross section of a
papilla, with its
taste buds. An
individual taste bud
and its nerve are
shown in the
drawing at the
bottom. From
"Smell and Taste,"
by A. J.
Haagen-Smith,* Scientific
American, *1952,
186, 28–32.
Copyright © 1952
by Scientific
American, Inc. All
rights reserved.
Reprinted by
permission.*

sweet, sour, bitter, and salt. According to Guyton (1971), the stimuli that produce these four primary tastes are as follows.

The sour taste is caused by acids, and the intensity of the sour sensation is roughly proportional to the logarithm of the hydrogen-ion concentration—that is, to the concentration of cations. In contrast, the taste sensation of salt is dependent upon the anions (for example, the Cl^- ions in common table salt, or $NaCl$) of the salts. It is an interesting finding that adding a bit of salt to a sour grapefruit will reduce the sourness. This is presumably because the anions of the salt combine with the cations of the grapefruit's acid to produce a more neutral experience.

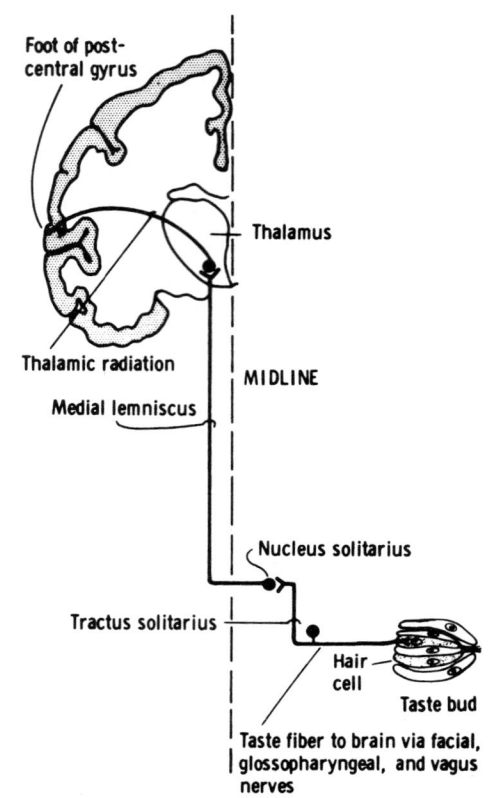

Figure 5-13
The taste pathways.
Adapted from
Review of Medical
Physiology, *(7th
ed.), by W. F.
Ganong. Copyright
1975 by Lange
Medical
Publications.
Reprinted by
permission.*

Neither the sweet nor the bitter taste is caused by a single class of chemicals, and the basis for these taste sensations is not nearly as clear as it is for sour and salt. In fact, some substances (such as saccharin) have a sweet taste when applied to the front of the tongue, where taste buds are selectively sensitive to the sweet sensation, but a bitter taste when applied to the back of the tongue, where taste receptors are most sensitive to the bitter taste. This quality makes saccharin objectionable to some people.

The bitter-taste sense is much more sensitive to stimuli than are the other taste qualities; in other words, a bitter taste can be detected at much lower concentrations. Further, the bitter taste at high intensities will usually cause a person or other animal to reject a food. This is an adaptive response on the part of the organism because many of the deadly toxins found in poisonous plants cause an intense bitter-taste sensation.

Adaptation of Taste. We are all familiar with the fact that taste sensations rapidly adapt. If we hold a substance in our mouth for a while, the taste will actually disappear. Furthermore, adaptation to one taste quality can significantly affect the taste sensation for a subsequently ingested substance. This latter phenomenon is called **cross adaptation.** For example, a sour food will taste much more sour than usual if the taste buds have been adapted just previously to a very sweet substance.

The neural mechanisms involved in both adaptation and cross adaptation have been the subject of much research. It has been found that the taste buds do not adapt enough, in terms of their receptor-potential outputs, to account for these phenomena. For this reason, it appears that these adaptation processes must occur in the central nervous system. Unfortunately, the central mechanisms responsible for physiological adaptation in the sensation of taste have yet to be uncovered.

Olfaction

Olfaction is the least understood of all of our senses. This is partly the result of the inaccessibility of the olfactory apparatus; it is high in the nose and hence difficult to study. This lack of understanding is also partly due to the fact that, in humans, as compared with many other animal species, the sense of smell is almost rudimentary. For example, a German shepherd dog's sense of smell is approximately one million times as sensitive as a human's. This does not imply that the sense of smell has lost its survival value for us. Quite the contrary is true. Poisonous substances, in addition to tasting bitter, frequently have unpleasant odors. The formation of harmful bacteria in spoiling food often produces very unpleasant, putrid odors, which serve as a warning signal to the otherwise unsuspecting potential eater.

As is true for taste, the olfactory receptors are chemoreceptors that are activated by molecules in solution. To be detected, odorous substances must be volatile (in the form of airborne particles) so that they can be sniffed into the nostrils. They must also be at least partly soluble in water so that they can pass through the nasal mucus to the olfactory cells. Finally, they must be soluble in lipids (fatty substances) so that they can pass through the lipid layer that forms the surface membrane of the olfactory receptors. Before examining the nature of the basic substances that can produce olfactory sensations, we must consider the anatomy of the olfactory system.

Olfactory Cells. In the human, the olfactory receptors are located in a small patch or olfactory membrane in the superior part of each nostril (see Figure 5-14). The olfactory membrane in each nostril has a surface area of approximately 5 square centimeters (Brown, 1975). The receptor cells for olfaction are called **olfactory cells.** Unlike most receptor cells of the senses, they perform both primary-reception and

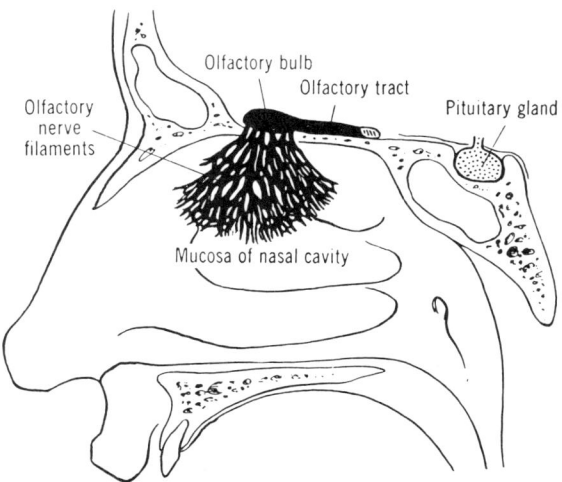

Figure 5-14 The olfactory structures in the nasal cavity. From Fundamentals of Neurology *(5th ed.), by E. Gardner. Copyright 1968 by W. B. Saunders Company. Reprinted by permission.*

conduction functions. There are approximately 100 million of these cells interspersed in the olfactory membrane.

As shown in Figure 5-15, each olfactory cell terminates in numerous fingerlike processes or cilia in the mucus. A single olfactory cell may have as many as 1000 of these processes. These cilia increase the receptive area of the receptors so that the 2.5-square-centimeter surface area is in effect increased to an area of 600 square centimeters. This factor undoubtedly is important in making the sense of smell so very sensitive. Another feature that contributes to the sensitivity of olfaction is the fact that

Figure 5-15
The olfactory membrane and the central projections of the olfactory receptors. Adapted from "The Sense of Smell in Man—Its Physiological Basis," by R. A. Schneider, New England Journal of Medicine, *1967, 277, 299–303. Reprinted by permission of the* New England Journal of Medicine.

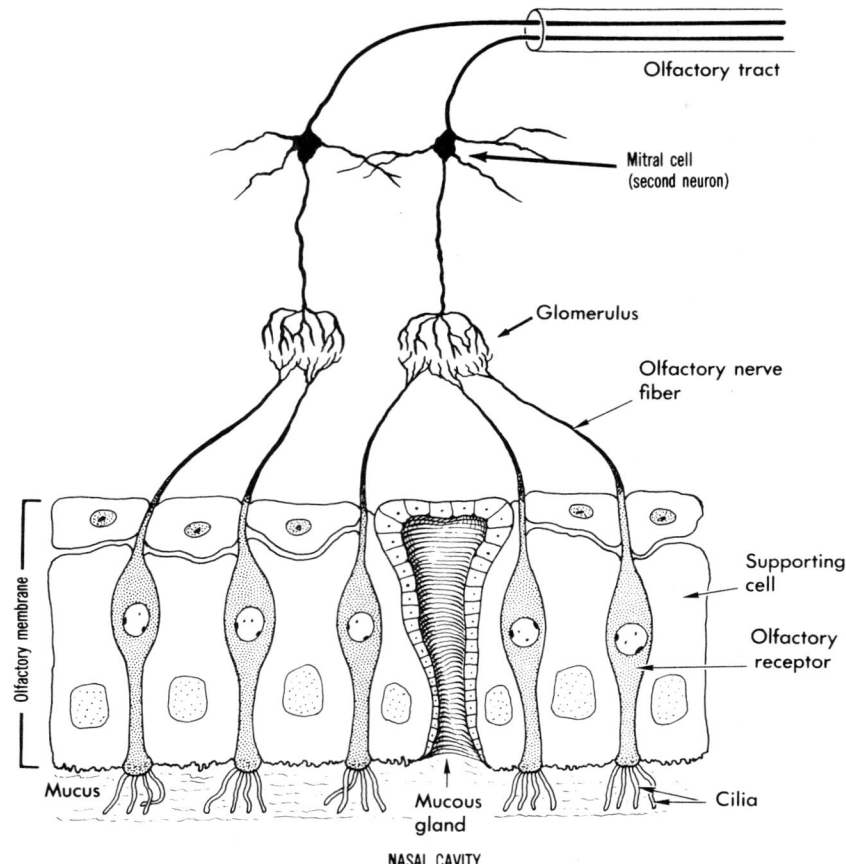

many thousands of receptors converge and summate on each second-order neuron in the olfactory system. The entire olfactory system apparently uses this summation process. In contrast, you'll remember, visual convergence was limited largely to the peripherally located rods. No olfactory fibers exhibiting the direct, one-to-one pathways of the cones in the fovea have been discovered. However, the fine analysis required in the visual system is not required in the processing of olfactory information.

Olfactory Pathways. The fine, unmyelinated axonal fibers of the olfactory receptors leave the nasal cavity by way of minute perforations in the bony **cribiform plate.** The axons of these receptor cells proceed into the **olfactory bulb** (see Figure 5-14), to end on dendrites from **mitral cells** in a structure called the **glomerulus** (see Figure 5-15). An average of 26,000 olfactory-cell axons converge on each glomerulus. Fibers from the olfactory bulbs travel posteriorly—as the olfactory tracts—to many rhinencephalic areas (see Chapter 3) and the hypothalamus. It would be an error to consider these higher levels to which the olfactory system projects to be exclusively concerned with processing olfactory information. The olfactory inputs to these regions are undoubtedly related to functions performed by these areas of eating, arousal and attention, and emotion, and they are perhaps related to learning. The olfactory system is the only sensory modality that is not represented in the thalamus, and there is no neocortical projection area for olfaction.

Adaptation in the Olfactory System. We have all experienced the phenomenon of rapid adaptation to a pungent smell. As is true for taste, olfaction exhibits cross adaptation. As is also true for taste, the psychological process of adaptation occurs much more rapidly and to a greater degree than would be predicted on the basis of electrophysiological recordings from the receptor cells. For this reason, it has been proposed, as it has for taste adaptation, that olfactory adaptation is mediated centrally.

Primary Odors and Their Coding. There has been much less agreement about the basic types of olfactory sensations than about the basic types of taste. This lack of consensus makes it particularly difficult for researchers to decide how these stimuli are coded. John E. Amoore and his associates have proposed seven **primary odors**: *camphoraceous* (mothballs), *musky, floral* (roses), *pepperminty* (mint candy), *putrid* (rotten eggs), *ethereal* (dry-cleaning fluid), and *pungent* (vinegar). Regardless of the basic odors that are settled on, the question remains as to how their stimulus qualities are coded. Two prominent theories that have been proposed to account for this process are the **radiation theory** and the **stereochemical theory.**

According to the radiation theory (Beck & Miles, 1947), stimulating particles differentially absorb and radiate heat and light energy, depending upon their molecular structure, and this feature is responsible for the different olfactory sensations. Research conducted by Ottoson (1956) questioned the validity of this theory. Ottoson showed that, if a thin membrane that transmits light and heat is placed over the olfactory receptor cells, the olfactory receptors cannot be activated by odor molecules.

The stereochemical theory of olfactory coding (see Amoore, Johnston, & Rubin, 1964) is based largely on Moncrieff's (1949) proposal that there are specific receptor cells for each primary odor and that molecules of odoriferous material produce their effects by fitting into the correct receptor "slots." Moncrieff's explanation is an application of the "lock and key" concept that has been useful in explaining the actions of enzymes with their substrates, of antibodies with antigens, and other, similar relationships.

Amoore and his associates were able to determine the molecular shapes of their seven primary odors. For example, it was found that the camphoraceous-odor molecules are more or less spherical. Thus, it was hypothesized that the receptor for this olfactory sensation must be shaped like a bowl. When molecules of the other primary odors were studied, it was found that an additional four of them had characteristic shapes that would thus fit into distinctly shaped receptor sites. These were musky, floral, pepperminty, and ethereal. Figure 5-16 shows the shapes of the molecules and receptors for these odors. No characteristic shapes were found for pungent and putrid odors, but fortunately it was found that a certain electrical charge is characteristic of each of these two remaining classes of odors. Pungent substances were found to carry a positive electrical charge, while putrid substances were found to be negatively charged. These electrical charges may attract these substances to oppositely charged receptor sites. This theory has received some empirical support in that it was possible to predict the odor characteristics of several newly synthesized compounds on the basis of their molecular shape (Amoore, Johnston, & Rubin, 1964; Johnston & Sandoval, 1960). At present, the stereochemical theory is the best explanation available for stimulus coding in the olfactory system.

Figure 5-16
Six primary-odor molecules and the hypothesized shapes of their receptors. The diagrams indicate the receptor dimensions as measured from above and from the side. From "The Stereochemical Theory of Odor," by J. E. Amoore, J. W. Johnston, Jr., and M. Rubin, Scientific American, *1964, 210, 42–49. Copyright © 1964 by Scientific American, Inc. Reprinted by permission.*

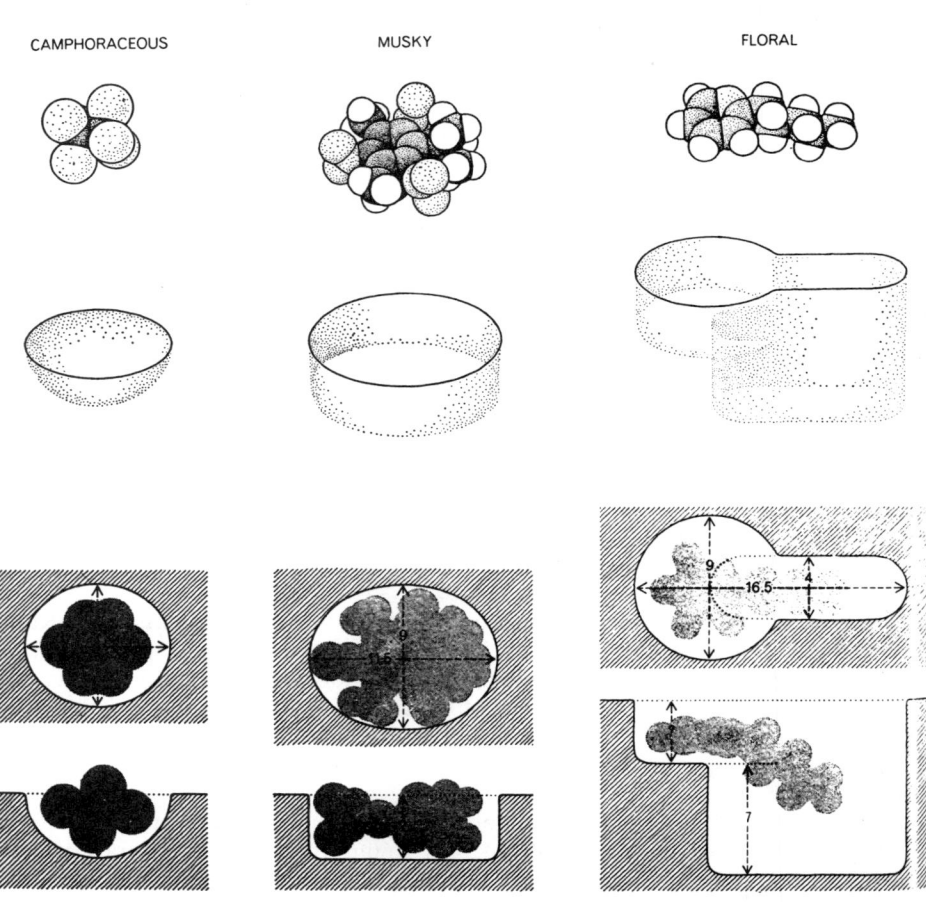

CAMPHORACEOUS   MUSKY   FLORAL

The Somatosensory System

The somatosensory system is the least specialized of all of our sensory modalities. The word *somesthesis* will be used here to refer to the sensations of pain, touch or pressure, cold, and warmth that arise from the skin, muscles, and viscera throughout the body. In the discussion below, the operations of this system will be illustrated through reference to the somesthetic senses of the skin, which are called the *cutaneous senses*. Pain, touch, cold, and warmth are often referred to as the **basic cutaneous senses.**

The skin is a very complicated structure with many important functions. One thing it of course does is keep us from falling apart into a mass of jelly. It also aids in temperature regulation and serves many crucial protective functions. For our purposes, it is important to note that the skin serves as a repository for many different

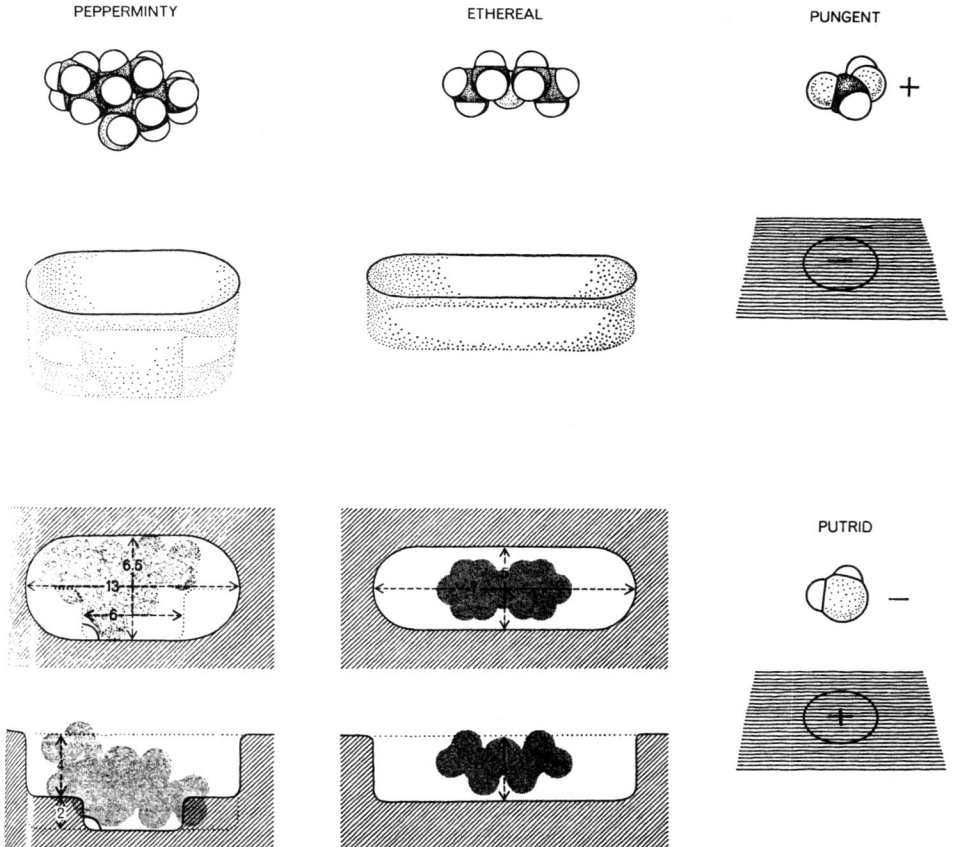

sensory organs. It appears that the skin's most important sensory function is to signal the presence of potentially harmful stimuli (Brown, 1975).

A cross section of the skin is diagramed in Figure 5-17. This illustration depicts the two main layers of the skin: the outer **epidermis** and the inner **dermis.** The epidermis can in turn be subdivided into an outer, dead layer versus an inner, living layer. The outer layer contains neither nerve fibers nor blood vessels. The inner layer also contains no blood vessels but does have some cutaneous receptors called *free nerve endings.* As you can see in Figure 5-17, the dermis, in contrast, contains a rich supply of free nerve endings, cutaneous somatosensory receptors, cutaneous glands, blood vessels, and so on. The dermis merges into the subcutaneous tissue without any distinct border.

Figure 5-17
The nerve supply of skin with sparse hair. Not all the endings shown are to be found in any one skin area. The heavy lines are myelinated fibers, the light lines nonmyelinated fibers. From Fundamentals of Neurology *(5th ed.), by E. Gardner. Copyright 1968 by W. B. Saunders Company. Reprinted by permission.*

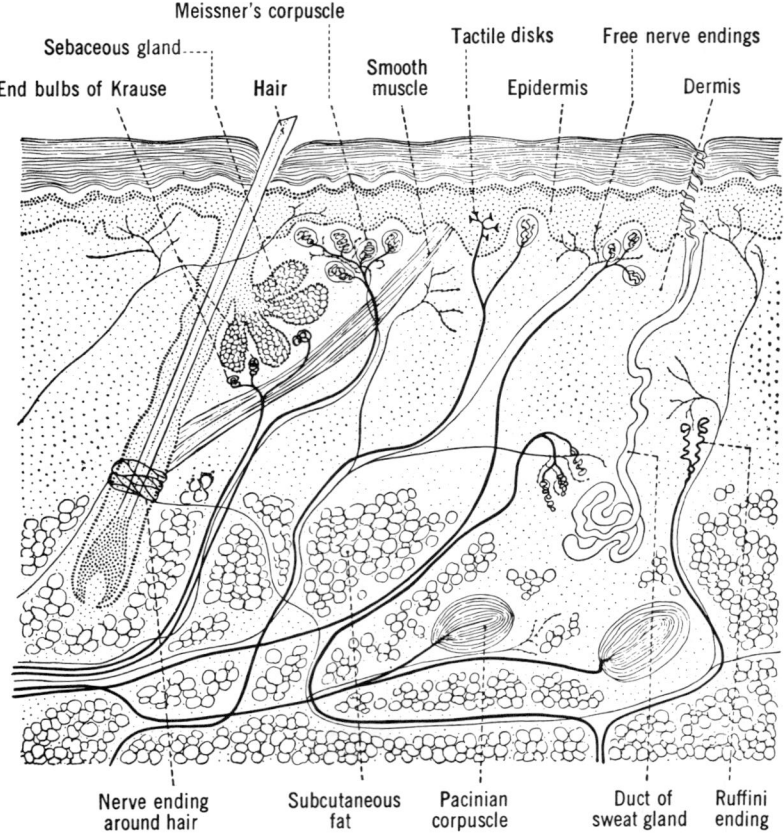

Meissner's corpuscle

Sebaceous gland

Tactile disks   Free nerve endings

End bulbs of Krause   Hair   Smooth muscle   Epidermis   Dermis

Nerve ending around hair   Subcutaneous fat   Pacinian corpuscle   Duct of sweat gland   Ruffini ending

For the past almost 100 years, a popular experimental exercise has been to attempt to discover four specific cutaneous receptors that mediate the four basic cutaneous sensations—namely, pain, touch, cold, and warmth. Unfortunately, the data arising from these inquiries were often contradictory, and no specific receptors were found definitely to mediate any of the cutaneous sensations exclusively. Another problem confronting researchers interested in this endeavor was the discovery that more than the expected four types of receptors existed. Finally, it was determined that some receptors are sensitive to more than one category of cutaneous stimuli. A healthy cornea, for example, is sensitive to all of the varieties of cutaneous sensations, yet it contains only one type of cutaneous receptor: the free nerve endings. Taken together, these pieces of information argued against the view that specific cutaneous sensations arise from the activation of sensation-specific receptors. In spite of these somewhat discouraging findings, some meaningful relationships between cutaneous sensations and the various types of receptors have emerged (Brown, 1975; Christman, 1971; Guyton, 1971). These will be summarized next.

Cutaneous Pain. Pain is a protective mechanism; it seems to arise whenever there is potential or actual tissue damage. It is fairly generally agreed that cutaneous pain is mediated by **free nerve endings**—the most widespread somatosensory receptors in the skin and throughout the body. It has been further theorized that intense, pain-eliciting stimuli activate these free nerve endings via a chemical process Mountcastle, 1968; Weddell & Verrillo, 1972). Support for this notion comes from the observation that extracts from damaged tissue will cause intense pain when injected into normal skin. Two prime candidates for a pain-mediating chemical are **bradykinin** and **histamine.** Both of these substances are found in the skin after painful stimuli are applied, and they can both be extracted from damaged tissue. Further, very minute amounts of these substances will elicit intense pain if injected into normal skin.

Touch or Pressure. At least six categories of tactual receptors exist: free nerve endings, **Meissner's corpuscles, tactile discs, hair nerve endings, Ruffini endings,** and **pacinian corpuscles.** These receptors were illustrated in Figure 5-17. The free nerve endings can detect light touch and pressure. I indicated above that these endings are also thought to mediate pain. How would pain, versus a tactual sensation, be conveyed by the efferent fibers from these receptors? Probably by the rate of nerve impulses. A low rate would signal touch or pressure information, while a very rapid rate would signal either potential or actual tissue damage.

Meissner's corpuscles are very abundant in the fingertips, the lips, and other areas of the skin where the touch modality is particularly sensitive. They probably perform important functions in our ability to detect the texture of objects touched. Further, they adapt very rapidly to an object that is allowed to continuously stimulate them, and so they are probably very sensitive to objects being moved across the skin's surface. Tactile discs have a distribution similar to that of Meissner's corpuscles and also appear to be involved in fine tactual sensitivity. In contrast to the Meissner's corpuscles, which adapt to a stimulus in a second or so, the tactile discs do not adapt rapidly to continued stimulation. Therefore, activation of the tactile discs probably transmits long-lasting signals that allow us to be cognizant of continuous contact of objects with the body.

Hair nerve endings are stimulated by any movement of the hair around which they are entwined. These receptors adapt rapidly, like the Meissner's corpuscles, and probably similarly detect information about an object moving across the surface of the skin.

Ruffini endings and pacinian corpuscles are located in the deeper layers of the dermis and also in the deeper tissues of the body. Ruffini endings adapt very slowly to continuous stimulation. For this reason, they are thought to be important in detecting and transmitting information regarding continuous states of deformation of deeper tissue and heavy, continuous pressure. Pacinian corpuscles, on the other hand, adapt very rapidly (in only a small fraction of a second) to tactile stimuli. They are excited only by very rapid movement of the tissues. They seem to be important for detecting rapid deep touch or pressure sensations. The pacinian corpuscles are also very important in detecting vibrating stimuli, and, by their discharge rate, they can code tissue vibrations occurring at rates of up to 700 Hz.

Temperature. There seem to be two types of temperature receptors, according to electrophysiological studies of postreceptor nerve fibers. One group of receptors apparently responds maximally to temperatures that are slightly above our normal body temperature of 37° C. These are called *warmth receptors,* and they respond maximally at a temperature of 37.5–40° C. A second group of temperature receptors, called *cold receptors,* shows a maximal rate of discharge to temperatures in the range of 15 to 20° C—a temperature range that is well below normal body temperature.

Attempts have been made to distinguish the cold receptors from the warmth receptors. The early suggestion of Max von Frey (1895) that the Ruffini endings are possibly the thermoreceptors for warmth while the **end bulbs of Krause** detect cold has never been verified. Other attempts to denote the specific receptors for these temperature sensitivities have been equally disappointing.

An interesting phenomenon occurs when we experience the sensation of hot. If the temperature stimulus applied to the skin goes above 45° C, the warmth receptors stop discharging. Paradoxically, the cold receptors begin to respond again. Further, it is thought that pain receptors also now begin to increase their discharge rate. Therefore, the sensation of heat apparently results from the combined discharge of the cold and the pain receptors.

Neural Pathways of the Somatosensory System

The cell bodies of the cutaneous receptor cells are located in **dorsal root ganglia,** which lie outside the spinal cord. Upon entering the spinal cord, the efferents from these receptors become organized into two systems: the **medial lemniscal** and the **spinothalamic.** The pathways of these two systems are diagramed in Figure 5-18.

The Medial Lemniscal System. Upon entering the spinal cord, the fibers of the medial lemniscal system enter the *dorsal columns* and progress toward the brain. Within the dorsal columns, ascending fibers from the legs and lower trunk travel in a fiber bundle called the **fasciculus gracilis,** and fibers from the arms and upper trunk travel to the brain stem by way of the **fasciculus cuneatus.** These tracts synapse in the dorsal medulla in the **nucleus gracilis** and the **nucleus cuneatus,** respectively. Axons then carry impulses to the contralateral side of the medulla and subsequently ascend to the thalamus via the **medial lemniscus.** The specific thalamic region to which these fibers travel is the posteroventral nuclear complex. The thalamic neurons in turn send their axons to the somatosensory cortex of the postcentral gyrus (areas 3, 2, and 1). The thalamic and neocortical components of the somatosensory system were diagramed in Figures 3-9, 3-10, and 3-11.

The functions of the medial lemniscal system have been clarified by the investigation of the effects of damage to the dorsal columns on somatosensory processes. It has been shown that damage to the dorsal columns produces a loss in

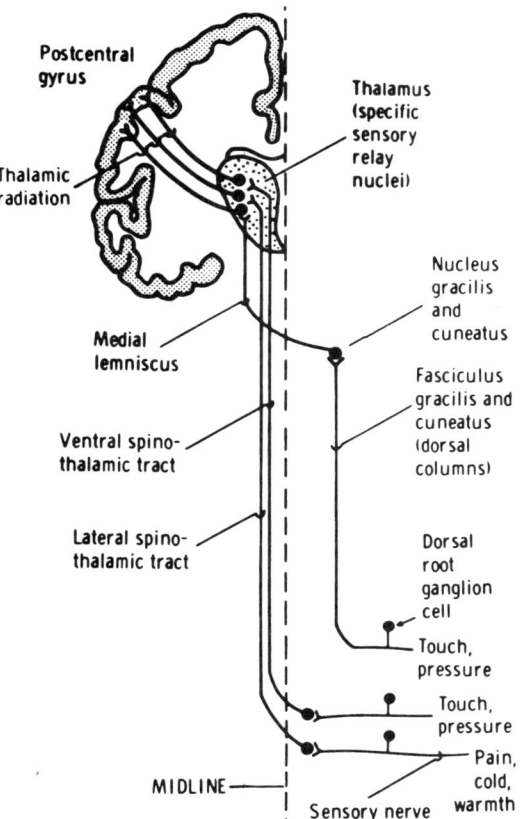

Postcentral
gyrus

Thalamic
radiation

Medial
lemniscus

Ventral spino-
thalamic tract

Lateral spino-
thalamic tract

MIDLINE

Thalamus
(specific
sensory
relay
nuclei)

Nucleus
gracilis
and
cuneatus

Fasciculus
gracilis and
cuneatus
(dorsal
columns)

Dorsal
root
ganglion
cell

Touch,
pressure

Touch,
pressure

Pain,
cold,
warmth

Sensory nerve

Figure 5-18
*The touch, pressure,
pain, and
temperature
pathways. From*
Review of Medical
Physiology *(7th
ed.), by W. F.
Ganong. Copyright
1975 by Lange
Medical
Publications.
Reprinted by
permission.*

certain aspects of fine touch sensitivity, in the ability to distinguish where the skin has been touched, in the ability to perceive vibration, and in the ability to know the position of the limbs without looking (Brown, 1975).

The Spinothalamic System. Fibers of the spinothalamic system travel over two fiber tracts: the ventral and the lateral **spinothalamic tracts.** Upon entering the spinal cord, fibers that are to compose both of these tracts cross to the contralateral side of the cord, where they synapse with second-order neurons. These second-order neurons project to the thalamus, where they synapse in the posteroventral nuclear complex. As was described earlier, this thalamic relay in turn sends projections to the somato-sensory cortex on the postcentral gyrus. The ventral spinothalamic and lateral spinothalamic tracts are distinct in function, in terms of the types of somatosensory information that they convey to the cortex. Analysis of the effects of damage to these two tracts has shown that the lateral spinothalamic tract conducts information regarding pain and temperature (Brown, 1975) and that the ventral spinothalamic tract conveys gross sensations of touch and pressure (Ganong, 1975).

Cortical Representation of the Somatosensory System. The arrangement of the thalamic radiations to the postcentral gyrus is such that the parts of the body are represented in order along the postcentral gyrus, with the legs at the top and the head at the bottom of this gyrus. This arrangement is shown in the *sensory homunculus* pictured in Figure 5-19. Those areas of the human body that have the greatest sensitivity have the largest representation in the cortex. For example, the cortical areas for sensations from the trunk and back are small, while large areas are devoted to the hands and parts of the mouth concerned with speech. Since the somatosensory fibers cross over to the contralateral side of the nervous system prior to reaching the cortex, the somatosensory cortex on the right side of the brain receives sensations originating from the left side of the body.

Figure 5-19
A sensory homunculus, drawn on a coronal section through the postcentral gyrus. From The Cerebral Cortex of Man, *by W. Penfield and T. Rasmussen. Copyright © 1950 by the Macmillan Co. Reprinted by permission.*

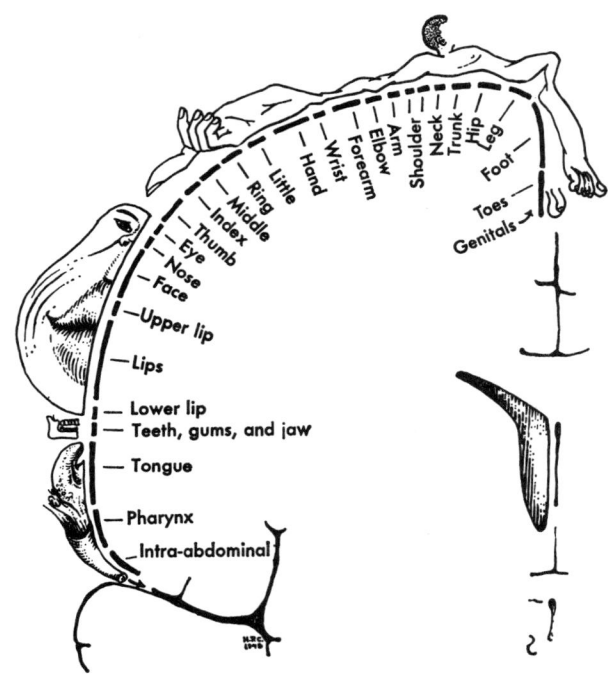

Chapter Summary and Conclusions

We are continually being bombarded by stimuli in our environment. For us to respond adaptively to this stimulus barrage, the information must be transmitted to the central nervous system for processing. The transmission of information to the central nervous system is the function of our sensory systems. In this chapter, we examined the performance of these functions, from the receptor level to the neocortex, by the visual, auditory, olfactory, taste, and somatosensory systems.

The receptors of the visual system are the rods and the cones. The rods function primarily at low levels of illumination but are insensitive to fine detail and color. In contrast, the cones are sensitive to fine detail and color but cannot function at low levels of illumination. Visual cortical neurons, which are highly organized into receptive fields, are crucially involved in distinguishing the shape of objects in the visual field.

The human ear is a marvelously engineered system for bringing sound from the environment to the receptor hair cells of the inner ear. Distortion of the hair cells by uneven movements of the basilar and tectorial membranes, in response to vibrations of the fluid medium of the inner ear, evokes neural impulses in the auditory pathway.

Auditory stimuli vary along two dimensions: amplitude and frequency. Theories regarding how these two qualities are coded by the auditory system were considered. It was concluded that, at low frequencies (up to 5000 Hz), pitch is coded according to the number of impulses in the auditory system. At higher frequencies, pitch is coded first by the place of vibration along the basilar membrane and later by the locus of activation in the auditory pathway. Loudness is coded by the rate of discharge of fibers in the auditory system and by the total number of fibers activated. Cortical involvement is not required for the perception of either loudness or pitch, but both the ability to discriminate patterns of auditory stimuli and the ability to localize a sound require an intact auditory cortex.

The chemical senses of taste and olfaction were considered together because of the similarity of their transduction processes (both senses respond only to molecules of substances that are in a dissolved state) and because both senses are intimately concerned with eating. Flavor is to a large extent determined by a combination of taste and smell. The basic tastes and smells were described, as were possible explanations regarding how these experiences are received and coded by the chemical sensory systems.

The last sensory system described was the somatosensory system. *Somesthesis* refers to the sensations of pain, touch or pressure, cold, and warmth. The operations of this system were illustrated through the example of the somesthetic senses of the skin. The few known relationships between cutaneous sensations and the various types of cutaneous somesthetic receptors, which have emerged from research conducted over the past 100 years, were summarized. As with the other sensory systems, the neural pathways mediating the somatosensory system were described. It was shown that the entire surface of the body is represented on the somatosensory cortex of the postcentral gyrus.

6
Movement

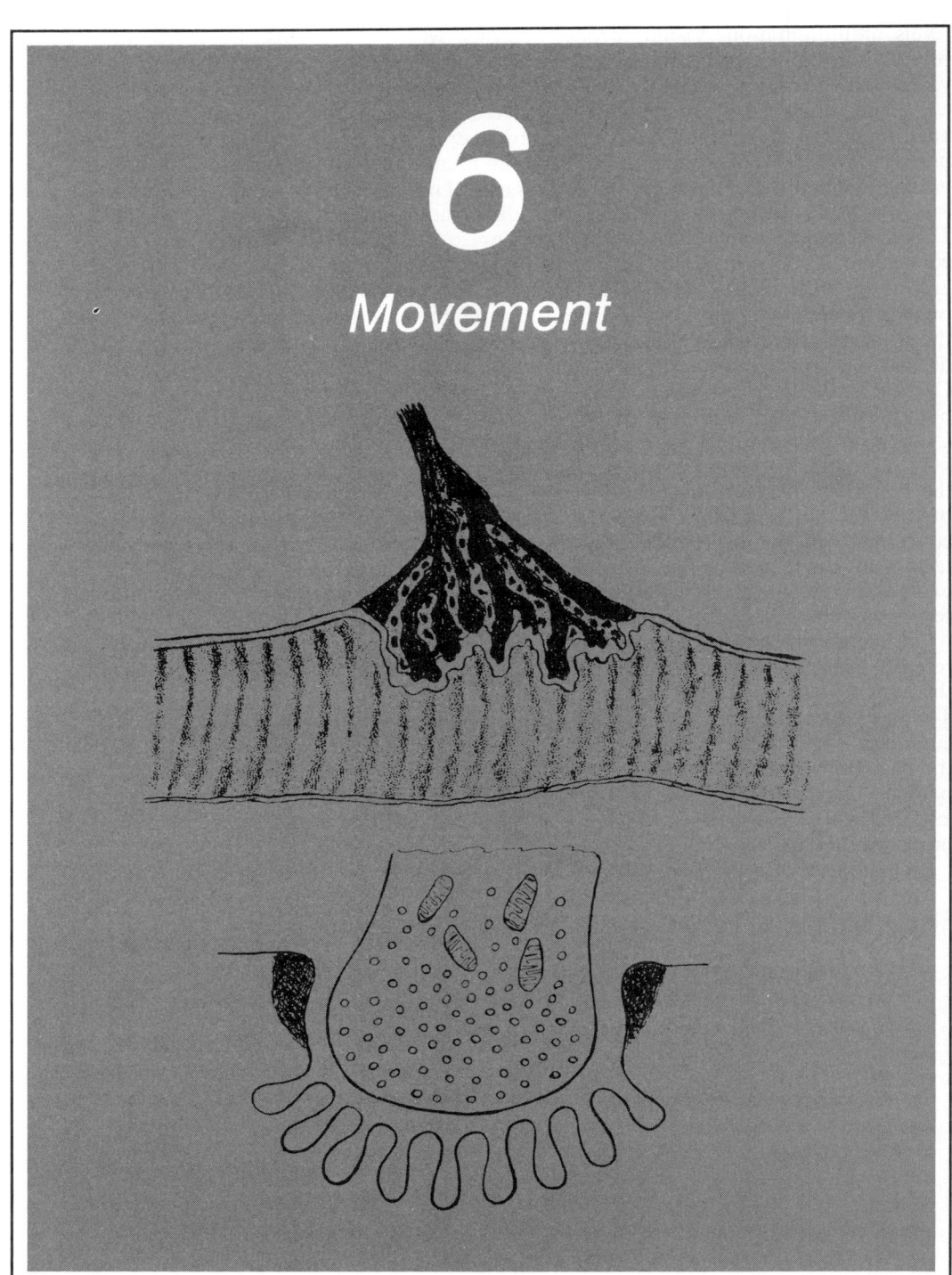

In Chapter 5, we examined the neural mechanisms involved in the reception and processing of stimuli. In this chapter, I'll discuss neural mediation of the output side of behavior—that is, movement. We will consider the various levels of control exerted over movement by the nervous system, and some examples of pathological conditions that interfere with normal, smooth execution of movement patterns will be detailed.

Movement is the product of muscle activity—specifically, activity of the **skeletal** or *striated* **muscles.** There are actually three kinds of muscle tissue in the body, each with a different structure. In addition to the skeletal musculature, which controls movements and postural reflexes, there are **smooth** and **cardiac muscles.** The smooth muscles are primarily involved in regulating visceral activity, and cardiac muscle makes up the bulk of the heart. Skeletal muscle is sometimes called *voluntary muscle* because it regulates movement, while smooth and cardiac muscle functions are referred to as *involuntary.* This is basically a valid distinction, but there are some exceptions. For example, certain postural adjustments occur automatically and thus do not require conscious mediation, but they are under the control of skeletal muscles. Another exception to this general rule is bladder control. Bladder control is governed by smooth muscles, yet it is under voluntary control. Finally, evidence (for example, Miller, 1969) indicates that heart rate can, under certain conditions, be voluntarily controlled to some extent, and heart rate is mediated by cardiac muscle.

The Reflex Arc

The simplest mechanism regulating the expression of movement is the **reflex arc,** an example of which is diagramed in Figure 6-1. Suppose that you touch your hand to a very hot surface. This painful stimulus will normally elicit the reflex withdrawal of your hand. The stimulus will activate axons that travel toward the spinal cord and synapse in the dorsal-horn gray matter of the spinal cord. From this point, a second group of neurons (**interneurons,** or *internuncial neurons*) conducts the nerve impulses to the ventral horn of the spinal cord, where they synapse with relatively large neurons called *ventral-horn cells* or **alpha motor neurons.** The axons of the alpha motor neurons leave the spinal cord and travel directly to the skeletal muscles of the arms. Activation of these muscles yields the withdrawal reflex. An even simpler example of a reflex movement is the knee-jerk reflex, which we're all familiar with. The knee-jerk reflex is elicited by tapping the tendon of the quadriceps femoris muscle just below the kneecap. In this instance,

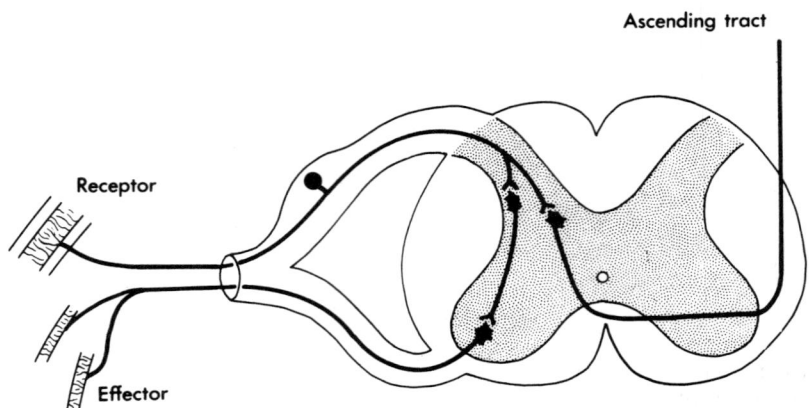

Figure 6-1
How impulses from
a cutaneous receptor
reach an effector
(skeletal
muscle)—by a
three-neuron arc.
Impulses also reach
the cerebral
hemisphere, by way
of an ascending
tract. From
Fundamentals of
Neurology *(5th*
ed.), by E. Gardner.
Copyright 1968 by
W. B. Saunders
Company.
Reprinted by
permission.

the reflex is mediated without interneurons. The receptor neurons synapse directly with the motor neurons in the ventral gray matter of the spinal cord.

Reflexes represent the simplest form of movement, and they do not require the integrity of the brain for their occurrence. Reflexes will occur after the spinal cord has been transected above the level at which the reflex is mediated. In spite of their apparent simplicity, however, reflex actions require some sophisticated processes for their execution (Gardner, 1968). For example, if a knee jerk, which involves activation of the extensor muscles, is to occur, the opposing muscles (flexors) must relax. The production of this relaxation is a function of the gray matter of the spinal cord. The stimulus eliciting the knee jerk results in impulses being conducted from the receptors to the motor neurons that activate the extensor muscles to yield the reflex. However, branches from the dorsal-root receptor fibers also reach *inhibitory interneurons* (Figure 6-2), whose axons in turn reach the motor cells supplying the flexor muscles. The flexor muscles are thereby relaxed or inhibited. This process is referred to as **reciprocal inhibition** or *Sherrington's inhibition.*

The Neuromuscular Junction

As indicated, axons of the ventral-horn cells, or alpha motor neurons, conduct impulses from the spinal cord directly to the skeletal muscles. Each axon entering a muscle divides into a number of branches. Each of these branches ends on the surface of a single muscle fiber, forming a specialized ending called the *motor end plate* or **neuromuscular junction.** At the tips of the branches in the neuromuscular junction are **sole feet.** Figure 6-3 shows both the neuromuscular junction and the junction between a sole foot and a muscle-fiber membrane. This junctional region is called a **neuromuscular synapse** and has properties similar to those exhibited by excitatory synapses in the central nervous system.

The transmission of impulses from the motor neuron to the muscle is similar to the transmission of impulses across excitatory synapses in the central nervous system. The electrical impulse arriving at the end of the motor neuron yields the release of the transmitter acetylcholine, which is stored in vesicles contained in the

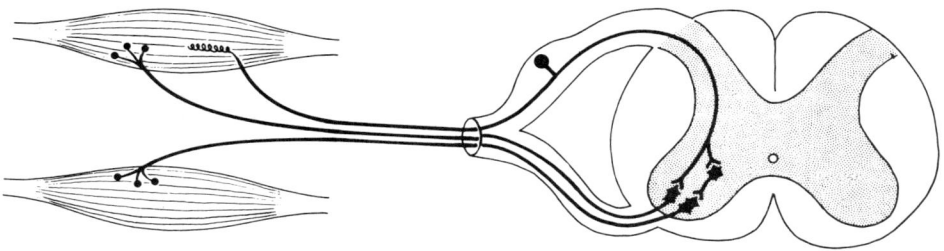

Figure 6-2
How the knee-jerk reflex (a two-neuron reflex) works. The extensor muscles (the upper muscle in the diagram) must be activated and the opposing flexor muscles (the lower muscle in the diagram) must be relaxed. To produce the flexor relaxation, a collateral from the dorsal-root receptor fiber synapses with an inhibitory interneuron. The axon from the interneuron in turn reaches motor fibers of the flexor muscle and signals them to relax—a process called reciprocal inhibition. *From* Fundamentals of Neurology *(5th ed.), by E. Gardner. Copyright 1968 by W. B. Saunders Company. Reprinted by permission.*

sole feet. The acetylcholine increases the permeability of the underlying membrane of the muscle fiber to sodium ions. This results in a partial depolarization of the muscle fiber, which may be recorded as an **end-plate potential.** The end-plate potential has properties similar to those of an excitatory postsynaptic potential. If the end-plate potential attains the threshold of about 40–50 mv depolarization, an action potential is generated. The muscle action potential, in turn, initiates muscular contraction. The action of the acetylcholine on the postsynaptic muscle fiber is short-lived because of the presence of the enzyme acetylcholinesterase, which inactivates the transmitter.

A disease known as **myasthenia gravis,** which occurs in humans, is presumably the result either of the inability of the sole feet to secrete or produce adequate amounts of acetylcholine or of a loss of sensitivity to acetylcholine on the part of the postsynaptic membrane. In this disorder, when the muscles are used they become weak and, for all intents, paralyzed (Gardner, 1968; Guyton, 1971). After a period of rest, activity can be resumed, but weakness will again set in. If the disease is severe enough, the patient will die of paralysis—in particular, paralysis of the respiratory muscles. However, drug therapy, involving medications that inactivate acetylcholinesterase and thereby allow a prolongation of the effects of acetylcholine, can provide some relief from these symptoms.

The Motor Unit

The axon of a single motor neuron supplies a number of skeletal-muscle fibers. The motor neuron and the muscle fibers supplied by it are collectively called a **motor unit.** The number of muscle fibers per motor unit depends upon the precision of movement mediated by that particular muscle. A muscle with many motor units for a given number of muscle fibers is capable of performing more precise movements than is a muscle with fewer motor units for the same number of muscle fibers. For example, the muscles of the thumb have a large number of small motor units, and the thumb is thereby allowed many precise and discrete movements. In contrast, some of the muscles involved in postural reflexes have a large number of muscle fibers in each motor unit, and relatively few motor units control the muscles' activity. We will next examine how different levels of the brain control or modify the activity of motor units to produce movements, which constitute the behavior of organisms.

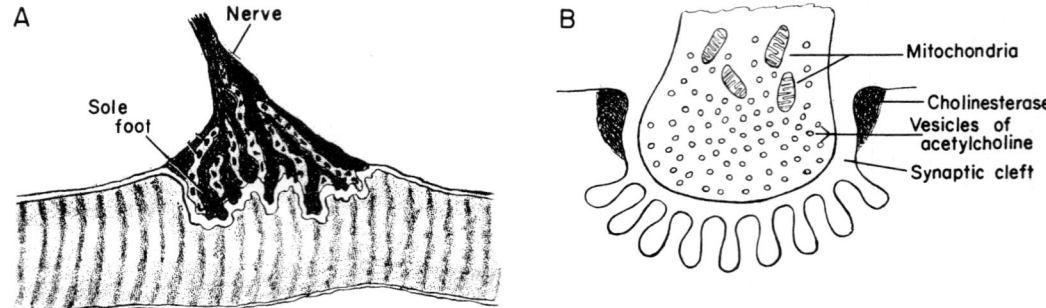

Figure 6-3
(A) The
neuromuscular
junction. (B) A
neuromuscular
synapse. Adapted
from Textbook of
Medical Physiology
(4th ed.), by A. C.
Guyton. Copyright
1971 by W. B.
Saunders Company.
Reprinted by
permission.

Voluntary Movement

As we all know, animals not only respond reflexively to environmental stimuli but also initiate voluntary movements. Although the spinal cord and alpha motor neurons are involved in voluntary movements, these responses, which form the basis of behavior, are initiated and mediated by regions in the brain. The levels of control above the spinal cord include the reticular formation of the brain stem, the cerebellum, the basal ganglia, and the cerebral cortex. For convenience, and because of differences in the type of motor control exerted, neural systems controlling complex, voluntary movements are classified as belonging to either the **pyramidal motor system** or the **extrapyramidal motor system.** In the discussion below, we will examine the anatomical components of these systems, the types of influences they exert over movement, and disorders of movement resulting from injury or pathological destructions of these regions.

The Pyramidal Motor System

The pyramidal system controls precise voluntary movements, such as those involved in writing, using a typewriter, playing a piano, fielding a baseball, and talking. Most of the cell bodies in the pyramidal system originate in the precentral gyrus, or area 4, of the frontal lobe (see Figure 6-4). Axons leave this primary motor

Figure 6-4
The approximate
locations of the
motor areas on the
lateral surface of the
frontal lobe. From
Fundamentals of
Neurology (5th
ed.), by E. Gardner.
Copyright 1968 by
W. B. Saunders
Company.
Reprinted by
permission.

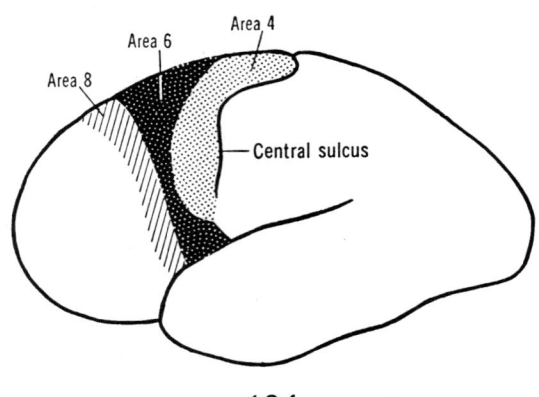

cortex and descend directly to the spinal cord, where they synapse either directly with alpha motor neurons or, as in the majority of cases, with interneurons that then synapse with alpha motor neurons. In humans, approximately 90% of the descending fibers synapse with interneurons (Ganong, 1975). As you'll remember, the alpha motor neurons are the cells whose axons control the output or efferent side of the reflex arc by conducting impulses to muscle fibers. Since the alpha motor neurons ultimately mediate all movements, whether reflexive or voluntary, they are often called the *final common pathway.*

When the descending fibers of the pyramidal system reach the level of the medulla in the hindbrain via the pyramidal tract, approximately 80% of them cross the midline in the **pyramidal decussation** to form the **lateral corticospinal tract.** The remaining 20% of the fibers descend as the **anterior corticospinal tract,** and they decussate, or cross, the midline just prior to their termination (Ganong, 1975). The end result is that the control of limb musculature is largely contralateral; that is, the right cerebral cortex controls limb movements on the left side of the body, and the left cerebral cortex controls limb movements on the right side. The decussations of the corticospinal tracts of the pyramidal motor system are shown in Figure 6-5.

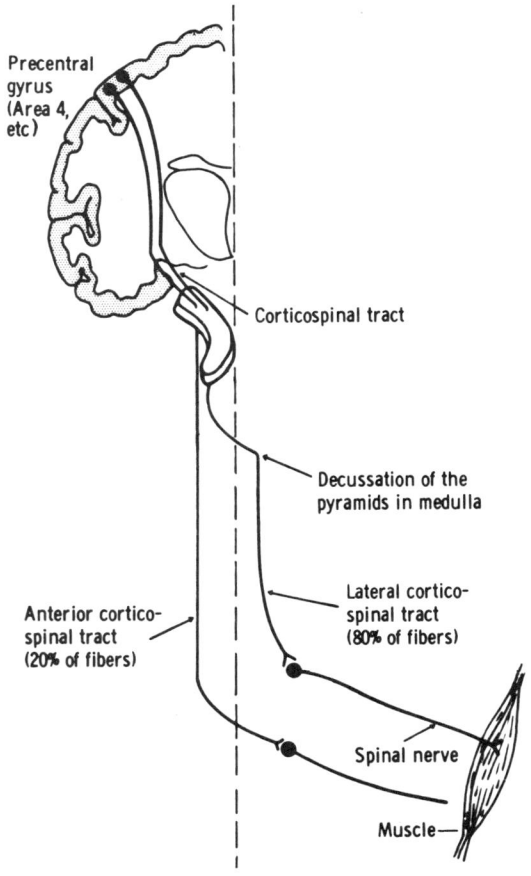

Precentral gyrus (Area 4, etc)

Corticospinal tract

Decussation of the pyramids in medulla

Anterior cortico-spinal tract (20% of fibers)

Lateral cortico-spinal tract (80% of fibers)

Spinal nerve

Muscle

Figure 6-5
The corticospinal tracts of the pyramidal motor system. Adapted from Review of Medical Physiology *(7th ed.), by W. F. Ganong. Copyright 1975 by Lange Medical Publications. Reprinted by permission.*

Organization of the Precentral Gyrus. Experiments with human patients undergoing brain surgery have contributed a good deal to our understanding of the organization of the precentral gyrus. By means of electrical stimulation, it has been possible to map out how the body regions are represented on the precentral gyrus. Such a map results in a *motor homunculus,* as shown in Figure 6-6. There are two noteworthy things about this map. First, the representation of movements is inverted, such that the feet are controlled by neurons located at the top of this gyrus and the face by neurons at the bottom. A second notable aspect of the homunculus is that the cortical representation of each body part is proportional in area to the degree of motor control that we have over that body part; that is, it is proportionate in size to the relative skill or precision with which a body part is used in voluntary movement. For example, the muscles involved in speech and in hand movements are particularly well represented in the precentral gyrus. In contrast, a body part such as the back, which is subject to little discrete motor control, has a relatively small area devoted to it.

Figure 6-6
The motor homunculus superimposed on a section of the precentral gyrus. The broken lines represent the relative amounts of cortical tissue controlling the muscles of parts of the body. Surrounding the section is a caricature of the body in the same relative proportions. From The Cerebral Cortex of Man, *by W. Penfield and T. Rasmussen. Copyright © 1950 by the Macmillan Co. Reprinted by permission.*

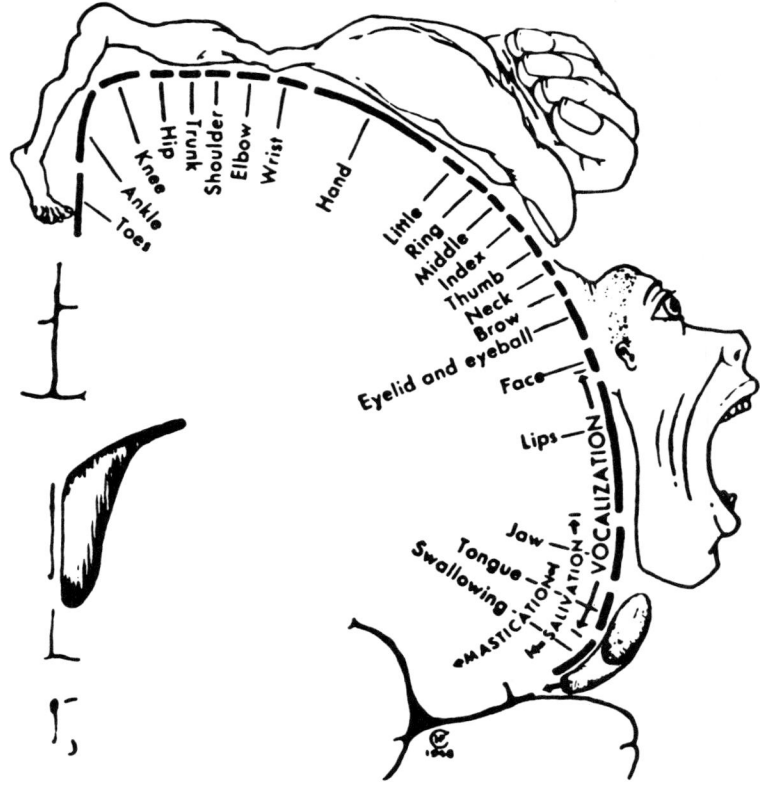

The characteristics of the motor movements that result from electrical stimulation of the precentral gyrus depend upon the intensity and duration of the stimulating current. If a stimulus barely above threshold is applied for a short duration, a single muscle contraction may result. If, on the other hand, an intense stimulus of long duration is applied to the motor cortex, an organized movement, such as an arm or finger flexion, may occur. Coordinated movements occur when long-duration, intense stimulating currents are applied, because a wider area of the cortex is activated. Gardner (1968) indicates that the type of movement elicited by electrical stimulation depends not only on the intensity and duration of the electrical stimulus but also on the frequency or pulses per second of the current. Contraction may occur in one group of muscles during stimulation at one frequency, while another frequency may yield contractions in a different muscle group. Finally, the effects of stimulating the precentral gyrus also depend upon posture. If a limb is placed in a certain position, the effects of stimulation may be different from those that would occur if that same limb were situated in another position. However, regardless of the initial position of the limb, it always ends up in the same final position (Guyton, 1971).

Supplementary Motor Area. The supplementary motor area is located on the medial wall of the cerebral hemispheres and superior to the cingulate gyrus. It lies just anterior to the precentral gyrus. The supplementary motor area apparently has a separate motor homunculus representing the muscles of the body. Stimulation of the supplementary motor area produces movements that are qualitatively different from those elicited by stimulation of the precentral gyrus. Movements mediated by the supplementary area are slower in execution and resemble postural adjustments. For example, when stimulation is applied to this region, a limb will move relatively slowly, and, after the stimulation is ended, it will maintain its final position for a number of seconds. Further, in many instances the movements produced will be bilateral rather than occurring only on the side contralateral to the one stimulated, as results from precentral-gyrus stimulation.

Premotor Area (Area 6). As you can see in Figure 6-4, Brodmann's area 6, which has traditionally been called the *premotor cortex* or **premotor area,** is located just anterior to the precentral gyrus (area 4). Stimulation of the premotor area produces movements that are of a different nature from those elicited by precentral-gyrus stimulation. Stimulation in area 6 produces gross movements involving many muscles, in contrast to the more discrete movements produced by stimulation of the primary motor cortex of area 4. Stimulation of area 6 can produce such movements as gross rotation of the eyes, head, and trunk to the side opposite to their resting position. The fact that movements resulting from stimulation of this region seem more coordinated than those arising from other areas does not imply that the premotor cortex is a center for higher or highly coordinated movements. Rather, these findings simply indicate that the musculature represented in this region is different from that represented on the precentral gyrus.

Frontal Eye Field (Area 8). Referring back to Figure 6-4 again, you can see that area 8 is located anterior to area 6. Stimulation of this area produces eye movements, which is why this region is called the **frontal eye field.** The most common response to stimulation of this region is movement of the eyes in the same direction (**conjugate eye movements**), but pupillary dilation and **nystagmus** (rapid side-to-side movements of the eyeballs) have also been observed. It has been suggested that this portion of the cortex is concerned with the control and coordination of eye movements. That such a large area of cortex should be concerned with such a specialized function is reasonable in light of the importance of our visual system in our processing of information from our environment.

The available evidence indicates that the pyramidal system, which provides a direct path from the cerebral cortex to the spinal cord via the pyramidal and corticospinal tracts, is phylogenetically new. Hence, it is most prominent in primates. Its influences appear to be primarily excitatory, and it controls the execution of skilled movements. It gets its name from the fact that its fiber tracts are shaped like pyramids in the lower brain stem. Other components of movement patterns, such as the relaxation of opposing muscles and postural adjustments associated with the performance of skilled movements, are coordinated by the extrapyramidal system. The extrapyramidal system is made up of fibers that mediate movement but that reach the spinal cord via routes other than the pyramidal and corticospinal tracts. Several levels of extrapyramidal control will be discussed below.

The Extrapyramidal Motor System

As you've seen, the pyramidal motor system is concerned with the initiation of skilled, precise, voluntary movements. The extrapyramidal motor system is involved in the process of facilitating or "smoothing out" patterns of movement that are initiated by the pyramidal system. Destruction of portions of the extrapyramidal system results in a pattern of jerky, uncoordinated movements, as will be detailed below. There are several levels of control or integration in the extrapyramidal system: (a) cortical neurons, which are diffusely organized and lack functionally distinct areas, (b) the basal ganglia, (c) the cerebellum, and (d) the reticular formation of the brain stem. We will examine the functions of the subcortical regions of the extrapyramidal system next.

Reticular Formation. As shown in Figure 6-7, the reticular formation extends from the top of the spinal cord into the hypothalamus and even upward through the central portion of the thalamus. In the anatomy chapter, I indicated that there are two aspects of reticular-formation influence. First, the ascending reticular activating system is involved in behavioral arousal, a function that will be considered in Chapter 7. The second aspect of reticular-formation activity concerns its functions as part of the extrapyramidal motor system. By stimulating different regions of the reticular formation, it is possible to either facilitate or inhibit movement.

With regard to its influence over motor functions, most of the reticular formation is excitatory. This is especially true for the pontile (located in the pons), mesencephalic, and diencephalic portions of the reticular formation as well as for the lateral regions of the reticular formation in the medulla. Collectively, these excitatory regions of the reticular formation are referred to as the **bulboreticular facilitatory area.** Depending upon the parameters and location of stimulation, activation of the bulboreticular facilitatory area produces an increase in muscle tone either throughout the body or in a specific area (Guyton, 1971). There is also a small segment of the reticular formation that exerts inhibitory influences over motor functions. Located in the ventromedial portion of the medulla, this division of the reticular formation is called the **bulboreticular inhibitory area.** Stimulation of this region results in decreased muscle tone throughout the body (Guyton, 1971).

The bulboreticular facilitatory area is intrinsically excitable. This means that, if this region is not inhibited by signals arising from other portions of the brain, it tends to send continuous nerve impulses to skeletal muscles located throughout the body. However, in the normal organism this excitatory activity is regulated or dampened by

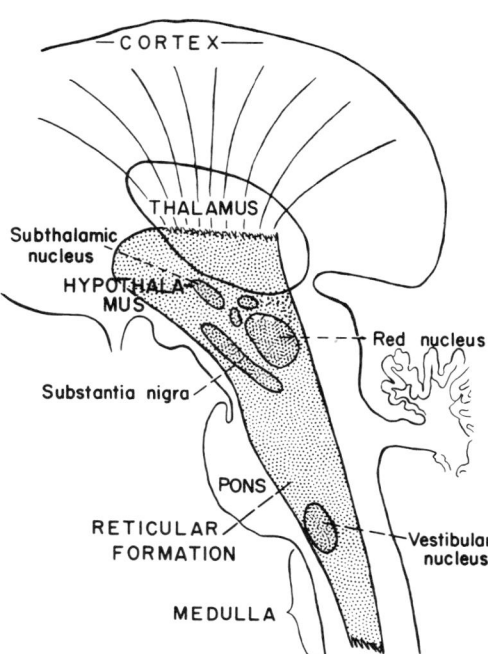

Figure 6-7
The reticular formation and associated nuclei. Adapted from Textbook of Medical Physiology *(4th ed.), by A. C. Guyton. Copyright 1971 by W. B. Saunders Company. Reprinted by permission.*

inhibitory signals that arrive from the basal ganglia and the cortex. These influences prevent the bulboreticular facilitatory area from becoming overactive (Guyton, 1971).

Transection of an animal's brain between the superior and inferior colliculi of the midbrain is the classic *decerebrate preparation.* This surgical procedure, diagramed in Figure 6-8, interrupts the normal inhibitory influences over the reticular facilitatory area by the basal ganglia and cortex. This interruption allows the

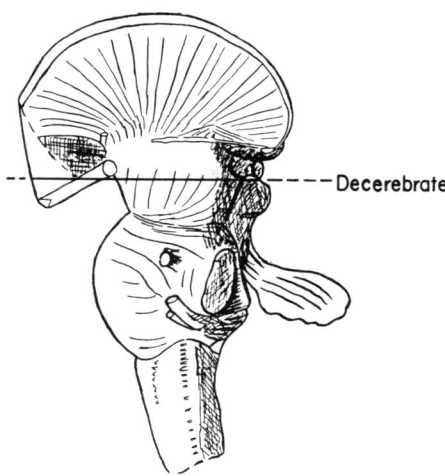

Figure 6-8
Where the brain is transected in decerebrate surgery. Adapted from Textbook of Medical Physiology *(4th ed.), by A. C. Guyton. Copyright 1971 by W. B. Saunders Company. Reprinted by permission.*

bulboreticular facilitatory area to become very active. Extensive excitatory impulses are then directed toward the skeletal musculature, and a condition of extreme muscle rigidity results. This syndrome is called **decerebrate rigidity.** The extensor muscles, especially, are maintained in a state of strong tonic contraction (Guyton, 1971). In contrast, if the brain stem is cut at a level slightly below the vestibular nucleus (see Figure 6-7), the descending influences of the bulboreticular facilitatory area are blocked, and, as a result, almost all of the skeletal musculature becomes totally flaccid.

The nature of the reticular influences that have been described thus far suggests that the reticular formation causes a gross increase or decrease in muscle tone throughout the body. Such is not necessarily the case, because electrical stimulation of the reticular formation can also produce specific facilitation or inhibition of ongoing movement. Further, stimulation of discrete loci in the reticular formation can at times produce discrete muscle contraction or inhibition of contraction in specific body parts. These findings indicate that there are two broad categories of reticular-formation influences over motor functions. First, the reticular formation appears to mediate diffuse alterations in muscle tone throughout the body. Second, the reticular formation is capable of controlling specific motor responses.

Basal Ganglia. In Chapter 3, when I discussed the anatomy of the brain, I indicated that the principal structures of the basal ganglia are the caudate nucleus, the putamen, and the globus pallidus. I pointed out that the amygdala is also often classified as belonging to the basal ganglia because it merges with the tail of the caudate nucleus. However, functionally speaking, the amygdala should not be classified as one of the basal ganglia, since the amygdala is not concerned directly with motor functions. The basal ganglia were shown from several views in Figure 3-15.

Certain brain-stem nuclei, which lie outside of the boundaries of the primary structures of the basal ganglia, appear to operate in conjunction with the basal ganglia in mediating motor functions. For this reason, they are considered part of the basal-ganglia system for motor control. These nuclei include the **lateral ventral nucleus of the thalamus** (Figure 3-10), the **subthalamus,** the **substantia nigra,** and the **red nucleus** (Figure 6-7).

The interconnections of the basal ganglia are very complex. Some important features of these pathways are the following (Jung & Hassler, 1960). There is a feedback loop that begins by projecting from the motor cortex to the caudate nucleus and putamen. From here, fibers pass to the globus pallidus. From the globus pallidus, numerous fibers course to the lateral ventral nucleus of the thalamus. Finally, from this thalamic nucleus, connections travel back to the motor cortex. This circular pathway thus provides a feedback loop connecting the motor cortex, the basal ganglia, and the thalamus. In addition to projecting to the thalamus, the globus pallidus also sends fibers to the subthalamus, red nucleus, substantia nigra, and midbrain reticular formation.

As will be seen later in this chapter, the motor cortex also sends signals to the pons, which sends signals to the cerebellum. In turn, impulses are transmitted from the cerebellum back to the motor cortex by way of the lateral ventral nucleus of the thalamus. As you saw, impulses from the basal ganglia are also transmitted to the motor cortex via this thalamic nucleus. This circuit thereby allows for an integration of the basal-ganglia and cerebellar feedback signals.

Functions of the basal ganglia. In lower species such as birds and reptiles, which have a poorly developed or essentially absent motor cortex, the basal ganglia are highly developed and serve the functions normally carried out by the cerebral cortex, including control of voluntary movement. However, in mammalian species, the basal ganglia appear to be primarily involved in the production of gross, stereotyped movements, such as walking, that we normally perform subconsciously. While it is wrong to assign a unitary function to the basal ganglia, it does appear that one general function of this neural region is to inhibit muscle tone. This is accomplished by the transmission of inhibitory signals to the bulboreticular facilitatory area and excitatory impulses to the bulboreticular inhibitory area (Guyton, 1971). As indicated, if basal-ganglia influences are blocked by transection of the brain at the collicular level, the excitatory region of the reticular formation becomes overactive and the inhibitory region becomes underactive. This produces muscular rigidity, which is characteristic of the decerebrate preparation.

Information regarding more specific functions of the basal ganglia has come from experiments in which these nuclear complexes were either electrically stimulated or destroyed. The caudate nucleus and putamen function together to regulate gross, intentional movements that we normally perform subconsciously. They accomplish this by inhibiting movements that are initiated by the motor cortex. Stimulation of the caudate nucleus in an awake, unrestrained animal will often inhibit ongoing motor activity. In contrast, bilateral destruction of this area in cats will produce a motor pattern called **obstinate progression.** This disorder also follows subthalamic lesions. In obstinate progression, the animal can walk in an almost completely normal fashion. However, if a barrier is placed in its path, the cat will simply butt its head against it and try to keep walking.

It is thought that the purpose of the globus pallidus is to produce background muscle tone for voluntary movements. This would be true for movements initiated in either the motor cortex or the striate body. Electrical stimulation of the globus pallidus, yielding an increase in muscle tone, will often cause a cessation of movement. The animal will hold the position in which it found itself at the time stimulation began. It will remain in this position until the stimulation ends. It is thought that this function may enable us to hold our limbs still in a certain position while we perform delicate skills with our hands (Guyton, 1971).

Diseases of the basal ganglia. A good deal of our knowledge about the functions of the basal ganglia has come from the study of human clinical cases in which the basal ganglia have been destroyed through disease processes. The resulting movement aberrations have been examined during the disease process, and the loci of the basal-ganglia lesions have been determined through histological study of the brains of these patients after death. Two general types of motor disorders occur as a result of basal-ganglia pathology in humans: **hyperkinetic** and **hypokinetic.** The hyperkinetic syndromes, which involve excessive and abnormal movement, include *chorea, athetosis,* and *ballism. Parkinson's disease* (*paralysis agitans*) has both hyperkinetic and hypokinetic components. The hypokinesis involves difficulty in initiating voluntary movements and associated movements—a loss of normal, unconscious movements such as swinging the arms when walking (Ganong, 1975). A more detailed description of these syndromes than is possible here is provided by Guyton (1971) and Ganong (1975).

Chorea is correlated with degeneration of the striate body. It is characterized by continuous random, uncontrolled "dancing" movements caused by contractions of different muscle groups throughout the body. Normal progression of movements cannot occur.

In the disease *athetosis,* continuous slow writhing movements occur in the peripheral parts of one or more of the limbs. These rhythmic movements often preclude voluntary movements in the affected limb. The damage in athetosis is usually located in the outer portion of the globus pallidus or in this outer portion plus the putamen.

Ballism is characterized by an uncontrollable succession of intense, flailing, violent movements. This disorder occurs as a result of subthalamic damage, and the violent movements may occur once every few minutes or as frequently as every few seconds. In this disorder, an entire leg might suddenly jerk to full flexion or an arm might suddenly be violently extended. Ballism of the legs or trunk will cause a walking person to fall to the ground. Even when lying in bed, the afflicted individual is tossed violently by these powerful movements. Unfortunately, attempts to perform voluntary movements often elicit ballistic movements in these afflicted individuals.

Parkinson's disease, named after the English physician James Parkinson (1755–1824), who first described it, is probably the best known of the basal-ganglia disorders. It was a common late complication of a type of influenza that was rampant during World War I, and it frequently occurs in patients with cerebral arteriosclerosis. Parkinsonism, also called *paralysis agitans,* almost invariably results from widespread destruction of the substantia nigra and globus pallidus. The disease is characterized by rigid muscles that strongly resist attempts by individuals other than the patient to move them, tremor in these same muscles when they are at rest, difficulty in initiating voluntary movements, and a loss of associated movements. The tremor that is present at rest disappears when voluntary movements are performed. The tremor occurs at a frequency of 4–8 cycles per second and results from contractions of antagonistic muscles. When a person afflicted with Parkinson's disease attempts to perform a discrete voluntary movement with the hands, the normally automatic associated postural adjustments do not occur. Further, the patient has a masklike face, demonstrating almost no variation in expression.

Several treatment regimens have been employed to alleviate the tremor associated with this disorder. Interestingly enough, further destruction of the basal ganglia will often bring about clinical improvement. The most prevalent neurosurgical treatment to relieve the tremor is destruction of the ventrolateral nucleus of the thalamus. This is accomplished by electrical ablation of this nucleus or by injection of alcohol to yield a chemically induced lesion. Drug therapy has now replaced surgery for many patients. When administered in large doses, L-dopa alleviates most of the symptoms of Parkinson's disease in about two-thirds of the sufferers. It is believed that dopamine, which is a derivative of L-dopa and is also the immediate precursor of norepinephrine, is secreted by neurons whose cell bodies are in the substantia nigra and whose projections reach the basal ganglia. These are the areas implicated in Parkinson's disease. Thus, the L-dopa is converted to dopamine in the brain and substitutes for the transmitter substance not secreted by the degenerated neurons. In accord with this view, it has been shown that the dopamine content of the basal ganglia of patients with Parkinson's disease is only about 50% of normal, and peripheral administrations of L-dopa produce an increase in brain dopamine levels (Ganong, 1975).

Cerebellum. The cerebellum is the last portion of the extrapyramidal motor system that we'll consider. As I said in Chapter 3, the cerebellum is a phylogenetically old structure. During the course of evolution, the cerebellum was the first brain region to be specialized for sensory-motor coordination. It functions to coordinate, adjust, and smooth out movements. The cerebellum ultimately receives input from all sensory systems and can influence both reflex and voluntary movements. I'll confine my discussion to its functions in mediating voluntary movements.

The cerebellum is situated on the brain stem in a position just above the medulla and behind the pons (see Figure 6-9). It is attached to the rest of the brain by three pairs of bilateral fiber bundles: the *superior, middle,* and *inferior cerebellar peduncles.* Nerve tracts entering and leaving the cerebellum form the peduncles. Afferent fibers to the cerebellum and efferent fibers leaving the cerebellum provide interconnections with a variety of regions. These include the spinal cord, the reticular formation, the vestibular nucleus (a nucleus in the medulla concerned with balance; see Figure 6-7), and, via the lateral ventral nucleus of the thalamus, the basal ganglia and cerebral cortex.

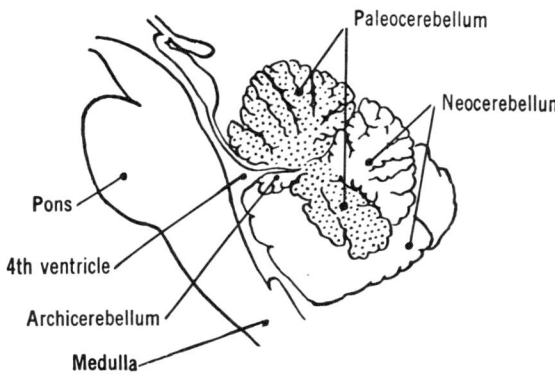

Figure 6-9
A median section of the brain stem and cerebellum. The neocerebellum, which forms the bulk of this organ, is only partially visible in this view. Adapted from Fundamentals of Neurology *(5th ed.), by E. Gardner. Copyright 1968 by W. B. Saunders Company. Reprinted by permission.*

The cerebellar cortex is highly convoluted. In fact, the cerebellar hemispheres are even more extensively folded than the cerebral cortex. While the cerebellum weighs only about 10% as much as the cerebral cortex, its surface area is almost 75% of the area of the cerebral cortex (Ganong, 1975). Like the cerebral cortex, the cerebellum is made up of an outer layer of gray matter (cell bodies), which surrounds the cerebellar tracts, or white matter. The cerebellum can be functionally divided into three regions, as shown in Figure 6-9. The smallest division is the *archicerebellum.* The archicerebellum is involved in the control of postural adjustments and balance. The archicerebellum is probably relatively unimportant in humans, and, for this reason, the human cerebellum is usually subdivided into simply the *paleocerebellum* and the *neocerebellum.* The neocerebellum is so called because it is most extensively developed in primates, especially humans. As was indicated in Chapter 3, the elaboration of the cerebellum has probably resulted from two factors: the assumption of an upright posture in locomotion and the discrete movements made possible by the evolution of the hands—particularly the development of the opposable thumb.

The cerebellum is crucial in the control of voluntary movement, but it only functions to mediate motor activities initiated by other regions of the motor system. The pathways involved in cerebellar control of voluntary movement are illustrated in Figure 6-10. As shown in this figure, when an impulse is transmitted downward from the motor cortex to the spinal cord via the corticospinal tract to initiate voluntary movement, collateral impulses are sent simultaneously into the cerebellum. When the muscles respond to the motor signals, feedback signals are transmitted upward into the cerebellum and arrive at the same locus as did the impulses from the motor cortex. Thus, signals descending from the motor cortex can be integrated with signals arriving from the muscles that expressed the voluntary-movement patterns. After this integration occurs, signals are sent back up to the place in the motor cortex where the signal originated. The return pathway is by way of the lateral ventral nucleus of the thalamus, which also receives inputs from the basal ganglia and thereby provides a station for the integration of basal-ganglia and cerebellar feedback signals (Guyton, 1971).

Figure 6-10
The pathways for cerebellar control and correction of voluntary movements. From Textbook of Medical Physiology *(4th ed.), by A. C. Guyton. Copyright 1971 by W. B. Saunders Company. Reprinted by permission.*

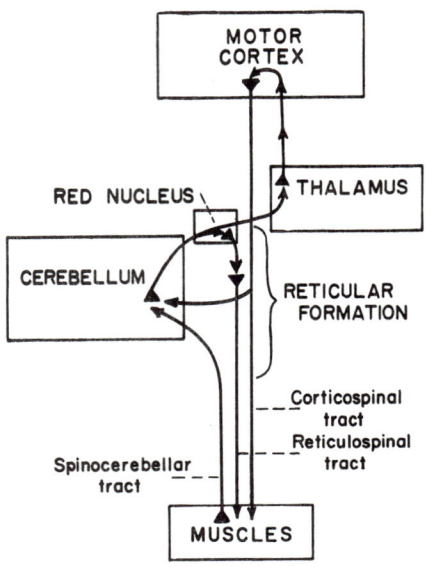

The circuit described provides a complicated feedback circuit that is the basis for the cerebellum's functions in coordinating, adjusting, and smoothing-out movements. The system provides a mechanism by which the cerebellum can compare the orders from the cortex with what is happening in the peripheral musculature. If there is a mismatch—that is, if an error has occurred—then the cerebellum can make corrections. For example, if the cortex has signaled that an arm be moved to a specific place but the arm is being moved so rapidly that it will overshoot its intended destination, then the cerebellum can initiate inhibitory signals to slow down the arm so that it stops in the correct place. To accomplish this operation, the cerebellum must calculate the rate of movement of the limb and the duration of time that will be required to move the limb to the desired location. It must then transmit the proper inhibitory impulses to the muscles that are moving the arm and excitatory impulses to the muscles that will oppose this movement so that the arm reaches the exact intended position (Guyton, 1971). In an individual with cerebellar damage, this braking function is lost. As a result, the person overshoots the intended destination whenever a limb is moved to a new position. When this happens, other brain regions detect this overshoot and initiate movement back in the opposite direction. Again, however, the limb overshoots its intended position, and corrective movements are again initiated. As a result, the limb will oscillate for several passes until it reaches its intended position. This disability is called an **intention tremor** or *action tremor*.

The inability of the individual with cerebellar damage to perform a simple action such as moving the arm to a desired point underscores the severe deficit that such a patient encounters in attempting to engage in a complex-motor-skill sequence. Earlier I noted that the cerebellum is critically involved in motor coordination. This function is particularly important for movement patterns involving a succession or progression of movements. When the cerebellum is damaged, the individual loses his or her ability to progress from one movement to the next in an orderly fashion. The result is that a succeeding movement may begin too early or too late. As a result, complex skill patterns, such as running, writing, or talking, become almost totally uncoordinated.

When this disability affects talking, it is called *dysarthria*. Talking requires a rapid and orderly succession of muscular movements by the larynx and tongue. When the ability to coordinate these movements is lost, speech is almost unintelligible. The verbal output of the person is jumbled. Some syllables are long, some short, some loud, and some soft. This disorder provides one of the most striking illustrations of the importance of the cerebellum in coordinating and smoothing out precise patterns of movement.

Chapter Summary and Conclusions

Movement is the output side of behavior, and in this chapter the various levels of control exerted over movement by the nervous system were considered. The simplest level of movement control is the reflex arc, or spinal reflex. In the reflex arc, the receptor neurons synapse either directly with motor neurons, as in the knee-jerk reflex, or with an interneuron that then connects to the motor neuron. Reflexes are the least complicated form of movement, and they do not require neural integration. In spite of their apparent simplicity, however, reflexes do require some sophisticated processes, and these were discussed in the text.

Animals do not only respond reflexively to their environment; they can also initiate voluntary movements. Most of the chapter was concerned with the various neural mechanisms that mediate voluntary movements. Two systems mediate voluntary movements: the pyramidal system and the extrapyramidal system.

The pyramidal motor system, which originates in the neocortex and sends impulses downward through the corticospinal tracts, controls precise voluntary movements. Examples of behavior patterns under pyramidal control are writing, typing, fielding a baseball, and talking. Most of the pyramidal-tract fibers originate in the precentral gyrus, and it has been shown that this gyrus is organized into sectors that mediate movements performed by specific body regions or muscle groups. Pyramidal-system fibers are also contributed by the supplementary motor area, the premotor cortex, and the frontal eye field. The functions of these three regions were considered.

The extrapyramidal motor system is concerned with smoothing out patterns of movement that are initiated by the pyramidal system. I illustrated the importance of this function by describing several pathological motor syndromes that result from destruction of various regions of the extrapyramidal system. The various levels of control in the pyramidal motor system—the reticular formation of the brain stem, the basal ganglia, and the cerebellum—were discussed.

The mechanisms by which the pyramidal and extrapyramidal systems integrate their activities are very complicated. One must marvel at the precision achieved by these levels of motor control in such complex patterns of movement as speech and writing.

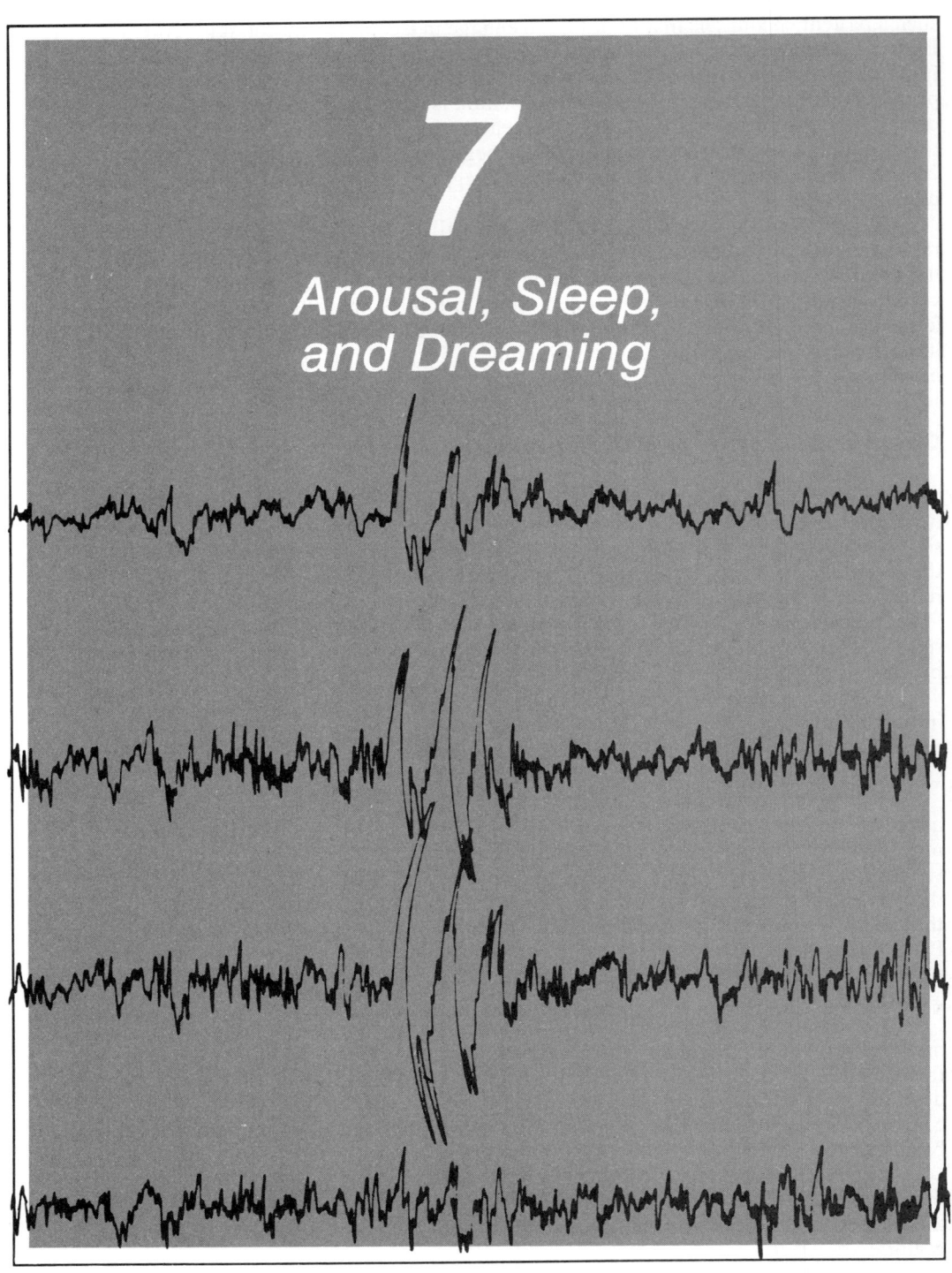

7

Arousal, Sleep, and Dreaming

Each night at an accustomed time people begin to set the stage for sleep with small rituals that lead to bed and darkness. A dusk of consciousness will fall like a curtain on the day and soon, from outside, the body will seem still but for a shallow and even breathing. A twisting, a groan, fluttering of the eyelids and perhaps muffled sounds may occasionally break the stillness, but for 7 or 8 hours the person seems to have departed, gone from the world into a silent internal communion from which he will rise like an amnesic [Luce, 1965, p. 9].*

Most of us spend about one-third of our lives in sleep, and we remember very little of what transpires during those periods. It is surprising how easily we accept this suspension from active life. Further, approximately 20–25% of each night's sleep is spent in active dreaming. Upon awakening the next morning, we rarely remember what we dreamed about. We all think we know what sleep is, and we generally equate this state with unconsciousness. This is a mistake; the brain is not inactive during sleep. Rather, there are changes in its electrical activity that correlate with the depth of sleep and the occurrence of that unique experience we call dreaming. Freud thought that dreaming is essential for psychological health, that it acts as a safety valve to allow so-called civilized humans to express their primitive drives. Was he correct? Information relevant to this question, obtained from experimental studies of dream deprivation, will be described later in this chapter. The general plan of this chapter is as follows. First, the nature of sleep will be described. Next, the stages of sleep that occur during the night will be defined and discussed. Finally, the effects of three types of sleep deprivation will be reviewed.

The Nature of Sleep

Sleep was once thought to be a passive process similar to a state of unconsciousness. The view that sleep is simply a cessation of an active condition of wakefulness has even persisted into modern theories of the nature of sleep (for example, Kleitman, 1963). According to this view, which is called the *reticular hypothesis of sleep* (Lindsley, 1960), sleep is the product of the cessation of ascending impulses in the ascending reticular activating system. Such a view seemed very plausible in view of the findings, reviewed in Chapter 3, that electrical stimulation of this system produced an EEG record characteristic of arousal (Moruzzi & Magoun, 1949) and that midbrain lesions interrupting these ascending influences resulted in a constantly stuperous, or sleeping, animal (Lindsley, Bowden, & Magoun, 1949).

*From *Research on Sleep and Dreams,* by G. G. Luce. National Institute of Mental Health, 1965.

However, a major shortcoming of the passive, or reticular, hypothesis was that it could not account for the experimental findings that sleep could be induced by stimulation of some regions of the brain and that selectively placed lesions could sometimes produce an animal that was constantly awake. A detailed discussion of these findings is presented by Jouvet (1967a). For our purposes, you should know that these findings suggest the existence of an active sleep-inducing, or hypnogenic, system extending from the base of the brain through the thalamus and into the neocortex. It may be that activation in this system contributes to the sleep process by exerting inhibitory influences over behavioral arousal.

These findings have led to the formulation of the *active theory of sleep.* According to this theory, sleep is not a passive process resulting from deactivation of the ascending reticular activating system. Rather, sleep is an active process produced by activation of a hypnogenic system. Proponents of this theory believe that different neural systems control the conditions of wakefulness and sleeping.

Sleep Stages

The study of sleep stages, or within-sleep patterns, has been made possible by the electroencephalogram (EEG). The early history of electroencephalography and the nature of brain waves were outlined in Chapter 4. As was indicated in that chapter, a major breakthrough for the physiological study of the sleep/wakefulness continuum occurred in the 1930s when Loomis and his colleagues discovered that brain waves of cortical origin showed distinct changes with the onset of sleep and continued to change throughout the sleep period. They devised a system for classifying these EEG patterns into five stages that were thought to represent increasing sleep depth.

In this discussion, I'll use a more recently evolved scheme for classifying stages of sleep. This is the Dement-Kleitman system, named after its founders (Dement & Kleitman, 1957a). Their system involves four stages of sleep depth (**Stages 1–4**) and a fifth stage—**Stage REM.** It is during Stage REM that vivid dreaming generally occurs. Dement and Kleitman's research served as a strong impetus for research on within-sleep physiological phenomena. A more detailed description of sleep stages than will be presented here can be found in Luce (1965) and in the Association for the Psychophysiological Study of Sleep scoring manual (Rechtschaffen & Kales, 1968). The APSS sleep-scoring manual is based on the Dement and Kleitman work.

Relaxed Wakefulness

Suppose that you've just jumped into bed. You're relaxed, and you close your eyes to surrender yourself to the state of sleep. The brain waves have shifted from the desynchronized pattern characteristic of an alert person into the rhythmic 8–12 Hz alpha activity. As was indicated in Chapter 4, alpha is the EEG correlate of **relaxed wakefulness.** If during this time you experience a bit of tension, try to solve a mental problem, or open your eyes to look around, the desynchronized pattern will again appear. However, if you allow yourself to drift into sleep, the alpha activity will gradually diminish also, and quite possibly you will experience dreamlike fragments as you hover on the border of sleep. If you succumb to sleep, you enter Stage 1. The EEG correlates of the various sleep stages are shown in Figure 7-1.

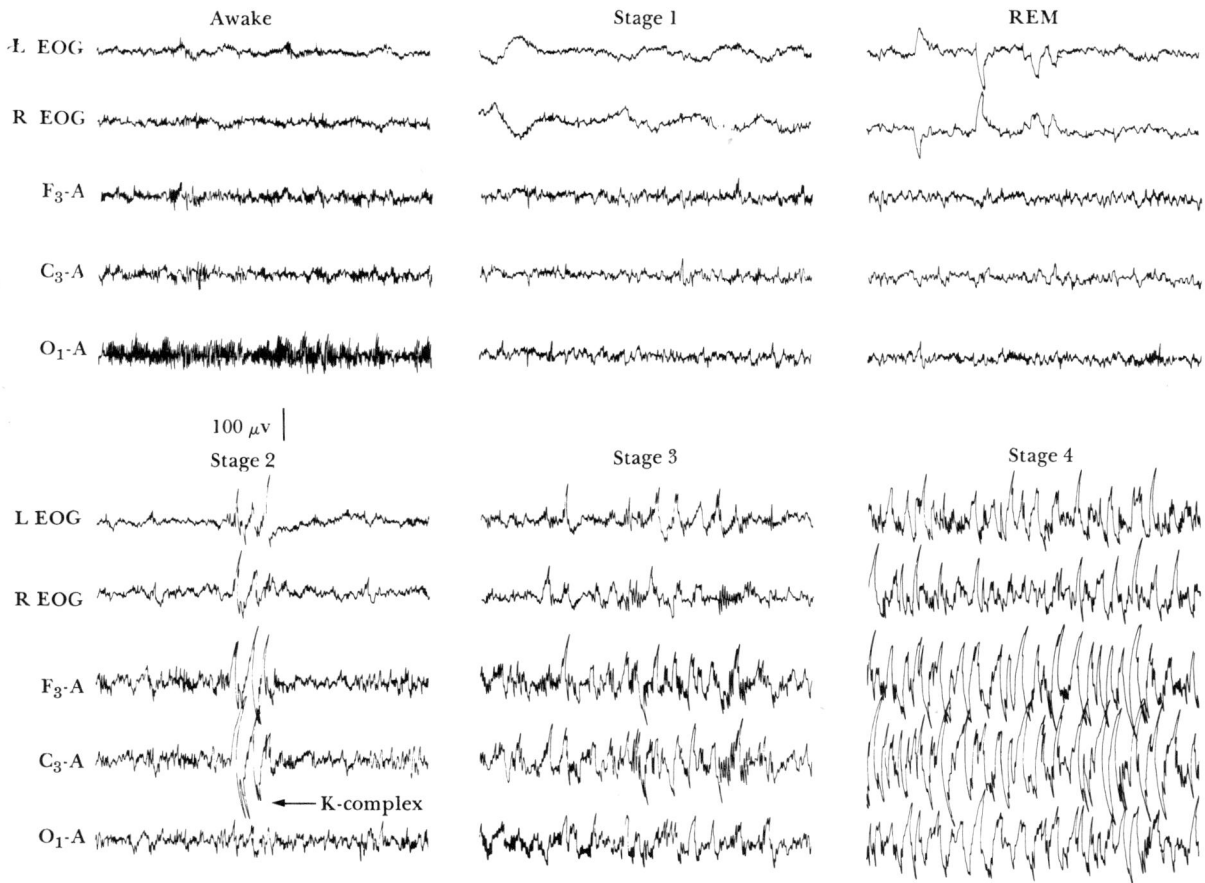

Figure 7-1

The EEG correlates of the various sleep stages. The L EOG and R EOG records indicate movements of the left and right eyes. The tracings labeled F_3-A, C_3-A, and O_1-A show electrical activity recorded from frontal, central, and occipital regions of the cortex. From "Are Stages of Sleep Related to Waking Behavior?" by L. C. Johnson, American Scientist, *1973, 61, 326–338. Reprinted by permission,* American Scientist, *journal of Sigma Xi, The Scientific Research Society of North America.*

Stage 1

The electrical activity of the brain during Stage 1 is desynchronized, as it is during the alert state, but this low-amplitude activity has a strong component of activity in the 2–7 Hz range. Stage 1 is the transition from drowsiness to the deeper stages of sleep; it also follows body movements during sleep. The duration of this stage is usually relatively short: from one to seven minutes. During this stage, it is easy to awaken you with a noise. Your body is relaxing. Your muscle tone is diminishing, your heart rate is slowing down, and your breathing is becoming deeper and more regular.

Stage 2

During Stage 2, brief bursts (two seconds or less in duration) of EEG waves appear against a background of desynchronized activity. These are called **sleep spindles,** and they have a frequency of approximately 12–15 Hz. The appearance of wave patterns called **K-complexes** (see Figure 7-1) is also a clear indicator of Stage 2. When in this stage, you are soundly asleep yet can still be easily awakened.

Stage 3

Large-amplitude delta waves begin to be interspersed with the spindles and background irregular activity at the onset of Stage 3. Stage 3 is defined by an EEG record in which at least 20% but not more than 50% of the record consists of delta waves with a frequency of 2 Hz or less. The amplitude of these waves may be as high as 300 μv, as compared with the 60 μv amplitude of the alpha rhythm during drowsiness. It will take a relatively loud sound to awaken you when you are in Stage 3—perhaps the repetition of your name. Your blood pressure, body temperature, muscle tone, and heart rate are all decreasing. Your breathing is deeper and more even.

Stage 4

Stage 4 is often referred to as deep sleep. This stage is defined by an EEG record in which more than 50% of the record consists of delta waves of 2 Hz or slower, but in general Stage 4 records show slow-wave activity almost continuously. When you are in Stage 4, your muscles are very relaxed, you rarely move, and it is very difficult to wake you up. If you are awakened, you will come into focus slowly. We normally spend about 15% of the night's sleep in Stage 4. If we are prevented, by some annoyance or tension, from getting our 15% quota, we will make up for it on subsequent nights by spending more time in Stage 4. This compensation may reflect a physiological necessity to spend a certain amount of time in Stage 4.

A possible physiological function of Stage 4, as well as Stage 3, has been proposed by Sassin, Parker, Mace, Gotlin, Johnson, and Rossman (1969). They found that there was a significant relationship between the release of **human growth hormone** and the occurrence of Stages 3 and 4 of sleep. Human growth hormone is secreted by the pituitary of individuals of all ages, and it promotes growth of tissues throughout the body. Sassin and his associates found that, if a person was kept awake all night, no growth hormone was released during the periods when Stages 3 and 4 would normally have occurred. If the sleep/wakefulness cycle was reversed, the growth hormone was released during the daytime when the individual engaged in Stage 3 and 4 of sleep. Hence these two phenomena, the occurrence of Stages 3 and 4 and the release of human growth hormone, are apparently highly correlated and are probably mediated by identical brain pathways.

Stages 1–4 are sometimes referred to collectively as **non-REM sleep,** to contrast them with Stage REM, which will be discussed below. We have examined sleep stages in humans thus far, but they can also be detected in the sleep patterns of infraprimate species, such as the cat. However, because these stages are less distinct in lower animals than they are in humans, some researchers who study animals (for example, Jouvet, 1967a, 1970) prefer to simply describe non-REM sleep stages collectively under the rubric **Slow-Wave Sleep (SWS).** Jouvet has contributed greatly to our understanding of the physiological basis of SWS. He has proposed that a collection of nuclei called the *nuclei of raphe,* on the midline of the caudal portion of the brain stem (see Figure 7-2) are involved in SWS (Jouvet, 1967a, 1970). Specifically, he argues that these nuclei produce **serotonin,** which acts to suppress the normal alerting effects of the ascending reticular activating system. Jouvet was able to induce SWS by artificially increasing brain serotonin levels.

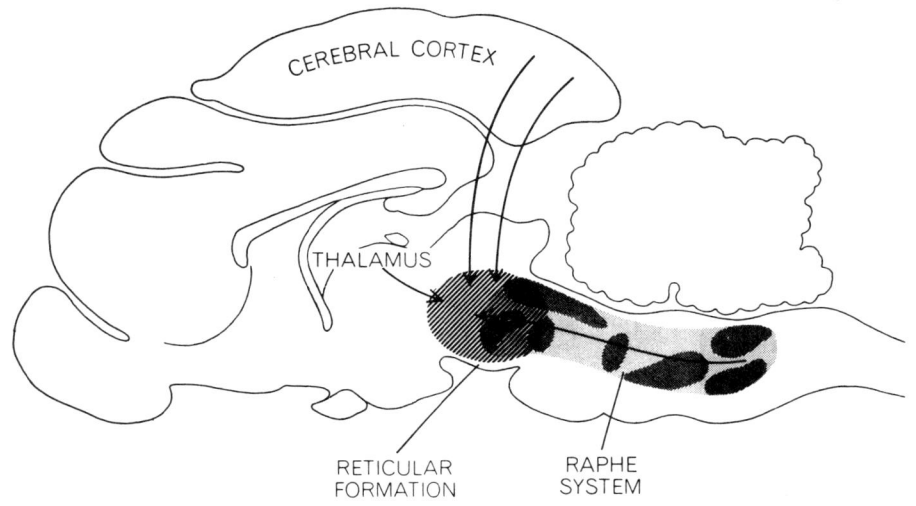

CEREBRAL CORTEX

THALAMUS

RETICULAR FORMATION

RAPHE SYSTEM

Figure 7-2
The location of the raphe system, which may bring about Slow-Wave Sleep by producing serotonin. Serotonin suppresses the alerting effects of the ascending reticular activating system. From "The States of Sleep," by M. Jouvet, Scientific American, *1967, 216, 62–72. Copyright 1967 by Scientific American, Inc. Reprinted by permission.*

Stage REM

Physiological Indexes. If you are allowed to sleep uninterrupted, after about an hour or so of sleep, you begin to drift back from Stage 4 into Stage 3 and Stage 2. As your sleep pattern, reflected by the EEG tracings, shifts from Stage 2 into Stage REM, a new phenomenon occurs: two pens that pick up movements from your eyes become activated. The pens will stop for a while and then begin moving again. These rapid eye movements are called **REMs,** and they signal a phase of vivid dreaming. The appearance of the Stage 1 EEG pattern in combination with REMs means that you have entered Stage REM, a unique state of consciousness. Although the EEG pattern is like that of Stage 1, it will be much more difficult to arouse you from Stage REM than it would be from Stage 1.

During Stage REM, many pronounced changes occur in the body. These have been separated into *tonic* and *phasic phenomena* (Dement, 1969; Grosser & Siegal, 1971). The tonic phenomena are the Stage 1 EEG pattern, the presence of theta waves throughout the hippocampus, and a striking loss of muscle tone. For example, the muscles of the neck and chin relax so completely that the mouth drops open. The tonic phenomena provide the background against which certain phasic phenomena occur.

The phasic phenomena are the REMs, **ponto-geniculo-occipital (PGO) waves,** myoclonic twitches, and short-term fluctuations of autonomic activity. The PGO waves are sharp spikes in the EEG record that originate in the pons, travel to the lateral geniculate body of the thalamus, and arrive at the occipital cortex. In cats, the PGO waves are closely associated with REMs (Jouvet, 1970). REMs are seen during Stage REM sleep in blind humans (Gross, Feldman, & Fisher, 1965) and in kittens immediately after birth, when their eyes have not yet opened (Valatx, Jouvet, & Jouvet, 1964).

Myoclonic twitches are small twitches or jerks in the body muscles. We have all seen our dogs lying on the floor asleep and apparently oblivious to everything around them. Suddenly, they start emitting slight barking sounds, and their legs show small jerking movements. When we see this, we probably all wonder what rabbit they are dreaming about chasing.

Dreaming During Stage REM. The most striking aspect of Stage REM is the now well-substantiated finding that this is a period of vivid dreaming in humans. If awakened during this sleep stage, humans will almost invariably report that they have been dreaming. However, if humans are awakened even a few minutes after all signs of this phase of sleep have ended, the dream will often have been forgotten. This explains why we so frequently are unaware of the fact that we dream every night. In fact, most of us will spend a total of almost five years of our lives in vivid dreaming but remember very little of it.

The discovery of the occurrence of dreaming during Stage REM was made by Aserinsky and Kleitman (1953). They found that, when they awakened their human subjects during REM, about 74% of the time their volunteers would report that they had been dreaming. When these same individuals were awakened during non-REM periods, only about 17% of them reported dreams. Subsequent studies by Dement and Kleitman (1957b) and Kales, Hodemaker, and Jacobson (1963) found dream reports in 83–88% of REM awakenings and 6–7% following non-REM awakenings. In general, most sleep researchers have found that REM awakenings result in a high incidence of dream recall, but there have been discrepant findings regarding the incidence of dream-like experiences reported following awakening from non-REM periods. In one study, Foulkes (1966) found 74% dream recall following non-REM periods! Fortunately, Foulkes himself has offered an explanation for these divergent findings.

Foulkes suggested that two types of mentation can occur during sleep. According to Foulkes, non-REM mentations are less well recalled, more thoughtlike, less vivid, less visual, less bizarre, and less emotional than reports obtained from REM awakenings. Dream reports following REM awakenings, on the other hand, have a well-integrated structure. They are what we normally think of as dreaming. They have a well-integrated story line. Thus, it appears that the phase of sleep called Stage REM represents the period in our sleep cycle during which we dream.

The Anatomy of Stage REM. The neuroanatomy of the REM state has been studied by a number of investigators—most notably Jouvet and his colleagues (Jouvet, 1967a, 1970). Their research has led them to conclude that the mechanisms that mediate Stage REM are contained in the pons. Activation of this triggering system leads to the induction of Stage REM. When Jouvet destroyed this system, the animals no longer exhibited this phase of sleep. Furthermore, Jouvet and his fellow investigators have shown that a small cluster of cells called the **nucleus locus coeruleus,** within the pontile area concerned with Stage REM sleep, is responsible for the inhibition of muscle tone that accompanies the onset of REM sleep. Perhaps this inhibition stops us from acting out our dreams. When Jouvet destroyed this tiny nucleus in cats, he found that an animal in the midst of REM sleep moved around a great deal, as if it were "acting out a dream."

If the pons contains the trigger for the onset of Stage REM, then what pulls the trigger? Jouvet has suggested that REM sleep is biochemically mediated. Earlier, I indicated that Jouvet has proposed that serotonin mediates the onset of SWS. He has further hypothesized that the transition from SWS to REM sleep is mediated at the pontile level by the breakdown of serotonin. The onset of the tonic phenomena of Stage REM is subsequently triggered by cholinergic mechanisms (pathways using acetylcholine at their synapses) at the pontile level. Finally, the occurrence of phasic phenomena during REM sleep is mediated by noradrenergic mechanisms (pathways using norepinephrine at their synapses) in the pons. Thus, the REM state "depends upon a relatively fail-safe mechanism since it necessitates at least three different 'keys' to be started" (Jouvet, 1970, p. 22).

A Total Night of Sleep

Sleep is a succession of repeating cycles. There are wide individual variations in patterns of sleep, but generally we as adults dream about every 90 minutes and show a full cycle of sleep stages approximately every 90–120 minutes. We spend about the same proportion of each night in SWS and REM sleep (about 20–25% of the night in each). (In humans, *SWS* refers to Stages 3 and 4 combined.) Most (up to 75%) of the total Stage 4 sleep occurs during the first third of the sleep period, while a greater incidence of REM sleep occurs during the last third of the night.

Variations in Sleep Patterns with Age

In discussing sleep patterns thus far in this chapter, I've been giving you information about patterns of sleep in the average adult. There are alterations in sleep patterns as a function of age—most notably in Stages 4 and REM. Regarding Stage 4 sleep, Webb and Agnew (1971) found that there was a decrease in the percentage of total sleep time spent in Stage 4 as a function of age. To obtain these data, they examined the sleep patterns of humans ranging in age from 21 months to 69 years. Their results are graphed in Figure 7-3. As you can see by examining this graph, the

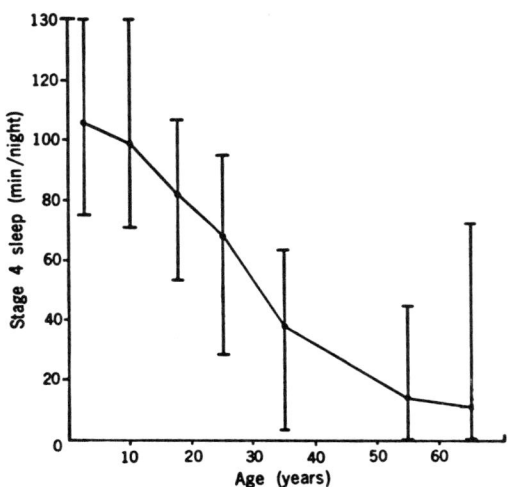

Figure 7-3 Stage 4 sleep per night in seven age groups. The dots represent the mean for each age group, and the vertical lines indicate the range of individual times. From "Stage 4 Sleep: Influence of Time Course Variables," by W. B. Webb and H. W. Agnew, Jr., Science, 1971, 174, 1354– 1356. Copyright 1971 by the American Association for the Advancement of Science. Reprinted by permission.

average total amount of Stage 4 during a night ranged from approximately 105 minutes in the youngest children to about 10 minutes in the oldest adults.

There are also differences between adults and young children in the characteristics of Stage REM. One notable difference is that in infants there is often almost a direct transition from wakefulness to the REM state, whereas in the normal adult non-REM sleep always precedes REM sleep for about 50–90 minutes (Roffwarg, Muzio, & Dement, 1966; Korner, 1968). As was the case with Stage 4, there is a decrease in the percentage of total sleep time spent in Stage REM as a function of age.

Very premature infants (that is, ten weeks premature) sleep during most of the 24-hour day, and 80% of their sleep time is spent in Stage REM. This indicates that we do not enter Stage REM in order to dream; the two events simply occur together in human adults. By early adulthood, time spent in REM has declined to 22–28% of an eight-hour sleep period. REM time remains at this level for the rest of life, although a slight drop has been noted in some very old people (over 80) by Williams, Karacan, and Hursch (1974). This finding has suggested to some investigators (for example, Roffwarg et al., 1966) that REM sleep performs functions first in maturation and then in maintenance of the central nervous system.

Phylogenetic Variations in Sleep Patterns

Jouvet and his colleagues (see Jouvet, 1965) have conducted several inquiries into phylogenetic variations in sleep patterns. They have examined the incidence of and the percentage of sleep time occupied by REM sleep at various levels of the phylogenetic scale. Jouvet reported that SWS has been demonstrated in all mammals studied and can also be observed in the sleep patterns of birds and reptiles. In contrast, REM sleep does not occur in reptiles (tortoises, for instance). Birds (for example, pigeons, chickens) show very short periods of REM sleep, lasting from 6–15 seconds; approximately 0.2% of bird sleep is spent in REM sleep. In mammals, REM sleep accounts for 6–30% of the sleep of adults, depending on the species.

The sleep patterns of the domestic cat have been studied more extensively than those of any other nonhuman species. In normal adult cats, REM sleep invariably occurs after a period of SWS. Its average duration is 6 minutes, but REM periods of 15–20 minutes duration are often recorded. REM thus takes up about 20–25% of a cat's sleep. Since cats sleep about 80% of the day, this means that they spend about 15–20% of their lives in Stage REM.

Sleep Deprivation

Total Sleep Deprivation

Studies of the behavioral and physiological effects of sleep loss have occupied a prominent position in experimental sleep research. Studies of sleep starvation, as these inquiries may be considered, began in the 1890s, and there has been a steady output of these studies since that time. Reviews of these investigations are presented by Kleitman (1963), Luce (1965), and Murray (1965). In general, these studies have found that distinct and predictable behavior changes occur over the course of a period of sleep deprivation.

It has consistently been noted that prolonged sleep deprivation results in "progressive unevenness of mental functioning, lapses in attention, growing fatigue, weariness, and a tendency to withdraw from the outside world" (Luce, 1965, p. 19). After 30–60 hours of sleep starvation, people begin to show difficulties with depth perception. Lights appear to be shrouded in a halo of fog, small objects dart out of place, and pieces of furniture change size (Luce, 1965). Many individuals will begin to experience hallucinations after about 90 hours of sleep loss. A striking example of the effects produced by sleep loss is provided by Luce (1965).

In January, 1959, the largely unaware public saw before its very eyes the kind of temporary psychosis that can be induced with sleep starvation. Under the supervision of doctors and scientists, Peter Tripp, a 32-year-old disc jockey, undertook to stay awake for 200 hours in a Times Square booth for the benefit of the March of Dimes. Throughout his marathon of over eight days, Tripp was given medical and neurological examinations, tests of performance, psychological tests, and was closely attended by Drs. Harold L. Williams, Ardie Lubin, Louis Joylon West, Harold Wolff, William C. Dement, and others. Although his experience was undoubtedly worsened by the tension of publicity and public conditions, some of the ordeals of Peter Tripp may indicate the kind of mental symptoms that can beleaguer the severely sleep starved.

Almost from the first, the desire to sleep was so strong that Tripp was fighting to keep himself awake. After little more than two days and two nights he began to have visual illusions; for example, he reported finding cobwebs in his shoes. By about 100 hours the simple daily tests that required only minimal mental agility and attention were a torture for him. He was having trouble remembering things, and his visual illusions were perturbing: he saw the tweed suit of one of the scientists as a suit of furry worms. After 120 hours he went across the street to a room in the Hotel Astor, where he periodically washed and changed clothes. He opened a bureau drawer and dashed out into the hall for help. The drawer, as he had seen it, was ablaze. Perhaps in an effort to explain this and other visions to himself he decided that the doctors had set the illusory fire, deliberately, to test him and frighten him. About this time he developed a habit of staring at the wall clock in the Times Square booth. As he later explained, the face of the clock bore the face of an actor friend, and he had begun to wonder whether he were Peter Tripp, or the friend whose face he saw in the clock. The daily tests were almost unendurable for Tripp and those who were studying him. "He looked like a blind animal trying to feel his way through a maze." A simple algebraic formula that he had earlier solved with ease now required such superhuman effort that Tripp broke down, frightened at his inability to solve the problem. Scientists saw the spectacle of a suave New York radio entertainer trying vainly to find his way through the alphabet.

By 170 hours the agony had become almost unbearable to watch. At times Tripp was no longer sure he was himself, and frequently tried to gain proof of his identity. Although he behaved as if he were awake, his brain wave patterns resembled those of sleep. In his psychotic delusions he was convinced that the doctors were in a conspiracy against him to send him to jail. On the last morning of his wakathon, Tripp was examined by Dr. Harold Wolff of Cornell. The late Dr. Wolff had a somewhat archaic manner of dress, and to Tripp he must have appeared funebrial. Tripp undressed, as requested, and lay down on the table for medical examination, but as he gazed up at the doctor he came to the gruesome decision that the man was actually an undertaker, about to bury him alive. With this grim insight, Tripp lept for the door, and tore into the Astor hall with several doctors in pursuit. At the end of the 200 sleepless hours, nightmare hallucination and reality had merged, and he felt he was the victim of a sadistic conspiracy among the doctors.

With some persuasion, Tripp managed to make a final appearance in the glass-windowed booth in Times Square, and after his broadcast he went to sleep for 13 hours. Although the record of his ordeal covers hundreds of pages, the few instances cited here may give some indication of the extreme distortions, mental agonies, and delusions he suffered, especially during his last 100 hours of sleeplessness. When he awakened after his first long sleep the terrors, hallucinations, and mental deterioration had vanished. He no longer inhabited an unstable visual world where objects appeared to change size, where a doctor's tie would jump out of place, and where it was a superhuman effort to solve a simple problem or remember an anecdote. In 13 hours of sleep the nightmare existence had been left behind, although for three months afterward Tripp suffered a mild depression. Quite aside from the quick apparent recovery from extreme symptoms, there had been two extremely striking patterns throughout the ordeal, periodicities that suggested that Tripp's times of strength and moments of worst symptoms followed some inner cycles. Throughout the ordeal Tripp had been able to organize and perform his daily broadcast. Temperature readings showed that he was at his peak at the broadcast time, the point of his highest daily temperature. His bursts of hallucination and strange behaviors, on the other hand, seemed to occur in 90–120 minute intervals, at times when he might normally have been dreaming [Luce, 1965, pp. 19–20].*

The chronicle of Peter Tripp's ordeal following long-term sleep deprivation represents an extreme example of the possible effects of sleep starvation. Five years after Tripp's marathon of wakefulness, a 17-year-old high school student named Randy Gardner set out to break the record. He accomplished his goal in the quiet setting of his own home, and, without the help of coffee or any other stimulants, he stayed awake for a total of 264 hours (Luce, 1965). Although Randy showed some irritability, memory lapses, and difficulties in concentration, he did not show the extreme psychological disturbances that Peter Tripp showed. Randy did suffer some neurological abnormalities during his last few days of wakefulness. For example, his vision was blurred, his right eye was making involuntary sideways movements, and his EEG pattern looked like that of a sleeping person, regardless of whether his eyes were open or closed (Johnson, Slye, & Dement, 1965; Ross, 1964).

After his 11-day marathon of wakefulness, Randy Gardner slept for over 14 hours and rebounded into a cheerful, psychologically healthy person. It is interesting to note that, during this initial recovery sleep, Stages 4 and REM dominated the sleep period. His ordeal was undoubtedly lessened by his being in his own home, but his resistance to the potentially debilitating effects of sleep loss was undoubtedly strengthened by his youth and "psychological stability." Research by Morris and Singer (1961) has shown that resistance to the adverse effects of sleep loss is roughly proportional to what we might loosely call "psychological stability," as indexed by interviews and psychiatric-test scores. Webb (1962) has shown that, in general, younger animals (rats, in his study) were more resistant to the detrimental effects of sleep loss than older animals.

In another study of sleep deprivation, Webb and Agnew (1965) restricted eight male college students at the University of Florida to three hours of sleep per night. This regimen was continued for eight successive nights, during which EEG recordings were made during sleep. On these nights of restricted sleep, the sleep patterns of the subjects were not simply miniatures of their normal sleep patterns. Rather, the students spent as much time as usual in the deep sleep of Stage 4, at the expense of the other sleep stages. During the recovery night, the early part of the sleep period was also dominated by Stage 4, even though this stage suffered the least deprivation during the eight-day restricted-sleep regimen. Only after this period of Stage 4 sleep did Stage REM sleep appear.

*From *Research on Sleep and Dreams,* by G. G. Luce. National Institute of Mental Health, 1965.

Thus far, we have examined the effects of total sleep loss. Other experiments have investigated the outcome of depriving subjects of specific sleep stages. The majority of these inquiries have studied the effects of Stage REM deprivation—deprivation of the stage of sleep associated with vivid dreaming in humans. One important study was W. C. Dement's in 1960.

In Dement's research, volunteer human adults under strict instructions not to take any alcohol, drugs, or naps, were allowed to sleep their usual sleep in the laboratory—except for Stage REM. Whenever Stage REM was entered, the subjects were awakened and then allowed to go back to sleep. This procedure continued for five successive nights. Although these individuals still got about six hours of sleep each night, they showed irritability, anxiety, and difficulty in concentrating. These adverse reactions were not experienced by control subjects who received the same number of awakenings as the REM-deprived subjects but during non-REM periods.

This finding created a great deal of excitement by suggesting that we have a need to dream. It is very important to note, however, that this finding has not been reliably replicated by other investigations. Although this finding is often cited in introductory psychology textbooks, Dement, in later studies, and many other researchers (for example, Kales, Hodemaker, Jacobson, & Lichtenstein, 1964) have failed to demonstrate any marked psychological changes in humans even after more extended Stage REM deprivation. For this reason, it has been concluded that Stage REM deprivation does not necessarily produce psychological disturbances.

In his initial investigation, Dement also found that his subjects attempted to enter Stage REM more frequently during each successive deprivation night. Further, after their deprivation regimen had ended and they were allowed to sleep undisturbed in the laboratory, they spent about 60% more time in REM sleep than they had during baseline nights preceding deprivation. They appeared to be making up for the lost Stage REM sleep. This phenomenon is called the **REM-rebound effect.** The REM-rebound effect was subsequently verified many times in humans (for example, Clemes & Dement, 1967; Dement, 1965; Dement, Greenberg, & Klein, 1966; Kales et al., 1964; Sampson, 1966) and in animals, including the rat (Morden, Mitchell, & Dement, 1967), mouse (Cohen & Dement, 1968), rabbit (Khazan & Sawyer, 1963), cat (Dement, Henry, Cohen, & Ferguson, 1967; Jouvet, 1967a), and monkey (Berger & Meier, 1966).

Stage 4 Deprivation

Shortly after Dement (1960) demonstrated the REM-rebound effect, a complementary study by Agnew, Webb, and Williams (1964) demonstrated a similar rebound phenomenon following Stage 4 deprivation. They used a different procedure with their subjects. Their volunteers were not awakened, but rather a tone was sounded, which moved the subjects into a lighter stage of sleep. In the final days of the experiment, it was necessary to use an electric shock to prevent Stage 4 from occurring. During recovery from this deprivation, there was an increase in the percentage of the night's sleep spent in Stage 4. No behavior changes resulted from this deprivation.

Each night we willingly accept suspension from active life and enter the silent world of sleep. It was once thought that the onset of sleep was a passive process resulting simply from a cessation of ascending impulses in the ascending reticular activating system. However, later research suggested that sleep is instead an active process that results from excitation of a sleep-inducing, or hypnogenic, system. This hypnogenic system extends from the base of the brain through the thalamus and into the neocortex. Activation of this system may contribute to the sleep process by exerting direct inhibitory influences over behavioral arousal.

Sleep has been divided into stages: Stages 1–4, which represent increasing depths of sleep, and Stage REM, which is correlated with dreaming in humans. These sleep stages are defined by certain EEG patterns and other physiological indexes. Stage 1 is characterized by a desynchronized EEG pattern with a strong component of electrical activity in the 2–7 Hz range. The appearance of sleep spindles announces the beginning of Stage 2; the frequency of the spindle bursts is approximately 12–15 Hz. Large-amplitude delta waves begin to be mixed with the spindles at the onset of Stage 3. Stage 3 is defined by an EEG record in which at least 20% but not more than 50% consists of delta waves of a frequency of 2 Hz or less. The EEG records obtained during Stage 4 sleep are dominated by an almost continuous train of slow-wave delta activity, although this stage is defined by a record in which more than 50% of the EEG activity consists of delta waves of 2 Hz or slower. About 20–25% of the night's sleep is spent in SWS (Stages 3 and 4 combined); a similar amount of time is spent in Stage REM. Stage REM is characterized by electrical activity similar to Stage 1, intermittently accompanied by rapid eye movements (REMs). This stage of sleep is correlated with vivid dreaming in humans. Tonic and phasic phenomena accompanying Stage REM were described.

The anatomy and chemistry of sleep stages were also considered. Research by Jouvet and his colleagues has indicated that the nuclei of raphe in the caudal portion of the brain stem yield sleep by producing serotonin, which acts to suppress the alerting effects normally exerted by the ascending reticular activating system. Jouvet has further asserted that the transition from non-REM sleep to REM sleep is mediated at the pontile level by the breakdown of serotonin. The onset of tonic phenomena of Stage REM is subsequently triggered by cholinergic mechanisms at the level of the pons, and, finally, the occurrence of phasic phenomena during Stage REM is regulated by pontile noradrenergic mechanisms.

Variations in sleep patterns as a function of age and species were discussed. Percentage of sleep time spent in both Stage 4 and Stage REM decline as a function of increasing age in humans. The percentage spent in Stage REM increases as the phylogenetic scale is ascended. REM sleep does not occur in reptiles. It is very short in birds, accounting for only about 0.2% of sleep. However, in mammals it accounts for 6–30% of sleep, depending on the species.

The effects of total sleep deprivation were illustrated by a case history of an individual who engaged in a sleepless marathon of 200 hours. In general, it has been shown that sleep loss produces predictable deficits in performance and perception that become more pronounced as the deprivation continues. Resistance to the adverse effects produced by sleep deprivation is roughly negatively correlated with age and positively correlated with what we might loosely call mental stability.

Selective deprivation of specific sleep stages was the final topic considered. Deprivation of Stage REM was at first shown to produce psychological disturbances and the REM-rebound phenomenon. *REM-rebound* refers to the fact that, when the deprived subjects were allowed to sleep undisturbed following the end of deprivation, they spent more time than adults normally spend in Stage REM, apparently making up for this lost REM time. The REM-rebound effect has been demonstrated many times in human and animal studies, but it has not been possible to replicate the finding of debilitating psychological effects of REM deprivation in humans. Deprivation of Stage 4 in humans yields a rebound effect similar to that found following REM deprivation and no psychological disturbances.

Experimental studies of sleep have allowed scientists to probe into a realm of human existence that was before only the province of armchair psychiatric theorists. As our knowledge of normal sleep phenomena increases, so will the possibility of understanding various sleep disorders. It may be possible, by examining sleep patterns, to diagnose the state of the human infant's developing nervous system long before behavioral tests are possible. Finally, an understanding of the nature of and need for sleep may help us as adults to better schedule our periods of work and rest.

8

Neural Mechanisms of Emotion

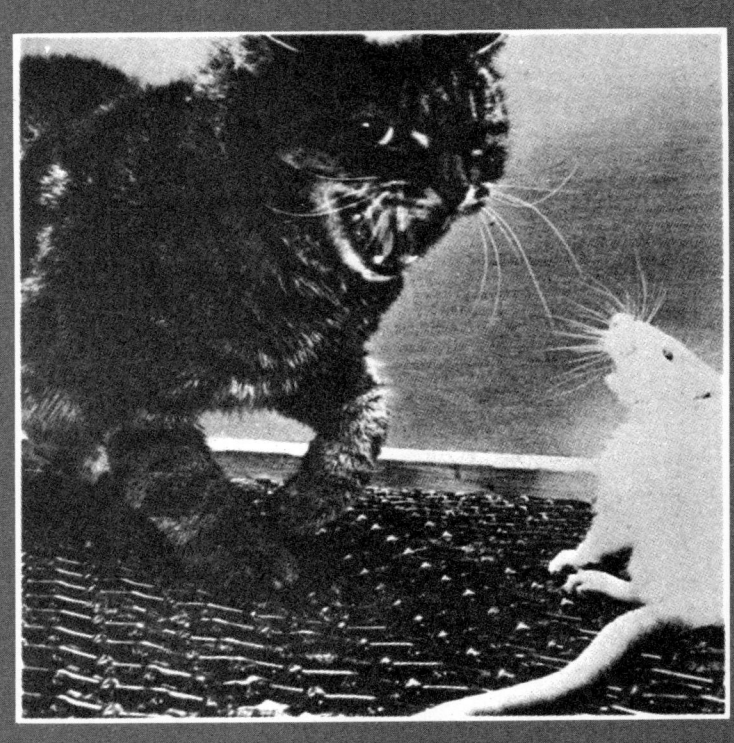

Although we use the words *emotion* and *emotionality* quite often in our everyday language, the exact meaning of these words is hard to decide on. Does emotion refer to the way we "feel," or the way we act, or the way we look? Is it some combination of all of these things? The difficulty of defining emotion makes it very hard to determine how the brain regulates this process. The researcher interested in brain-behavior relationships is continuously plagued by the problem that the behaviors for which he or she is attempting to determine neural mechanisms simply have not been adequately defined. Until different categories of behavior have been clearly distinguished by the behavioral psychologist, it will continue to be difficult for the physiological psychologist to determine the physiological substrates of these behaviors.

Drawing on the early writings of Papez (1937) and the later work of Flynn and his associates (Flynn, Vanegas, Foote, & Edwards, 1970), the term *emotion* can be applied to three types of phenomena. First, *emotion* can be used to refer to a *subjective feeling*. The only way we can study this type of emotion is by examining our own introspections or by asking some other human about his or her feelings. There is very little information available regarding how the brain mediates this aspect of emotion. Presumably, though, the cortex mediates it.

Whereas we cannot assess the subjective-feelings component of emotion simply by watching the behavior of an organism, the other two aspects of emotion can be directly observed. One of these aspects of emotion is the organism's *way of acting*—that is, its *emotional expression.* Emotional expression may or may not be accompanied by the subjective feelings of emotion. The angry facial expression of an enraged individual is accompanied by strong subjective feelings, but the scowl of an actor on a stage may not be. A blind, nondirected expression of emotion will still occur if *all* of the brain tissue above the hypothalamus is removed (Bard, 1928, 1934); the hypothalamus is apparently the essential region in the mediation of emotional expression.

Finally, as Flynn and his associates (1970) have pointed out, certain *complex behaviors* that occur during an *animal's interactions with its environment* are often regarded as emotional. Fighting, fleeing, and sexual behavior are examples of this third aspect of emotion. The second and third types of emotion can be easily studied in animals. Over the years, many excellent studies have extended our knowledge about the neural mechanisms mediating emotional behaviors. This work has also greatly enhanced our understanding of how different parts of the brain interact to mediate complex patterns of behavior in general.

In this chapter, I will first describe some of the classic work that provided much of the impetus for current interest in neural mechanisms of emotion. You'll see that many of the early findings were conflicting and confusing. I'll then outline a model that resolves these conflicts and accounts for neural mediation of emotion. You'll see how different brain structures cooperate or interact, according to this model, to mediate emotional expression and complex emotional responses. The chapter will end with a consideration of the use of psychosurgery in the treatment of human behavior disorders.

Early Studies of the Brain and Emotion

Although Bard (1928) and Hess (1928), among others, had demonstrated the importance of the hypothalamus in emotional expression and thereby laid the foundation for later studies on the neuroanatomical substrates of emotion, most of the current interest in the role of brain mechanisms in emotional, or **affective,** behavior can be traced to the publication of two papers in 1937. One of these was the anatomist James W. Papez's now classic article attempting to define a neuroanatomical system concerned with emotional expression. The other important paper of 1937 was the historic report by a pair of University of Chicago investigators—Heinrich Klüver and Paul C. Bucy. This report, based on data obtained on two rhesus monkeys, focused attention on the functions performed by temporal-lobe structures in mediating emotion. The authors' preliminary findings were amplified in a report published two years later (Klüver & Bucy, 1939). We'll examine the writings of Papez and of Klüver and Bucy in the discussion that follows.

The Papez Circuit

In an article entitled "A Proposed Mechanism of Emotion," Papez (1937) proposed a neuroanatomical model of limbic-system mediation of emotion. As was indicated in Chapter 3, the limbic system includes the hypothalamus, parts of the thalamus, the amygdala, the septal area, the cingulate gyrus, and the hippocampus. Many of these regions were at one time thought to be exclusively concerned with processing olfactory information, and for this reason they were grouped together as the rhinencephalon. However, it is now accepted that their primary function is not olfactory. Rather, these structures are crucially involved in the expression of such behavior processes as emotion, motivation, and learning.

Papez proposed that "the hypothalamus, the anterior thalamic nuclei, the cingulate gyrus, the hippocampus, and their interconnections comprise a mechanism which may elaborate the functions of central emotion as well as participate in emotional expression" (p. 743). In discussing his circuit, Papez distinguished between subjective feelings of emotion and emotional expression. He suggested that subjective emotional experience requires the participation of the cortex. In contrast, emotional expression depends on the integrative activity of the hypothalamus. Impulses initiating the chain of events that occurs in the generation of emotion could occur in either the cerebral cortex or the hypothalamus.

According to the Papez model, emotional experiences of cortical origin pass first to the hippocampus and then, via a fiber tract called the fornix, to the mammillary bodies of the posterior hypothalamus. From the mammillary bodies, impulses next travel to the anterior thalamic nuclei via the mammilothalamic tract and then to the cingulate gyrus by way of the medial thalamocortical radiations. Papez suggested that the cingulate gyrus be considered the receptive region for experiencing emotion which results from impulses arriving from the hypothalamus, in much the same way as the primary visual cortex is considered the receptive region for visual signals arising from the retina. The flow of the emotional processes to other cortical areas would add "emotional coloring" to the subjective experience.

Emotional expression of hypothalamic origin, in the Papez circuit, actually begins with the arrival of sensory information at the specific sensory relay nuclei of the thalamus. From these sensory nuclei, some of the arriving information is relayed to the primary sensory receiving areas of the neocortex. Another part of the sensory information is conducted by short fiber tracts to portions of the hypothalamus concerned with emotional expression. From these regions, information is relayed to the mammillary bodies of the hypothalamus and then to the anterior thalamic nuclei. From here, as detailed above, information travels to the cingulate gyrus, where emotional experience is added. From the cingulate gyrus, impulses are carried to the hippocampus via the cingulum bundle. The hippocampus then organizes this information and relays it back to the mammillary bodies.

Papez based his circuit primarily on a few human clinical observations that were available in the literature. He also considered the few experimental animal studies that had been conducted up to that time. For example, the hippocampus was given an important position in his circuit because, in rabies, a disease characterized by, among other things, strong emotional rages, brain lesions occur predominantly in the hippocampus (although they also occur in other brain regions). One of the case histories he cited in his discussion of the cingulate gyrus reported irritability and emotional outbursts associated with degeneration of this region.

In spite of the paucity of information on which the Papez circuit was built, his observations were remarkably accurate and served as a strong impetus for animal experiments designed to delineate the functions of brain structures in emotion. Later research suggested that some areas that had been neglected in Papez's early formulations are intimately involved with emotional expression. Most notable among these areas are the septal region and the amygdala. Other investigators have attempted to clarify the ways in which different structures or nuclear groups in the limbic system interact in mediating emotion. Despite any shortcomings that characterize the Papez circuit, we must remember the remarkable job that Papez did with so little available information. His circuit deserves a high position in the annals of neuropsychological research. His was the first attempt to describe a neuroanatomical system mediating behavior.

The Klüver-Bucy Syndrome

In a preliminary report published in 1937, Klüver and Bucy described a striking set of observations of the behavioral effects of bilateral removal of the temporal lobes in rhesus monkeys. Their subsequent expanded investigation, the report on which was published in 1939, is another one of the classics in the brain-research literature (Klüver & Bucy, 1939). The extraordinary behavior changes they noted following bilateral temporal lobectomy have since come to be referred to as the *Klüver-Bucy Syndrome*. It's very interesting to note that many of the features of this syndrome were described years earlier by Brown and Schaefer (1888), who also examined the effects of bilateral temporal lobectomy in a monkey. However, they did not recognize the significance of their findings, attributing them instead to "idiocy" induced by general cortical damage. Thus, it was 50 years later that Klüver and Bucy finally electrified the scientific community with the significance of these behavior alterations as indicative of temporal-lobe functions in behavior.

Prior to conducting the historic work, Klüver had been aware of the fact that human epileptics whose seizure activity was originating in the temporal lobes were likely to experience visual hallucinations during their attacks. At the time he was also interested in the effects of mescaline and other hallucinogenic drugs. Since hallucinogenic drugs produce visual hallucinations, Klüver wondered whether the hallucinogenic experience might be the effect of the action of these drugs on temporal-lobe structures. He and Bucy therefore prepared some monkeys by creating temporal-lobe lesions. As I said, the striking behavior alterations they noted are now called the Klüver-Bucy Syndrome. The primary features of this syndrome can be divided into two classes: reactions to environmental stimuli and changes in sexual and emotional behavior.

Reactions to Environmental Stimuli. Following recovery from surgery in which the temporal lobes were bilaterally removed, the monkeys showed marked alterations in their reactions to objects in their environment. The animals displayed a strong tendency to examine all objects immediately, closely, and repeatedly, regardless of whether they were animate or inanimate. This strong approach tendency was even directed toward objects that had previously produced avoidance responses accompanied by strong emotional responses. The monkeys were just as eager to examine a lighted match or a hissing snake as a piece of food. They seemed to have lost their memory for the significance of objects and would even try to eat inedible objects, such as pieces of metal. Klüver and Bucy gave the name **psychic blindness** to this tendency to respond indiscriminately to various objects.

Another interesting aspect of the bilateral temporal lobectomized monkeys' interactions with their environment was their method of examining objects. They showed strong and compulsive tendencies to examine all objects by mouth (**oral tendencies**). Klüver and Bucy reported that they found no object the animals were not prone to examine orally. In general, the monkeys were extremely responsive to all environmental stimuli. The behavior pattern of the lobectomized animals appeared to be dominated by a compulsive, or irresistible, impulse to attend and react immediately to every object in their environment—a tendency referred to as **hypermetamorphosis.**

Changes in Sexual and Emotional Behavior. In addition to these modifications in the manner in which the animals reacted to objects in their environment, the bilateral temporal lobectomy produced alterations in sexual behavior and in emotion. The changes in sexual behavior first appeared three to six weeks after the operation. The monkeys became hypersexual, not only as measured by their marked increases in sexual activity, but also as indexed by the wide variety of objects toward which sexual responses were now directed.

In terms of emotional reactivity, the monkeys were made placid by the operation. From the time of surgery, the previously wild, fierce, aggressive rhesus monkeys could be handled with little danger. They demonstrated a total lack of aggressiveness both in their home cages and in testing situations. This finding was all the more remarkable in view of the fact that Klüver and Bucy had taken care to use only wild, aggressive monkeys for their subjects.

The temporal lobectomy performed by these investigators, in addition to removing the temporal-lobe neocortex, resulted in the removal of several temporal-lobe structures—namely, the amygdala, the hippocampus, and the uncus. Much of the subsequent work generated by their observations was devoted to assigning particular aspects of the Klüver-Bucy Syndrome to specific temporal-lobe structures. For example, as will be discussed in Chapter 10, psychic blindness was later shown to result from destruction of the temporal-lobe neocortex (Blum, Chow, & Pribram, 1950; Mishkin, 1964; Mishkin & Pribram, 1954).

In the discussion that follows, I'm going to describe research that has attempted to assign alterations in emotionality to specific temporal-lobe structures. I want to warn you in advance that the results will often be conflicting. However, out of the opposing findings will emerge an explanation. I'll then apply this explanation to the development of a model that describes how different brain regions regulate emotion.

Further Studies of the Effects of Temporal-Lobe Lesions on Emotion

The amygdala was a favorite target for subsequent research attempting to assign specific aspects of the Klüver-Bucy Syndrome to particular temporal-lobe regions. An astounding finding was that, although dogs (Fuller, Rosvold, & Pribram, 1957) and rats (Anand & Brobeck, 1951, 1952) were found to be friendly after bilateral injury to the amygdala, cats with similar lesions became savage (Bard & Mountcastle, 1948; Spiegel, Miller, & Oppenheimer, 1940). It should be pointed out that, although the main target for the lesions in these studies was the amygdala, the destruction usually encroached upon the surrounding cortex and some adjacent structures, including the hippocampus. The importance of possible variations in the extent and locus of the ablations will be discussed later in this chapter.

In a very comprehensive inquiry, Schreiner and Kling (1953) attempted to account for these discrepancies. They found that bilateral removal of the amygdala in cats produced an immediate shift toward greater docility. However, within 30–60 days after surgery, the cats became very aggressive. *The onset of this aggressiveness accompanied the appearance of hypersexuality.* The hypersexuality involved behavior elements that are not present in the sex patterns of unoperated cats. Their hypersexuality was not restricted to cats of the opposite sex or even to other cats. The amygdalectomized cats would attempt to copulate with any partner presented them, including cats, monkeys, dogs, agoutis (large Central-American rodents), and an old hen. In view of the fact that the onset of aggressiveness accompanied the development of hypersexuality in their amygdalectomized cats and the fact that sexual behavior in cats normally involves combative behavior, Schreiner and Kling proposed that the savageness might be a part of the hypersexuality syndrome.

In support of this possibility, these investigators made several observations. First, it was found that those cats that displayed only minimal increases in sexual activity remained docile. Second, castration of amygdalectomized males produced a decrease in sexuality and a return to the tameness shown just after surgery. Finally, cats that were castrated either prior to or during amygdalectomy never developed either hypersexuality or increased aggressiveness. Hence, the evidence quite strongly supported the theorists' contention that the aggressiveness noted in their subjects was highly correlated with the hypersexuality syndrome. However, this explanation doesn't account for the aggressiveness noted by Bard and Mountcastle (1948) and by Spiegel and his associates (1940) following amygdala ablations.

In the latter inquiry, the cats were savage immediately upon awakening from the ether anesthesia; they reacted to the slightest provocation with an outburst of well-directed rage. The behavior of these animals was studied only during the immediate postoperative period. In the research conducted by Bard and Mountcastle, the behavior responses of cats were studied for several months after surgery. The investigators found the gradual increase in aggression that was later noted by Schreiner and Kling, but their animals never became hypersexual!

An explanation for the discrepancy in results has been offered by Green and his associates. Green and his colleagues (Green, Clemente, & de Groot, 1957a, 1957b) argued that the aberrations in emotional and sexual behavior observed by Schreiner and Kling were not due to destruction of the amygdala but rather reflected inadvertent damage to other brain regions, near the amygdala. With regard to sexual behavior, they reported that bilateral destruction of the amygdala alone did not produce detectable changes in sexual behavior. However, if the lesion additionally encroached upon the cortex overlying the amygdala, hypersexuality did result (Green et al., 1957a). A similar finding emerged regarding the effects of temporal-lobe lesions on emotional behavior. If the extent of the bilateral lesions was limited to the boundaries of the amygdala, no alterations in emotionality were observed. In contrast, if the extent of the lesions was such that portions of the nearby hippocampus were involved, and, further, if the lesioned animals developed periodic epileptic seizures, then an increase in emotional behavior occurred (Green et al., 1957b). Thus, the altered emotional state may have been part of an epileptic syndrome.

Are alterations in emotional and sexual behavior produced only by lesions outside of the amygdala? Not according to a study published a year later by Wood (1958). Wood investigated the effects on behavior of lesions to discrete nuclei of the amygdala.

Before I review Wood's research, let me describe the anatomy of the amygdala in greater detail. The amygdaloid complex can be divided into several subnuclei, which can be identified in all mammalian brains. These are usually grouped into two nuclear complexes: the *basolateral complex* and the *corticomedial complex* (Gloor, 1960). A diagram of the amygdala in the right hemisphere is shown in Figure 8-1. The *basolateral nuclear complex* includes the *lateral nucleus,* the *basal lateral nucleus,* and

Figure 8-1
A cross section of the amygdaloid complex. Adapted from "Behavioral Changes Following Discrete Lesions of Temporal Lobe Structures," by C. D. Wood, Neurology, *1958, 8, 215–220. Copyright 1958 by the New York Times Media Company, Inc. Reprinted by permission.*

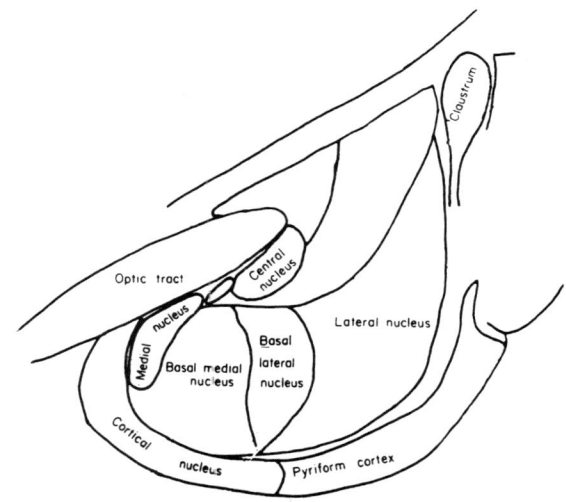

the *basal medial nucleus.* The *corticomedial nuclear complex* includes the *central, cortical,* and *medial nuclei.*

Wood reported that alterations in sexual and emotional behavior resulted when discrete lesions were bilaterally directed at certain of these amygdala nuclei. Hypersexuality was produced if, and only if, the lateral nucleus was bilaterally destroyed. Increased aggressive behavior was observed if bilateral lesions were made in either the basal or central amygdaloid nuclei. Thus, Wood was able to demonstrate distinct changes in both emotional and sexual behavior in the absence of damage to brain regions outside the border of the amygdaloid complex—a finding directly contrary to the data reported by Green and his associates. If we look at all of the findings I've reviewed, we are confronted with a giant conflict. Why? The following is a possible explanation.

Neural Mediation of Emotion: A Model

The Mechanism

The data that were reviewed, concerning the effects on emotion of lesions to temporal-lobe structures, were often contradictory. It is likely that these divergent results were in part due to variations in the lesioning procedures used by the various investigators. An exception would be those cases in which altered emotion was a secondary symptom of a lesion-induced neural disorder—for example, the epilepsy observed by Green and his associates (1957a, 1957b). In those studies that attempted to clarify the functions of the amygdala in emotion, variations in lesioning procedures would have resulted in different portions of the amygdaloid complex, surrounding areas, and adjacent structures being damaged.

Within the temporal-lobe region, we could expect to find regions that exert opposite influences over the expression of emotional behavior. More specifically, we could expect to find both excitatory and inhibitory mechanisms, the functions of which are normally coordinated. However, a brain lesion might differentially affect their activities. When brain lesions produce a decrease in emotional reactivity (that is, a docile animal), it is likely that normally excitatory influences over emotional behavior have been differentially disrupted. The animal's tolerance to annoying stimuli has been considerably raised. On the other hand, if a brain lesion yields a savage beast, an inhibitory mechanism has been interrupted. The animal's tolerance to annoying stimuli has been significantly lowered. It has lost its ability to inhibit an emotional outburst to a trifling, innocuous stimulus.

The evidence to be reviewed below argues for the existence of *two neural systems that mediate emotion: an excitatory system and an inhibitory system.* The same concept can be used to describe how the brain mediates all overt behaviors, as will be seen in later chapters. The use of the term *system* rather than *center* to describe brain control of behavior is important in that it emphasizes some principles of neural organization that were presented in Chapter 3. In that chapter, I indicated that the brain is a dynamic organization of distinct but highly interrelated structures. Further, I suggested that neural structures are organized into a hierarchy or "chain of command," with different levels profoundly affecting the activity of other levels. The lowest levels of the brain are those that developed first in the course of evolution, and they are responsible for the basic expression of behavior. Higher levels in the brain function to make the behavior more goal oriented or stimulus directed. The higher levels "polish" behavior.

The functions of excitatory and inhibitory systems are coordinated under normal circumstances. For the occurrence of an emotional behavior or some other behavioral response, increased activity in the excitatory system is required. It would be maladaptive for this system to operate at full capacity at all times, regardless of the intensity of the stimulus. Thus, the influence of an inhibitory or regulatory system is required. The inhibitory system serves to regulate the amount of activation of the excitatory system. The end product of the interactions between the excitatory and inhibitory systems is the observed behavior of an organism. This process of interaction, which yields a net expression of behavior, is probably analogous to the process that occurs at the synaptic level—**central summation.** As was indicated in Chapter 2, central summation refers to the algebraic summation of EPSPs and IPSPs on the postsynaptic membrane. If the sum is above the threshold level required to fire the neuron, an action potential will be generated. At the more global level of excitation versus inhibition, if the level of activity in an excitatory system significantly surpasses the influences exerted by the inhibitory system, then behavior will occur. The strength of the behavior response will depend upon the difference in the activity of these systems.

We'll next examine the evidence that supports the existence of neural systems regulating the initiation and inhibition of emotion. We will move up through a series of neural levels, or steps in the chain of command. When I indicate that stimulation produces a certain effect, remember that stimulation is generally equivalent to increasing the activity or influence of a system. In contrast, a lesion disrupts the functions of a system. Thus, stimulation of the excitatory system will yield an expression of emotion, while disrupting its normal functions by lesioning a portion of this system will produce an animal whose ability to express emotional behavior is impaired. In contrast, if an experimenter stimulates the inhibitory system to increase its influences, ongoing emotional behavior will be inhibited. Destroying a portion of the brain that normally exerts inhibitory influences over emotion will yield an animal that is incapable of effectively inhibiting emotional expression and that therefore reacts to the most inconsequential stimulus with a violent rage response.

Research Findings

Hypothalamus. The importance of the hypothalamus in emotional behavior was established when Hess, in 1928, showed that a display of rage could be elicited in otherwise normal cats by stimulation of the hypothalamus. This finding was later independently made by Ranson (1934). At about this same time, Bard (1928) demonstrated that emotional expression could still be elicited in cats after all brain tissue rostral, dorsal, and lateral to the hypothalamus had been removed. Emotional behavior failed to occur, however, if the brain stem was truncated at any level below the caudal hypothalamus. Although the rage response observed by Bard contained both visceral and behavioral components, nevertheless the behavior outburst was poorly coordinated and directed. This observation indicated the importance of higher brain levels in the elaboration of emotional behavior.

Bard's observations shed light on the functions performed by the hypothalamus in mediating behavior. It is generally agreed that the hypothalamus regulates the expression of basic drive states and related behaviors that are necessary for survival of the individual and the species. It does this in two ways. First, the hypothalamus plays a part in the expression of observable behavior responses. As Bard's analysis of hypothalamic control of emotional expression indicated, the function of this structure in mediating behavior is gross control yielding relatively undifferentiated expressions of behavior. Higher brain levels elaborate on and refine these expressions of behavior to make them more stimulus directed, or goal oriented.

The second contribution of the hypothalamus to behavior processes is made through its action as the highest integration level for the autonomic nervous system. The **autonomic nervous system** is the part of the nervous system that controls visceral functions of the body. Autonomic activities include the regulation of arterial pressure, cardiac output, gastrointestinal functions, urinary output, sweating, body temperature, endocrine-gland functions, and many other activities. The hypothalamus, through its control of the autonomic nervous system, prepares the organism, physiologically, to engage in a particular behavior pattern.

With regard to this second function, we can think of the hypothalamus as translating instructions from higher brain levels into the physiological correlates of the behavior being exhibited. For example, under high stress such as would occur during emotion or during an emergency, hypothalamic influences result in increased secretion of epinephrine (adrenalin) and norepinephrine into the blood stream from the *medulla* of the *adrenal glands*. The circulating epinephrine and norepinephrine have diffuse effects on various tissues of the body. These effects are all adaptive for emotional behavior in that they prepare the animal for performing overt responses such as attacking or fleeing.

To prepare the organism for action, there is an immediate increase in heart rate and respiration, and the bronchioles of the lungs are dilated so that more oxygen is absorbed into the bloodstream. Blood flow is increased to the muscles and to the brain so that these organs can function more effectively. Sweating increases to cool the body. The eyes dilate, and the body hair stands on end. Moreover, bodily processes that do not contribute to preparedness for action are inhibited by the adrenal secretions. Digestive and eliminative processes, for instance, are shut off.

The anatomy of the hypothalamus was pictured in Figure 3-13. It will be helpful to you to refer back to that figure while reading the discussion that follows.

A number of investigations have attempted to define the functions of different hypothalamic regions in emotion. Early research by Ingram, Barris, and Ranson (1936) and Ranson (1939) demonstrated that lesions in the caudal hypothalamus of monkeys produced a loss in emotional responsiveness as well as a generally somnolent state (decreased level of arousal). As you may remember from previous chapters, the posterior hypothalamus contains fibers of the ascending reticular activating system. Hence, the primary effect of the lesion may have been to produce a lowered state of arousal; chronically drowsy animals can't be very ferocious.

Another classic study on the role of the hypothalamus in control of emotional behavior was conducted by Wheatley (1944). Wheatley reported that discrete bilateral lesions of the ventromedial hypothalamic nuclei produced extremely savage behavior in cats. From Wheatley's description of his subjects' postoperative behavior, the reader gets a very vivid picture of these "savage beasts" hotly pursuing the experimenters around the lab. In interpreting the significance of his findings, Wheatley essentially hypothesized that he had destroyed an inhibitory region for emotional behavior. He suggested that the resultant behavior may have been due to the unbalanced, or unregulated, activity of the lateral hypothalamus. As you'll see in the next chapter, a similar interaction between the ventromedial and lateral hypothalamus has been proposed to account for the regulation of eating and drinking.

Wheatley's hypothesis that the lateral hypothalamus contains pathways involved in the initiation of emotional expression was confirmed by electrical-stimulation studies. For example, Wasman and Flynn (1962) demonstrated that electrical stimulation of the lateral hypothalamus of chronically implanted cats produced effective and well-directed attack behavior. Wheatley's suggestion that interactions between the ventromedial and lateral hypothalamus are intimately involved in emotional behavior was also verified by later researchers. Several studies have shown that severing the fiber pathways between the ventromedial and lateral hypothalamus produces heightened emotionality in rats (Paxinos & Bindra, 1972, 1973; Sclafani, 1971).

Although these results all indicate that basic emotional expression is apparently organized at the hypothalamic level, nevertheless, the integrity of this region is not absolutely essential for the expression of complex emotional behaviors. Ellison and Flynn (1968) reported that cats on which knife cuts had been used to isolate the hypothalamus and create a "hypothalamic island" were still able to display aggressive responses when provoked by a pinch on the tail or the sight of a mouse. This finding underscores the fact that there is simply no single area of the brain that has complete control over any behavior.

Research by John P. Flynn and his associates over the years has done much to clarify our understanding of the interactive influences of different levels of the brain on complex emotional responses. In their elegant series of experiments, the following procedure was employed. For their experimental subjects, only cats that would not attack rats spontaneously were used. Most of their laboratory cats fell into this category. When a rat was placed into a cage with an unstimulated cat, the cat remained quiet. However, as soon as the hypothalamus was stimulated in these chronically implanted cats, the cat approached and either struck or bit the rat. The attack stopped as soon as the current was turned off. In their research, Flynn and his associates have accomplished two major aims. First, they have detailed the characteristics of the attack response elicited by hypothalamic stimulation, and, second, they have demonstrated the influences of higher neural levels on this hypothalamically elicited attack behavior. Their work is reviewed by Flynn (1967) and by Flynn, Vanegas, Foote, and Edwards (1970). We will consider the influences of higher levels on hypothalamically elicited attack later in this chapter. The characteristics of this elicited attack response are as follows.

Flynn and his colleagues have described two quite different forms of directed attack that may be elicited by hypothalamic stimulation: **affective attack,** in which the animal shows full-blown rage and attacks, and **quiet biting attack,** in which the cat quietly stalks the rat, pounces, and kills. Flynn observed that quiet biting attack resembles normal predatory behavior of the cat. These two forms of attack are pictured in Figure 8-2. The following passage from Flynn et al. (1970) clearly describes these two forms of attack.

> Affective attack is characterized by a pattern of pronounced sympathetic arousal commonly regarded as indicative of feline rage. The response invariably begins with behavioral alerting and dilation of the pupils. At lower stimulus intensities, alerting constitutes the extent of the response, even if one stimulates for as long as 2 minutes.
> As one increases the stimulus intensity up to attack threshold, in addition to the initial alerting, piloerection becomes prominent, especially along the midline of the back. The

tail becomes bushy and fluffed out. Occasionally the ears go back. Hissing occurs alternately with low growls. Urination often occurs on the first trial of a session. If sitting, the animal leaps to its feet and begins to move with head low to the ground, back arched, claws unsheathed, hissing and/or snarling, sometimes salivating profusely, and breathing deeply. The cat either comes up to the rat directly or circles to the rear of the cage and then approaches the rat. The cat stands poised, appearing to watch the rat intensely, while the affective aspect of the reaction becomes still more pronounced. After a second or two, the cat raises a paw with claws unsheathed and then strikes with its paws in a series of swift, accurate blows. Any sudden movement of the rat serves to trigger the attack, but attack will occur even if the rat remains motionless. In some instances, the

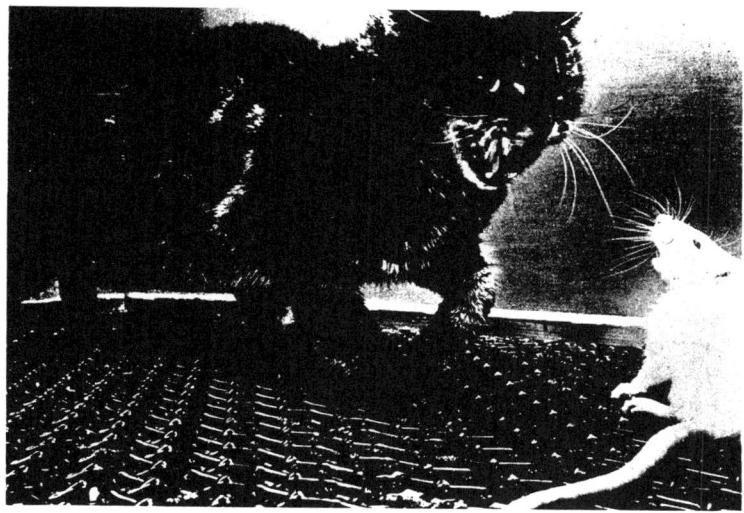

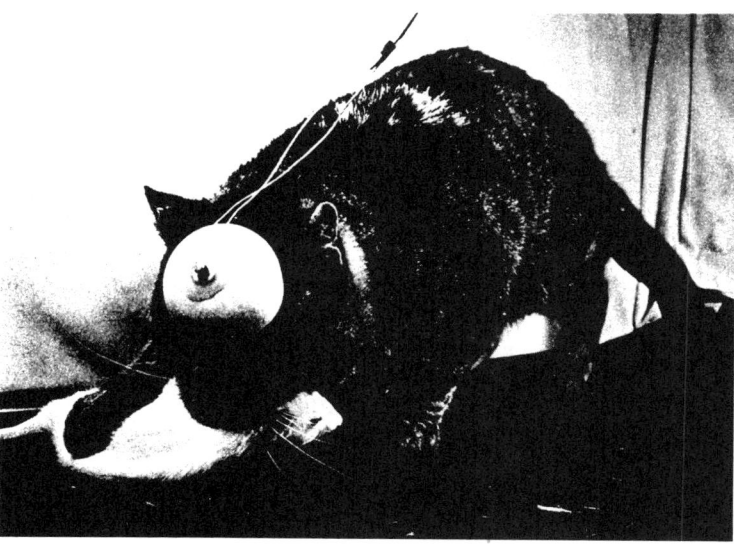

Figure 8-2 Affective attack, involving a display of rage, is shown at the top. Quiet biting attack is shown in the lower photograph. From "The Neural Basis of Aggression in Cats," by J. P. Flynn. In D. C. Glass (Ed.) Neurophysiology and Emotion. *Copyright 1967 by the Rockefeller University Press and the Russell Sage Foundation. Reprinted by permission.*

cat, instead of delivering discrete blows with a single paw, springs at the rat with a high-pitched scream and pounces, tearing at the rat with its claws. If the stimulus is continued, the cat will savagely bite the rat, although the initial part of the attack is clearly with its claws.

The second form of attack pattern [quiet biting attack] reminds observers of an animal stalking a prey. At lower intensities, the alerting response, accompanied by mydriasis, is quite sudden and discrete. The cat often leaps to its feet almost with the onset of the stimulus and attentively looks about from side to side. If the stimulus is continued, it will walk about the cage but will ignore the rat. At higher stimulus intensities, above attack threshold, the cat moves swiftly with its nose low to the ground and hair slightly on end.

Sometimes the cat's nose twitches slightly, as if it were sniffing. The cat usually goes directly to the rat and bites viciously at its head and neck. The cat uses its paws primarily to knock the rat on its back in order to get at its throat. The paws are used neither to deliver discrete blows nor to rake the rat with the claws. Although the cat will sometimes bite the rat's stomach or back first, biting is ultimately aimed at the head and neck. On some trials, the cat circles around the observation box a few times, ignoring the rat or sniffing at it in passing. In the course of circling, the cat will suddenly pounce on the rat and savagely tear at it with its mouth. This circling behavior does not constitute a stereotyped motor response, in that it does not occur regularly nor is it always in the same direction for a given animal, although there is a tendency for it to be the side contralateral to the one stimulated.

The stalking attack is characterized, especially at low stimulus intensities, by only minimal signs presumed indicative of feline rage. Piloerection is present down the midline. The animals never growl, emit high-pitched screams, nor salivate profusely. The cat's movement around the cage, however, is quicker and more persistent. Although this prowling or stalking behavior is never as dramatic as the presumably "enraged" attack, it is, in reality, more effective and deadly, as far as the rat is concerned [pp. 138–139].*

Flynn and his associates report that on occasion mixed behaviors, with some elements of both affective and quiet biting attack, will occur. Some cats will show affective arousal and a biting mode of attack while others will show a stalking attack with an occasional hiss or snarl. Some research has also been conducted to determine the selection of an object of attack. Flynn and his associates found that, if cats are faced with a choice of attacking either horsemeat or an anesthetized rat, they will regularly choose the rat. Levison and Flynn (1965) found that seven of nine cats given a choice of an anesthetized rat, a stuffed rat, and, as a third object, a hairy toy dog, a foam-rubber block, or a styrofoam block never bit the foam-rubber or the styrofoam blocks when hypothalamic stimulation was applied. Furthermore, eight of the nine cats regularly chose either the stuffed or the anesthetized rat. Finally, if cats are starved for 72 hours and then given their first food in a cage with a rat present, they will stop eating to attack the rat when stimulated (Flynn, 1967).

In summary, the data obtained by Flynn and his colleagues clearly showed that hypothalamic stimulation activates neural mechanisms or portions of a system concerned with the patterning of attack behaviors that represent complex emotional responses. Although the two forms of attack may be elicited by stimulation of closely adjacent brain regions and although mixed patterns sometimes occur, nevertheless it appears likely that there are two separate pathways traveling through the lateral

*From "Neural Mechanisms Involved in a Cat's Attack on a Rat," by J. P. Flynn. In R. E. Whalen, R. F. Thompson, M. Verzeano, and N. M. Weinberger (Eds.), *The Neural Control of Behavior.* Copyright 1970 by Academic Press. Reprinted by permission.

hypothalamus that mediate these two response patterns (Chi & Flynn, 1971). The
pathway mediating quiet biting attack travels through the lateral hypothalamus,
while the pathway involved in affective attack lies close to the midline of the brain.
Another accomplishment of Flynn and his associates has been to determine the
effects of higher neural levels on hypothalamically elicited attack. We will consider
that work later in this section.

Lateral hypothalamic stimulation has also been shown to elicit mouse killing in
both rats (King & Hoebel, 1968; Panksepp, 1971) and opposums (Roberts, Steinberg,
& Means, 1967). These findings provide additional support for the view that the
lateral hypothalamus is normally involved in attack behavior. Other studies have
investigated mouse killing by rats in an attempt to determine how this behavior is
chemically coded in the brain. Two types of rats were used in these inquiries:
normally nonkilling rats and killing rats. The results of these studies at least suggested
that this form of predatory behavior is cholinergically mediated—that is, that fibers
that either secrete or are sensitive to the cholinergic synaptic transmitter acetylcholine
mediate this behavior pattern.

Smith, King, and Hoebel (1970) reported that central injections of cholinergic
but not adrenergic agents into the lateral hypothalamus elicited mouse killing in
normally nonkilling rats. In contrast, the injection of the cholinergic blocking agent
atropine into the lateral hypothalamus suppressed killing of mice by killer rats.
Bandler, using lower drug doses, was able to demonstrate a facilitation of killing (that
is, an increase in the speed of attack) when cholinergic agents were injected into the
lateral hypothalamus of killer rats but was unable to replicate the conversion of non-
killers to killers (Bandler, 1969, 1970, 1971a, 1971b). Neither of the results originally
reported by Smith and his associates was replicated in a more recent study, using
still lower drug doses, by Lonowski, Levitt, and Larson (1973). In fact, Lonowski
and his associates found that cholinergic agents actually inhibited killing, while
atropine had no effect on this behavior. The reason for these conflicts is not immediately apparent. It is undoubtedly related in some way to drug doses, but the exact
relationship is unclear. Nevertheless, these experiments represent some attempts
to unravel the chemical coding involved in the neural systems mediating complex
emotional behavior patterns.

Thalamus. Studies of the functions of the thalamus followed Papez's proposal
that the anterior thalamic nucleus was part of the neural system controlling emotion.
(The major thalamic nuclei were diagramed in Figures 3-9 and 3-10.) In accord with
the Papez model, Schreiner, Rioch, Pechtel, and Masserman (1953) found that lesions
carefully restricted to the anterior thalamic nuclei produced a decrease in emotional
reactivity in cats. This finding was later replicated by Masserman and Pechtel (1956).
However, Brierley and Beck (1958) were unable to confirm these findings; they found
no changes in emotion in either cats or monkeys following lesions to the anterior
thalamic nuclei. Thus, the data are suggestive but not conclusive that the anterior
thalamic nuclei are involved in the initiation of emotional behavior.

The dorsomedial thalamic nucleus has also been implicated in emotion.
Schreiner and his associates (1953) found that cats with bilateral lesions to this
nucleus showed increased irritability and rage, but Brierley and Beck (1958) reported
that similar lesions caused a loss of emotional reactivity and fear reactions in
monkeys. Other researchers, using rats as their subjects, have noted no alterations in
emotionality after dorsomedial thalamic lesions (for example, Eichelman, 1971;

Means, Huntley, Anderson & Harrell, 1973). Although some of these results suggest that the dorsomedial nucleus is involved in emotion, the nature of that involvement is unclear.

Research by MacDonnell and Flynn (1964) and by Siegel, Bandler, and Flynn (1972) has helped to explain the discrepancies found in these studies. They found that stimulation of sites in the midline portion of the dorsomedial nucleus would produce attack behaviors similar to those observed following hypothalamic stimulation. If this stimulation was combined with hypothalamic stimulation, then attack was facilitated. These results support the existence of fiber pathways concerned with the initiation of emotion in the dorsomedial thalamic nuclei. In contrast, other points were found in the dorsomedial nuclei that, when stimulated, would suppress or inhibit hypothalamically elicited attack. Thus, it appears that there are pathways traveling through this region that mediate both the initiation and inhibition of emotional behavior. The discrepant findings may therefore have reflected slight differences in the extent of the dorsomedial lesions—differences that would have resulted in the two systems being unequally disrupted.

Amygdala. In the findings reviewed earlier regarding the effects of bilateral amygdalectomy on emotion, you saw that some investigators reported that savage behavior followed such lesions while others reported placidity. As I noted, it is likely that the amygdala exerts both excitatory and inhibitory influences over emotion—that is, that both systems are present within this structure. There is evidence available to support this conclusion, and some of it provides an excellent example of the interactions that occur among brain levels in the regulation of behavior processes. The basic subdivisions and nuclei of this structure were described earlier in this chapter and appear in Figure 8-1.

Data supporting a dual role of the amygdala in emotion have been published by Egger and Flynn (1962, 1963, 1967), who examined the effects of concurrent amygdaloid stimulation on hypothalamically elicited attack. In these studies, hypothalamic stimulation was used to induce cats to attack rats. When amygdala stimulation was superimposed on the hypothalamic stimulation, the attack response was either suppressed or facilitated depending upon which region of the amygdala was stimulated. A marked and consistent suppression of attack was produced by stimulation of either the basal medial nucleus or the anterior and medial portions of the lateral nucleus. In contrast, stimulation of the dorsolateral section of the posterior portion of the lateral nucleus facilitated hypothalamically elicited attack, although the facilitating effect was much less pronounced than was the inhibitory effect.

Amygdaloid stimulation has also been shown to modify hypothalamically elicited flight. Like aggressive responses, flight, or escape behavior, can be elicited by hypothalamic stimulation (Hunsperger, 1956; Roberts, 1958; Stokman & Glusman, 1969). In a study examining the effects of amygdala stimulation on hypothalamically elicited flight, Stokman and Glusman (1970) found that electrical stimulation of the basolateral nuclear group of the amygdala in cats significantly facilitated flight. This observation was in accord with Ursin and Kaada's (1960) finding that electrical stimulation of the lateral amygdala nucleus produced flight responses in cats and Ursin's (1965a) finding that lesions to this same nucleus significantly reduced flight behavior.

Cingulate Gyrus and Septal Area. We will consider the cingulate gyrus and the septal area together here and again in Chapter 10 ("The Anatomical Locus of

Memory"), because these two neural regions appear in many instances to exert equal but opposite influences over behavior patterns. This point will be elaborated on in Chapter 10, but for now let me indicate that many studies have shown that in general the cingulate gyrus performs an excitatory or facilitating function while the septal region exerts inhibitory influences over behavior. With regard to emotion, for example, Siegel and Skog (1970) found that septal stimulation increased the speed of hypothalamically elicited attack.

Siegel and Chabora (1971) investigated the effects of stimulation of the cingulate gyrus on hypothalamically elicited attack and found results inconsistent with the idea that the cingulate gyrus serves an excitatory function in the mediation of behavior. They reported that stimulation of the anterior cingulate region suppressed hypothalamically elicited attack. In one cat, a site in the posterior cingulate gyrus was found in which stimulation significantly facilitated attack, but this was an isolated observation. It is possible, however, that both types of influences exist in the cingulate gyrus. It may be hard to demonstrate the existence of a facilitating effect of such a high level of neural organization on a relatively primitively organized form of behavior expression. Future research like Siegel and Chabora's will have to further clarify the functions of this region. The following data represent the predominant findings regarding the influences exerted by the cingulate gyrus and septal area in emotion.

Bilateral anterior cingulate gyrus ablations in monkeys were reported by Smith (1944) and Ward (1948) to produce behavior changes in the direction of greater tameness and a decrease in fear and rage responses to humans. Glees, Cole, Whitty, and Cairns (1950) generally confirmed these observations, but they reported that the decreased emotional reactivity was short-lived, disappearing after six weeks to three months. Mirsky, Rosvold, and Pribram (1957) and Pribram and Fulton (1954) have also emphasized the limited duration of such taming effects. Similar lesions in psychotic humans reportedly lead to reductions in aggression and compulsive fear (Le Beau, 1954; Whitty, Duffield, Tow, & Cairns, 1952). More recently, Ursin (1969) found that cingulate lesions altered neither flight nor defensive behavior, but these behaviors may be so primitively organized that the cingulate region does not contribute greatly to their elaboration.

The effects of septal lesions on emotional behavior have received a lot of experimental attention. Rats with lesions limited to the septal region usually show dramatic increases in rage reactions and become hyperemotional immediately after surgery (Brady & Nauta, 1953, 1955; King, 1958). These emotional changes are often called the **septal rage syndrome.** They disappear over time, usually persisting for about two to four weeks. In agreement with this finding, it has been reported by several authors that septal lesions will also produce an increase in shock-induced fighting in rats (Ahmad & Harvey, 1968; Eichelman, 1971; Miczek & Grossman, 1972). Shock-induced fighting is what occurs when two animals are placed together in an arena that does not permit escape and an electric shock is delivered to their feet (Ulrich & Azrin, 1962). Septal lesions increased the number of attacks following the administration of shock in this situation.

Although the septal syndrome is easily observed in rats, it is more difficult to observe in other species, if it occurs at all. Sodetz, Matalka, and Bunnell (1967) were unable to produce the septal syndrome in hamsters, and Buddington, King, and Roberts (1967) were unable to demonstrate this phenomenon in monkeys. Although Moore (1964) found some hyperemotionality in cats following septal lesions, Bond, Randt, Bidder, and Rowland (1957) reported that bilateral septal ablations in cats resulted in no increase in rage reactions.

A number of investigators have attempted to clarify further the nature of the septal syndrome in rats. Gotsick and Marshall (1972) reported that the passage of time is not the only factor resulting in a lessening of the septal syndrome. They found that, if the septally lesioned animals were handled daily, normal levels of emotionality could be regained as early as six days after surgery. The age of the animals at the time of surgery also affects the duration of the septal syndrome in rats. Phillips and Lieblich (1972) found that lesions made shortly after weaning when the rats were approximately 20–25 days old produced only transient hyperemotionality. However, if the lesions were made when the rats were 55–65 days old, the alterations in emotion were of much greater duration. Finally, even after the hyperemotionality abates, septal animals retain some of their increased sensitivity to stimulation. Lints and Harvey (1969) and Lubar, Brener, Deagle, Numan, and Clemens (1970) found that "recovered" rats still showed enhanced reactions to shocks administered to the feet.

Hippocampus. Investigations of the role of the hippocampus in emotional behavior have produced conflicting results. For example, Orbach, Milner, and Rasmussen (1960) reported that bilateral hippocampal lesions produced marked and chronic ferocity in monkeys. Earlier in this chapter, I indicated that Green and his associates (1957a, 1957b) had found that lesions encroaching on the hippocampus yielded increased emotionality, but, in their cats, the behavior alterations were apparently a secondary symptom of a lesion-induced epileptic condition. In contrast, Fuller and his associates (1957) observed that bilateral hippocampal lesions caused a loss of social dominance in dogs, and Kim, Kim, Kim, Kim, Chang, Kim, and Lee (1971) reported a decrease in fear and aggressiveness in hippocampectomized rats. Similarly, Eichelman (1971) found that hippocampal lesions yielded significant decreases in shock-induced fighting in rats. Finally, Allen (1948) observed no emotional changes in dogs following bilateral removal of the hippocampus.

My own rather informal, anecdotal observations of the effects of bilateral hippocampal lesions on the emotional responsiveness of rats have led me to believe that there is simply not a consistent effect. Sometimes the lesioned animals show either no change or a slight decrease in emotionality. Sometimes the hippocampal ablations yield a very aggressive, savage rat. It's likely that the hippocampus has a dual role in the control of emotional behavior—that is, that it exerts both facilitating and inhibitory influences. Differential disruption of these influences will produce either tameness or increased emotionality. There is both anatomical and behavioral evidence to support the idea that the hippocampus serves two functions in emotion.

Anatomically, the hippocampus is interconnected with the cingulate gyrus, via the cingulum bundle, and the septum, via the fornix. In the last section, you saw that the septum exerts primarily inhibitory influences while the cingulate gyrus has facilitatory influences on emotion. Thus, the hippocampus may produce or modify both inhibitory and excitatory effects on emotion through its interconnections with these and other regions.

Behavioral evidence to support a dual function of the hippocampus in emotion comes from work conducted by Flynn and his associates. Siegel and Flynn (1968) examined the modulatory role exerted by different hippocampal regions over hypothalamically elicited attack behavior in the cat. The hippocampus of the cat is an apostrophe-shaped structure, and for convenience it is often divided into the dorsal and ventral sectors (see Figure 11-2). Siegel and Flynn found that, when the dorsal hippocampus was stimulated at the same time as the hypothalamus, normal attack toward a rat was delayed. On the other hand, stimulation of a region in the ventral hippocampus led to facilitation; that is, it speeded up the attack. Additional localization studies are needed to clarify the functions of the hippocampus in emotion; nevertheless, the available evidence suggests that this structure may exert both excitatory and inhibitory influences over this form of behavioral expression.

Prefrontal Cortex. The functions of the frontal pole—that is, the prefrontal association cortex—in the regulation of emotional behavior have received a lot of attention from both experimental brain researchers and human neurosurgeons since Fulton and Jacobsen (1935) reported that bilateral prefrontal lesions of a chimpanzee apparently reduced reactions to frustrating situations. Fulton and Jacobsen's observations served as a basis for legitimating and rationalizing the use of psychosurgery in the treatment of human behavioral disorders. Moniz (1936), a Portuguese neurosurgeon, pioneered the procedure of surgically undercutting the frontal lobes of psychotic patients displaying aggressive reactions, with some promising results. Later, several neurosurgeons replicated his findings (for example, Freeman & Watts, 1950; Scoville, 1960), while others did not (for example, Mettler, 1952). I'll elaborate on this and related work in the next section.

Animal lesion studies conducted since Fulton and Jacobsen's work have not yielded consistent effects on emotion following prefrontal ablations. Brody and Rosvold (1952) found that removal of this brain region produced an increase in intraspecific aggression in monkeys, but the same surgery had no effect on aggressiveness in male cats. In contrast, prefrontal ablations reduced the number of aggressive responses made by female cats. Warren (1964) has reported similar effects of prefrontal lesions on the behavior of female cats. In summary, these findings suggest that the effects of prefrontal lesions may be both species and sex specific. However, the sex difference was not replicated in a more recent study by Siegel, Edinger, and Lowenthal (1974).

Siegel and his associates employed the Flynn model, in which the effects of stimulation of various brain regions on hypothalamically elicited attack is evaluated. They examined the effects of prefrontal stimulation on hypothalamically elicited attack, on hypothalamically elicited flight, and on spontaneous attacks on a rat by killer cats. They used cats of both sexes for their subjects. As was indicated above, Siegel and his associates didn't note any differences in their findings according to the sex of their subjects. Their results indicated that the medial aspect of the prefrontal cortex exerted a powerful inhibitory influence over both hypothalamically elicited and spontaneous, naturally occurring, attack. Either significant increases in attack latency or a complete blockage of hypothalamically induced attack were found to occur following stimulation of a number of medial prefrontal sites. If a naturally occurring attack was in progress when prefrontal stimulation was begun, the attack was terminated immediately. A few loci were found that would slightly facilitate hypothalamically elicited attack, but the effect was not significant. No points of stimulation were discovered that would facilitate naturally occurring attack. Finally, no points were found in the prefrontal cortex that would consistently affect hypothalamically induced flight responses.

Another interesting aspect of the Siegel et al. study was the attempt to determine the principal diencephalic target nucleus of the medial regions of the prefrontal cortex that inhibit attack behavior. Lesions were made in the medial prefrontal cortex, and the pathways of degenerating axons were traced. It was found that the overwhelming majority of the fibers ended in the rostral half of the lateral segment of the dorsomedial thalamic nuclei—an area that MacDonnell and Flynn (1968) and Siegel and his associates (1972) were able to stimulate to produce inhibition of hypothalamically elicited attack. Thus, it appears that the major projection system by which the cat's medial prefrontal cortex inhibits the hypothalamus travels by way of the dorsomedial thalamic nucleus. The combination of stimulation and anatomical analysis used by Siegel and his associates is a technique that will aid greatly in clarifying the neural systems or pathways mediating behavior.

Psychosurgery

Psychosurgery refers to the use of brain surgery to treat disorders that are primarily behavioral in nature. It is difficult to discuss this topic in an objective way, since the idea of destroying parts of the brain stirs up such strong feelings. This is certainly understandable, in view of the fact that the brain mediates our capacity to learn and to express emotions. There are also many political and social ramifications of the use of psychosurgery to effect a change in personality and thereby control behavior. For a comprehensive, scientifically accurate, and very readable treatment of the topic of psychosurgery, the reader should consult an excellent book by Elliot S. Valenstein entitled *Brain Control.* This book is the primary source for the discussion that follows.

The Emergence of Psychosurgery as a Therapeutic Tool

When Jacobsen spoke to an assembly of scientists and physicians at the Second International Neurology Congress in London in the summer of 1935 about the calmative effects of frontal-lobe ablations on one of the chimpanzees he and Fulton had been studying, a Portuguese neuropsychiatrist named Egas Moniz was in the audience. After Jacobsen's presentation, Moniz asked whether Jacobsen and Fulton thought this surgical procedure could be applied to humans to alleviate psychotic symptoms. Moniz had missed the main point of the presentation, which was that frontal lesions produce a delayed-response deficit, which will be described in Chapter 10. The calmative effect, which was noted in only one subject, was only an incidental finding. Nevertheless, Moniz grasped at this straw, and, with the aid of Almeida Lima, he performed the first human lobotomy in Lisbon on November 12, 1935. Moniz was awarded the Nobel Prize in Medicine in 1949 for developing his radical treatment procedure.

The first human lobotomy performed by Moniz was accomplished by injection of alcohol into the frontal lobes, but later he developed a technique of cutting six cores of tissue out of the frontal cortex on each side. In reporting on his first 20 patients, Moniz stated that all had survived, 7 were recovered, and 7 were improved over their preoperative condition. The other 6 did not improve. He also reported that his best results were achieved with agitated depressed patients, whereas operated schizophrenics did not improve (Valenstein, 1973). Moniz did only about 100 such operations, because he wanted to assess the long-term effects of this operation before proceeding on a larger scale. Also, he was rendered a hemiplegic by a bullet in the spine incurred during an assault by one of his lobectomized patients.

The lobotomy technique was introduced into the United States by Freeman and Watts in 1936. They developed a different method for assaulting the frontal lobes—one that involved the use of skull landmarks to locate predetermined areas of the frontal lobes that were to be severed from the remainder of the brain (see Figure 8-3). Depending upon how much of the frontal lobes was separated from the remainder of the brain, Freeman and Watts called their operation *minimal, standard,* or *radical lobotomy.* If the minimal or standard lobotomy did not achieve the desired behavior alterations, a radical lobotomy was often undertaken.

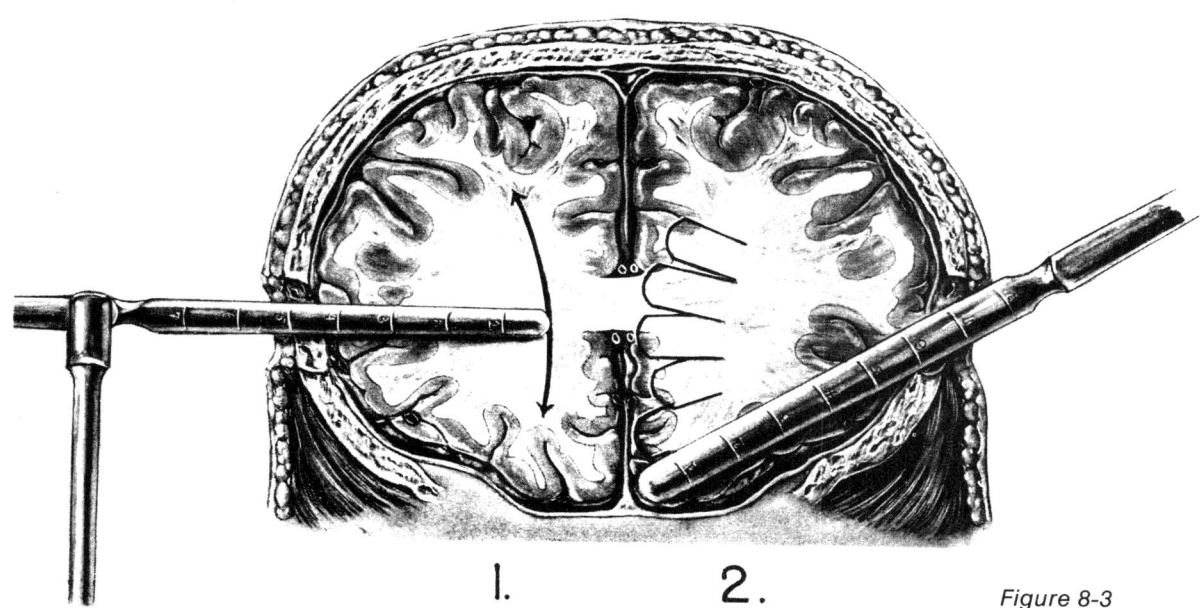

1.   2.

Figure 8-3
*The method of
Freeman and Watts.
After the sweeping
incisions have been
made with the
precision leucotome
(1), they are
deepened with a
somewhat wider
blunt knife called a*
radial stab incisor
(2). From
Psychosurgery in
the Treatment of
Mental Disorders
and Intractable
Pain *(2nd ed.), by
W. Freeman and
J. W. Watts, 1950.
Courtesy of Charles
C Thomas,
Publisher,
Springfield, Illinois.*

Freeman introduced the **transorbital leucotomy** to the United States in 1948. This procedure, which was originally devised by Fiamberti in Italy, consisted of driving a **transorbital leucotome** (surgical ice pick) through the bony cavity above the eye into the base of the frontal lobes. The handle of the leucotome was then swung to sever the fibers in the frontal lobes (see Figure 8-4). Due to the simplicity of this procedure, a great number of these operations were performed. Some were even conducted in a physician's office rather than in a hospital. According to Valenstein (1973), Freeman was reported to have once remarked that "an enterprising neurologist could perform 10–15 supraorbital lobotomies in a morning" (p. 316). Other surgical techniques for accomplishing frontal lobotomies, were to evolve around the world, and from 1945 to 1955 an untold number of psychiatric patients were subjected to this radical treatment procedure. It has been estimated that, in the United States alone, approximately 40,000 to 50,000 prefrontal lobotomies of one type or another were performed.

The wave of psychosurgery was generated by the extreme overcrowding in mental institutions and the lack of effective treatment procedures. With the introduction of psychoactive drugs in the mid-1950s and with growing public awareness of some of the abuses in the use of psychosurgery, the practice of this form of therapy rapidly declined. At present, psychosurgery is still employed, but on a very

Figure 8-4
Diagram showing
the position of the
transorbital
leucotome for
transorbital
leucotomy. From
Psychosurgery in
the Treatment of
Mental Disorders
and Intractable
Pain *(2nd ed.), by*
W. Freeman and
J.W. Watts, 1950.
Courtesy of Charles
C Thomas,
Publisher,
Springfield, Illinois.

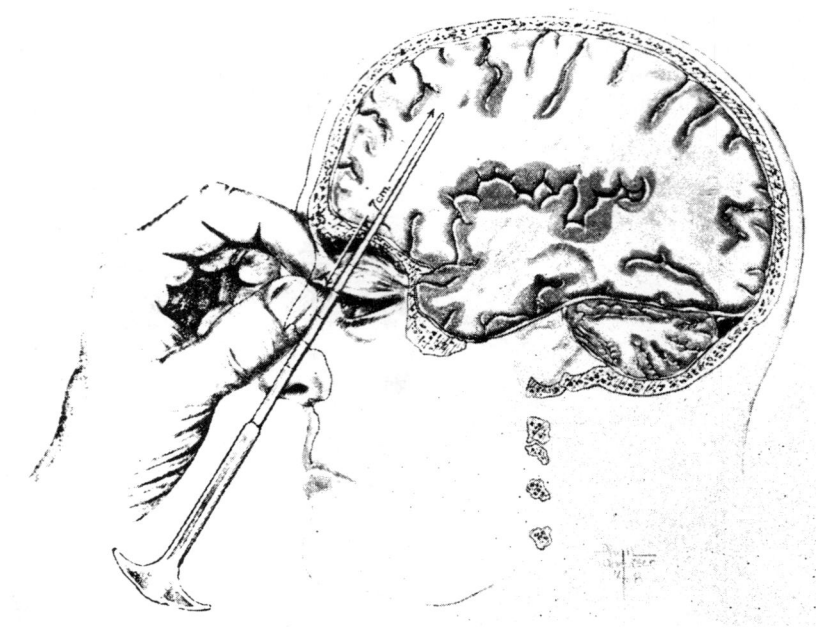

limited basis. Probably no more than 300–400 brain operations for purely psychiatric purposes are performed in the United States each year. Most of these surgeries involve limited lesions and are done by the stereotaxic technique. I will discuss some of these later in this chapter.

Another reason for the decline in popularity of the frontal lobotomy was that it simply did not have consistent effects on behavior. It did not, as some individuals have charged, reduce the patient to a mental "vegetable." On the other hand, it did not, as some of its advocates have argued, produce a miracle cure. Some individuals improved to the point where they could return to society, others became manageable in the institution to which they were confined, and others showed no improvement or actually became worse. Still, with no alternative procedures available at the time, it was in some cases the only method that might produce an improvement in behavior, at least to the point where a dangerously aggressive individual could be managed.

In some cases, the prefrontal lobotomy did cause an intellectual impairment, but it was argued that at least the patients could function in and interact with their environment in a more adaptive fashion than was possible before surgery (Greenblatt & Solomon, 1953). It is difficult to decide, however, whether a patient's mental state could have been improved via some treatment less drastic than brain surgery (Valenstein, 1973). Further, it is difficult to assess whether those people who did improve after psychosurgery would have improved anyway. There has been a striking lack of properly controlled observations attempting to assess the outcome of psychosurgery as a tool for treating mental illness. That is, very few studies have contrasted the results produced by psychosurgery with behavioral changes that occurred over an equivalent period of time in unoperated patients suffering from similar symptoms.

When psychosurgery was first done, the only people selected for this form of treatment were chronic psychotic patients who had not responded to any form of therapy and were therefore considered hopeless in terms of their ability to ever function in society. Some psychosurgeons have commented that it is too late to help an individual who has reached this state and that, if psychosurgery is to help patients, it must be undertaken much earlier in the course of the disorder. As a result, the patients considered today to be the best candidates are individuals suffering from such symptoms as depression, compulsions, obsessions, debilitating anxiety, and extreme aggressive tendencies.

The type of surgeries recently attempted have for the most part involved destruction of structures in the Papez circuit, but limited cutting of the fibers connecting the prefrontal cortex to the rest of the brain is still practiced and recommended by some neurosurgeons. The most popular nonfrontal regions for the psychosurgeons to ablate are the cingulate gyrus, the thalamus, the amygdala, and the hypothalamus. Even with these modern approaches, the question remains as to the effectiveness of this radical procedure. It is easy to find in the literature instances of significant improvement, examples of almost no effect, and instances of the condition worsening after surgery. The following case is an example of a dramatic recovery.

Heimberger, Whitlock, and Kalsbeck (1966) have concluded that bilateral or unilateral amygdalectomy is often successful in treating patients who were not benefited by more traditional forms of therapy, including psychotherapy and drug therapy. They cite several case histories in support of this conclusion, including the one that follows. This patient was suffering from epilepsy and associated hostility and aggressiveness. Much of the time she was locked in solitary confinement because of aggressive and destructive behavior. Although this girl's aggressiveness seemed to be part of her epileptic syndrome, let me emphasize that the actual relationship between epilepsy and violence is quite low.

> Case 26:
> A 15-year-old girl from a broken home was permanently committed to an institution after several months of drug therapy and psychotherapy failed to control her psychomotor seizures or her hostile, aggressive, destructive behavior. She has had no seizures nor behavioral abnormality during the ten months since her right amygdaloid nucleus was destroyed. She has returned to her regular high school and is well accepted [Heimberger et al., 1966, p. 169].

Instances in which an individual who undergoes psychosurgery is later able to return to society, as in the case above, are rare. Usually, the patient is rendered simply "more controllable" or "less agitated" in an institutional setting. In most instances psychosurgery is still used only when all other forms of therapy have failed. It is often hard for the reader of case histories to decide whether the patients are significantly better than they were before surgery. If the criterion is simply that they be less destructive, psychosurgery can often succeed.

The Animal-Research Basis for Psychosurgery

As Valenstein (1973) points out, almost every new technique used in psychosurgery has been directly stimulated by animal experimentation. It is a further fact, although an unfortunate one, that in every case in which psychosurgery methods have evolved from animal experimentation, it is quite clear that the psychosurgeons paid selective attention to only a small part of the animal literature. We saw this to be the case when Moniz was inspired to perform his frontal-lobe assaults on the basis of some incidental remarks made by Jacobsen. There are many other examples of this sort. A striking—and frightening—example of the selective use of small bits of data to support the development of a new psychosurgical technique is the work of Roeder, Orthner, and Müller (1972) of the University of Göttingen in Germany.

For a number of years, these individuals have treated "sexual deviants"—primarily *pedophilic homosexuals*. Pedophiles are men who seek out sexual encounters with young or teenage boys. At the First International Congress for Neurological Sciences, held in Brussels in 1957, Roeder and his associates happened to see Schreiner and Kling's film picturing sexual abnormalities produced by bilateral amygdala lesions. Schreiner and Kling's findings were discussed earlier in this chapter. As you'll remember, the lesioned animals exhibited extreme hypersexuality toward conspecifics of either sex and toward animals of other species. For some reason, Roeder and his colleagues thought that this cat behavior closely resembled "human sexual perversions." They were also struck by the finding that this observed hypersexuality disappeared after supplemental destructions of the ventromedial hypothalamic nuclei. They wrote that "this film convinced us that there were solid reasons for undertaking a therapeutic stereotaxic procedure" (p. 88). As you can probably guess by now, their therapeutic procedure is lesioning of the ventromedial hypothalamic nucleus.

Roeder and his associates also justified their work on the basis of some very controversial and tenuous data published by Dörner, Döcke, and Hinz (1969) that purportedly demonstrated the existence of distinct "male" and "female" "sex centers" in the rat hypothalamus. Supposedly, these centers are related such that one is dominant over the other, depending on the sex of the animal. If one is destroyed, the other will take over. Based on their work with rats, Dörner and his colleagues argued that, if the ventromedial hypothalamic "female sex center" is destroyed, male sexual behavior will become dominant, provided that male sex hormone is available.

As I've indicated before, the concept of centers that regulate behavior has been discarded by modern neuropsychological theory in the face of overwhelming evidence against such a notion. No behavior is dependent on a single brain structure. Systems of interconnected brain regions are responsible for behavior expression. Further, for the human organism, whose sexual orientation and behavior is thought to be almost exclusively the product of learning and experience, it is unlikely that a brain operation could radically affect sexual orientation. Nevertheless, the data presented by Schreiner and Kling and by Dörner and his co-workers provided all the justification Roeder, Orthner, and Müller needed to perform ventromedial hypothalamic lesions on pedophiles and others characterized as sexually "deviant." Their patients have either sought help voluntarily or been referred to them by the courts. In most cases, the ventromedial hypothalamic ablation was unilateral, but in one case a bilateral destruction was performed.

Although their short case histories indicate that some of their patients "were able to stay out of trouble after the operation and experienced a social recovery" (p. 109), there is really very little in their findings to justify such an extreme psychosurgical intervention or the confidence they express about their procedure. The ventromedial nucleus is crucially involved in certain endocrine and visceral functions, and, as you've seen, experimental reports have indicated that bilateral destruction of this nucleus can produce incurably savage behavior. As will be reported in the next chapter, the region of the ventromedial nucleus is also intimately involved in eating and drinking behaviors. Even students with the most elementary knowledge of neural functions would question the wisdom of destroying this portion of the brain. Who knows what neuroendocrine disturbances were produced by these lesions—disturbances that may not become evident for years. This is a clear example of the unwarranted adoption of a psychosurgical procedure from the animal literature on the basis of a partial assessment of only a small portion of the available data.

Overall Evaluation

At the outset, let me emphasize that in most cases psychosurgery is undertaken only after more conventional forms of therapy have been exhaustively employed to no avail. However, abuses have occurred, and for this reason it is essential that review committees composed of psychiatrists, neurosurgeons, lawyers, ministers, scientists, and lay persons be set up (Valenstein, 1973). These committees must be as independent as possible from those recommending the psychosurgical procedure so that the rights and best interests of the patient are clearly not violated.

Brain surgery is not like other forms of therapy. If a mistake is made, the physician cannot go back and repair the damage. The therapist cannot simply discontinue the operation and move on to a new procedure. A brain operation is irreversible and may produce permanent intellectual impairments and physiological disturbances, some of which may not be evident for years. For example, in the case of amygdala lesions, there is a tendency to describe the postoperative behavior of the patients simply in terms of an alleviation of the symptoms, such as hostility and aggressiveness, that were disturbing others. Less attention is paid to alterations in intellectual and emotional capacity. The psychologist Ruth Anderson (1972) describes the behavioral effects of unilateral amygdalectomy (bilateral in two cases) on 13 patients.

> Typically the patient tends to become more inert, and shows less zest and intensity of emotions. His spontaneous activity tends to be reduced, and he becomes less capable of creative productivity, which is independent of the intelligence level [p. 182].

Thus, it is apparent that psychosurgery can have far-reaching consequences for the patient. I would have to conclude that it should be used only on those people who are extremely dangerous to themselves or others and only after all alternative forms of traditional psychotherapy and drug therapy have been seriously attempted. Even at that point, final approval must rest in the hands of a review panel because, once psychosurgery has been completed, there is no turning back.

Chapter Summary and Conclusions

The functions of the brain in regulating emotional behavior were considered in this chapter. The chapter began with a description of some of the classic papers that sparked current interest in neural control of emotion. It was shown that subsequent attempts to clarify these initial results often produced highly conflicting findings.

It was proposed that the basis for the divergent results was the fact that different researchers used different lesioning techniques. These differences resulted in different lesions in the brains of the experimental animals. It was further proposed that neural control of emotion and behavior processes in general is accomplished through the interaction of excitatory and inhibitory influences by neural structures or parts of structures that are organized into systems at different levels of neural integration. These opposing systems normally coordinate their activities in a dynamic fashion analogous to the process of central summation, which occurs at the synaptic level. According to this theory, different lesioning techniques would result in differential disruption of these systems and hence would account for opposite findings following lesions to the same general region or structure. Experimental evidence supporting the existence of response initiation and inhibition systems that control emotion was reviewed. It was seen that opposite influences are often located in different loci within the same structure.

The chapter was concluded with a discussion of the use of psychosurgery as a treatment procedure for human behavioral disorders. The history of psychosurgery and the types of psychosurgical procedures currently being used were reviewed. It was shown that most psychosurgical procedures have been inspired by experimental animal research but that, unfortunately, the initiators of the various methods have based their rationale for using a certain surgical procedure on a partial assessment of only a small portion of the available experimental literature.

Caution in the use of psychosurgery was stressed. A brain operation is irreversible, and the diverse side effects produced by such a procedure may not become apparent for years. Psychosurgery should be employed only after an exhaustive attempt has been made to use all forms of conventional psychotherapy and drug therapy. Further, before such a radical treatment is embarked upon, it should be approved by a review committee whose object is to protect the rights and best interests of the patient.

9
Motivation

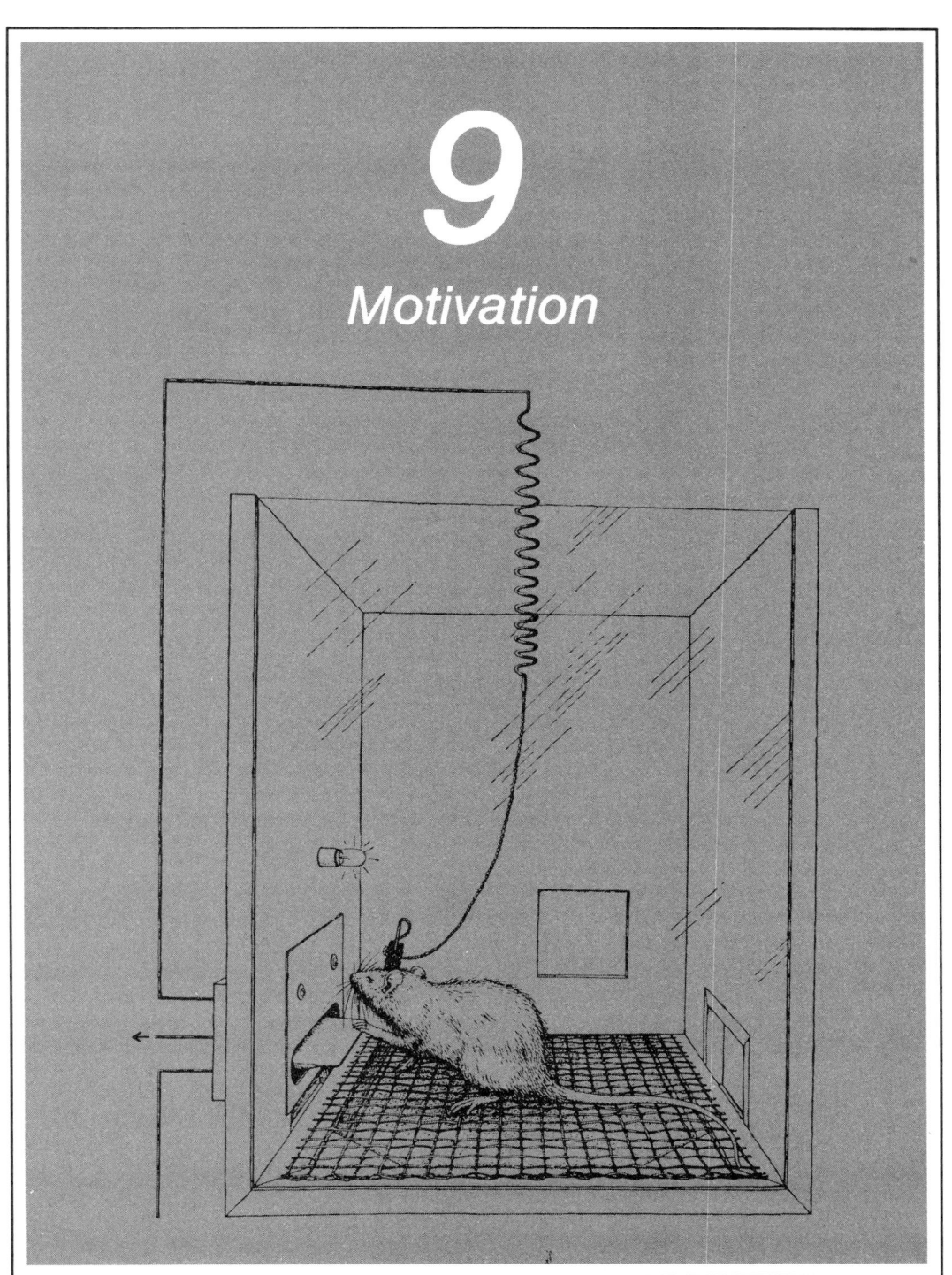

To survive in our environment, we must fulfill certain bodily, or biological, needs. This involves doing such things as eating and drinking, eliminating wastes, breathing air, and regulating our body temperature. If our species is to survive, we must also copulate. Motivation is the driving force, or energizer, of behavior that causes us to act in such a way that these biological needs will be fulfilled. We also say that organisms are motivated to act in a **hedonistic** way; that is, we approach pleasant things and avoid unpleasant ones. This second broad category of motivated behaviors often encompasses emotion, which was discussed in the last chapter.

In this chapter, we'll examine the neural mechanisms and physiological bases for some of these motivated behaviors. The chapter will begin with a description of the neural basis for the **hedonic system**—the system that apparently mediates our experiences of pleasure and pain, or displeasure. As indicated, this topic has to do with both emotion and motivation. It will therefore serve as a good bridge between the two topics. We'll next examine the physiological bases of hunger and thirst, to see how motivation is energized to fulfill bodily needs. Finally, the biological substrates of sexual behavior—behavior that, besides being hedonistic, has the purpose of ensuring survival of the species—will be described.

The Hedonic System: Electrical Self-Stimulation of the Brain

In 1954, James Olds and Peter M. Milner published a paper detailing a remarkable discovery they had made in the fall of 1953—a discovery that was to precipitate a deluge of research. They found that animals will actively seek to deliver very mild electric shock to their brains, just as rats will learn to seek out food. For example, whenever a behavior, such as choosing one of the arms of a T-maze or pressing a bar in an operant apparatus, was followed by electrical stimulation of the brain (ESB), the rat began repeating the response with increasing frequency. The same phenomenon was soon observed in many other species, including the goldfish, pigeon, gerbil, rabbit, cat, dog, goat, monkey, porpoise, and human. It appeared that a "pleasure center" had been discovered. Verbal reports from humans receiving ESB have generally confirmed the hypothesis that ESB is pleasurable. According to Heath (1963), who used ESB as a treatment for persons with a variety of physical and psychological disabilities, the patients reported that ESB resulted in experiences that were generally pleasurable and sexual in nature.

The discovery of the potent effects of ESB was accidental. It is a credit to Olds and Milner that they were able to recognize the potential significance of an incidental observation and quickly zero in on it. Olds (1955) later described how it happened.

> In the Fall of 1953, we were looking for more information about the reticular activating system. We used electrodes permanently implanted in the brain of a healthy, behaving rat. . . . Our systematic aim at the time was to stimulate the reticular formation in a maze to find whether such stimulation might increase attention and learning. . . . Quite by accident, an electrode was implanted in the region of the anterior commissure [a transhemispheric fiber bundle near the septum].
>
> The result was quite amazing. When the animal was stimulated at a specific place in an open field (a large square-shaped arena), he sometimes moved away but he returned and sniffed around that area. More stimulations at that place caused him to spend more of his time there.
>
> Later we found that this same animal could be "pulled" to any spot in the maze by giving a small electrical stimulus *after* each response in the right direction. This was akin to playing the "hot and cold" game with a child. Each correct response brought electrical pulses which seemed to indicate to the animal that it was on the right track.
>
> Still later, the same animal was placed on an elevated T maze. As there was an initial right turn preference, he was forced to the left and stimulated at the end of the left arm. After three such trials, he proceeded to make 10 consecutive runs to the left for electrical stimulation alone, with decreasing running times. Then the stimulus was stopped on the left, and 6 runs were forced to the right with electrical stimulation in the right arm. After this, the animal made 10 runs to electrical stimulation in the right arm. Up to this point, no food had been used in the maze at all.
>
> Afterwards, the animal was starved for 24 hours. Food was put in both arms of the T maze. The animal was given two forced runs to each arm. After this, he made 10 runs to the left, *stopping at the point of stimulation and never going on to the food* [pp. 83–84].*

Following these initial inquiries, experiments were conducted with an operant-conditioning chamber, in which the rat could stimulate its own brain by simply pressing a lever (see Figure 9-1). This allowed the experimenters to translate the animal's desire to receive electrical stimulation of the brain into a measure of response rate. Most of the subsequent research on the ESB phenomenon has been conducted in this type of operant apparatus. In later studies, researchers attempted to define the anatomical substrates of the "reward system" and to determine the similarities between the behavior produced by ESB and that produced by natural rewards such as food and water.

The Anatomical Locus of the Reward System

On the basis of many studies that have been designed to delineate areas of the brain where electrical excitation will sustain self-stimulation, it has generally been concluded that the region of the lateral hypothalamus and medial forebrain bundle is the most active locus—at least for the rat (Gallistel, 1973; Olds & Olds, 1965; Valenstein, 1966). A detailed description of these findings is provided in an excellent review of the self-stimulation literature by Gallistel (1973). As was

*From "Physiological Mechanisms of Reward," by J. Olds. In M. R. Jones (Ed.), *Nebraska Symposium on Motivation,* (Vol. 3). Copyright © 1955 by University of Nebraska Press. Reprinted by permission.

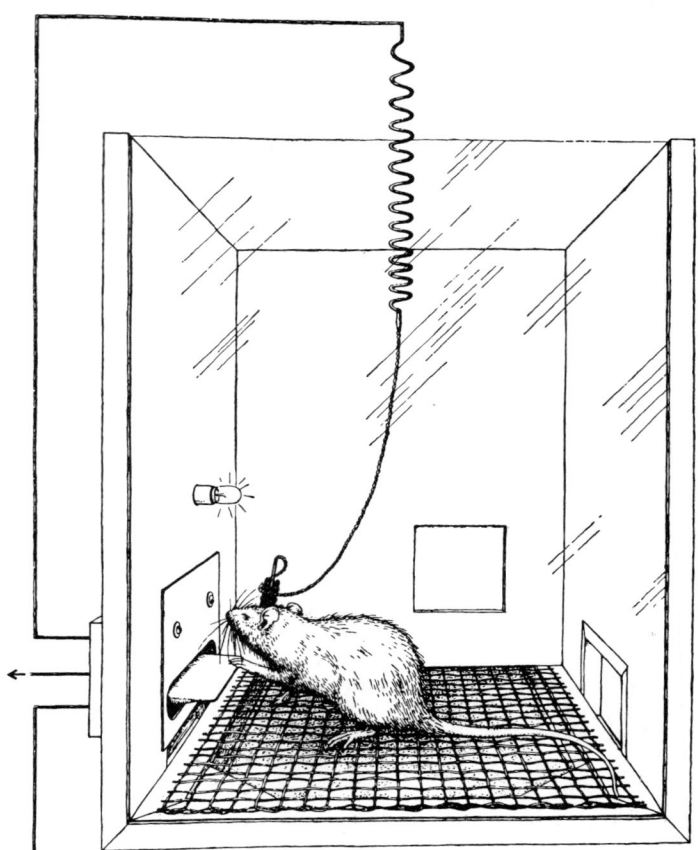

Figure 9-1
A rat in an operant-conditioning chamber. When the rat presses the treadle, it triggers an electric stimulus to its brain and simultaneously records the action via the wire shown at left. From "Pleasure Centers in the Brain," by J. Olds, Scientific American, *1956, 195, 105–116. Copyright © 1956 by Scientific American, Inc. All rights reserved. Reprinted by permission.*

indicated in Chapter 3, the medial forebrain bundle joins the anterior and lateral hypothalamic regions with various loci of the rhinencephalon and limbic regions. Although the ease of producing self-stimulation behavior varies somewhat across species, researchers have been able to demonstrate self-stimulation-producing loci in the amygdala (Brady, 1960; Hodos, 1965; Valenstein & Valenstein, 1964; Wurtz & Olds, 1963), the olfactory bulbs (Phillips & Mogenson, 1969; Routtenberg, 1971; Routtenberg & Olds, 1966), the hippocampus (Routtenberg, 1971; Ursin, Ursin, & Olds, 1966), the septum (Olds & Milner, 1954; Olds & Olds, 1963; Routtenberg, 1971), the cingulate gyrus (Olds & Milner, 1954; Olds & Olds, 1963; Routtenberg, 1971), the thalamus (Cooper & Taylor, 1967; Grastyán & Angyán, 1967; Lilly, 1960), and the caudate nucleus and globus pallidus of the basal ganglia (Brady, 1960; Olds, 1960; Justesen, Sharp, & Porter, 1963; Routtenberg, 1971).

As you can see, self-stimulation can be demonstrated with stimulating electrodes located in most parts of the limbic system. As was indicated, it's generally agreed that the most active loci appear to be in the region of the medial forebrain bundle. However, although the medial forebrain bundle is the most active locus, this pathway does not have to be intact for self-stimulation to occur. Valenstein (1966) concluded that the fiber pathways mediating self-stimulation must be extremely diffuse because he found that extensive lesions in the medial forebrain bundle rostral or caudal to the stimulating electrode had little effect on self-stimulation (Valenstein & Campbell, 1966). Similar results have been published by Lorens (1966). Lorens, too, found that lesions placed simultaneously both caudal and rostral to the stimulating electrode yielded only slight decreases in self-stimulation.

Aversive Effects of ESB

About the same time as Olds and Milner were making their important discovery, Delgado, Roberts, and Miller (1954) reported behavior effects of ESB that seemed to indicate that an aversive state had been produced. Hungry animals would avoid food that had been associated with ESB, and stimulation through these electrode placements could be used, much in the same way as shock, to motivate animals to learn an avoidance task. It was shown, for instance, that cats would learn to turn a wheel to end or avoid the onset of ESB; they would also learn to escape from a compartment in which they had previously been stimulated (Miller, 1961).

An interesting finding is that, with electrodes placed at certain sites, animals will work to turn on ESB and then work to turn it off if it's left on long enough (Bower & Miller, 1958; Roberts, 1958). In the Roberts study, electrodes were placed in the posterior hypothalamus. Cats learned to enter one arm of a three-armed maze to turn on the stimulation and to move into another arm to turn it off. As the intensity of the stimulation increased, they were more likely to stop the ESB when it was on than to turn it on when it was off. The important point here, though, is that both pleasurable and aversive reactions could be produced by stimulation of the same site. It is possible that such an electrode placement activated elements of both a pleasure, or reward, system and an aversive, or punishment, system.

Studies on what anatomical points will produce aversive effects when stimulated have shown that the aversive points are often very close to rewarding sites. Stimulation of points in the midbrain, ventromedial hypothalamic nucleus, thalamus, amygdala, and hippocampus can yield aversive effects (Olds & Olds, 1963; Wurtz & Olds, 1963). An interesting finding is that the pathways mediating aversive ESB reactions overlap a great deal with specific brain loci from which emotional behaviors such as flight, attack, and defense can be elicited with electrical brain stimulation (for example, de Molina & Hunsperger, 1959, 1962; Hess, 1954). Brain loci producing rewarding and aversive effects in the rat brain are shown in Figure 9-2.

Characteristics of Self-Stimulation Behavior

The most striking characteristic of rats' bar-pressing or performing some other learned response to obtain ESB is their apparently insatiable drive for electrical stimulation. Once self-stimulation is initiated, it is extremely intense and persistent. There are many reports in the literature of animals bar-pressing to receive ESB at rates up to 5000 presses per hour, continuing until exhaustion sets in (for example, Olds, 1958b; Ray, Hine, & Bivens, 1968). This phenomenon is graphically portrayed in Figure 9-3. The only natural reward that produces a similar behavior persistence and lack of satiation is a mixture of saccharine and very dilute glucose (Valenstein, Cox, & Kakolewski, 1967).

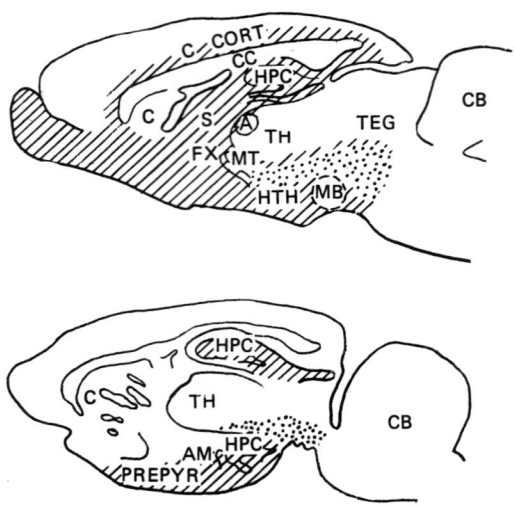

Another notable feature of behavior such as bar-pressing, which is motivated by rewarding ESB, is that, as soon as the reward is no longer given, the animal will almost immediately stop the behavior (Howarth & Deutsch, 1962; Olds, 1955; Seward, Uyeda, & Olds, 1959). This is very different from what occurs when rats or other animals are trained to press a bar for a food or water reward. In this latter case, the animals will usually continue to bar-press for a long time after reinforcement for the response has been discontinued. However, under some conditions, rewarding ESB has been shown to produce as much response persistence after reinforcement has been discontinued as conventional reinforcers do (Gibson, Reid, Sakai, & Porter, 1965; Thompson & Webster, 1974). In the Gibson et al. study, groups of rats were trained to press a bar to make a water dipper come up. For one group, licking the dipper resulted in their obtaining a sugar solution; the other group received rewarding ESB for licking the dipper. When pressing the bar no longer resulted in the dipper being presented, the two groups continued to press the bar for equivalent periods of time.

Because of the rapid decline in responding that usually follows cessation of rewarding ESB, it is often necessary to "prime" an animal during the next training session if bar-pressing is to be shown again (for example, Olds & Milner, 1954; Wetzel, 1963). Priming involves giving the animal a "free stimulation." This is an interesting finding; it's the opposite of what happens with natural rewards. Prefeeding hungry rats about to run a maze for food will cause the animals to run slower (Bruce, 1938; Morgan & Fields, 1938). Priming is not always necessary to initiate responding. Kent and Grossman (1969) found that some "nonpriming" rats never required priming to begin lever-pressing at the beginning of a session. It appeared that the electrodes in the nonprimers were more centrally located in the medial forebrain bundle than were the electrodes of those animals requiring priming.

In giving an overall assessment of the self-stimulation literature, I would have to conclude that positive electrical stimulation of the brain has a very potent effect in energizing behavior, particularly when the ESB is delivered to the region of the lateral hypothalamus and medial forebrain bundle. Positively reinforcing brain stimulation

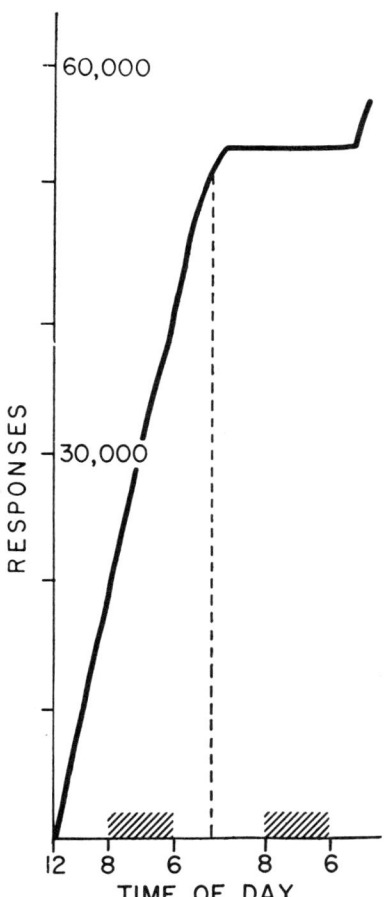

Figure 9-3
A graph of self-stimulation over a 48-hour period. Cumulative response totals are plotted along the ordinate; hours are plotted along the abscissa. The experiment started at noon; crosshatching indicates darkness from 8 P.M. to 6 A.M. The animal (with an electrode implanted in the anterior medial hypothalamus) stimulated itself at a rate of more than 2000 responses an hour for 26 hours, then slept, and then resumed self-stimulation at the same rate. From "Self-Stimulation of the Brain," by J. Olds, Science, *1958, 127, 315–324. Reprinted by permission.*

appears to have effects that are similar to the behavior effects of natural rewards such as food and water. For this reason, the study of the self-stimulation phenomenon may clarify our understanding of how natural rewards affect the central nervous system (Gallistel, 1973). Aversive brain stimulation may similarly have potent motivational effects on behavior. Clarification of aversive brain stimulation may aid our understanding of how punishment affects behavior.

Hunger and Thirst

Many times during the day we say that we're hungry or thirsty, without really being cognizant of the "reasons" why we feel that way. Learning undoubtedly plays a part in these sensations since most of us normally eat three times a day and become hungry partly because it is a normal eating time. When talking about physiological control of hunger and thirst, most physiological psychologists refer to two broad categories of factors that can influence hunger and thirst: *peripheral* factors and *central* factors. Peripheral factors include such things as the composition of the blood, the state of digestive processes, body temperature, and the amount of food currently in the stomach. Central factors are the brain mechanisms that mediate hunger and thirst. As you'll see later in this chapter, central mechanisms have come to mean the hypothalamus and associated subcortical regions. We will examine possible peripheral and central mechanisms in the control of hunger and thirst in the following pages.

Peripheral Mechanisms of Hunger

The Stomach. Peripheral theories of hunger have their roots in the 18th century, when Haller proposed that hunger arises when stomach contractions excite sensory nerves in the stomach. The relation of "hunger pangs" to hunger regulation was put to experimental test in a famous experiment by Cannon and Washburn (1912). In this study, Washburn swallowed a balloon and then inflated it in his stomach. His stomach contractions and his subjective feelings of hunger were then simultaneously recorded, as shown in Figure 9-4. As you can see by examining this figure, there was a high correspondence between the occurrence of stomach contractions and Washburn's subjective feelings of hunger. Washburn did not report feelings of hunger when his stomach was not contracting. As a result of these findings, Cannon and Washburn concluded that the adequate stimulus for hunger is contractions of the stomach.

Figure 9-4
The top record represents intragastric pressure (the small oscillations due to respiration, the large to contractions of the stomach). The second record is the time in minutes (10 minutes). The third record is Washburn's report of hunger pangs, and the lowest record is respiration. From Bodily Changes in Pain, Hunger, Fear and Rage, *by W. B. Cannon. Copyright 1963. Reprinted by permission of the Estate of W. B. Cannon.*

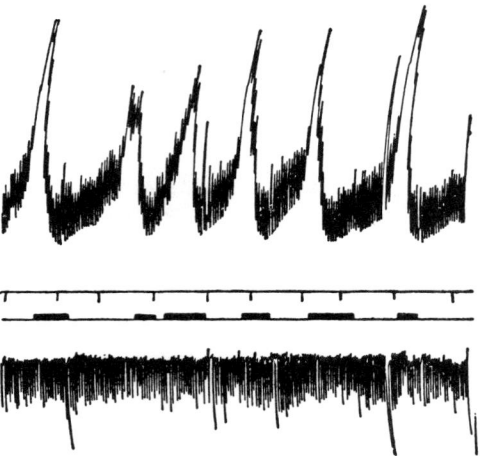

Cannon and Washburn's experimental findings were confirmed in other investigations, but later research found that the stomach contractions they observed were artifacts of the recording method. Davis, Garafalo, & Kveim (1959) recorded stomach contractions using abdominal electrodes rather than a balloon in the stomach. They found results the opposite of those obtained with the inflated-balloon technique. Specifically, they reported that stomach motility was at its lowest when the stomach was empty. Further, they found no correlation between the occurrence of stomach contractions and the subjective experience of hunger. As a result, they suggested that Cannon and Washburn's results may have been an artifact of placing an inflated balloon in the stomach.

Another gastric factor that has been suggested as important in hunger is **stomach distension.** We have all experienced this one—the Thanksgiving glut, as I often call it. Our stomach becomes so full that, even though we would like to eat a third serving of everything on the table, it lets us know that it's time to stop. It seems unlikely, except at extreme degrees of stomach distension such as the Thanksgiving glut, that stomach distension is a major factor regulating hunger. A number of years ago it was shown that, when rats were fed a diet that had been altered so that the food had a nonnutritive but filling material such as cellulose added to it, the rats still maintained a relatively constant caloric intake (Adolph, 1947). This occurred despite the fact that the animals experienced an unusually high degree of stomach distension.

The role of stimuli arising from the stomach in the control of hunger has been brought into further question by studies using animal preparations and human ulcer patients with either parts or all of their stomach removed or the nerve supply to and from their stomach removed by severance of the vagus nerve. The animals still eat, and the human ulcer patients still report sensations of hunger and regulate their diets reasonably well.

Oral Factors. Stimuli arising from the mouth have also been suggested as important peripheral mechanisms regulating hunger. Some very clever experiments by Epstein and Teitelbaum (1962) ruled out the possibility that oral stimuli are critical for the regulation of hunger. In these experiments, oral stimulation was completely bypassed; the animals pressed a lever that delivered a liquid food directly to their stomachs through a tube. The apparatus used for this procedure is shown in Figure 9-5. Under these conditions, the rats would regulate food intake to maintain their

Figure 9-5
(a) The apparatus for intragastric self-injection by the rat. The rat presses the bar in order to activate the pipetting machine, left, and thus deliver a liquid diet from the reservoir, left foreground, through the chronic gastric tube directly into its stomach. (b) The nasopharyngeal gastric tube through which the food is delivered. From "Regulation of Food Intake in the Absence of Taste, Smell, and Other Oropharyngeal Sensations," by A. N. Epstein and P. Teitelbaum, Journal of Comparative and Physiological Psychology, *1962, 55, 753–759. Copyright 1962 by the American Psychological Association. Reprinted by permission.*

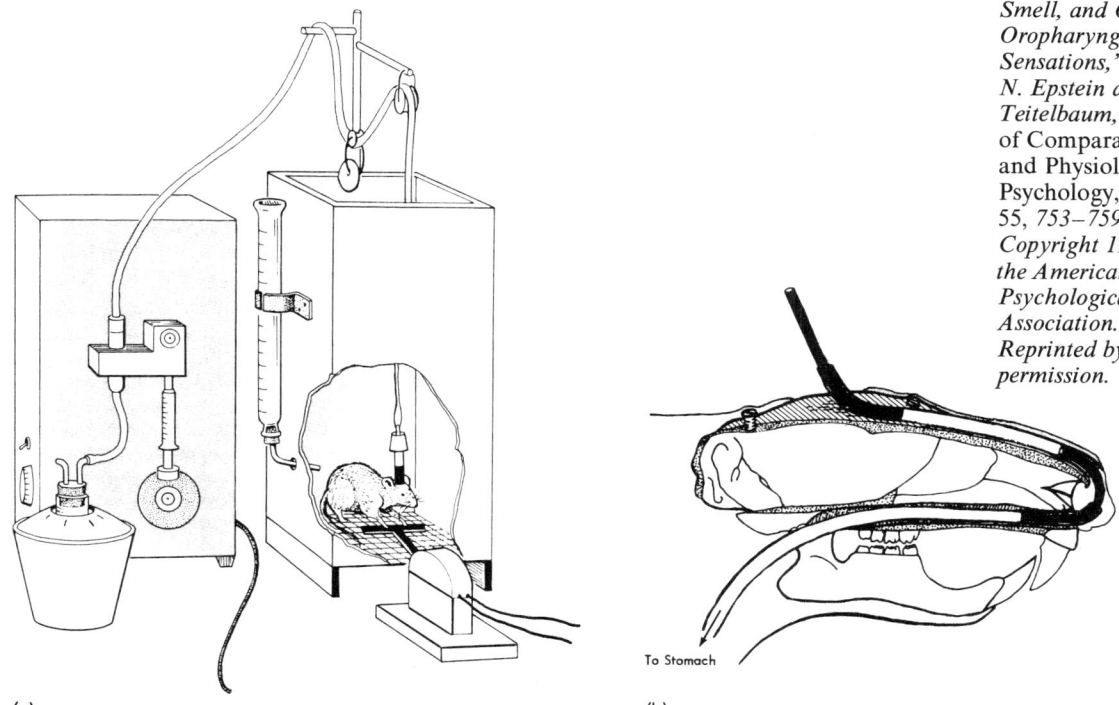

(a)

To Stomach

(b)

body weight. Furthermore, they varied their bar-pressing to compensate for experimental variations in the concentration of the injected food. As Epstein and Teitelbaum indicate, the fact that oral stimulation is not necessary for food regulation does not necessarily mean that oral stimuli do not contribute to this process. As was indicated in Chapter 5, taste and smell perform important functions in the selection of food and in the location of food in the environment.

Body Temperature. In 1948, Brobeck proposed a **thermostatic theory** of hunger regulation. According to this view, hunger arises in response to a decrease in body temperature, and animals eat in order to keep their body temperature from decreasing further. They stop eating when they become warm. The property of food that brings about a temperature increase was called its "specific dynamic action." Support for this theory was obtained from data that showed that eating protein, which quickly produced satiation, increased body temperature and from findings that indicated that low body temperatures increased eating while high body temperatures decreased food intake (Sundsten, 1969; Stevenson, 1969). Although these data imply that temperature can affect food regulation, they do not necessarily indicate that it is the major factor influencing hunger. Most researchers have concluded that hunger is mainly regulated by other factors.

The Lipostatic Theory. Proposed by Kennedy (1953), the **lipostatic theory** suggests that animals are sensitive to the overall fat stored in their bodies, presumably through some biochemical mechanism. Evidence to support this theory comes from the observations of Teitelbaum (1964). He reported that rats can maintain themselves within very close limits of their body weight, and they will reestablish their previous weight after they have been artificially fattened. The lipostatic theory has a good deal of merit in accounting for long-term weight regulation, but it probably cannot explain the short-term regulation of day-to-day eating.

The Glucostatic Theory. According to the **glucostatic theory,** hunger reflects an attempt on the part of an organism to keep glucose levels constant in the body. Mayer (1955) has argued that it is not the absolute level of glucose that is monitored by glucose-sensitive receptors, but rather it is the difference in glucose between the arteries and the veins that is important. Where are these receptors located? According to Mayer and Marshall (1956), they are located in the ventromedial hypothalamic nuclei. Specifically, these researchers suggest that a decrease in the blood-sugar level in the circulatory system produces a decrease in brain sugar usage and that this factor in turn stimulates brain mechanisms that regulate food intake. I will discuss central control of eating later in this chapter.

In support of the glucostatic theory, Stunkard, Van Itallie, and Reis (1955) have found arteriovenous glucose differences and hunger to be correlated. Herberg (1960) has shown that injections of small quantities of glucose into the ventricles of rats depress food intake. Although glucose levels and hunger are correlated, restoration of the glucose level to its optimal level is apparently not the mechanism that yields the cessation of eating in satiated animals. Koopmans (cited in Deutsch & Deutsch, 1973) demonstrated this in a very creative study using parabiotic rats whose intestines had been partially crossed. **Parabiotic** rats are two highly inbred rats who have been surgically joined together. They are, essentially, artificial Siamese twins. The fact that they are closely inbred minimizes the possibility of tissue rejection by the two animals.

In Koopmans' research, part of the small intestine of one of the rats was connected to the small intestine of the other animal. As a result, when one of the rats (the donor) ate, part of the food crossed over to its partner and was partially absorbed by the recipient's digestive system. By using this procedure, Koopmans was able to demonstrate that the amount eaten did not depend upon the blood-glucose levels. Although the recipient had absorbed large amounts of glucose from the food consumed by the donor, there was no decrease in the amount eaten by the recipient rat at various periods of time after the donor rat had eaten.

Although there appear to be a number of peripheral mechanisms that influence food intake, none of them are critical, because both experimental animals and humans still exhibit manifestations of hunger after these influences have been selectively interrupted. Therefore, peripheral factors are not the only determinants of hunger. Rather, they influence what foods will be eaten, when eating will occur, and the amount that will be ingested. The critical mechanisms mediating eating behavior are centrally located. We will examine these later in this chapter, but, before we do, peripheral factors influencing thirst will be discussed.

Peripheral Mechanisms of Thirst

Oral Factors. Attempts to explain why we have the urge to drink date back to the writings of Aristotle, Galen, and Hippocrates. All of these early writers emphasized the role of dryness of the mouth and throat in the production of thirst. In modern scientific writings, this same view is associated with Cannon (1918). Cannon equated thirst with local sensations of dryness arising from the mouth and throat. According to Cannon, these sensations arise because body dehydration results in a decrease in salivary flow. Cannon's views stimulated a great deal of interest in the possible role of peripheral mechanisms in thirst regulation. Unfortunately, the upshot of the majority of the subsequent research was that Cannon's theory had to be abandoned.

Although sensations of dryness arising from the throat may contribute to the regulation of thirst, these signals are not essential for this regulatory process. After complete removal of the salivary glands, dogs are able to maintain normal water intake (Montgomery, 1931). Humans without salivary glands still report thirst sensations and are able to regulate their intake of water according to their bodily needs (Steggerda, 1941).

Cellular Dehydration. **Osmosis** is the movement of water through a membrane in response to an unequal distribution of solutes on the two sides of the membrane; the concentration of solutes on either side of the membrane can be expressed in terms of **osmolality.** There are cells in the anterior hypothalamus (lateral preoptic area) that respond to changes in the osmolality of the extracellular fluid of the body. They are called **osmoreceptors.** These receptors appear to be sensitive to the concentration of solutes in the blood. When an animal has been deprived of water, the solutes in the blood will become more concentrated than normal, reflecting cellular dehydration in the periphery. The reaction of the osmoreceptor cells to this state may initiate water intake.

More specifically, it appears likely that, when the osmolality of the blood increases, water is pulled out of the osmoreceptors in the hypothalamus, which causes them to initiate a series of actions by which the dehydration is compensated for. In contrast, when the osmolality of the blood is low, water moves into the osmoreceptors, causing them to swell, and their rate of discharge decreases. Activation of the osmoreceptors compensates for thirst in two ways. First, drinking behavior is stimulated, and, second, antidiuretic hormone is released into the blood.

Antidiuretic hormone (ADH) is secreted into the blood by the hypothalamicohypophyseal axis. After being released into the blood from the pituitary, this hormone increases water reabsorption by the kidneys. When no ADH is secreted into the blood, the amount of water passing into the urine is 5 to 15 times normal. In contrast, when large quantities of ADH are secreted, water is reabsorbed to an extreme degree, with the result that the volume of urine formed may be as little as one-third of the normal output (Guyton, 1971). According to Guyton (1971), the osmoreceptor system is so sensitive that an overconcentration of the extracellular-fluid solutes of only 1–2% will result in a marked increase in water retention. A similar decrease in the concentration of extracellular solutes will produce a rapid water loss.

Extracellular Fluid Volume. In addition to the osmolality of the extracellular fluid, the absolute volume of the extracellular fluid, such as the amount of circulating blood, may be a peripheral factor in the regulation of thirst. When a large amount of water is consumed, the volume of intravascular fluids (fluids inside the circulatory system) increases. This condition is called **hypervolemia.** In contrast, prolonged water deprivation leads to a decrease in intravascular fluids, or **hypovolemia.** Stricker and his colleagues (Stricker, 1966; Stricker & Jalowiec, 1970; Stricker & Wolf, 1966, 1969) have published data supporting the possibility that there are receptors that are indeed sensitive to these volume changes. The volume receptors appear to be located in the kidneys (Fitzsimons, 1966, 1967, 1969, 1971).

Hypovolemia results in the secretion of **renin** into the bloodstream by the kidneys. Renin is an enzyme that catalyzes the conversion of one of the plasma proteins into **angiotensin.** The circulating angiotensin has two effects on thirst regulation. First, it results in increased water retention by the kidneys, and, second, angiotensin appears to have a direct excitatory action on the hypothalamic regions controlling drinking (Booth, 1968; Epstein, Fitzsimons, & Rolls, 1970). Thus, two factors appear to stimulate the brain to either initiate or stop drinking: the concentration of solutes in the blood and the volume of intravascular fluid. These factors can act independently of each other or can have an additive effect on drinking when activated together (Fitzsimons, 1971).

Neural Mechanisms of Hunger and Thirst: The Hypothalamus

Just as we saw with emotional behavior, the primary mechanisms for the mediation of hunger and thirst are located at the hypothalamic level. Regions that interconnect with these hypothalamic mechanisms polish, modify, or elaborate the hypothalamic influences. The hypothalamic influences over the behavioral aspects of eating and drinking are of two types: excitatory and inhibitory. The interactions of excitatory and inhibitory systems in controlling behavior were discussed in the preceding chapter. Let me emphasize again that dominance of the excitatory system results in the initiation of behavior (in this case, eating and drinking), while sufficient inhibitory influences will produce either a diminution or cessation of behavior.

In view of the fact that so much central overlapping occurs in the systems controlling hunger and thirst, they will be considered together. They are also considered together because eating and drinking are so highly correlated under normal, everyday conditions. If animals are experimentally subjected to food deprivation, they will voluntarily curtail their water intake. Similarly, animals subjected to water deprivation will eat less food. The findings discussed below will show that inhibitory control over eating at the hypothalamic level is primarily located in the region of the ventromedial hypothalamic nucleus. Excitatory influences on eating are exerted by the lateral hypothalamic area. It is interesting that these same regions perform analogous functions in mediating emotion (see Chapter 8). The major nuclei and areas of the hypothalamus were shown in Figure 3-13. For your convenience, they appear again in Figure 9-6. It will be helpful for you to refer to this figure in the discussions that follow in the remainder of this chapter.

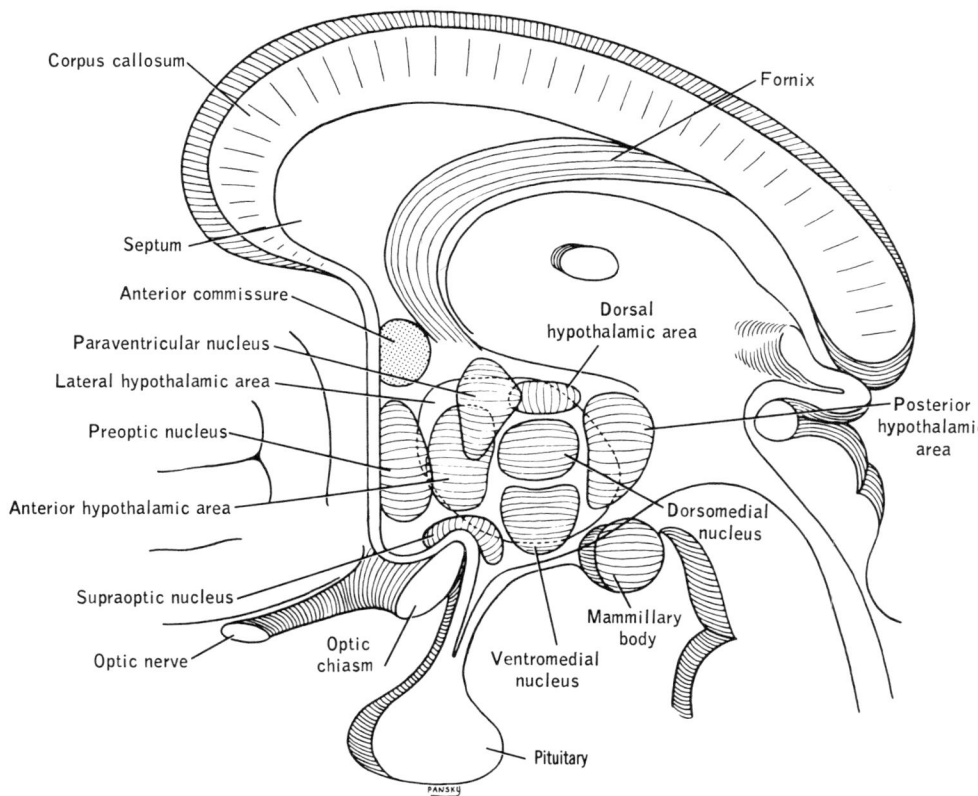

Figure 9-6
The hypothalamic nuclei. From A Functional Approach to Neuroanatomy, *by E. L. House and B. Pansky. Copyright 1967 by McGraw-Hill, Inc. Reprinted by permission.*

The Ventromedial Hypothalamic Satiety Mechanism. The ventromedial hypothalamic nuclei have long been thought to be involved in satiation. Electrical stimulation of the ventromedial hypothalamus produces a cessation of eating in food-deprived animals (Anand & Dua, 1955; Morgane, 1961; Smith, 1956). Bilateral destruction of the ventromedial nuclei is followed by a dramatic increase in food intake that persists for periods of up to 40 or 50 days and leads to extreme obesity (Brobeck, Tepperman, & Long, 1943; Hetherington & Ranson, 1940, 1942; Teitelbaum, 1961). This syndrome is called **hypothalamic hyperphagia.**

These results have been interpreted as indicating that the lesion removes the normal inhibitory control exerted by the ventromedial satiety region over the adjacent lateral excitatory region. Normal activation in the lateral region results in the initiation of eating; presumably, the ventromedial region acts to regulate or inhibit these excitatory influences. In support of this theory, several researchers have shown that bilateral cuts between the ventromedial nuclei and the lateral hypothalamic nuclei, severing the connections between these regions, will reliably produce hyperphagia (Albert & Storlien, 1969; Grossman & Grossman, 1971; Jansen & Hutchison, 1969; Paxinos & Bindra, 1972, 1973; Sclafani, Berner, & Maul, 1973). Grossman (1971) has shown that transverse cuts made either anterior or posterior to the ventromedial nucleus also yield hyperphagia. Taken together, these results indicate that neural fibers projecting from the ventromedial hypothalamic nuclei, which conduct inhibitory impulses over eating, project rostrally, caudally, and laterally to various brain regions.

Recent research by Gold and his colleagues has brought into question the view that it is destruction of the ventromedial nucleus per se that produces hyperphagia (Gold, 1973; Kapatos & Gold, 1973). These investigators have suggested that hyperphagia results from disruption of the ascending **ventral noradrenergic bundle,** which is adjacent to the ventromedial nuclei. In their studies, they found that lesions to the ventromedial nucleus alone, sparing this fiber tract, did not produce hyperphagia. To produce hyperphagia, hypothalamic lesions had to bilaterally interrupt the ventral noradrenergic bundle. This pathway ascends from midbrain nuclei to limbic-system regions, including several hypothalamic nuclei. It is of interest to point out, however, that this tract sends relatively few projections to the ventromedial nuclei. Gold's findings do not alter the model described above of hypothalamic control of eating; they simply localize the effective site of the lesion to a greater extent than has been done by previous researchers.

The general effects produced by ventromedial hypothalamic lesions on eating behavior have usually been interpreted as signifying a decrease in the effectiveness of a satiety mechanism. Nevertheless, there are several behavioral and physiological results of these ablations that argue against any simple effect of these lesions. For instance, ventromedial-lesioned animals are more finicky about the taste of their food than are normal animals. If their food is even slightly adulterated by some unpalatable substance, such as quinine, they will quickly reject the food, even though the quinine is present at levels that will not prevent normal animals from eating (Corbit & Stellar, 1964; Teitelbaum, 1955). Ventromedial hypothalamically lesioned rats also tend to accumulate more body fat than normal animals, even if the lesions do not produce overeating (Han, 1967; Rabin, 1974).

Some preliminary reports on the willingness of animals with ventromedial-hypothalamic lesions to work to obtain food indicated that they would not work as hard as would normal subjects (Miller, Bailey, & Stevenson, 1950; Teitelbaum, 1957). However, it has been more recently shown that, if the body weight of ventromedially lesioned animals was restricted to its preoperative level or lower, they worked as hard or harder to obtain food as normal animals (Kent & Peters, 1973; Porter, Allen, & Arazie, 1974; Sclafani & Kluge, 1974; Wampler, 1973). When these same animals were tested at obese body-weight levels, they would not work as hard as normals. Wampler suggested that the obese body weight interfered with responding because the sheer bulk of the animal made it difficult for it to emit the response required to obtain food. These findings suggest that ventromedially lesioned animals are indeed hungrier than nonlesioned control subjects but that this difference will only emerge under appropriate testing conditions.

The Lateral Hypothalamic Feeding Mechanism. As was indicated earlier in this chapter, the lateral hypothalamic area appears to be involved in the initiation of eating. The lateral hypothalamic area is not a nuclear group as is the ventromedial hypothalamic nucleus; that is, the lateral area does not represent a grouping of cell bodies with a fairly distinct border. Nevertheless, it is still possible to produce distinct behavioral effects by either electrically stimulating or lesioning this area.

It has long been established that electrical stimulation of the lateral region produces immediate eating in animals that have just eaten to satiation (Brügger, 1943; Larsson, 1954; Smith, 1956). Conversely, bilateral electrolytic destruction of the lateral hypothalamic region produces **aphagia** (cessation of eating) and **adipsia** (cessation of drinking), which lead to death unless the animal is maintained by tube feeding (Anand & Brobeck, 1951; Anand, Dua, & Schoenberg, 1955; Teitelbaum & Epstein, 1962; Teitelbaum & Stellar, 1954). These same effects are produced by transecting the fibers that enter or leave the lateral hypothalamus along its lateral border (Grossman & Grossman, 1973).

If the lesioned animals are tube fed after the operation, they will eventually eat food and drink water again. Usually, eating reappears before drinking. Teitelbaum and Epstein described a series of four stages in the recovery of eating and drinking following lesions to the lateral hypothalamus, and they named this recovery process the **lateral hypothalamic syndrome.** The recovery stages can be summarized as follows (see Figure 9-7).

In the first stage of recovery (*aphagia and adipsia*), animals with lateral hypothalamic lesions refuse all food and do not drink water. They will die unless

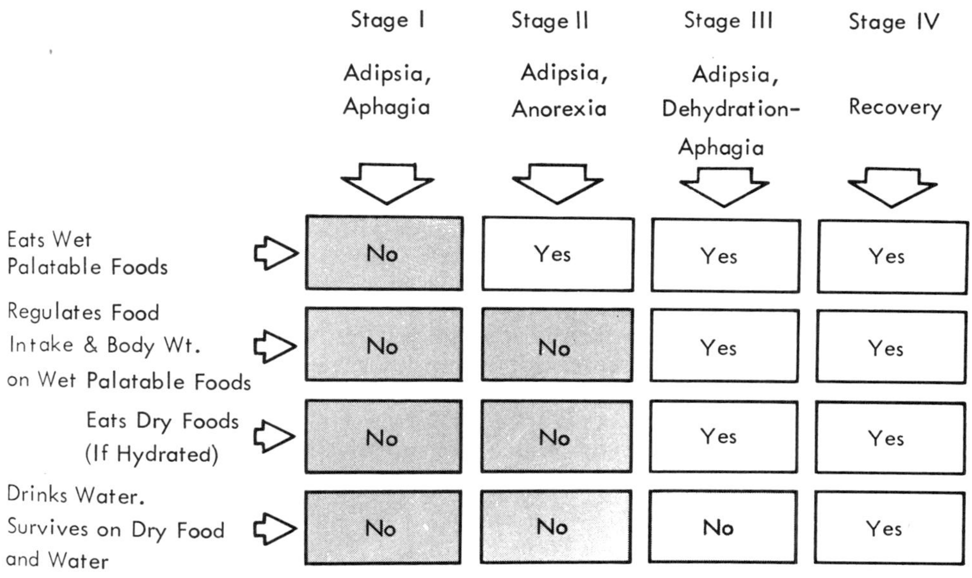

	Stage I Adipsia, Aphagia	Stage II Adipsia, Anorexia	Stage III Adipsia, Dehydration– Aphagia	Stage IV Recovery
Eats Wet Palatable Foods	No	Yes	Yes	Yes
Regulates Food Intake & Body Wt. on Wet Palatable Foods	No	No	Yes	Yes
Eats Dry Foods (If Hydrated)	No	No	Yes	Yes
Drinks Water. Survives on Dry Food and Water	No	No	No	Yes

Figure 9-7
The stages of recovery seen in the lateral hypothalamic syndrome. The critical behavioral events that define the stages are listed on the left. From "The Lateral Hypothalamic Syndrome: Recovery of Feeding and Drinking After Lateral Hypothalamic Lesions," by P. Teitelbaum and A. N. Epstein, Psychological Review, *1962, 69, 74–90. Copyright 1962 by the American Psychological Association. Reprinted by permission.*

artificial feeding and watering are carried out. The animals actually resist contact with food. If food is placed directly into their mouth, they will spit it out and try to wipe it off their face. They act as if contact with food were aversive. In general, the severity of this disorder is correlated with the size of the lesions (Teitelbaum & Epstein, 1962).

During the second stage of the lateral hypothalamic syndrome (*anorexia and adipsia*), animals consume wet and very tasty foods, such as eggnog, cookies, and milk chocolate, but they do not eat enough to maintain their body weight. They still depend on tube feeding for maintenance and will die if it is discontinued. The animals are therefore **anorexic**; they eat but not enough to keep alive. They still refuse dry food and do not drink water.

Animals whose recovery has proceeded to stage three (*adipsia with a secondary dehydration-aphagia*) will regulate their caloric intake when wet and palatable foods are available, but they still refuse to drink water. However, they will drink water if it is artificially sweetened with a nonnutritive substance such as saccharin. If the animals are allowed access to an artificially sweetened solution or are tube fed water, they will even eat dry laboratory chow. However, if given the standard diet of tap water and lab chow, they refuse to drink the water, their food intake drops to zero in two or three days, and starvation ensues. In this third stage of recovery, adipsia is apparently the primary cause of the remaining disturbance of the food-regulation process. This contrasts markedly with the first two stages, during which hydration of food does not prevent the appearance of aphagia.

The fourth stage of the lateral hypothalamic syndrome is called *recovery*. This refers to the finding that most rats with lateral hypothalamic lesions eventually arrive at the point where they will maintain their weight on a dry-food diet with water as the only fluid. However, more sensitive tests indicate that water regulation is only superficially normal. This is indicated by two facts. First, when these seemingly recovered rats were artificially dehydrated by injections of hypertonic salt solutions into their peritoneal cavity, they did not drink water as normal animals will. Second, when "recovered" rats were offered water for only two hours each morning, they did not compensate by drinking their total daily water requirements during that period as normal animals do. Teitelbaum and Epstein reported that these animals only drank water when they ate. Apparently these animals were only drinking water to wet their mouths. This phenomenon, in which drinking is only secondary to eating, is called **prandial drinking.** The "recovered" rats were still hypersensitive to the taste qualities of their food and water. They refused food and water if it was only slightly adulterated with quinine, even at levels that would not begin to deter normal rats. This latter finding closely resembles the finicky eating observed in obese rats following ventromedial hypothalamic lesions.

The recovery shown by the lateral hypothalamically lesioned animals is at least contributed to by the undamaged tissue surrounding the lesion. This was demonstrated by Teitelbaum and Epstein (1962). They found that additional lesions adjacent to the original ones resulted in a return to aphagia and adipsia. The animals then showed an orderly pattern of recovery following the same sequence of stages described earlier. In one animal, this recovery process was repeated four times.

It is also interesting to note that it is possible, with large lesions covering both the ventromedial and lateral areas, to produce an animal capable of showing both the lateral hypothalamic syndrome and hypothalamic hyperphagia (Teitelbaum & Epstein, 1962; Williams & Teitelbaum, 1959). Animals prepared in this fashion are initially aphagic and adipsic. When caloric intake becomes reestablished during stage three, these same rats become hyperphagic if adequately hydrated. However, artificial watering is essential; the animals will again become aphagic if artificial watering is discontinued. This is an important finding because it demonstrates that the lateral hypothalamic feeding mechanism is not absolutely necessary for the production of hyperphagia. However, it undoubtedly contributes to this phenomenon in the intact animal.

An interesting alternative interpretation of the effects of lateral hypothalamic lesions on eating has been offered by Keesey and Powley (1975). They suggested that animals with lateral hypothalamic lesions become aphagic and adipsic not because neural control over eating has been lost but rather because the lesion results in a reduction in the regulation level, or set point, for body weight. The reason why an animal becomes aphagic and adipsic following lateral hypothalamic lesions is because, they suggest, "curtailing food intake is the most effective means at its disposal of bringing weight into adjustment with the reduced set point" (p. 561). In support of this hypothesis, they have reported that, if rats were starved prior to being lesioned, so that their body weight was severely reduced, they actually became hyperphagic after surgery until they attained their new, although lower than prestarvation, weight level. The level they attained was similar to that reached by similarly lesioned animals that were lesioned when at normal body weight. Keesey and Powley also reinterpreted the effects of ventromedial hypothalamic lesions in a similar light. They proposed that ventromedial hypothalamic lesioned animals become hyperphagic not because of the loss of a satiety mechanism but rather because the set point for weight regulation has been raised.

The Independence of the Mechanisms Controlling Eating and Drinking. In studies of the lateral hypothalamic syndrome, we saw that the lesions disrupted both food and water intake. It was also shown that the rates of recovery of eating and drinking were different. This latter observation suggests that the alterations in food intake may have been independent of the effects on water intake. Thus, it is possible that there are two independent systems controlling eating and drinking and that these systems are located close together in the hypothalamus. Destruction of these two overlapping systems would produce the full set of deficits seen in the lateral hypothalamic syndrome.

The independence of the neural systems mediating eating and drinking was firmly established by an exhaustive series of studies conducted by Grossman (1960, 1962a, 1962b). As was indicated in Chapter 4, these inquiries emphasized the potential for intracranial chemical stimulation as a brain-research tool. In these experiments, crystalline chemicals were repeatedly applied to the lateral hypothalamic area through chronically implanted cannulas, and the effects on behavior were observed. Grossman's findings implied that the feeding systems of the brain used adrenergic transmitters while the neural systems mediating drinking used cholinergic neurotransmitters.

Grossman reported that implantation of crystals of adrenergic substances, such as epinephrine and norepinephrine, caused rats that had just eaten and drunk to satiation to start eating again. This finding has been replicated by other investigators (for example, Booth, 1967, 1968; Davis & Keesey, 1971; Herberg & Franklin, 1972; Slangen & Miller, 1969). Myers and his colleagues have demonstrated adrenergic feeding in primates (Myers, 1969; Myers & Sharpe, 1968). Grossman also found that adrenergic stimulation of the lateral hypothalamus caused satiated rats to work at a learned bar-press response to obtain food—a finding that was later replicated by Coons and Quartermain (1970). Finally, Grossman found that injection of an adrenergic blocking agent (ethomoxane) into the lateral hypothalamus produced an incomplete but substantial blockage of normal eating. Taken together, these data provide compelling evidence for the view that eating is adrenergically coded.

In his examinations of the neurochemical coding of drinking, Grossman implanted crystals of cholinergic substances (acetylcholine and carbachol) through the same cannulas of these chronically implanted rats at exactly the same site that had previously elicited eating. The effect of this cholinergic stimulation was to produce drinking and pressing of a different bar in the operant apparatus—one that delivered water. When a cholinergic blocking agent (atropine sulfate) was applied to these same brain areas, ingestion of water was significantly reduced. Cholinergically induced drinking in rats has been reproduced in laboratories throughout the world. However, it has not been possible to generalize this phenomenon to a wide range of species (Myers, 1969).

The hypothalamic thirst mechanism is sensitive to hypertonic salt solutions. This sensitivity has been demonstrated in rats (Blass & Epstein, 1971), rabbits (Peck & Novin, 1971), and goats (Andersson, 1952). Andersson's discovery of this phenomenon was described in Chapter 4. Angiotensin injections into the hypothalamus will also elicit drinking (Epstein et al., 1970). In conclusion, the weight of the evidence suggests that there are independent neural systems mediating hunger and thirst. Although these two processes are highly interrelated, they are apparently coded differently.

Extrahypothalamic Mechanisms of Hunger and Thirst

The functions of hypothalamic regions in regulating hunger and thirst are modified by other brain structures to which the hypothalamus either directly or indirectly connects, including, among others, the globus pallidus, the amygdala, the septal area, and the hippocampus. Lesions in the globus pallidus of the basal ganglia, for instance, produce effects on food and water consumption that are essentially identical to those seen after lateral hypothalamic lesions (Marshall & Richardson, 1974; Morgane, 1961). The similar outcomes produced by these lesions probably indicate that lateral hypothalamic and globus pallidus lesions disrupt common pathways. In support of this notion, Grossman and Grossman (1971, 1973) have shown that severing the fibers between these two structures yielded the lateral hypothalamic syndrome even though neither structure was itself damaged.

The amygdala participates in the regulation of food and water intake. Both excitatory and inhibitory influences are exerted by this structure, but they have not yet been precisely localized. Amygdala lesions have been reported to produce both aphagia (Fonberg, 1966) and hyperphagia (Anand & Brobeck, 1952; Grossman & Grossman, 1963). Continuous bilateral electrical stimulation of the transitional zone between the corticomedial division of the amygdala and the adjacent cortex has been shown to depress food intake in deprived rats (White & Fisher, 1969). This effect was blocked by bilateral lesions to the ventromedial hypothalamic nucleus, indicating that the suppressive effects produced by amygdala stimulation were serving to activate the ventromedial satiety mechanism. Both excitatory and inhibitory influences of the amygdala over water intake have been demonstrated in the rat by Grossman and Grossman (1963) using electrical stimulation. Cholinergic stimulation of the cortical nucleus of the amygdala will augment water intake in rats elicited by cholinergic stimulation of the lateral hypothalamus (Singer & Montgomery, 1969). In their study, Singer and Montgomery also found that hypothalamically elicited drinking was reduced to normal levels if the anticholinergic agent atropine sulfate was injected into the amygdala cortical nucleus. Hence, both electrical- and chemical-stimulation, as well as lesion, studies of the amygdala point to a dual (excitatory and inhibitory) control function over eating and drinking.

Several studies have reported that septal lesions are followed by an increase in water consumption (Donovick & Burright, 1968; Harvey & Hunt, 1965; Lubar, Boyce, & Schaefer, 1968). However, there are findings in the literature that argue against our concluding that the septum is directly involved in thirst regulation. It has been suggested that the effect of septal lesions is to alter animals' reactivity to tastes such that their approach tendencies to pleasant tastes and their aversion to unpleasant tastes are enhanced (Beatty & Schwartzbaum, 1968; Donovick, Burright, & Gittleson, 1969). In support of this interpretation, Carey (1971) reported that his septally lesioned rats drank less quinine-adulterated water but more water with saccharin in it than did normal animals.

The effects of bilateral removal of the hippocampus on eating and drinking have also been considered by several researchers. In general it has been shown that hippocampal lesions either produce no effect or only a slight elevation of food and water consumption in rats (Boitano, Lubar, Auer, & Furnald, 1968; Kimble & Coover, 1966). Similarly, lesions to the cortex adjacent to the hippocampus produce only a transitory hyperphagia in cats (Entingh, 1971). Thus it appears that, at the level of the hippocampus, only a slight modulatory control of eating and drinking is exerted.

In summary, these findings indicate that the neural systems mediating eating and drinking are independently organized. There is evidence to indicate that the feeding system is adrenergically coded while the drinking, or thirst, system is cholinergically coded. The primary mechanisms involved in hunger and thirst are organized at the hypothalamic level. Activity in these hypothalamic regions is modified by structures with which the hypothalamus is interconnected.

Sexual Behavior

Sexual behavior is different from other motivated behaviors along several dimensions. For example, unlike hunger and thirst, sexual behavior is unnecessary for survival of an individual member of the species. However, survival of the species is of course dependent on sexual behavior. Another difference between sexual behavior and other motivated behaviors is the dependence of sexual behavior on hormonal mechanisms.

The glands that secrete hormones into the blood—glands such as the pituitary, thyroid, adrenal, and gonads—make up the **endocrine system.** In the male, the gonads are the testes. The female gonads are the ovaries. The sex hormones secreted by the gonads have two primary functions in the control of sexual behavior. First, they mediate the development and differentiation of both the internal and external reproductive structures. Second, sexual hormones are involved in the development and differentiation of brain mechanisms that control reproductive cycles and sexual behavior. In this section of the chapter, we'll first examine basic endocrine mechanisms of sexual and reproductive behavior. Next, the effects of hormones on the development of sexual behavior will be considered. Finally, the loci of brain regions involved in sexual behavior and the influences that these areas appear to exert will be described.

Basic Endocrine Mechanisms of Reproductive Behavior

The sexual motivation of the male and the sexual receptivity of the female are, particularly in infrahuman species, controlled by sexual hormones. Learning plays such an important role in human sexual behavior that the importance of sex hormones for both male motivation and female receptivity is greatly diminished. One notable difference between the patterns of sexual behavior in infrahuman species of different sexes is that the receptivity of the female waxes and wanes as a function of cyclic hormonal changes. In contrast, the sexual motivation of the male remains fairly stable after puberty. This is because the hormone levels in the male do not show cyclic fluctuations.

The principal sex hormones in the female are **estrogen** and **progesterone**; they are secreted by the ovaries. In the male, the principal sex hormones are the **androgens testosterone** and **androstenedione,** both of which are secreted by the testes. However, the quantity of circulating testosterone is so much greater than androstenedione that testosterone can be considered the hormone responsible for the hormonal effects produced by the testes. The secretory activities of the gonads are in turn under the control of hormones released by the anterior pituitary (adenohypophysis). These hormones released by the adenohypophysis are called **gonadotrophic** hormones. Finally, the activities of the adenohypophysis are controlled by regions of the hypothalamus that are sensitive to circulating levels of hormones secreted by the gonads; thus, there is a feedback loop. Secretions from the adenohypophysis are elicited by *hypothalamic neurosecretory hormones,* or **hypothalamic releasing factors.** Releasing factors are synthesized in the hypothalamus and then sent through the **hypothalamic-hypophyseal portal vessels** to the adenohypophysis, where they cause pituitary hormones to be released into the blood. With one possible exception, there is a hypothalamic releasing factor for each hormone secreted by the pituitary. The hypothalamic-hypophyseal portal system is shown in Figure 9-8.

*Figure 9-8
The hypothalamic-hypophyseal portal system. Adapted from* Textbook of Medical Physiology, *by A. C. Guyton. Copyright 1971 by W. B. Saunders Company. Reprinted by permission.*

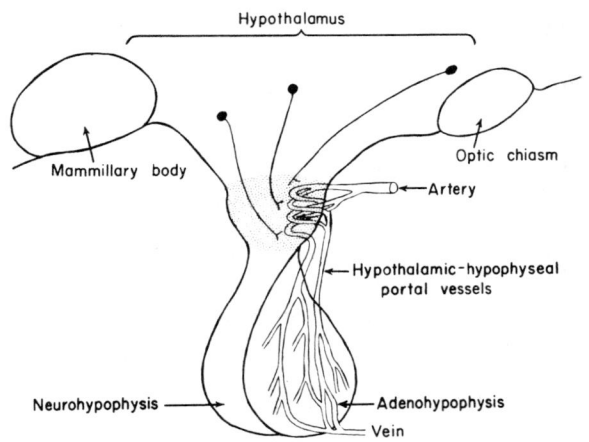

Endocrine Control of Female Receptivity. In the female, the primary pituitary gonadotrophic hormones concerned with sexual behavior are **follicle-stimulating hormone (FSH)** and **luteinizing hormone (LH).** They interact with gonadal hormones as follows. The adenohypophysis secretes FSH at the beginning of an ovarian cycle and the FSH stimulates the growth of follicles in the ovaries. Each follicle contains an ovum or egg. The follicles then begin to secrete estrogen, which acts on the hypothalamic mechanisms that produce LH releasing factor. The LH releasing factor next causes the release of LH by the adenohypophysis. The LH travels to the ovaries, where it acts together with the FSH to accelerate growth of the follicular tissues. In humans, for unknown reasons, usually only one follicle is singled out for complete development.

Eventually, the enlarged follicle ruptures, and the ovum is expelled into the abdominal cavity. This is the process of **ovulation.** The **ovum** is picked up by the hair-like endings of the fallopian tubes and transported into the uterus. Unless fertilization occurs, the egg proceeds on out through the vagina. In many species, ovulation occurs independently of copulation; in others, it is triggered by copulation.

The follicle that ruptures undergoes a series of changes, beginning within a few hours after expulsion of the ovum, and becomes the **corpus luteum.** The corpus luteum secretes primarily progesterone but also large amounts of estrogen. The combined action of these hormones modifies the tissues of the uterus in preparation for implantation of a fertilized egg. If pregnancy occurs, the corpus luteum persists and there are no more cycles until after birth of the offspring. If there is no pregnancy, the corpus luteum degenerates, and the secretions of estrogen and progesterone consequently decrease. In the human female, this lowering in hormone level leads to the sloughing off of the lining of the uterus and menstrual bleeding, which persists for four to five days.

The end of menstrual bleeding is followed in humans by a preovulatory stage of about seven to ten days duration, which is terminated by ovulation. The ovum must be fertilized within 24 hours after ovulation if pregnancy is to result. Probably most sperm remain viable in the female reproductive tract for no more than 24 hours also. Therefore, for fertilization of the egg to take place, copulation must occur between one day prior to ovulation and one day after ovulation.

In all subprimate species, female sexual receptivity is almost always restricted to the period just before and after ovulation. This interval of heightened receptivity is called **estrus.** Nonhuman primates tend to concentrate their sexual activity in the estrus period, but a female will often receive a dominant male when not in estrus. Few studies correlating human female receptivity with the stage of the menstrual cycle have been conducted, and the available evidence suggests that human females may feel more sexually aroused during the period around ovulation. In general, however, human females do not show much variation in receptivity as a function of hormonal cycling, probably because learning plays such an important function in the human female sexual response.

Endocrine Control of Male Receptivity. As was indicated earlier, the sexual motivation of the male does not show cyclic fluctuations as does that of the female, because the male's hormone levels remain fairly stable after puberty. Male sex hormones do not show cyclic variations because testosterone inhibits the hypothalamic mechanisms responsible for the cyclic release of gonadotrophic hormones in the female. Testosterone is produced by the testes only when the testes are stimulated by **interstitial cell-stimulating hormone (ICSH)** from the adenohypophysis, and the quantity of testosterone secreted varies as a function of the amount of ICSH available.

ICSH in the male is the same hormone as LH in the female. FSH is also important in male sexual functions. Its interaction with ICSH results in the complete formation of the spermatozoa, which fertilize the female's ovum.

Removing the influence of sex hormones by castrating either males or females (removing the testes or ovaries) does not make it impossible for either sex to engage in copulation, but both sexes normally show a decrease or complete cessation of sexual activity. There are wide species, as well as individual, differences in the effects of castration on sexual behavior. In general, the effects are less severe as one ascends the phylogenetic scale. In humans, particularly the female, castration will often result in no changes in sexual motivation. When decreases in sexual receptivity do occur in either sex of any species, copulatory behavior can be restored with injections of sex hormones. For comprehensive reviews of these findings, the reader should consult Beach (1971) and Sawyer (1960).

Hormones and the Development of Sexual Behavior

The most exciting finding to emerge from the vast research literature dealing with sexual behavior is the possibility that gonadal hormones may influence the development of brain regions that mediate distinctly male and female patterns of sexual responding. Beach (1971, 1975) has published excellent reviews of these data. The issue of the possible effects of sex hormones on neural organization was brought to the forefront by the publication of articles by Goy, Bridson, and Young (1964) and Phoenix, Goy, Gerall, and Young (1959).

In these studies, it was shown that, if a single dose of testosterone proprionate (a synthetic male sex hormone) was administered to pregnant guinea pigs between the 30th and 35th day of gestation, the female offspring responded poorly or not at all to injections of estrogen and/or progesterone that normally bring anestrus (not in estrus) females into estrus. That is, the animals were partially *defeminized.* The index of decreased estrus was a decrease in lordosis behavior. **Lordosis** is the response shown by a female when she is mounted from the rear by a male and consists of arching the back and raising and exposing the genitalia. Further, these early-androgenized genetically female guinea pigs, when ovariectomized and given testosterone proprionate injections as adults, showed more male behavior as adults than did normal females (see also Gerall, 1966), indicating a degree of *masculinization.* The components of male sexual behavior include mounting a female, intromission, and ejaculation. "Intromission and ejaculation" in these early-androgenized females does not mean that either vaginal penetration or seminal expulsion occurred. Rather, the use of these terms refers to the fact that the overt behavioral responses that normally accompany these events in male rodents were made.

In summary, as a result of prenatal treatment with male sex hormones, female guinea pigs showed less behavior characteristic of female sexual responses but more behavior characteristic of male sexual responses under appropriate conditions of hormonal stimulation during testing. For this reason, the females were said to have been masculinized or defeminized by the early androgen stimulation. Effects similar to those produced by early androgen stimulation of female guinea pigs have been demonstrated in other rodent species, including mice (Edwards, 1971; Edwards & Burge, 1971), rats (Harris & Levine, 1965; Hendricks, 1969; Ward & Renz, 1972; Whalen & Edwards, 1967; Whalen, Edwards, Luttge, & Robertson, 1969), and hamsters (Carter, Clemens, & Hoekema, 1972; Doty, Carter, & Clemens, 1971; Paup, Coniglio, & Clemens, 1972, 1974; Swanson & Crossley, 1971). However, in the mouse, rat, and hamster (which all have much shorter gestation periods than the guinea pig), the critical period for these effects to result from treatment with male sex hormones is somewhere between birth and 10 days of age rather than prenatal.

The studies described thus far all indicate that the presence of male sex hormones during some critical period of development will yield masculine patterns of sexual behavior in adult rodents of either sex. What would happen if androgen were not present? Would it lead to female sexual patterns of behavior in both males and females? To answer this question, several researchers have examined the effects of early castration of male rodents on later sexual behavior. Castration results in the removal of male sex hormones during early development. Such inquiries have generally shown that removal of the male sex hormones has feminizing effects. Male rats castrated within five days after birth (Grady, Phoenix, & Young, 1965; Hendricks, 1969; Thomas & Gerall, 1969; Whalen & Edwards, 1967) and male hamsters castrated at birth (Eaton, 1970; Johnson & Tiefer, 1972) show female sexual behavior—that is, lordosis—more frequently when estrogen and progesterone are administered in adulthood than normal, untreated, intact males. The quality of the lordoses shown by these neonatally castrated animals was inferior to that of normal females, but Ward (1972) suggests that this may have been due to the defeminizing effect of endogenous prenatal androgens.

Taken together, all of these data indicate that there is a critical development period during which neural mechanisms mediating either male or female patterns of responding are either organized or sensitized. These neural mechanisms are essentially female. Male sex hormones act to defeminize and masculinize the neural systems of the genetic male. The absence of male sex hormones during this critical period allows the neural system mediating female sexual responses to develop normally (Phoenix, Goy, Gerall, & Young, 1959).

Histological evidence supporting the existence of different neural systems regulating male and female patterns of reproductive behavior has come from research by Raisman and Field (1973). Through electron-microscope analysis of hypothalamic areas involved in controlling secretory activity of the pituitary gland, they have shown that differences exist between newborn male and female rats in the connections of nerve cells. Their research has further indicated that these fine differences can be reduced or even eliminated by early postnatal hormone manipulations. These treatments must occur, however, within the first few days of life for an effect on neural organization to take place. If female rats were administered androgen treatments during this critical period, their brains were permanently changed to assume the structural characteristics of a male's brain. In contrast, males deprived of their early androgen supply by castration on the day of birth failed to develop "male" brains; instead, their brains assumed the organization of female brains. As adults, the altered male and female rats showed pituitary gonadotrophic secretory activity corresponding to their brain organization rather than to their genetic sex.

The theory stressing the importance of early hormone stimulation in the development of patterns of reproductive behavior is a good one for accounting for sexual behavior in lower mammals. It probably has some merit for human behavior as well. However, it should be pointed out again that most aspects of human sexual behavior are learned, and humans do not show the high correlation between hormonal levels and degree of sexual arousal that is so common in lower animals. To carry this point a bit further, consider the fact that homosexual men will not suddenly become heterosexual if we give them a massive dose of testosterone proprionate. Instead, they will simply become more active homosexuals (Milner, 1970). Another important point that should be stressed is that, although androgens may be *necessary* for the development of patterns of male sexual activity, they are *not sufficient* for the emergence of these patterns in adults. Adult male copulatory activity also depends on early social experience with conspecifics. Male guinea pigs (Valenstein, Riss, & Young, 1955), rats (Gerall, Ward, & Gerall, 1967), and monkeys (Mason, 1960) reared in social isolation are unable to copulate effectively as adults.

Neural Mechanisms of Sexual Behavior

Hypothalamus. Earlier, you saw that hormonal mechanisms concerned with sexual motivation are regulated by hypothalamic regions. Considerable evidence also suggests that many of the behavioral aspects of sexual and reproductive behavior are integrated at the hypothalamic level. As was the case with other motivational and emotional systems regulating behavioral expression, the influence of hypothalamic mechanisms on sexual behavior is further regulated by other regions to which the hypothalamus projects.

Two broad categories of effects on sexual behavior result from lesioning specific hypothalamic loci. First, if hypothalamic regions concerned with the regulation of gonadotrophic hormone are destroyed, the gonads (ovaries or testes) become nonfunctional. Sexual behavior then decreases or totally ceases because the hormone levels required for normal sexual motivation are no longer present. The effect on mating behavior is thus indirect, arising from an inadequate hormonal level. It can be reversed, and normal mating behavior can be reestablished, through hormone-replacement therapy. The second effect on sexual behavior following hypothalamic lesions is a total cessation of all mating behavior even though adequate supplies of circulating sex hormones are still present. Administering sex hormones in this case will not reverse the effects of the brain lesion. This latter type of lesion effect probably indicates that the region destroyed was involved in translating signals arising from hormonal stimulation into the neural activity that produces sexual behavior.

Research by Sawyer and his colleagues can be used to illustrate these two effects. Sawyer (1957), using rabbits as his subjects, found that small bilateral lesions in the mammillary region of the hypothalamus (see Figure 9-6) induced permanent anestrus, which could not be reversed by hormone-replacement therapy. In contrast, lesions involving the arcuate and the base of the ventromedial nuclei resulted in a decrease in sexual receptivity, but this latter effect could be reversed by administration of sex hormones to the operated animals.

There appear to be species differences in the exact loci that will produce these two categories of effects on mating behavior. Using cats as their subjects, Sawyer and Robison (1956) found that small electrolytic lesions of the anterior hypothalamus rostral to the ventromedial nuclei resulted in permanent anestrus resistant to hormone-replacement treatment. On the other hand, lesions in the mammillary region or in the ventromedial nuclei also abolished mating behavior, but the effect was reversed by hormone therapy.

The region of the preoptic nucleus of the hypothalamus (see Figure 9-6) has also been implicated in the control of reproductive behavior. Several researchers have shown that electrical stimulation of this region increases sexual activity in male rats (Malsbury, 1971; Van Dis & Larsson, 1971; Vaughn & Fisher, 1962). In contrast, lesions to this area have generally been reported to produce a decrease in receptivity (Giantonio, Lund, & Gerall, 1970; Heimer & Larsson, 1967; Hitt, Bryon, & Modianos, 1973; Larsson & Heimer, 1964; Singer, 1968). These effects are apparently independent of alterations in circulating sex hormones.

Some of the most interesting data on the functions of the preoptic region in reproductive behavior have come from Fisher's laboratory (Fisher, 1956, 1961, 1964). Using intracranial chemical stimulation, Fisher found that injections of testosterone into the lateral preoptic region elicited vigorous male sexual patterns of responding in both male and female rats. This effect has more recently been replicated in male rats by Kierniesky and Gerall (1973). Injection of estrogen through these same cannulas had the same effect, although not quite so dramatic.

When the cannulas were situated slightly differently, so that they were instead located in the medial preoptic region, testosterone injections elicited components of maternal behavior in male and female rats, including nest building, carrying of infants to the nest, and grooming of litters of young rat pups. Again, estrogen had a similar but less potent effect in animals of both sexes. The importance of the medial preoptic area in regulating maternal behavior has recently been reaffirmed by Numan (1974). Numan found that severing the lateral connections of the medial preoptic area disrupted maternal behavior.

Fisher's findings are fascinating. They demonstrate that the neural systems mediating male copulatory behavior and female maternal activities are organized at the hypothalamic level in both sexes. The fact that both patterns can be elicited by injection of either male or female sex hormones is puzzling. These hormones are structurally similar. It may be that testosterone can be converted to estrogen and vice versa when injected into appropriate brain regions. It is also possible that the high concentrations of one hormone that occur in chemical stimulation activate neural regions that are maximally sensitive to the other hormone.

Extrahypothalamic Influences. In Chapter 8, I indicated that one of the most striking features of the Klüver-Bucy syndrome, produced by bilateral temporal lobectomy in rhesus monkeys, was extreme, indiscriminate sexuality (Klüver & Bucy, 1937, 1939). Their work thus emphasized the possible importance of temporal-lobe structures in the regulation of sexual behavior. Schreiner and Kling (1953) later noted that similar alterations in sexual behavior could be produced by lesioning the amygdala in cats—a finding that Kling (1968) later replicated using monkeys. Investigations by Harris and Sachs (1975) and Wood (1958) showed that hypersexuality could be produced by lesioning the basolateral nuclear complex of the amygdala. Harris and Sachs also found that lesions limited to the corticomedial nuclear complex of the amygdala yielded a transitory decrease in sexual activity. These findings suggest that both facilitating and inhibitory influences over sexual behavior are organized at the amygdala level. The amygdala has also been implicated in sexual activity by the findings that amygdala ablations in young rats will produce precocious puberty (Critchlow & Bar-Sela, 1967) and that the amygdala is the only extrahypothalamic region of the brain that stores sex hormones (Stumpf, 1968; Zigmond & McEwen, 1970).

The cerebral cortex is unnecessary for the maintenance of mating behavior in most female mammals (Sawyer, 1960). On the other hand, the cortex does appear to be necessary for the initiation of mating behavior in most male mammals (Sawyer, 1960). In the rat, for example, Beach (1940) found that, while removal of 20% of the cortex did not reduce the percentage of males exhibiting copulatory activity, no male showed mounting behavior if more than 60% of his cortex was destroyed. However, no particular part of the cortex seemed to be specifically related to sexual behavior; the critical factor in the decrease in mounting behavior was the total amount of cortical tissue removed.

In the cat, too, Goldstein (1957) found that large cortical ablations decreased male mounting and copulatory activity. However, after detailed inspection of his lesioned subjects, Goldstein concluded that the effect of the lesions was to impair sensory and motor activity related to copulation rather than to depress the male's interest in the female. The role of the cortex in mediating sexual behavior is therefore probably one of regulating sensory feedback and precise motor coordination. Because the female performs a passive role in the sexual patterns of most infrahuman species, cortical lesions will not disrupt the female reproductive pattern. The motor responses and sensory feedback required for the male to gain successful intromission are, on the other hand, relatively complex and require cortical mediation.

Chapter Summary and Conclusions

Motivation is the energizer or driving force of behavior, and in this chapter we examined the neural bases for specific categories of motivated behaviors. The chapter was begun with a discussion of the neural basis for the hedonic system—that system that processes information related to our experiences of pleasure and displeasure. The physiological bases of hunger and thirst were next described, and the chapter was ended with a consideration of the biological substrates of sexual and reproductive behavior. We saw that the basic expression of behaviors related to these motivational systems was integrated at the hypothalamic level. Regions that connect with the hypothalamus modify these hypothalamic influences on behavior.

The discovery of the self-stimulation phenomenon was outlined. *Self-stimulation* refers to the finding that animals will actively seek to deliver very mild electric shock to their brains. The anatomical distribution of brain regions from which self-stimulation can be elicited and the characteristics of this behavior were reviewed. It was concluded that electrical stimulation of the brain can be a very potent energizer of behavior. It was also indicated that, from different points in the brain, mild electrical stimulation will have aversive effects. Animals will actively seek to terminate aversive electrical stimulation, much as they will learn to escape or avoid a punishing stimulus. Investigations of self-stimulation and avoidance of aversive brain stimulation may clarify our understanding of how natural rewards and punishment affect the central nervous system and behavior.

Peripheral and central factors thought to influence hunger and thirst were described. Proposed peripheral factors affecting hunger are stimuli arising from the stomach and mouth, body temperature, amount of body fat, and body glucose levels. Peripheral mechanisms important in thirst have likewise been proposed. Some of these are stimuli arising from the mouth, cellular dehydration, and extracellular fluid volume. Many of these peripheral factors participate in hunger and thirst regulation, and they affect eating and drinking by acting on neural regions that mediate these behaviors. A good working model to account for hypothalamic mediation of hunger and thirst centers around the existence of initiating, or excitatory, versus inhibitory systems that control these processes. The region of the ventromedial hypothalamic nuclei appears to exert inhibitory influences over eating and drinking, while the lateral hypothalamus is apparently involved in the initiation of these behaviors. Other hypothalamic areas also contribute to the control of these processes, as do extrahypothalamic brain mechanisms. Although the anatomical systems mediating eating and drinking overlap a great deal, they are not identical. This point has been demonstrated by studies that have mapped the feeding and drinking systems using intracranial chemical stimulation.

Sexual behavior is unique among motivated behaviors along several dimensions. It is unnecessary for survival of the individual and is very dependent on hormonal mechanisms. In this last section of the chapter, basic endocrine mechanisms of reproductive behavior were described. Most infrahuman females show cyclic sexual activity that is closely tied to ovulation. Human females do not show this cyclicity to any great extent, probably because learning performs such an important role in patterns of human sexual responding. Males of all mammalian species, in contrast, show constant high levels of receptivity, and this has been related to stable levels of circulating testosterone. In addition to controlling receptivity in postpubertal animals, gonadal hormones may affect the development of brain regions that mediate distinctly male and female patterns of responding. Data bearing on this possibility were reviewed. Finally, the neural systems involved in the control of patterns of reproductive behavior and the types of influences they exert were considered.

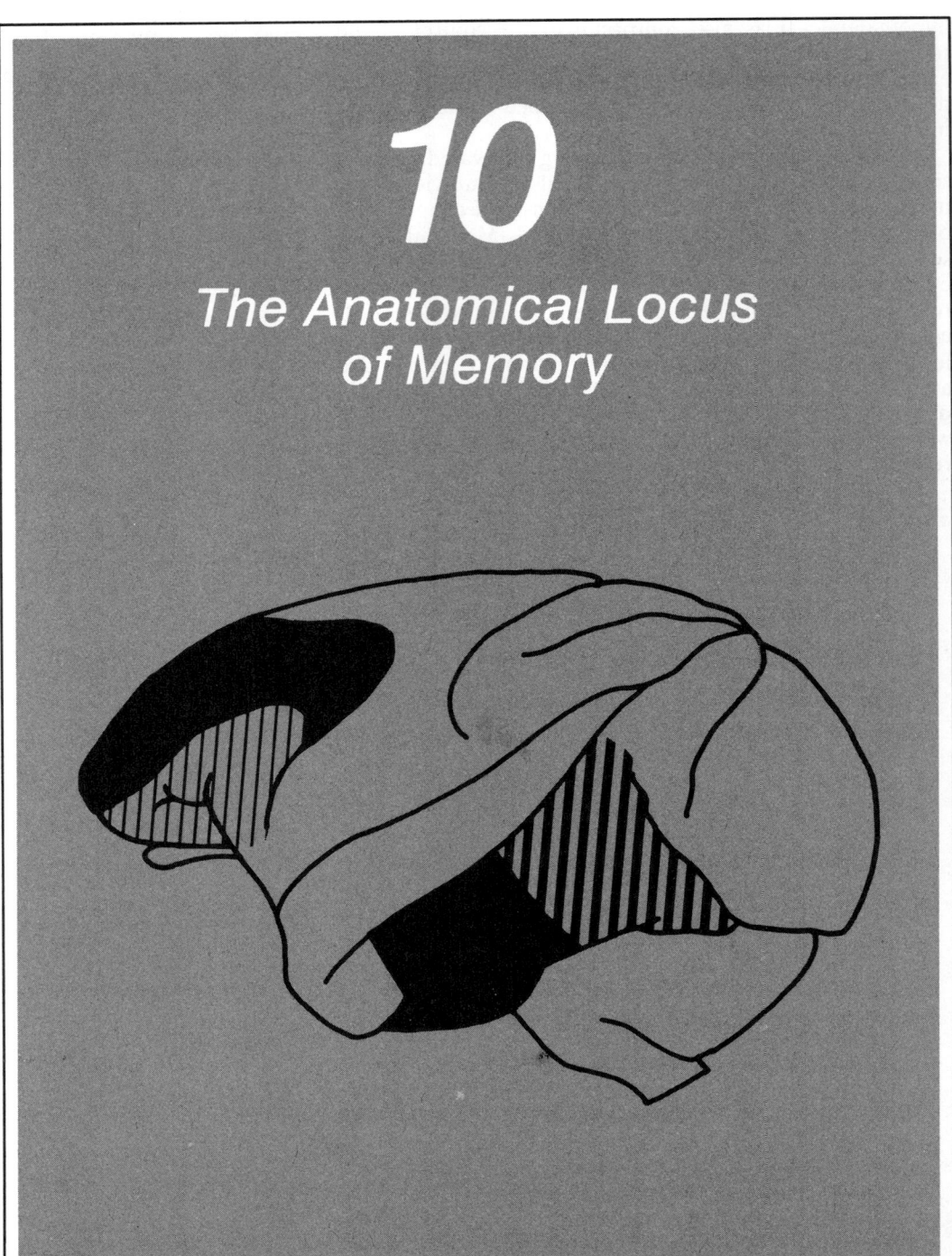

10

The Anatomical Locus of Memory

The idea that memory is located in a specific structure or locus of the brain has had a long history in the neurosciences, and this view has usually coexisted with the more general notion that specific behavior processes are mediated by specific neural centers. In the eighth century B.C. for example, Nemesius proposed that memory is located in the posterior ventricle, intellect in the middle ventricle, and perception in the anterior ventricle of the brain. This view was still accepted in the Middle Ages.

The specific-localization-of-function hypothesis was again given impetus when a school of psychology called **phrenology** began to emerge, in the 18th century. Phrenology's proponents suggested that the brain could be separated into different centers or organs, each controlling a separate behavior process or faculty. These theorists suggested, for instance, that memory is located in the cerebral cortex while reason and imagination are located in the underlying white matter. Phrenology reached its summit in the writings of Gall and his student Spurzheim, published during the early and middle 19th century. These investigators proposed no fewer than 37 "powers of the mind," governed by an equal number of cortical "organs of the mind," the development of which caused enlargements of the skull. The protrusions on the skull allow for a quantitative analysis of these powers or faculties, according to phrenological doctrine. A map of the skull, denoting the exact location of each faculty, was devised, as shown in Figure 10-1.

In contrast to these early formulations, which lacked an empirical foundation, clinical reports published in the 19th century seemed to confirm the idea that specific behavior functions, such as speech, are located in specific cerebral regions (for example, Broca, 1861; Wernicke, 1874). In the years that followed, clinicians were to propose the existence of many centers in the brain. Based on human clinical evidence involving the effects of brain lesions caused by either accident or pathology, centers were described for many complex behavioral and cognitive functions (John, 1971).

Paralleling human clinical observations, experimental inquiries using lower animals were suggesting that memory processes might be located in specific brain structures (for example, Bianchi, 1895; Ferrier, 1876; Hitzig, 1874). These early researchers, in their search for the location of the memory trace, or **engram,** confined their observations for the most part to the most recently evolved portions of the brain—that is, to the neocortex. The rationale for this orientation was as follows.

There are two characteristics of organisms that become increasingly evident as the phylogenetic scale is ascended. First, **encephalization of function** occurs. This means that the cerebral cortex—particularly the neocortex—becomes much more elaborate and tends to assume some of the functions once totally under the control

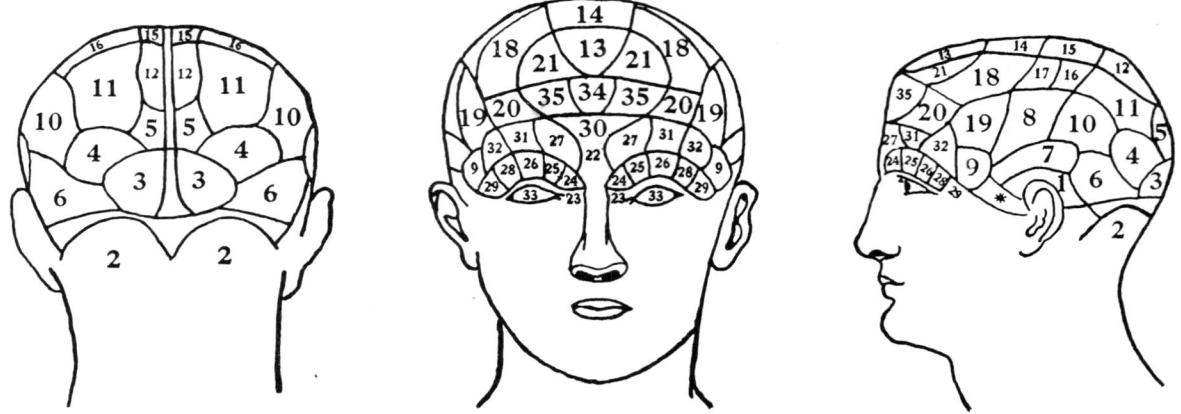

AFFECTIVE FACULTIES

PROPENSITIES	SENTIMENTS
? Desire to live	10 Cautiousness
* Alimentiveness	11 Approbativeness
1 Destructiveness	12 Self-Esteem
2 Amativeness	13 Benevolence
3 Philoprogenitiveness	14 Reverence
4 Adhesiveness	15 Firmness
5 Inhabitiveness	16 Conscientiousness
6 Combativeness	17 Hope
7 Secretiveness	18 Marvelousness
8 Acquisitiveness	19 Ideality
9 Constructiveness	20 Mirthfulness
	21 Imitation

INTELLECTUAL FACULTIES

PERCEPTIVE	REFLECTIVE
22 Individuality	34 Comparison
23 Configuration	35 Causality
24 Size	
25 Weight and Resistance	
26 Coloring	
27 Locality	
28 Order	
29 Calculation	
30 Eventuality	
31 Time	
32 Tune	
33 Language	

Figure 10-1
The locations of the "organs of the mind," according to the phrenologists. From A History of Experimental Psychology *(2nd ed.), by E. G. Boring, as adapted from Spurzheim, 1834. Copyright © 1950 by Appleton-Century-Crofts. Reprinted by permission of Prentice-Hall, Inc., Englewood Cliffs, New Jersey.*

of lower brain regions. Second, behavior becomes much more complex as we look at animals higher and higher on the phylogenetic scale. As for the relationship between these two factors, there is a strong positive correlation between the degree of encephalization of function and the complexity of behaviors that an organism can emit. Very complex behavior patterns such as those exhibited by humans require sophisticated memory processes. Since the neocortex is so very prominent in humans, it appeared plausible that the cortex was involved in these memory functions.

The cortex also seemed a likely candidate for the anatomical locus of memory because it receives sensory impulses from all of the sensory systems and has a region devoted to motor functions. This anatomical arrangement might provide the anatomical substrate for complex sensory-motor associations. Finally, the cortex was postulated to be the seat of memory because only the cortex has the wealth of interconnections that would be necessary for the storage of huge amounts of information. Within the neocortical mantle, several researchers have suggested, particularly in humans, memories are stored in sensory association areas that border specific sensory projection regions of the cortex (for example, Hebb, 1949; Konorski, 1948).

The brain-lesion technique has been the most widely used method in attempts to determine structures or pathways that might be responsible for learning and memory functions. The problems encountered in attempting to interpret the effects of brain lesions were described in Chapter 4. Let me reemphasize one of these that must be kept in mind in evaluating the research described below. This problem involves determining the basis of a lesion-induced behavior deficit. Specifically, it is often difficult to decide whether a learning deficit actually reflects a disruption of mechanisms specifically related to memory processes or whether the deficit has occurred as a result of the disruption of complex sensory, motor, emotional, and/or motivational functions essential to the expression of behavior, independent of memory processes.

Many excellent analyses of the functions of the neocortex in learning and memory have been conducted over the years. Some representative ones will next be reviewed. I will begin my discussion of this research with the classic work of Karl Lashley. His program of study represents one of the finest endeavors ever conducted in brain research.

Cortical Functions in Learning and Memory

Lashley's Search for the Engram

In summing up the results of 30 years of research, Karl Lashley (1950) was forced to conclude that memory did not appear to be located in any single region of the cortex. He wrote:

> I sometimes feel, in reviewing the evidence on the localization of the memory trace, that the necessary conclusion is that learning just is not possible. It is difficult to conceive of a mechanism which can satisfy the conditions set for it. Nevertheless, in spite of such evidence against it, learning does sometimes occur [p. 477–478].

We'll now review the findings that led him to these conclusions. A detailed review of these findings is presented in Lashley's (1950) classic paper, entitled "In Search of the Engram."

Some of Lashley's earliest work involved refuting the hypothesized conditioned-reflex circuits that Pavlov (1927) had proposed as mediating associative processes. (*Associative processes* refers to the learning of associations between stimuli and responses. For example, an animal might learn to associate the response "stop" with the stimulus "red light." Association is the basis of learning.) Pavlov had hypothesized that associations between stimuli and responses were formed by pathways extending from sense organs to specific sensory projection areas of the cerebral cortex, then through adjacent association areas to the motor cortex, and finally down to the motor cells of the medulla and spinal cord. To test this hypothesis, Lashley trained animals in a variety of tasks and then examined the effects of various sorts of brain-surgical interventions on either original learning or retention. His experimental subjects were mostly rats and monkeys, although a few chimpanzees were also used.

One of his findings was that such well-defined conditioned-reflex paths simply did not exist. In fact, the motor cortex was found to be unnecessary for the retention of either sensory-motor associations or complex, skilled, manipulative patterns of responding. Neither cutting the fiber pathways between sensory and motor regions nor ablating the motor cortex abolished these habits.

Similarly, the association cortex bordering specific sensory areas—at the restricted areas supposedly concerned with each sensory modality—did not appear to be the repository for specific memories. Memory disturbances for simple tasks occurred only after destruction of almost the entire association cortex, in all species studied. Even if this extensive surgery was done, animals could still learn these problems, although at a slower rate. Thus, these data suggested that the association cortex is not absolutely necessary for memory consolidation and recall processes.

Since neither the motor nor association cortical regions appeared necessary for basic memory functions, Lashley examined the functions of specific sensory areas of the cortex in sensory-motor associations. From this work his notion of **equipotentiality** evolved. To be mastered, certain tasks related to a sensory system, such as learning to discriminate visually between a triangle and a circle, require an intact sensory region for the modality involved. In one series of experiments, Lashley and his associates attempted to determine the smallest amount of visual cortex that was able to mediate the learning of a pattern (triangle versus circle) discrimination. It was found that pattern discriminations were still possible when only 1/60th of the visual cortex remained. Further, any small part within the primary visual cortex was equally capable of maintaining the discrimination ability. There was no specific localization; all small regions appeared to contribute equally to the visual discrimination. This equipotentiality has also been shown to be true for other sensory modalities (for example, Allen, 1945; Diamond & Neff, 1957). It's important to note that the principle of equipotentiality was used to describe the action of specific sensory cortical regions in mediating discriminations based on that particular sense modality. It did not imply, as some people have mistakenly thought, that the whole cortex is equipotent for all of its functions.

A second general principle that evolved from the investigations of Lashley and his co-workers was the concept of **mass action.** This notion was based on observations of the effects of cortical ablations on the retention of a maze task by rats. The mass-action principle argued that the effect of cortical lesions is dependent on their size. Essentially, it is the total volume of cortical tissue available that affects performance. Further, according to mass action, it does not matter which part of the cerebral hemispheres is destroyed as long as the destruction is roughly symmetrical— that is, the same in the two hemispheres. The principle of mass action was based primarily on the effects of cortical destruction on maze learning and retention in rats. For this reason, one might want to qualify the generality of its applicability to higher memory processes. However, it should be pointed out that similar findings were reported by Lashley and his associates regarding the effects of cortical ablations on the learning and retention of a fairly complex task by monkeys. Hence, the principle has some applicability to higher behavior processes.

Mass action is illustrated by the following example. If rats are trained on a maze and then undergo cortical lesions, the following results are obtained. If the lesion is small, involving only 5–10% of the cortex, the loss in retention may be almost negligible. In contrast, if 50% or more of the cortex is ablated, the maze habit is completely lost, and relearning may require much longer than did original learning. When the amount of training required to relearn the maze is plotted as a function of the extent of the lesion (see Figure 10-2), it is seen that these two variables are directly related.

Lashley was aware that there were difficulties in interpreting the meaning of this relationship. Since, in learning a maze, the rat utilizes a variety of sensory cues—visual, tactual, kinesthetic, olfactory, and so on—it was possible that the observed effects simply reflected the loss of more and more sensory functions.

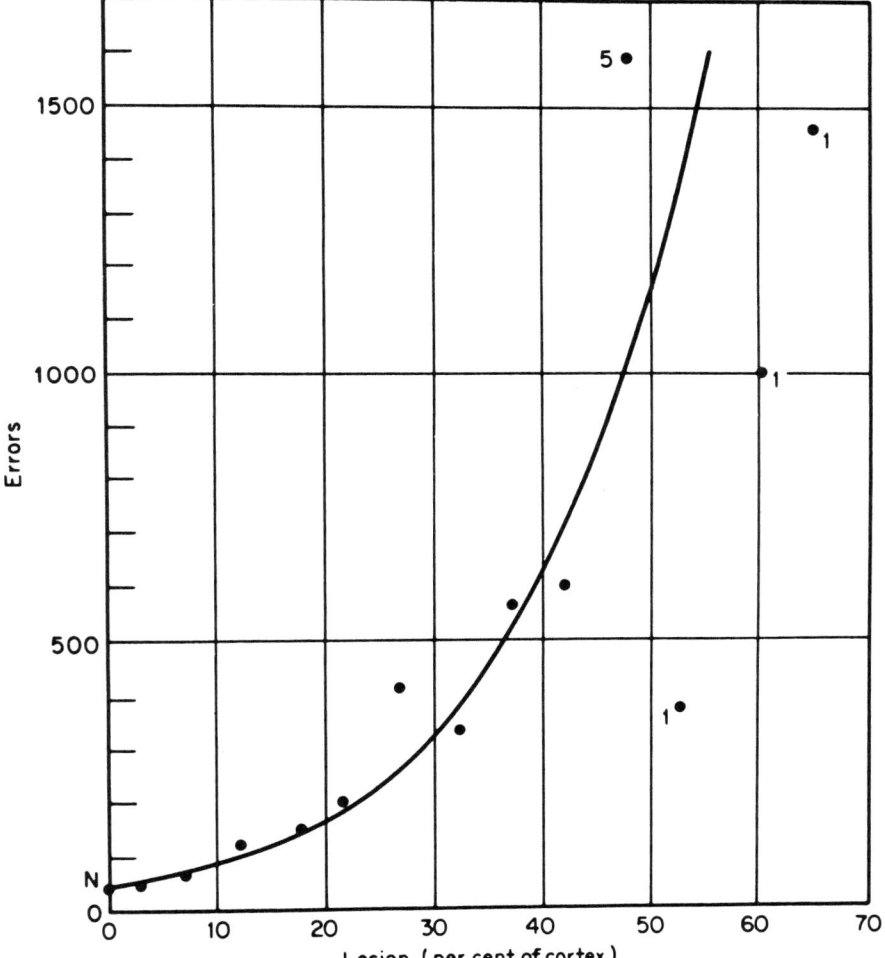

Figure 10-2
The relation of errors in maze learning to the extent of cortical damage in the rat. For lesions destroying more than 45% of the cortex, the number of cases (indicated by numerals on the graph) is too small for reliability. From "In Search of the Engram," by K. S. Lashley, Society for Experimental Biology, 1950, Symposium No. 4, 454 – 482. Copyright 1950 by Academic Press, Inc. Reprinted by permission.

However, sensory loss could not explain all of the retention deficit, and Lashley published data demonstrating that cortical lesions interfered with performance more than any specific sensory loss did. Lashley showed that, when blind animals were trained in a maze, the removal of the primary visual cortex still produced a severe performance loss and difficulty in relearning. Tsang (1934) also demonstrated that rats reared blind from birth showed a loss of the ability to run a maze following lesions to the visual cortex. Later research, using rats, cats, and monkeys as subjects, increased the generalizability of the finding that the visual cortex exerts significant influences on the learning of tasks that aren't clearly dependent upon vision (for example, Orbach, 1959; Perachio & Lubar, 1970; Saavedra, Pinto-Hamuy, & Oberti, 1965).

On the basis of his very intensive investigations, Lashley was forced to conclude that the memory trace, or engram, is not located in any single structure. As an alternative, he proposed that the memory trace represented a diffuse "reorganization of a vast system of associations involving the interrelations of hundreds of thousands or millions of neurons" (p. 475). This view persists in modern theoretical accounts of the locus of the memory trace. Although Lashley's work brought into question the idea that the cortex serves as the storehouse for memory, his research and that of his contemporaries demonstrated that specific learning and performance deficits resulted from cortical lesions. A large research literature has been generated by attempts to clarify the nature of cortical-lesion-produced deficits; we'll turn to this issue next.

The Frontal Lobes

For many years the frontal association cortex has been assumed to be involved in the mediation of the highest intellectual functions in humans. For this reason, the frontal association area has been a favorite target for neuroscientists attempting to determine the functions of the neocortex in the regulation of behavior. Current interest in the functions of the frontal lobes can be traced back to research conducted by Jacobsen in the 1930s. At the risk of oversimplification, I'll say at this point that no general deficit in memory processes occurs following ablations of the frontal association cortex. Rather, deficits in performance occur when animals are required to select a response on the basis of information presented earlier in testing (delayed response) or when they are required to change their pattern of responding by inhibiting a previously rewarded way of responding and performing in a new way (response inhibition).

Delayed-Response Deficit. In a classic study by Jacobsen (1936), an attempt was made to investigate the role of the frontal lobes in memory. He found that, while monkeys with large frontal-lobe ablations were normal in their ability to perform discriminations and puzzle-box problems, they were severely deficient on *delayed-response* problems. In a simple delayed-response problem, an animal is shown a piece of food, which is then placed under one of two identical cups in front of the animal. After a delay, the animal is allowed to choose one of the cups. Normal monkeys learn this problem easily even when the delay interval is several minutes, but primates with frontal lesions show a clear deficit on this task with delays as short as five seconds (for example, French & Harlow, 1962). Similar disruptions of performance have been reported following frontal lesions in cats (Lawicka & Konorski, 1961; Warren, 1964) and in dogs (Lawicka, 1957; Lawicka & Konorski, 1959). However, the severity of the deficit in these two species is often not as pronounced as it is in primates.

Jacobsen's initial findings suggested to him that the frontal association cortex was necessary for short-term, or immediate, memory. Many independent laboratories subsequently replicated his findings. As more data were collected, however, it became increasingly apparent that the observed deficits were not specifically related to memory processes. For example, Malmo (1942) showed that, if the monkeys were kept in the dark during the delay period, they performed normally. Finan (1942) found that, if frontally lesioned monkeys were allowed to make a rewarded response before the delay began, they also showed no deficit in delayed-response performance. This latter result suggested that part of the frontal monkey's problem in performing this task was that it did not pay enough attention to the task stimuli when they were presented.

Growing out of these and other studies was the idea that the effect of the frontal lesion was to make the animal hyperactive and easily distractable. In support of such an interpretation, Wade (1947) and Pribram (1950) reported that monkeys and baboons with frontal lesions improved on delayed-response tasks when given small doses of barbiturates, which had tranquilizing effects. Unfortunately, the view that hyperactivity was the primary reason for the frontal monkey's deficit has been questioned by other experimental evidence. New-world monkeys (for example, squirrel monkeys) show a marked deficit in delayed-response performance but are not hyperactive following frontal lesions (Miles & Blomquist, 1960). Warren and Konorski and their associates have similarly shown that frontal lesions make neither cats nor dogs hyperactive.

Response-Inhibition Deficit. Response perseveration is another characteristic of the behavior alterations produced by frontal lesions. The frontal animals are deficient in the ability to inhibit previously rewarded patterns of responding and to perform in a new and different way. As will be shown later in this chapter, this behavior change is very similar to the behavior deficits produced by hippocampal lesions in infrahuman species. This deficit was reported by many early investigators of frontal-lobe functions (for example, Harlow & Dagnon, 1943).

Perseverative responding by frontal animals has been studied under several different experimental paradigms. A popular way to study this phenomenon has been to employ either spatial- or object-reversal problems. In a spatial-reversal problem, the animal is required to choose an object located on the side opposite that of the object previously rewarded. In an object-reversal problem, the animal must switch its pattern so that the previously nonrewarded object is chosen. A spatial-reversal problem was employed by Warren (1964) to study frontal-lobe functions in cats.

In Warren's research, cats were trained preoperatively on an alternation problem in which a white object always presented on the left and a black stimulus always presented on the right were alternately rewarded during successive testing days. The cats were tested for 20 days. Nine of the subjects then underwent frontal ablations. Learning curves showing the percent of correct responses as a function of trials are shown in Figure 10-3. Examining these curves, you can see that the unoperated controls performed similarly at the times when pre- and postoperative testing was being given to the frontal animals. The frontal animals, in contrast, made more errors postoperatively than they had preoperatively. Statistical analyses indicated that the frontal animals were significantly retarded in their postoperative reversal skills, as compared with both their own preoperative performance and the retest performance of the control animals. An even greater impairment was found in the frontal cats if the two objects were identical instead of black and white—especially if the cats were trained on three reversals per day. More recent observations of cats with frontal lesions have verified that they are impaired in tasks that require inhibition of previously acquired responses (for example, Brutkowski, 1965; Warren, Coutant, & Cornwell, 1969).

Figure 10-3
These curves show the performance of control (left) and frontally ablated (right) cats on an alternation problem requiring response inhibition. The curves compare performance before and after surgery. From "The Behavior of Carnivores and Primates with Lesions in the Prefrontal Cortex,"
by J. M. Warren. In J. M. Warren and K. Akert (Eds.), The Frontal Granular Cortex and Behavior. *Copyright 1964 by McGraw-Hill, Inc. Reprinted by permission.*

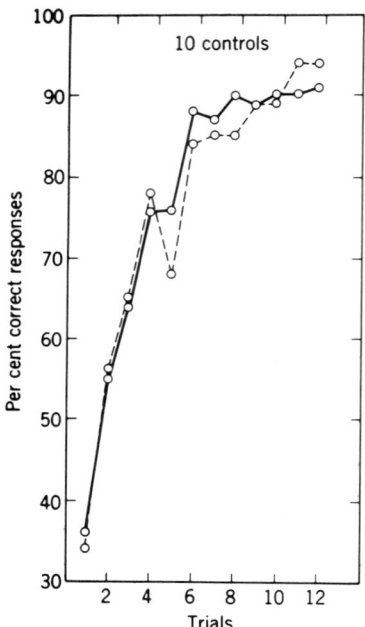

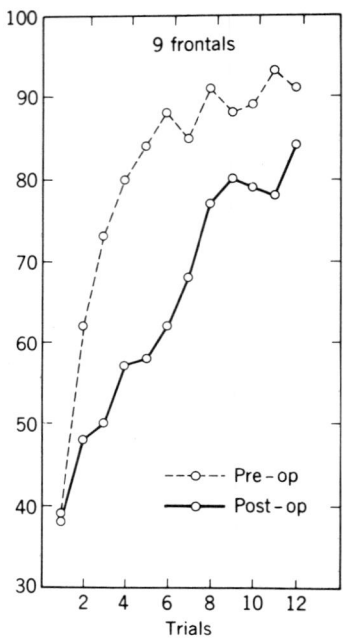

Mishkin (1964) has similarly shown a spatial-reversal deficit in monkeys subjected to frontal lesions. He also presented some interesting data on the effects of frontal lesions on object-discrimination reversal. In Mishkin's research, an object was presented alone for five trials, and the food cup below it either had a food reward in it every trial or had nothing in it every trial. In this way, the object was presumably made reinforcing for one group but not for the other. It was then paired with an indifferent object for ten discrimination trials. On some of the problems, the monkey was rewarded for showing its "acquired preferences"—that is, for approaching the rewarded object or avoiding the nonrewarded object. In the other problem, the opposite behavior pattern—avoiding the rewarded object or approaching the nonrewarded object—was rewarded. A new pair of objects was used for each problem administered to the monkeys, and each pair consisted of a training object and an indifferent stimulus. Forty problems—ten of each kind—were presented to each subject.

The results, shown in Figure 10-4, provide strong evidence for a perseverative tendency following frontal lesions. If the frontal monkeys' previously acquired preferences were reinforced in the object-discrimination problem, they performed almost as well as did the normal animals. In contrast, if the frontal animals had to suppress their previously acquired preferences, their performance was distinctly impaired. This impairment occurred regardless of whether they were required to suppress the tendency to approach the previously rewarded stimulus or the tendency to avoid the previously nonrewarded stimulus.

Mishkin interpreted these deficits of the frontal monkeys in terms of a perseverative tendency; that is, the frontal animals persisted with behavior responses that were no longer appropriate. They were not able to alter their response pattern when the reinforcement contingencies were altered. Mishkin further concluded that

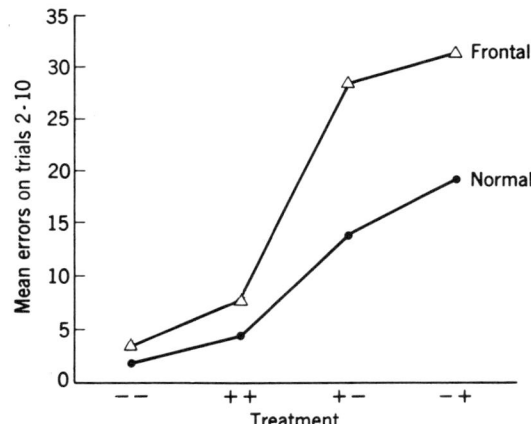

Figure 10-4
Mean errors on two forms of discrimination reversal (+ −, − +) and two forms of nonreversal (− −, + +). Errors on the first, or informing, trial have been excluded. From "Effects of Object Preferences and Aversions on Discrimination Learning in Monkeys with Frontal Lesions," by E. S. Brush, M. Mishkin, and H. E. Rosvold, Journal of Comparative and Physiological Psychology, *1961, 54, 319–325. Copyright 1961 by the American Psychological Association. Reprinted by permission.*

this perseverative tendency could not be invoked to account for the impaired performance of frontal animals on delayed-response tasks. Thus, it appears that there are two effects arising from frontal lesions: a delayed-response deficit and a perseverative tendency.

Several experiments have now shown that these two deficits associated with frontal-lobe resections result from lesioning different portions of the frontal association areas (for example, Butter, 1969; Mishkin, 1964; Mishkin, Vest, Waxler, & Rosvold, 1969). The locations of these different frontal lesions are shown in Figure 10-5. The orbital sector (*orf* lesion) of the frontal lobes appears to be involved in the inhibition of previously reinforced patterns of responding, and the dorsolateral section (*dlf* lesion) apparently mediates delayed-response performance.

As Peter Milner (1970) has suggested, the delayed-response deficit that occurs in frontal monkeys may not shed light on the functions of the frontal lobes to any great extent. As indicated, this deficit in some species, such as cats and dogs, is quite mild compared with the deficit in monkeys. Milner also indicated that the delayed-response deficit does not appear at all in humans, presumably because of verbal mediation during the delay. That is, a human can use covert verbal rehearsal to bridge the delay gap. In contrast, perseverative tendencies are very marked following frontal lesions in all infrahuman species studied, and Brenda Milner (1964) and others have demonstrated that humans with frontal lesions similarly have difficulty in altering their mode of responding when it ceases to be appropriate for the existing reinforcement contingencies.

The Posterior Association Cortex

Although not getting as much attention from neural researchers as the frontal lobes, the posterior association cortex has also undergone a good deal of experimental investigation. The posterior association cortex includes cortical association areas of the parietal and temporal lobes. Most investigations of the posterior association cortex have emphasized the temporal lobe. This emphasis is probably due in large part to Klüver and Bucy's (1937, 1939) dramatic discovery of **psychic blindness** in monkeys with temporal-lobe resections—a finding that was reviewed in Chapter 8.

Figure 10-5
Lateral view of the
monkey brain
indicating the
extent of dlf
(dorsolateral frontal
lesion), orf
(orbitofrontal
lesion), ifc *(inferior*
convexity of frontal
lobe), pos
(preoccipital
sulcus), pt *(posterior*
temporal lesion),
and at *(anterior*
temporal lesion).
From "Brain
Lesions and
Memory in
Animals," by S. D.
Iversen. In J. A.
Deutsch (Ed.), The
Physiological Basis
of Memory.
Copyright 1973 by
Academic Press, Inc.
Reprinted by
permission.

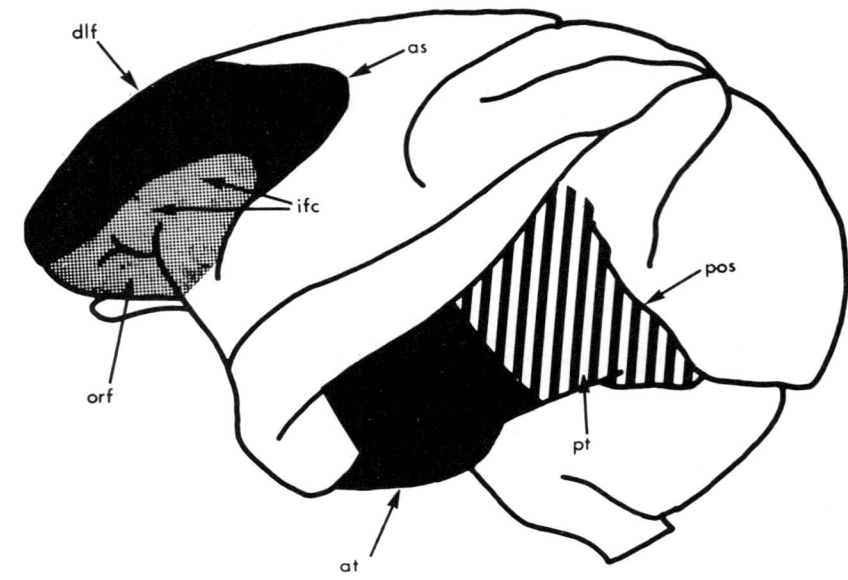

The inability of the temporal-lobectomized monkeys to recognize the significance of objects presented visually—that is, their psychic blindness—was later shown to result from the neocortical involvement of these lesions. This conclusion was based on the finding that discrimination deficits specific to the visual modality follow lesions to the temporal lobes (Blum, Chow, & Pribram, 1950). Later research restricted the effective site of this lesion to the ventrolateral portion of the temporal lobe (Mishkin, 1954; Mishkin & Pribram, 1954). This region of the temporal lobe of the monkey, which acts as a higher-processing area for the visual modality, is called the **inferotemporal cortex.** Posterior cortical association regions performing functions presumably analogous to those performed by the inferotemporal cortex of the monkey have been identified in the cat (for example, Hara, 1962; Hara, Cornwell, Warren, & Webster, 1974; Warren, Warren, & Akert, 1961) and the rat (Thompson, Lesse, & Rich, 1963).

The auditory, tactile, and olfactory senses similarly have discretely localized higher-processing areas in the posterior association cortex of the monkey (for example, Blum, 1951; Brown, Rosvold, & Mishkin, 1963; Neff, 1961; Wilson, 1957). However, these regions have been less intensively studied than the visual area. The importance of the discovery of these areas is that it demonstrates the existence of modality-specific loci, outside the primary sensory areas, that mediate sensory discrimination functions (Iversen, 1973). It is important to note that these regions do not appear to be involved in memory consolidation as a general process; rather, they act as processing regions for information concerned with specific modality-related responses.

Some differences between the effects of frontal- and of posterior-association-cortex lesions should be pointed out. First, in contrast to the posterior association cortex of the parietal and temporal lobes, the frontal lobes lack distinct modality-specific processing regions. For example, it has been shown that discrete dorsolateral frontal lesions, which yield visual-discrimination impairments, produce auditory-discrimination (Weiskrantz & Mishkin, 1958) and tactual-discrimination deficits as well (Iversen, 1967). Wilson (1957), on the other hand, found that lesions to the posterior association cortex of the parietal lobes resulted in tactile but not visual deficits, while inferotemporal lesions yielded the opposite effects.

Another difference between the effects of frontal- and posterior-association-cortex lesions is that posterior lesions do not produce a delayed-response deficit (Rosvold & Szwarcbart, 1964). In fact, monkeys subjected to removal of the anterior-temporal-lobe neocortex in addition to the association cortex of the frontal lobes do no worse on a delayed-response task than do subjects sustaining only frontal-lobe resections (Schiltz, Thompson, Harlow, Mohr, & Blomquist, 1973). Finally, posterior-association-cortex ablations, in contrast to frontal lesions, do not produce perseverative tendencies (Mishkin, 1964).

Data obtained from human clinical observations by Penfield and his associates at the Montreal Neurological Institute have stimulated interest in the functions of the temporal lobes in learning and memory processes. The most famous of their investigations of the temporal-lobe neocortex was published by Penfield and Rasmussen (1950). In this inquiry, the authors demonstrated that electrical stimulation of the temporal-lobe neocortex could at times elicit complex auditory and visual hallucinations and even activate complex memories. However, the integrity of the neocortex was subsequently shown to be unnecessary for the recall of past events because memories could still be elicited after the cortex was removed (Penfield, 1965; Penfield & Perot, 1963).

Data collected since Lashley's pioneering work have substantiated Lashley's view that no region of the neocortex is essential for learning and memory. Simple conditioning does not require the cortex, and even very difficult discrimination problems can be relearned following damage to cortical association areas. These results have led many brain researchers to propose that the actual formation of stimulus-response associations occurs at the subcortical level. As a result, a tremendous number of experiments have investigated the effects on learning and retention of discretely placed lesions to various subcortical structures. Attention to the functions performed in learning and memory processes by subcortical brain regions has also been dictated by the availability of subjects for neural research. The rat seems to have been the most popular subject for experimental investigations, and, although the rat's subcortex is relatively well differentiated, its cortex is not very sophisticated. The rat has very little association cortex; its cortex is devoted almost entirely to sensory and motor functions.

Subcortical Functions in Learning and Memory

The Hippocampus

Human Clinical Observations. Over the past 25 years, the subcortical structure that has been most intensively investigated for possible functions in the storage and retrieval of memory has been the hippocampus. Interest in this structure and its functions in associative processes was generated by human clinical observations. Case studies indicated that bilateral damage to the hippocampus of humans, as a result of tumor growth or vascular disturbances, resulted in severe deficits in the ability to add new information to permanent memory. These effects appeared to be specific to the memory-consolidation mechanism, because general intelligence and the ability to recall information acquired prior to surgery were, for the most part, unaffected. The location of the hippocampus in the human temporal lobe is shown in Figure 10-6.

A similar disturbance of memory-consolidation processes has been noted in clinical cases in which bilateral temporal-lobe excisions have been performed for the relief of temporal-lobe epilepsy or of psychotic personality disorders. These radical

Figure 10-6
Drawing of a dissected human hippocampus. The hemisphere has been partially removed, the midbrain is cut across, and the third ventricle is exposed. Adapted from "The Hippocampus," by J. D. Green. In J. Field (Ed.), Handbook of Physiology; Section I: Neurophysiology, *(Vol. 2). Copyright 1960 by the American Physiological Society. Reprinted by permission.*

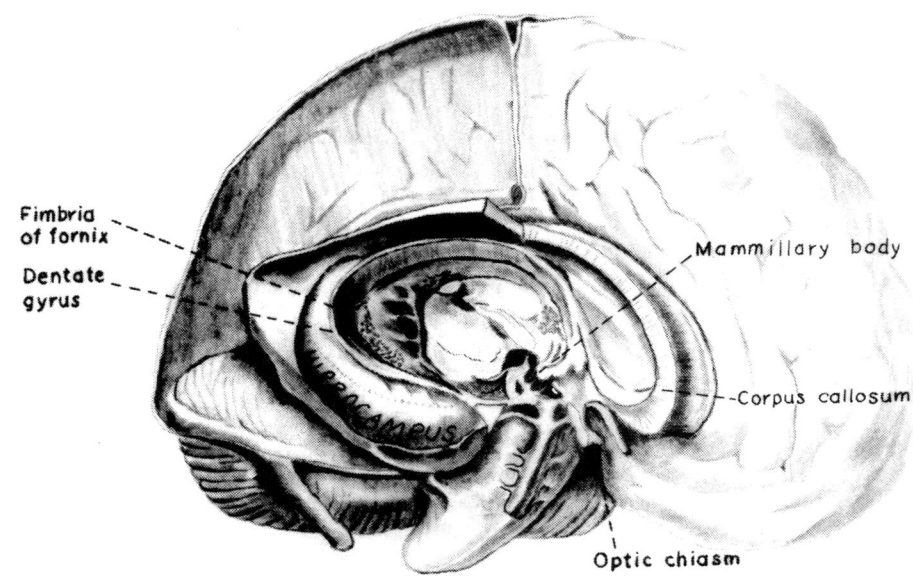

surgical procedures were undertaken only after more conservative types of treatments had proved ineffective. The surgical preparations, in addition to removing the anterior two-thirds of the temporal-lobe neocortex, approximately, ablated the amygdala and portions of the hippocampus. Of ten such patients studied by Scoville and Milner (1957), there was some disturbance in the ability to consolidate new information in all whose lesions extended far enough posterior to involve portions of the hippocampus bilaterally. The extent of the resulting deficit was roughly proportional to the amount of hippocampal damage. According to Milner (1966), no residual memory deficits occurred following lesions limited to the amygdala.

These observations led Penfield and Milner (1958) to propose that the initial recording of memory traces may be accomplished via hippocampal mechanisms. This observation was to precipitate a flood of investigations, using infrahuman species, on the functions of the hippocampus in learning and memory. These studies will be reviewed later in this chapter. It is important to emphasize that Penfield and Milner's formulations did not imply that the memory trace was located in either the hippocampus or the adjacent temporal-lobe neocortex. Their patients who were unable to form new permanent memories after surgical removal of the hippocampus could still recall events that had occurred prior to surgery.

Much of our present knowledge concerning memory deficits produced by hippocampal lesions in humans has come from extensive study of an epileptic patient

(H. M.), who was first reported on by Scoville (1954). This reliance on a single case is due to the fact that the psychotic patients have often not been well enough to be tested. In general, though, there have been no indications of any dramatic changes in the patients' basic intelligence following radical hippocampal damage.

An example of the drastic effects on memory consolidation of hippocampal lesions is provided in the following account by Scoville and Milner (1957) regarding the capabilities of H. M., whose hippocampus was removed bilaterally in 1954 to relieve intractible seizures associated with temporal-lobe epilepsy.

> After the operation, this young man could no longer recognize the hospital staff nor find his way to the bathroom, and he seemed to recall nothing of the day to day events of his hospital life. There was also a partial retrograde amnesia. His early memories were apparently vivid and intact [p. 14].

H. M. was able to retain a three-digit number or a pair of unrelated words as long as he was not distracted. However, as soon as his attention was diverted, he forgot the material. If, on the other hand, the information on which responses were based was made continuously available, difficult problem-solving tasks could be mastered (Milner, 1966). These results appeared to indicate an inability to add any new information to the long-term memory store. Evidence to support this view was provided by Milner's description, in 1966, of H. M.'s memory deficit. She wrote that "the remarkable memory defect persists, and it is clear that H. M. can remember extremely little of the experiences of the past twelve years" (p. 113). She concluded that the only way this patient could retain new information was by constantly verbally rehearsing it; H. M. immediately forgot new information if verbal rehearsal was prevented by the diversion of his attention to a new activity.

A few cases of global amnesia, similar to that observed in H. M. following bilateral hippocampal excisions, have resulted from unilateral temporal lobectomy. These operations were performed on patients as a treatment for temporal-lobe epilepsy in cases in which the epileptogenic factors were thought to be located on one side. Penfield and Milner (1958) attributed the occurrence of the global amnesia to the presence of a preoperatively unsuspected lesion of the opposite hippocampal formation. In support of this interpretation, these cases were later shown to exhibit an EEG abnormality postoperatively in the intact temporal lobe. One of these cases died of unrelated causes. Upon histological examination of her brain, Milner (1966) reported that the hippocampus in the unoperated right temporal lobe was "shrunken and pale and had lost its normal structure" (p. 119). This finding confirmed Penfield and Milner's contention that only patients with bilateral hippocampal damage are liable to develop severe memory defects. Further, they interpreted these findings as consistent with their view that the hippocampal region is essential for the transfer of new information to permanent memory in humans.

These clinical reports on the functions of the hippocampus in memory consolidation were based on relatively few subjects, and, with the exception of the case mentioned above, histological verification of the exact extent and locus of the lesions has not been obtained. Nevertheless, these findings have provided great impetus to researchers attempting to define the functions of the hippocampus. As with any type of neurological research involving human subjects, this research has had serious limitations. Thus, in order to further examine the functions of the hippocampus, investigators have turned to the use of infrahuman species as subjects.

Hippocampal Lesions and Learning in Infrahuman Species. The fact that humans with hippocampal lesions were severely impaired in the acquisition of new skills or information suggested that the concept of *recent memory* could not be clearly distinguished from *learning ability.* Operationally, both of these constructs imply an ability to consolidate new material into memory and to recall this material when necessary. Learning cannot be accomplished unless the subject has the capacity to permanently store relevant information. For this reason, tests of the proposed memory-consolidation function of the hippocampus have usually examined the effects of hippocampal ablations on the acquisition of novel learning tasks.

Much to the surprise of early researchers in this area, clear support for a memory-consolidation view of hippocampal functioning was not forthcoming from the animal hippocampal literature. In infrahumans, hippocampal lesions did not produce a global memory-consolidation deficit, as they appeared to do in humans. Rather, animals sustaining bilateral hippocampal destructions were found to be capable of learning some complex problems. Rats, cats, and monkeys were found to be normal in their acquisition and retention of a simultaneous-discrimination problem, regardless of whether the discrimination was between tactual stimuli (Teitelbaum, 1964; Webster & Voneida, 1964), spatial cues (Kimble & Kimble, 1965), or visual stimuli that varied in brightness, size, or shape (Douglas & Pribram, 1966; Kimble, 1963; Kimble & Pribram, 1963; Stein & Kimble, 1966; Thompson & Massopust, 1960; Truax & Thompson, 1969). Hippocampal lesions were found actually to facilitate learning and performance of a two-way active-avoidance problem in rats (for example, Antelman & Brown, 1972; Isaacson, Douglas, & Moore, 1961; Lovely, 1975; Olton & Isaacson, 1968; Rabe & Haddad, 1969), rabbits (Papesdorf & Woodruff, 1970), and guinea pigs (Ireland, Hayes, & Schaub, 1969; Weiss & Hertzler, 1973). (In a two-way active-avoidance problem, the animal is tested in a chamber divided into halves by a hurdle. At a signal, the animal must leap the hurdle and move to the other end of the apparatus to avoid shock. When the signal is again presented, the animal must move back over the hurdle to the side on which it started. The sequence then repeats itself, with the animal moving back and forth across the hurdle on successive trials.) In contrast, hippocampally ablated rats were generally found to be deficient in the acquisition of complex mazes (Hughes, 1965; Kaada, Rasmussen, & Kveim, 1961; Kimble, 1963; Kveim, Setekleiv, & Kaada, 1964; Madsen & Kimble, 1965; Means, Leander, & Isaacson, 1971; Niki, 1962; Spiegel, Hostetter, & Thomas, 1966; Stein & Kimble, 1966; Thomas, 1971), but, once they mastered the maze, they remembered it as well as did normal animals (for example, Jarrard & Lewis, 1967).

Taken together, studies of the effects of hippocampal lesions on infrahuman species have failed to confirm the memory-consolidation hypothesis of hippocampal functioning. This could be due to differences that have evolved in the role performed by this brain structure in mediating the behavior of humans. It seems more plausible, however, that the lack of supporting evidence has been the product of methodological differences between the human and the infrahuman experiments. The almost exclusive use of two-choice discrimination problems in the animal-lesion studies may have resulted in hippocampal investigators failing to tap the dimensions necessary to evoke evidence of a recent-memory deficit. In the majority of human studies, the testing involved recall of chains of verbal items or of complex events from the patient's daily life.

In an experiment conducted in my laboratory, we (Anton & Bennett, 1974) proposed that an alternative technique for assessing the memory-consolidation hypothesis of hippocampal functioning in rodents—a way perhaps more analogous to the testing regimen used with human hippocampal patients—was to require rats to utilize information acquired during their day-to-day activities, in a transfer-of-learning paradigm. Specifically, we examined the effects of hippocampal lesions on transfer of perceptual learning using the early-experience model of Gibson and Walk (1956). This paradigm has been used in a number of inquiries over the years to determine how early exposure to shapes affects subsequent discrimination of them (for example, Bennett & Ellis, 1968; Bennett, Anton, & Levitt, 1971; Gibson & Walk, 1956; Kerpelman, 1965).

In the early-experience paradigm, experimental animals are exposed to the to-be-discriminated forms (for example, circles and triangles) during rearing. At maturity, the animals are required to learn to discriminate between these shapes as a test of the effects of the early-experience conditions. It has generally been found that preexposed animals learn the discrimination problem significantly faster than do nonexposed control subjects. This paradigm requires the animals to acquire information in their daily living environments and to later transfer this information to a discrimination problem.

In our study, we hypothesized that the amount of information transferred to the subsequent discrimination problem by hippocampectomized animals might be an index more analogous to that employed in the human investigations and might thereby provide a better basis for assessing the view that the hippocampus is important for memory-consolidation processes in infrahuman species. Although some ambiguities existed in our results, our data appeared to support the memory-consolidation hypothesis of hippocampal functioning. Whereas normal animals profited from preexposure to the to-be-discriminated stimuli, animals that had had their hippocampi destroyed prior to preexposure fared no better on the later circle/triangle discrimination problem than did animals not preexposed to the stimuli.

In interpreting the significance of these data, it was unclear whether the observed deficits reflected impairment of memory consolidation and recall processes or whether, instead, the hippocampal lesions had altered the animals' ability to process information arising from the preexposure—an ability necessary for information storage. For example, the hippocampal lesions may have produced decreased attention to environmental stimuli. Such an interpretation is plausible in light of animal lesion findings (Jackson & Strong, 1965; Kimble & Kimble, 1970) and animal EEG findings (Bennett, 1971, 1975; Bennett, Hébert, & Moss, 1973), which have implicated the hippocampus in the processes of attention to environmental cues. As indicated earlier, a major problem in interpreting the significance of a lesion-induced deficit in learning is determining the basis for the deficit. This is why it is often so very difficult to discern whether a learning deficit reflects an actual disruption of memory consolidation and recall or a disruption of behavior processes involved in the performance of some response.

Perseverative Tendencies Resulting from Hippocampal Lesions. There has been one rather dramatic and consistent effect of hippocampal lesions on learning and performance reported in the experimental literature. In general, hippocampally lesioned animals are less likely than unoperated control subjects to stop doing something that has become either punishing or nonrewarding. That is, they seem to be deficient in the ability to inhibit previously reinforced responses and perform new, different responses. Earlier in this chapter, we saw that similar perseverative tendencies followed bilateral excisions of the orbital sector of the frontal lobes.

In the case of hippocampectomized animals (and frontal subjects, for that matter), acquisition of information appears to interfere with the learning of new information at some later time. Almost all demonstrated learning deficits following hippocampal ablations fall into this category of deficits due to response perseveration. On the basis of results obtained in some very carefully conducted experiments, Warrington and Weiskrantz (1973) have proposed that this phenomenon—proactive interference—may be the basis for the memory deficits observed in human clinical patients. They argue that the amnesic syndrome observed in these patients does not reflect, as is commonly assumed, a failure of the memory-consolidation mechanism. Rather, they suggest that the problem is one of information recall. In the human hippocampal subject, there is an excess of interference among stored items, and this interference produces an inability to recall information from memory. Basically, this view contends that information stored in the past interferes with the ability to recall information stored more recently. This is a very intriguing reinterpretation of the human hippocampal syndrome, and future research will determine its validity.

The perseverative tendencies exhibited by hippocampally lesioned infrahuman subjects may be observed in a number of situations. For a more detailed review of these data than is possible here, the reader should refer to Douglas (1967), Isaacson (1974), or Kimble (1968). One index of a hippocampal animal's perseverative tendency is the greater resistance to extinction of a variety of its responses in straight alley runway or operant situations. "Greater resistance to extinction" means that, once it has learned to emit a response to obtain a reward, the hippocampal animal will continue making this response much longer after reinforcement has been discontinued than will normal animals. Greater resistance to extinction has been reported in rats following acquisition of an approach response in a straight alley runway (Jarrard & Isaacson, 1965; Jarrard, Isaacson, & Wickelgren, 1964; Niki, 1962; Raphelson, Isaacson, & Douglas, 1966). (A straight alley runway is a long chamber. The animal runs from a start-box area to a goal-box area to secure a food reward. Approach in this situation involves running down the alley to the goal box to obtain the reward.) Increased resistance to extinction may also be observed following acquisition of an operant response, such as bar-pressing to secure a food reward, in rats (Amsel, Glazer, Lakey, McCuller, & Wong, 1973; Kimble & Kimble, 1965; Niki, 1965), cats (Peretz, 1965; Webster & Voneida, 1964), and monkeys (Douglas & Pribram, 1966). Closely related to increases in resistance to extinction are deficits in passive-avoidance learning in hippocampectomized rats. As with extinction, passive avoidance requires the animal to relinquish a previously rewarded response, but, in the case of passive avoidance, the incentive to give up the old response is provided by punishment for continuing this inappropriate response, in addition to the removal of the reward.

To test for passive avoidance, animals are first trained to make an approach response, such as running down a runway or entering a compartment, to secure a food reward. After acquiring this approach response, the subjects are shocked whenever they again attempt to obtain the food. Deficits in the animals' ability to inhibit the previously acquired approach response are used as an index of a passive-avoidance deficit, and a number of studies have demonstrated passive-avoidance deficits following removal of the hippocampus (Glick & Greenstein, 1973; Isaacson, Olton, Bauer, & Swart, 1966; Isaacson & Wickelgren, 1962; Kimble, 1963; Kimble, Kirkby,

& Stein, 1966; Nonneman & Isaacson, 1973; Papesdorf & Woodruff, 1970; Snyder & Isaacson, 1965; Stein & Kirkby, 1967; Teitelbaum & Milner, 1963).

Difficulty in discrimination reversal is a third measure that can be used to assess the hippocampal animal's perseverative tendencies. Subjects with hippocampal lesions show deficits in their ability to stop approaching a previously rewarded stimulus and instead approach the previously nonrewarded one. This deficit occurs even if the prereversal response was readily acquired. The discrimination-reversal impairment has been reported in a variety of infrahuman species, including rats (Kimble & Kimble, 1965; Niki, 1966; Olton, 1972; Racine & Kimble, 1965; Thompson & Langer, 1963), cats (Nonneman & Isaacson, 1973; Teitelbaum, 1964; Webster & Voneida, 1964), and monkeys (Douglas & Pribram, 1966; Rosvold & Szwarcbart, 1964).

Performance deficits due to response perseveration in hippocampally ablated subjects also occur when animals are shifted from a continuous- to an intermittent-reinforcement schedule. In a continuous (CRF) schedule, all bar-presses are reinforced, while, in an intermittent schedule, only specific responses are rewarded. For example, under an intermittent-reinforcement schedule, an animal might receive reinforcement for the first response that occurs on an average of 15 seconds after the last response (variable-interval schedule), or a rat might receive a reinforcement only if it waits at least 20 seconds *between* successive bar-presses. This latter example illustrates a schedule called DRL (differential reinforcement of low rates of responding), under which only those responses occurring a set interval apart are rewarded. For example, in a DRL 20-second schedule, only those responses occurring at least 20 seconds apart are reinforced. If the animal emits an incorrect response by pressing the bar before this interval has elapsed, the interval resets, or begins again, and reinforcement is thus postponed. There is no maximal interval before which the animal must respond. Hippocampectomized rats and cats have been shown to overrespond when they are shifted from a CRF to either an intermittent variable-interval (Jarrard, 1965) or a DRL schedule (Clark & Isaacson, 1965; Nonneman & Isaacson, 1973; Pellegrino & Clapp, 1971; Rickert, Bennett, Anderson, Corbett, & Smith, 1973; Schmaltz & Isaacson, 1966).

The Schmaltz and Isaacson study can be used to illustrate this type of perseverative deficit. Three groups of rats were employed: unoperated controls, hippocampally lesioned rats, which had had their hippocampus bilaterally removed via suction, and neocortically lesioned controls, which had had the neocortex over the hippocampus removed as a control for the effects of the neocortical destruction the hippocampals experienced. (Ablating the rat hippocampus via aspiration necessitates the removal of the overlying neocortical mantle.) The majority of rat hippocampal studies have used these three groups. In one of the experiments in the Schmaltz and Isaacson study, animals were shifted from a CRF to a DRL 20-second schedule of reinforcement. Animals learned to bar-press for food and were then given 20 daily sessions of CRF, during which all bar-presses were reinforced. On the 21st day, these animals were switched to a DRL 20-second schedule; only those bar-presses occurring at least 20 seconds apart were rewarded.

Although all groups performed similarly on CRF, differences among the groups emerged when they were shifted to the DRL 20-second schedule. These differences are graphed in Figure 10-7. The hippocampal rats were found to obtain fewer reinforcements per session, and the number of bar-presses they emitted that resulted in reinforcement was lower. This is because they overresponded on DRL, persisting

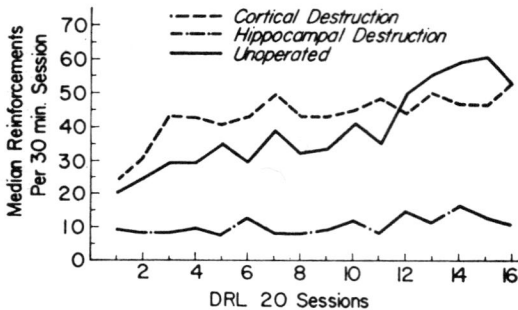 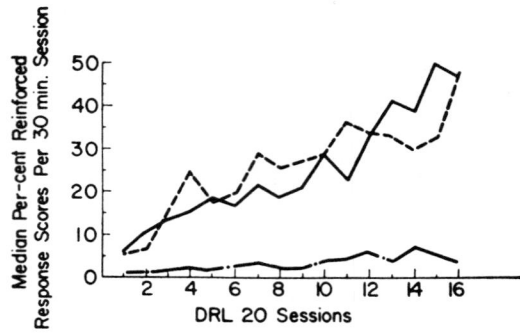

Figure 10-7
The performance of
cortical,
hippocampal, and
control rats, all with
prior experience on
CRF, on a DRL
20-second schedule.
From "The Effects
of Preliminary
Training Conditions
upon DRL
Performance in the
Hippocampectomized
Rat," by L. W.
Schmaltz and R. L.
Isaacson,
Physiology and
Behavior, 1966,
1, 175–182.
Copyright 1966 by
Brain Research
Publications, Inc.
Reprinted by
permission.

with a response pattern that had been appropriate during CRF. The rapid rate of bar-pressing that was acquired during CRF had proactively interfered with their ability to respond appropriately to the new contingencies of reinforcement imposed by the DRL schedule—that is, to press the bar no more frequently than every 20 seconds.

In a second experiment in their paper, Schmaltz and Isaacson verified that proactive interference was the factor underlying the observed DRL deficits. In this experiment, the rats were trained only on DRL 20 seconds, never experiencing CRF. Under these conditions of training, the hippocampectomized animals showed no deficits in terms of the number of reinforcements received per session or the number of reinforced responses emitted per session. These findings are graphically portrayed in Figure 10-8. Taken together, the results of the Schmaltz and Isaacson study clearly demonstrated that hippocampally lesioned animals tended to perseverate with behaviors that were acquired prior to a change in training conditions.

Research by Winocur and Mills (1970) has suggested that prior training will always interfere with the performance of hippocampally lesioned subjects, as long as the preceding task is in some way related to the current problem. Training on unrelated tasks will not produce perseverative tendencies. These findings suggest that the hippocampus may be responsible for the matching of expected and obtained consequences of responding. Without an intact hippocampus, an animal is unable to adjust its pattern of responding when a mismatch occurs.

What is the basis for this deficit? That is, what does the hippocampus do to mediate behavior in the intact animal? The perseverative tendencies exhibited by hippocampectomized subjects have led several researchers to suggest that the hippocampus is needed for inhibition of a prepotent response when a mismatch occurs between the expected and obtained consequences of responding (Douglas, 1967; Kimble, 1968; Schmaltz & Isaacson, 1966). An alternative interpretation of the perseverative tendencies is that hippocampally lesioned rats are deficient in their ability to process information concerning environmental change (Jackson & Strong, 1965; Kimble & Kimble, 1970; Kirkby, Stein, Kimble, & Kimble, 1967; Winocur & Mills, 1969). According to this latter view, the basis for the perseverative tendency lies in the inability of the hippocampectomized animals to perform an attention shift when reinforcement contingencies are altered.

There are data available, on the other hand, that would restrict the generality of either the response-inhibition or the attention-shift accounts for the hippocampal-lesion effect (Pellegrino & Clapp, 1971; Rickert & Bennett, 1972; Rickert, Bennett,

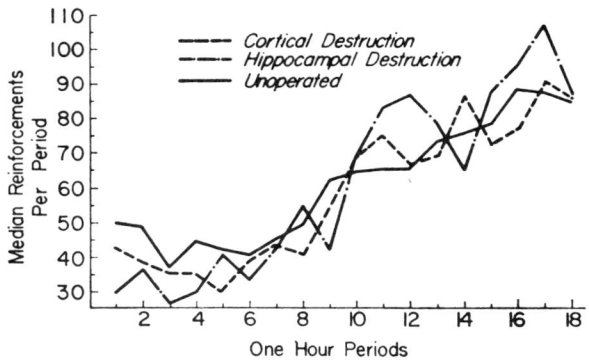
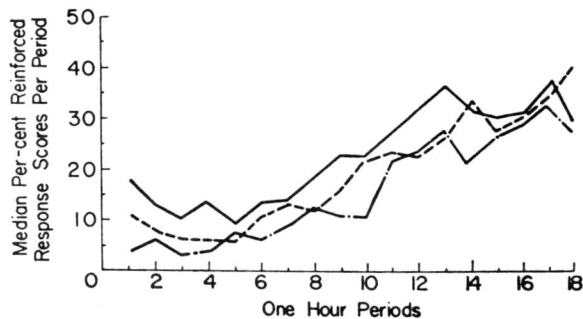

Figure 10-8
The performance of cortical, hippocampal, and control rats, all without prior experience on CRF, on a DRL 20-second schedule. From "The Effects of Preliminary Training Conditions upon DRL Performance in the Hippocampectomized Rat," by L. W. Schmaltz and R. L. Isaacson, Physiology and Behavior, 1966, 1, 175–182. Copyright 1966 by Brain Research Publications, Inc. Reprinted by permission.

Anderson, Corbett, & Smith, 1973). In one of the experiments in the Rickert et al. (1973) inquiry, we trained rats on CRF for 15 sessions and then shifted them to DRL for 20 sessions. DRL sessions varied according to the stringency of the DRL imposed; different groups of animals were shifted to DRL 10 seconds, DRL 20 seconds, or DRL 30 seconds. We reasoned that, if the basis of the DRL deficit were an inability to inhibit a previously reinforced pattern of responding, then shifting hippocampectomized rats to schedules that require different amounts of inhibition should produce different results. That is, the deficit of hippocampally lesioned subjects should increase as the DRL schedule length increases if the response-inhibition account is valid. Our results ran counter to the response-inhibition view of hippocampal functioning. The hippocampal rats were certainly deficient on DRL performance after experiencing a CRF schedule, but they did not show increased deficits, compared with control animals, as the stringency of the DRL increased.

In a second experiment in this same study, we replicated the conditions of our first experiment, but we modified the DRL tasks so that the end of the "time out" and the availability of reinforcement were signaled by the onset of a light. Under these conditions, the hippocampal rats acquired the DRL schedule at a normal rate. Similar findings have been reported by Pellegrino and Clapp (1971). These observations led us to propose that the role of the hippocampus might be one of processing information from response-produced, or proprioceptive, feedback, or stimulation. Thus, in terms of an attentional deficit, hippocampectomy produces a deficit in the ability of the animal to detect changes in the conditions of learning only when those changes require the utilization of response-produced stimulation for their detection.

An alternative interpretation of our data is that the addition of the light cue either altered the conditions of training to such an extent that proactive interference did not occur or made the conditions of reinforcement so distinctive that the animal's tendency to perseverate with inappropriate hypotheses was negated. Future research will have to further clarify the nature of this perseverative tendency. Regardless of its basis, proactive interference appears to be the most reliable effect of hippocampal lesions on learning and performance. In light of Warrington and Weiskrantz's reinterpretation of the human hippocampal literature and in view of the kinds of deficits exhibited by infrahuman species that have undergone hippocampal destructions, it might be profitable to conceive of the hippocampus' function in learning and memory as one of "stamping out" previously acquired but currently inappropriate information rather than "stamping in" or consolidating memory traces.

Several structures to which the hippocampus sends projections have also been implicated in processes of learning and memory. The fornix is the major efferent pathway from the hippocampus, and the fornix links the hippocampus with other regions of the subcortex. Specifically, nerve tracts from the hippocampus course downward via the fornix to the septum, the mammillary region of the hypothalamus, and the anterior nuclear complex and the medial nuclear group (dorsomedial nucleus) of the thalamus. All of these connections are reciprocal.

The Hypothalamus and Thalamus. The mammillary bodies and the medial thalamus have been implicated in memory because they (but not the hippocampus) are destroyed in the human clinical syndrome **Korsakoff's psychosis.**

Korsakoff's psychosis (Korsakoff, 1889; Victor & Yakovlev, 1955) is characterized by extreme memory deficits similar to those observed following bilateral hippocampal destructions in human patients. That is, patients suffering from Korsakoff's syndrome demonstrate an inability to store new information from the onset of the illness, but past memories are relatively well preserved. This disorder results from chronic alcoholism.

Careful studies of the brains of patients afflicted with Korsakoff's psychosis have revealed associated lesions involving the pulvinar, anterior, and dorsomedial thalamic nuclei, the mammillary bodies, and the terminal portions of the fornices (Brain & Walton, 1969). Medial thalamic and mammillary lesions were present more consistently than were lesions to the other loci (Adams & Sidman, 1968). The observed memory defect has often been attributed to the mammillary lesions, but recent evidence has suggested that changes in the dorsomedial thalamic nuclei are particularly critical to the memory loss (Alpers & Mancall, 1971). The lesions produced by this disorder consisted of sharply defined zones of brain-tissue degeneration involving nerve cells, axons, and myelin sheaths. At times, the lesions actually formed a cavity in the affected region.

Experimental lesions to the mammillary bodies of the hypothalamus or to the dorsomedial thalamic nuclei in infrahuman species have generally been shown to produce learning deficits (Delacour, 1971; Means, Huntley, Anderson, & Harrell, 1973; Thompson, 1969, 1974; Tigner, 1974; Vanderwolf, 1971). However, these lesions in infrahuman species do not produce the global amnesia seen in humans. A further complication is that lesions directed to the mammillary region or medial thalamus may also produce hyperemotionality in infrahumans. For this reason, one is often not able to determine whether the deficits in learning reflect an inability to consolidate information or rather the interference of a heightened emotional state with adaptive responding (Delacour, 1971; Vanderwolf, 1971).

This confounding effect was minimized in a study by Means and his associates (1973). These researchers investigated the effects of dorsomedial thalamic lesions on both the acquisition and the retention of a two-choice compound-stimulus problem. The animals learned to approach one of two compartments in a simultaneous-discrimination apparatus. One of the goal boxes had a smooth floor and was painted with black and white stripes; the other goal box had a wire-mesh floor and was painted gray. The goal boxes were randomly alternated from side to side as a function of trials.

One group of animals receiving medial thalamic lesions was operated on prior to original learning of this problem. Their performance was compared with that of a similarly trained group of rats that had received sham operations. The animals were run to a criterion of 90% correct choices for three consecutive days or a minimum of six days. The performance scores of these two groups of animals during the first six acquisition sessions are shown in Figure 10-9. These graphs show that the medial-thalamically lesioned rats were severely retarded on this problem.

To examine the effects of medial thalamic lesions on retention and reacquisition, Means and his colleagues again used two groups of animals—a thalamic group and a sham operated group. In this part of the experiment, the animals learned the task to criterion and were then subjected to either medial thalamic or sham operations. They were then allowed 14 days recovery before being retested. The

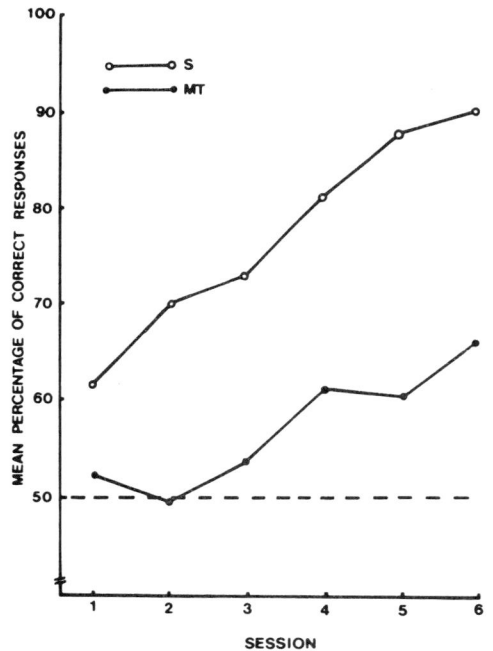

Figure 10-9 Comparison of the performance of sham-operated and medial-thalamically lesioned rats in learning a discrimination task. Adapted from "Deficient Acquisition and Retention of a Visual-Tactile Discrimination Task in Rats with Medial Thalamic Lesions," by L. W. Means, D. H. Huntley, H. P. Anderson, and T. H. Harrel, Behavioral Biology, *1973, 9, 435–450. Copyright 1973 by Academic Press, Inc. Reprinted by permission.*

results of this inquiry are graphically portrayed in Figure 10-10. These graphs show that the animals subjected to dorsomedial thalamic lesions experienced a severe postoperative loss of the discrimination habit and that the sham operatees did not. Further, the thalamically lesioned animals did not show much evidence of reacquisition during the first six postoperative training sessions.

An excellent feature of this study was that Means and his associates tested to determine whether the medial thalamic lesions additionally yielded changes in emotionality, motor activity, food consumption, or visual placing responses. (*Visual placing response* refers to the fact that an animal being held facing a surface such as a table will extend its legs when it is brought close to the supporting surface.) Because none of these changes were found to have occurred, the possibility of confounding effects obscuring an interpretation of their findings was significantly reduced. These results provide the strongest corroborative evidence yet, using infrahuman species,

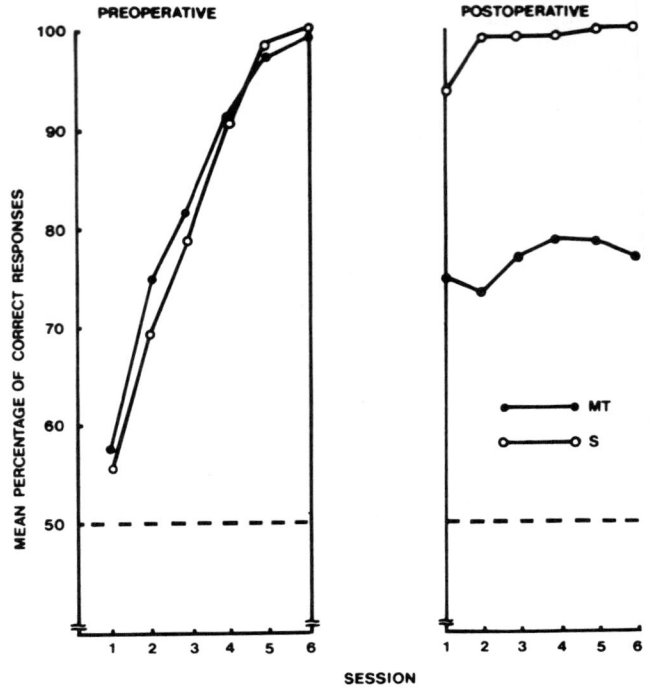

Figure 10-10
Comparison of the
performance of
sham-operated and
medial-thalamically
lesioned rats on the
same discrimination
task before and after
surgery. From
"Deficient
Acquisition and
Retention of a
Visual-Tactile
Discrimination
Task in Rats with
Medial Thalamic
Lesions," by L. W.
Means, D. H.
Huntley, H. P.
Anderson, and
T. H. Harrel,
Behavioral Biology,
1973, 9, 435–450.
Copyright 1973 by
Academic Press.
Reprinted by
permission.

that medial thalamic lesions can produce learning deficits. The basis for this disruption will have to be clarified by future research, although research by Means, Harrell, Mayo, and Alexander (1974) suggests that the basis may be an attentional deficit.

Another way to study the role of hypothalamic/thalamic mechanisms in learning and retention is to bilaterally destroy the mammilothalamic tract, which interconnects these two structures. The mammilothalamic tract connects the mammillary region of the hypothalamus with the anterior nuclear complex of the thalamus. From the anterior nuclei, impulses are conducted via the medial thalamo-cortical radiation to the cingulate gyrus, which will be considered shortly.

The effects of bilateral transections of the mammilothalamic tract in cats on both acquisition and retention of a two-way active-avoidance habit were examined by Thomas and his associates (Kriekhaus, 1964; Thomas, Frey, Slotnik, & Kriekhaus, 1963). The apparatus they used to test two-way active avoidance consisted of a chamber divided into halves by a hurdle. Following presentation of a signal, the animal leaped over the hurdle to the other side. When the signal was again presented, the animal jumped back to the other side, and it continued shuttling from side to side with successive trials. The results of the research indicated a clear loss in retention of preoperatively acquired two-way avoidance following transection of the mammilothalamic tract. In contrast, the effects produced by these lesions on postoperative learning of the task were mixed. Seven of the lesioned cats learned the task as fast as normals, but the other four ablated animals failed to learn the task at all.

Later research by Kriekhaus and his co-workers appeared to clarify the nature of the deficit produced by mammilothalamic-tract lesions (Kriekhaus, Coons,

Greenspon, Weiss & Lorenz, 1968; Kriekhaus & Lorenz, 1968; Kriekhaus & Randall, 1968). Their research indicated that the observed deficits were apparently related to the "willingness" of the animals to undertake the required response. Once the animals were induced to begin a behavioral sequence, they made as many correct choices as did normal subjects. Isaacson (1974) has suggested that the most significant effect of mammilothalamic lesions is deficiency in the ability to initiate behavior—an alteration that you will see is very similar to the effect of lesions to the cingulate gyrus.

The Septum and Cingulate Gyrus. There is really very little data, either of a clinical or of an animal-lesion nature, to suggest that brain structures other than the areas described thus far are involved in basic processes of memory consolidation or recall. Nevertheless, they probably do perform certain functions affecting learning and performance. As indicated above, the hippocampus is directly connected, via the fornix, to the septal region; it also has interconnections with the cingulate gyrus via the cingulum bundle. These two regions (the septum and the cingulate gyrus) will be discussed together because they often appear to exert opposite influences on behavior.

From the results of experiments that have examined the functions of the cingulate gyrus and the septal area on learning and performance, it appears possible that these neural regions exert equivalent but opposite effects on responding. Similar, antagonistic functions of these regions in mediating emotional behavior were proposed in Chapter 8. Taken together, these findings indicate that the effects of these regions in mediating behavior are not response specific but rather involve general processes of initiating and inhibiting behavior.

A number of researchers (see McCleary, 1966) have posited that the role of the septum in mediating learning and performance is one of response inhibition or suppression—a function that, as you've seen, has also been assigned by some researchers to the hippocampus. In contrast, the cingulate gyrus appears to exert a response-initiation function. In some species, such as the rat, these processes are responsible for the conflict, in avoidance situations, between "freezing," which the septum presumably initiates, and fleeing, which is under the control of the cingulate gyrus (Thomas, Hostetter, & Barker, 1968; Trafton, 1967).

The functions of the cingulate gyrus and septal region in learning and performance apparently do not involve laying down and recalling memory traces. Rather, their functions seem to be related to either the initiation (cingulate gyrus) or suppression (septum) of responding. For this reason, one would expect—and one does indeed find—cingulectomized animals to be deficient in learning tasks that require response initiation but superior (due to the unregulated activity of the septum) to normal subjects in the acquisition of a problem that requires response suppression. In contrast, one would expect—and find—septally lesioned animals to be superior in their acquisition of tasks that require response initiation. This presumably results from the unregulated influence of the cingulate gyrus. Septally lesioned animals should be found to be inferior on a training paradigm that requires response suppression.

Evidence for the opposing influences of the cingulate and septal regions comes from studies that have examined the effects of selective lesions to these structures on two-way active-avoidance and passive-avoidance tasks. Presumably, two-way active avoidance requires response initiation since the animal must leave the previously safe side of the apparatus and leap a hurdle to get to the other side. In contrast, passive avoidance requires response suppression because a previously rewarded approach response must now be inhibited. In accord with the proposed model, it has been demonstrated that cingulectomized animals are, as compared with normal subjects, retarded in their ability to learn a two-way active-avoidance problem. This is true regardless of whether rats (Kimble & Gostnell, 1968; Peretz, 1960; Thomas & Otis, 1958; Thomas & Slotnik, 1962, 1963; Trafton, 1967), cats (Lubar & Perachio, 1965; McCleary, 1966), or monkeys (Pribram & Weiskrantz, 1957) are used as the subjects. In contrast, cingulectomized animals are superior to normals in their ability to master a passive-avoidance problem (Lubar, 1964; McCleary, 1966).

The basis for the deficits observed in two-way active avoidance has been questioned. Lubar, Perachio, and Kavanagh (1966) proposed that the impairment may have been produced by damage to the visual cortical areas, which were inadvertently undercut when the cingulate-gyrus lesions were made. This explanation doesn't account for all of the effects produced by cingulate-gyrus lesions; Trafton, Fibley, and Johnson (1969) found that lesions of several different regions of the anterior cingulate gyrus, far removed from the visual neocortex, were still effective in producing an active-avoidance impairment.

The effects of septal lesions are the opposite of those observed following cingulectomy. As measured by passive-avoidance behavior, septally lesioned animals are inferior to normal subjects. This finding has been reported by many authors (Albert & Mah, 1973; Beatty, Beatty, O'Briant, Gregoire, & Dahl, 1973; Fried, 1969, 1971; Fox, Kimble, & Lickey, 1964; Kaada, Rasmussen, & Kveim, 1962; McCleary, 1966; Miczek, Kelsey, & Grossman, 1972; Middaugh & Lubar, 1970; Singh, 1973; Zucker, 1965). Further, it has been well substantiated that septal animals are superior in their acquisition of a task that requires response initiation—that is, a two-way active-avoidance problem (Buddington, King, & Roberts, 1967; Deagle & Lubar, 1971; Hamilton, 1972; Johnson, 1972; King, 1958; Kriekhaus, Simmons, Thomas, & Kenyon, 1964; Lovely, 1975; Lubar, Herrmann, Moore, & Shouse, 1973; Miczek et al., 1972; Schwartzbaum, Green, Beatty, & Thompson, 1967; Singh, 1973; Trafton, 1967). It is important to note that it is unlikely that the facilitated two-way avoidance learning observed in septally ablated animals is due to hyperemotionality produced by the lesion, as King proposed in 1958. Several researchers have found that increased irritability produced by septal lesions can be dissociated from the improved avoidance behavior (Kriekhaus et al., 1964; Schwartzbaum et al., 1967; Trafton, 1967).

Although the available data suggest that the cingulate gyrus and septal regions exert equivalent but opposite influences on responding, more work needs to be done on this question. In 1964, Lubar analyzed the avoidance behavior of cats with lesions that involved both the septal inhibitory and cingulate facilitation regions. He wanted to determine whether the effects of the lesions would cancel each other out. His subjects learned a passive-avoidance problem and mastered it at a normal rate. Thus, the effects of the cingulate lesion apparently offset the usual effects of the septal lesion on passive avoidance. It would be of interest to determine whether similar results would occur in more complex learning situations.

The loss of inhibition in septally lesioned animals is in many ways very similar to the perseveration observed in hippocampally lesioned subjects. Animals subjected to lesions in either of these locations demonstrate, as you've seen, enhanced two-way active-avoidance performance and deficient passive-avoidance learning. As was shown to be the case for hippocampectomized subjects, animals with septal lesions show greater resistance to extinction (Gray, Quintao, & Araujo-Silva, 1972; Henke, 1974; Raphelson, Isaacson, & Douglas, 1966; Schwartzbaum, Kellicutt, Spieth, &

Thompson, 1964), have more difficulty in learning a discrimination reversal (Gittleson & Donovick, 1968; Schwartzbaum & Donovick, 1968; Zucker, 1965), and overrespond on either an intermittent fixed-interval (Ellen & Powell, 1962) or a DRL schedule following practice on a continuous reinforcement (CRF) schedule (Burkett & Bunnell, 1966; Ellen & Aitken, 1973; Ellen & Braggio, 1973; Ellen & Butter, 1969; Ellen, Wilson, & Powell, 1964; Johnson, Beliauskas, & Lancaster, 1973; MacDougall, Van Hoesen, & Mitchell, 1969). There are some data available that indicate that septal animals, in contrast to hippocampal animals, will overrespond on the DRL in the absence of prior practice on CRF (Ellen, Aitken, & Stahl, 1973).

Regarding the similarities of the septal and hippocampal deficits in DRL responding, however, it has been reported that septal rats will learn to respond normally on DRL if the end of the time out and the availability of reinforcement are signaled by the onset of an environmental cue (Ellen & Butter, 1969). Earlier, we saw a similar phenomenon with hippocampally ablated animals. Another interesting and related finding is that overresponding on DRL is most pronounced in subjects whose lesions involve loci of the septum that project directly to the hippocampus (MacDougall et al., 1969). Taken together, these findings argue for the existence of a septo-hippocampal system or subsystem mediating response inhibition or attention processes. However, in light of the data published by Ellen, Aitken, and Stahl, 1973, regarding the contrasting importance of prior CRF experience in producing the DRL deficit in septally lesioned versus hippocampectomized animals, such a formulation may be unwarranted.

The Amygdala. The septum and cingulate gyrus are reciprocally connected with the amygdala—a rhinencephalic, temporal-lobe structure. Septo-amygdaloid influences are carried by the stria terminalis, and cingulo-amygdaloid impulses are conducted via the cingulum bundle. The amygdala interacts with the temporal-lobe neocortex by way of the amygdalotemporal fasciculus. The stria terminalis also conducts impulses between the amygdala and the hypothalamus. There is also strong evidence for the existence of connections between the amygdala and the dorsomedial nucleus of the thalamus. As indicated in Chapter 8, the amygdala has a long history of being implicated in the control of affective, or emotional, behavior (Fuller, Rosvold, & Pribram, 1957; Klüver & Bucy, 1937, 1939; Schreiner & Kling, 1953). For this reason, examinations of the amygdala's role in learning have generally centered around the learning and performance of various types of avoidance responses. On the basis of a number of investigations, one thing is clear: there is no global memory deficit or inability to acquire new behaviors following bilateral amygdalectomy.

As you saw to be the case for the cingulate gyrus and septum, there is evidence that the amygdala is involved in the initiation and suppression of responding. These opposing functions are apparently organized in different regions of the amygdala. A number of years ago, Kaada (1951), on the basis of experiments on the effects of amygdala stimulation on cats, suggested that the more lateral aspects of this structure—that is, the basolateral amygdala complex—are involved in response initiation while medial portions of the amygdala—the corticomedial complex—exert inhibitory influences over movement. In light of these opposing response, or motor, functions organized in different regions of the amygdala, the wisdom of making total-amygdala lesions must be questioned. I will generally confine my discussion of the functions of the amygdala in learning and performance to those experiments that have been based on a discrete-lesion approach—that is, experiments in which the effects of ablations of distinct amygdala areas have been assessed.

A report on one of the most carefully conducted and comprehensive investigations of the role performed by the amygdala in avoidance conditioning was published by Ursin (1965b). He examined the effects of lesions variously situated in the amygdala, and his data are of particular interest because he was able to separate the behavioral effects of laterally versus medially placed amygdala ablations. The avoidance deficits observed by Ursin corresponded nicely with Kaada's findings regarding motor facilitatory and inhibitory effects of amygdala stimulation.

Ursin found that a deficit in runway active avoidance occurred in cats whose lesions were confined to the lateral, or motor-facilitation, region of the amygdala complex. The effective site was the rostral part of the lateral nucleus—one of the nuclei of the basolateral complex. It is important to note that these animals were not simply less emotional than normal cats. Ursin reported that all of the operated subjects showed strong emotional and autonomic responses to both a conditioned avoidance signal and a shock. Their deficiency was due primarily to the fact that it took them longer to begin making active-avoidance responses; that is, the lesioned cats were deficient in their ability to initiate behavior. The similarity between this deficit and alterations produced by mammilothalamic-tract or cingulate-gyrus lesions is striking. Additional evidence supporting a response-initiation function of the basolateral amygdala complex was published by Horvath (1963). He reported that cats were impaired in two-way active-avoidance (shuttle-box) learning after basolateral-amygdala lesions.

In contrast, basolateral-amygdala ablations do not yield passive-avoidance deficits in cats (Horvath, 1963; Ursin, 1965b). Ursin found that a passive-avoidance deficit was produced only if the lesions were discretely located in the motor-inhibitory regions of the medial amygdala. For a deficit in passive avoidance, the effective site was the medial nucleus of the corticomedial amygdala complex. Passive-avoidance deficits also occurred if the fibers of the stria terminalis—the pathway connecting the medial amygdala to the septum—were interrupted. Thus, lesions of the medial amygdala nucleus yielded passive-avoidance deficits similar to those seen after hippocampal or septal ablations. Ursin's data, when added to other findings reported in this chapter, support the existence of discretely organized response initiation and response inhibition systems that mediate behavior.

A final experiment described in the Ursin paper examined the effects of discretely placed amygdala lesions on visual-discrimination behavior. The cats were trained on both brightness- and pattern-discrimination problems. Food was the reward for correct responses. It was found that the operated and control animals did not differ significantly on any of the measures used to assess visual-discrimination ability. This is an important finding because it indicates that amygdala lesions do not produce a general deleterious effect on learning processes.

Results of studies investigating the effects of discrete amygdala ablations on passive-avoidance or conditioned-suppression responses in the rat directly conflict with Ursin's cat data. Generally speaking, for the rat, the ability to inhibit a previously conditioned response is apparently mediated by the basolateral amygdala complex rather than by the corticomedial complex as is the case with the cat (Kemble & Tapp, 1968; Pellegrino, 1968; Pellegrino & Clapp, 1971; Thompson & Schwartzbaum, 1964). One possible explanation for these conflicting results is that species differences exist in the functional organization of the amygdala. Another possibility, as suggested by Kemble and Tapp, is that there is some difference between the species in the characteristics of the complex intraamygdala connections.

Another feature of the behavioral-inhibition deficit observed in amygdala-lesioned animals bears mentioning. Just as we saw with inhibition deficits associated
with septal and hippocampal ablations, the amygdala-produced deficit will disappear
if a visual cue is added to guide behavior. Although rats with bilateral lesions of the
basolateral complex show deficits in DRL performance following CRF practice and
in spatial alternation without cues, these deficits disappear when the animals are
given either a cued-DRL or a visually cued spatial-alternation problem (Pellegrino,
1968; Pellegrino & Clapp, 1971). The Pellegrino and Clapp (1971) research can be
used to illustrate this finding.

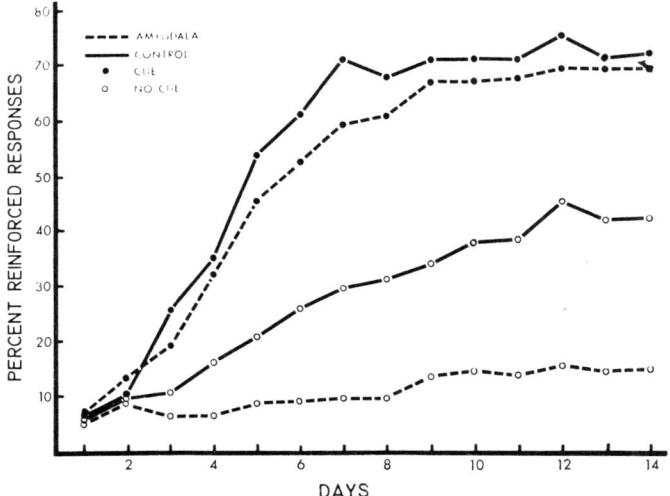

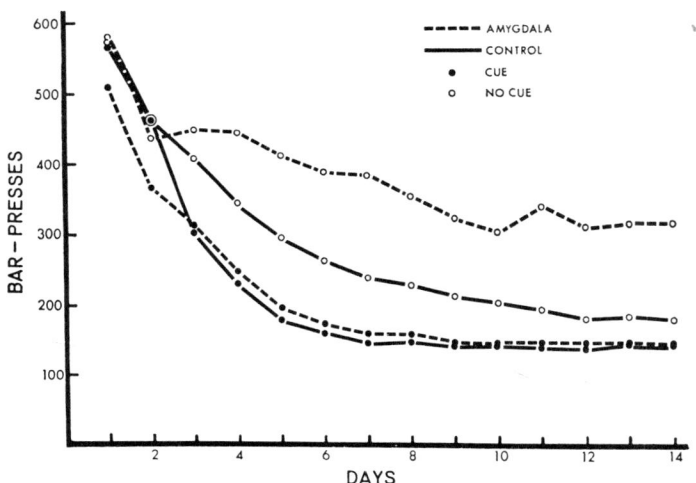

*Figure 10-11
Comparisons of
cued- and
uncued-DRL
performance by
basolateral-amygdala
and control rats.
From "Limbic
Lesions and
Externally Cued
DRL Performance,"
by L. J. Pellegrino
and D. R. Clapp,*
Physiology and
Behavior, *1971, 7,
863–868. Copyright
1971 by Brain
Research
Publications, Inc.
Reprinted by
permission.*

In this study, rats that either were nonlesioned or had been subjected to bilateral destructions of the amygdaloid nuclei were given practice on an operant continuous-reinforcement schedule for six days, receiving up to 150 reinforcements during each 30-minute training session. Half of the animals were then shifted to a noncued-DRL 20-second schedule, and the remaining animals were shifted to a cued-DRL 20-second schedule in which the onset of a cue light over the bar signaled the end of the time out and the availability of reinforcement for the next bar-press. The findings are graphed in Figure 10-11. It was found that, in the uncued condition, the amygdala-lesioned rats emitted more responses during each daily session and had a lower percentage of correctly timed responses than the control animals. These differences disappeared under the cued-DRL condition. During cued-DRL training, there were no significant differences between the group with basolateral-amygdala lesions and the control subjects on either the total number of responses emitted per session or the percentage of correctly timed responses.

Chapter Summary and Conclusions

Experimental attempts to discover a structure or pathway that is crucial for the consolidation of information into memory and for the subsequent recall of this information have been discouraging. Of all the regions and structures examined in this chapter, the hippocampus appears to perform the most pervasive functions in memory, particularly in light of the results of human clinical investigations that evaluated the effects of hippocampal ablations on the ability to store and recall complex memories. However, even if the hippocampus is indeed required for some higher memory processes in humans, this structure's integrity is apparently not essential for basic memory functions in nonhuman animals. Infrahumans are capable of mastering a variety of tasks in the absence of an intact hippocampus. Researchers must be cautious in evaluating the effects of brain-lesion-induced learning and performance deficits. Rather than representing global memory dysfunctions, deficits in original learning and retention that occur following lesions to a variety of neural structures may reflect a disruption of neural systems mediating processes such as attention, arousal, emotionality, response initiation, and response inhibition.

Analysis of the findings reported in this chapter has led many researchers in the neurosciences to conclude that memory is simply not located in any particular brain region or identifiable pathway (John, 1967, 1971; Lashley, 1950, 1958). As an alternative, John has proposed that memories reflect unique spatiotemporal patterns of discharge of electrical activity in neural systems that encompass most if not all of the brain. Experimental results bearing on this very plausible view will be reviewed in the next chapter.

11

Electrophysiological Correlates of Learning and Performance

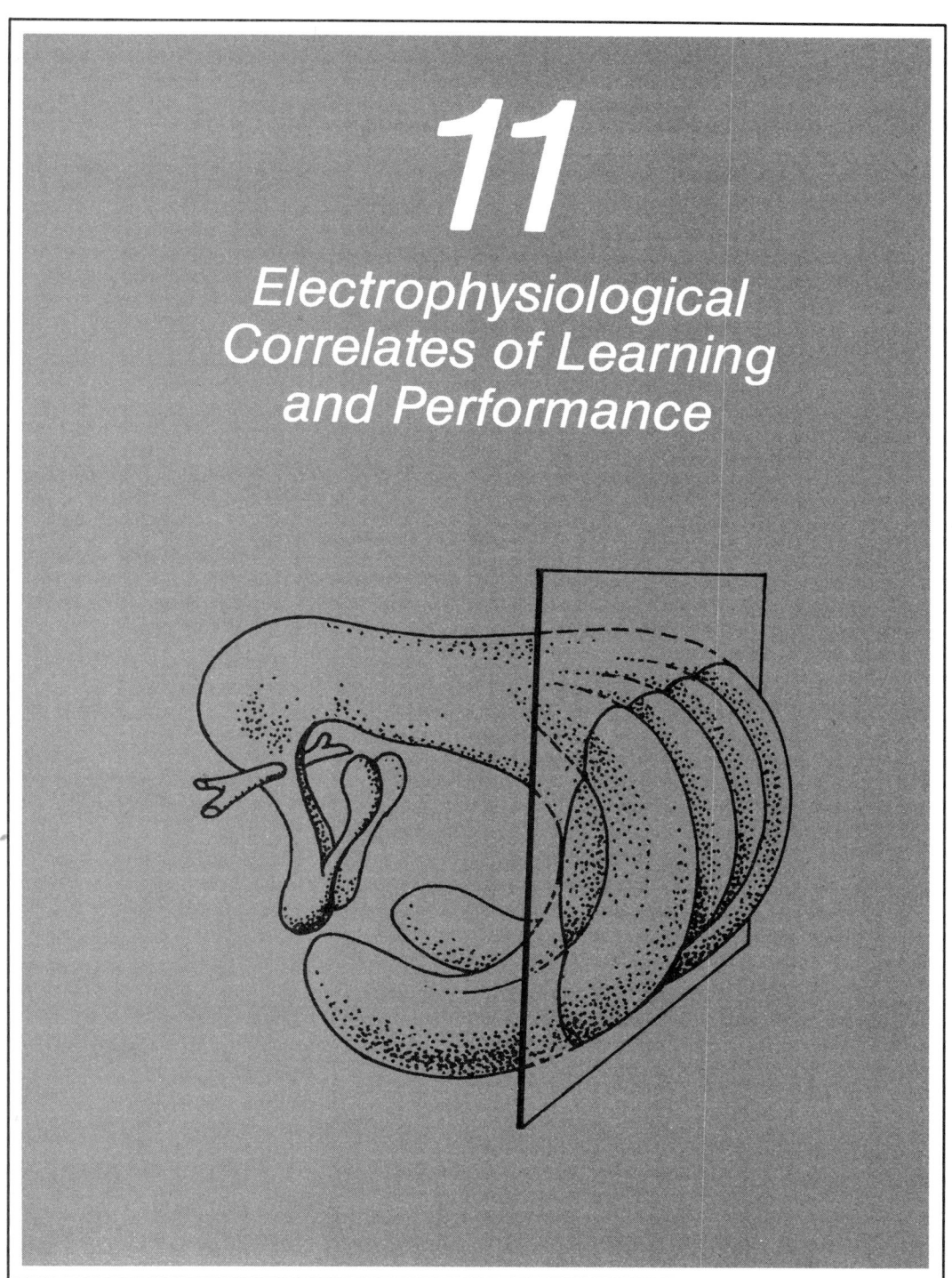

As you saw in Chapter 10, brain-lesion experiments have suggested that no specific structure is required for basic learning and memory processes. These observations have led many brain researchers to conclude that memory is simply not located in any particular part of the brain. An alternative view, proposed by John (1967, 1971, 1972), is that *memories reflect unique spatiotemporal patterns of discharge of electrical activity in neural systems that encompass most if not all of the brain.*

This view of the neural substrates of memory is based on the well-substantiated finding that most brain cells are incessantly active. It is possible that alterations in the average temporal pattern of firing serve as the basis for information coding. If so, different bits of information would not need to be coded as activity in different, specifiable neurons, as an anatomical, or localization-of-function, view would contend. Rather, different items of newly acquired information could be represented by the firing of the same group of cells in different spatio-temporal patterns.

Guided by the supposition that memory is diffusely organized, many neuroscientists have investigated the ongoing electrical activity of the brain with the hope of discovering changes in neural electrical activity that are correlated with information processing, memory consolidation, and recall. It has been shown that such changes do indeed occur. The problem that next confronts researchers is to determine whether the alterations in the electrophysiology of the brain do reflect learning and memory processes per se. If the answer to this question is "yes, " then the investigators often attempt to determine whether these electrophysiological changes are required for the processes that they seem to accompany. In this chapter, I'll review the results of these types of inquiries.

Electrical Activity of the Hippocampus

In light of its apparent role in memory processes, suggested by human clinical observations, and because of its easily distinguished and distinctive EEG patterns, the hippocampus has been a favorite target for investigators attempting to discover electrophysiological correlates of learning and memory. Changes in its bioelectric rhythms have been found to accompany memory consolidation and recall as indexed by improved performance of certain learned responses. Whether these bioelectric changes indeed reflect the role of this structure—or of a system of which it is a part—in memory processes has been debated.

There are species differences in the electrical rhythms, or patterns of brain waves, recorded from the hippocampus. These differences will be discussed later in this chapter. Since most of the research relating patterns of hippocampal electrical activity to memory processes has used the cat as the experimental subject, I will, for the present, confine my remarks to this species.

During depth recording from the dorsal hippocampus of chronically implanted, freely moving, unanesthetized cats, one normally records fast, low-amplitude electrical activity, called **hippocampal desynchronization,** that is identical in appearance to the EEG arousal pattern of the neocortex. At other times, as the animal moves about or performs a learned response, the bioelectric rhythm of the hippocampus shifts, and the desynchronized pattern is replaced by a much slower, high-amplitude (up to 500 μv or larger), synchronized wave train, which is called **hippocampal theta activity.** In Chapter 4, I indicated that synchronous wave trains have Greek-letter names denoting their frequency range. *Theta* refers to a synchronous wave train with an average frequency of 4–7 Hz—that is, 4 to 7 peaks, or waves, per second. *Hippocampal theta* refers to a synchronous wave train occurring in the hippocampus that has a frequency of 4–7 Hz. Researchers have attempted to determine the behaviors during which these hippocampal brain-wave patterns will occur. Samples of hippocampal desynchronization and hippocampal theta are shown in Figure 11-1.

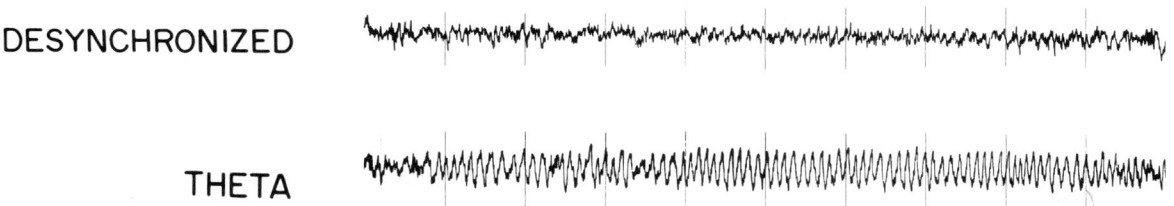

DESYNCHRONIZED

THETA

[500 μv
1 SEC

*Figure 11-1
Patterns of
electrical activity
recorded from the
dorsal hippocampus
of the cat.*

Two neural systems responsible for the occurrence of either hippocampal desynchronization or theta have been identified and delineated (Anchel & Lindsley, 1972), but the pathways mediating the theta rhythm have been studied much more extensively. The septal region has been shown to be extremely important for the occurrence of hippocampal theta activity. The occurrence of theta can be blocked by septal lesions or by sectioning of the fornix, which carries impulses from the septum to the hippocampus (Green & Arduini, 1954). Within the septal area, the activity of cells in the medial septal nucleus has been shown to act as a pacemaker for the hippocampal theta response (Petsche, Stumpf, & Gogolak, 1962). Lesions restricted to the medial septal nucleus abolish hippocampal theta activity (Brücke, Petsche, Pillat, & Deisenhammer, 1959; Mayer & Stumpf, 1958), as will injections of the anticholinergic agent scopolamine hydrobromide directly into this nucleus (Bennett, 1973). The theta-rhythm potentials recorded by macroelectrodes situated in the hippocampus probably arise as a result of synchronous postsynaptic potentials (PSPs) occurring in populations of neurons (Artemenko, 1972; Fujita & Sato, 1964), and the firing of cells may also contribute to this slow-wave pattern (Andersen, Bliss, & Skrede, 1971).

The hippocampus of the cat is shaped roughly like an apostrophe, as can be seen in Figure 11-2. A distinction is generally made between dorsal (top) and ventral (bottom) aspects of this structure, as shown in the coronal section through the hippocampus. The hippocampus has been further subdivided into fields by the anatomist Lorente de No. These are designated by the letters *CA*. *CA* signifies *cornu ammonis* (Ammon's horn) zones. The hippocampus is composed of two interlocking gyri—Ammon's horn and the dentate gyrus. The CA designations result in four subdivisions of the hippocampus, as shown in the coronal section in Figure 11-2. In the awake cat, theta is most prominent in the dorsal

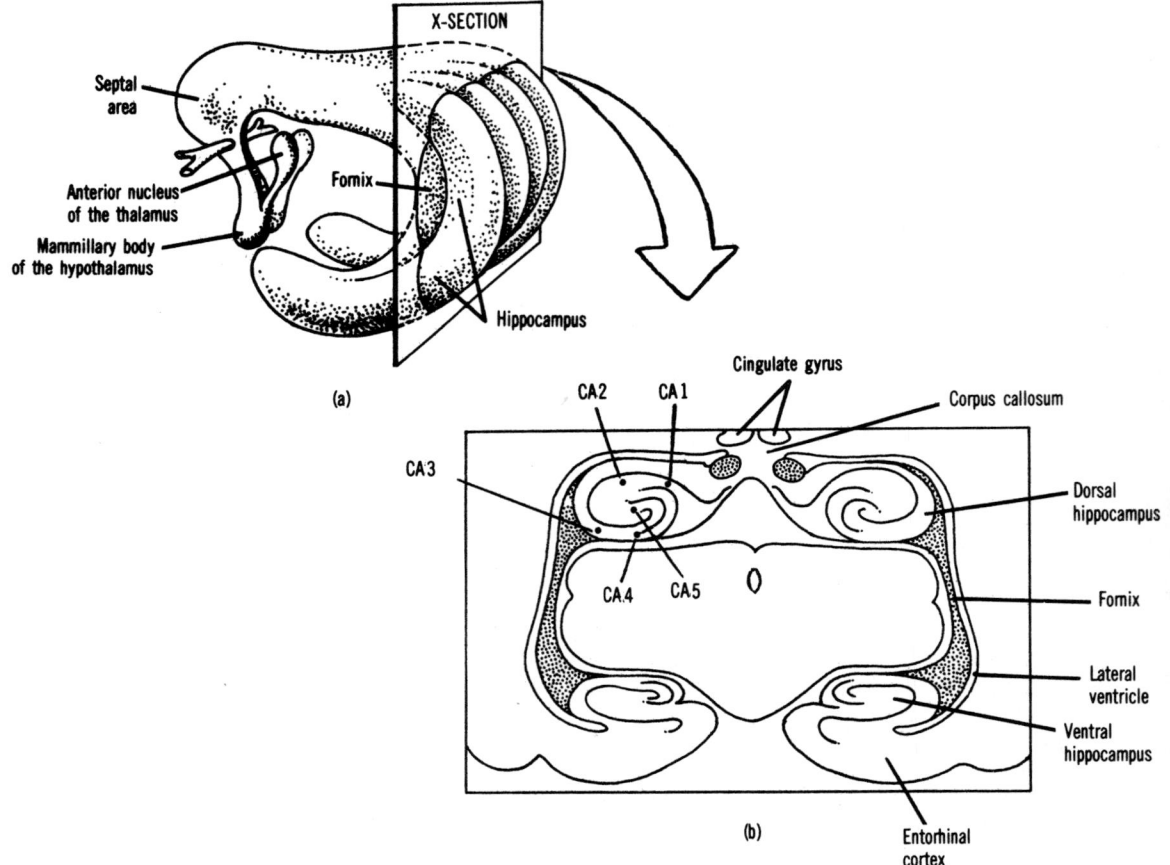

Figure 11-2
The hippocampus of the cat. (a) Dissection from the left side. (b) Cross section at level shown. The labels CA 1 *to* CA 5 *refer to different cellular regions of the dorsal hippocampus. Adapted from "The Hippocampus," by J. D. Green. In J. Field (Ed.),* Handbook of Physiology; Section I: Neurophysiology *(Vol. 2). Copyright 1960 by the American Physiological Society. Reprinted by permission.*

hippocampus—particularly in region CA 4 (Adey, Dunlop, & Hendrix, 1960). Trains of theta activity cannot usually be observed in recordings from the ventral hippocampus of awake animals, but, during Stage REM, theta occurs as a continuous train of activity in both the dorsal and ventral hippocampus (Jouvet, 1967a).

Over the years, several different theories have been proposed regarding the significance of the theta pattern as a correlate of the functions being performed by the hippocampus and by other brain regions to which the hippocampus relates. The appearance of the theta rhythm has been linked by different theorists to functions possibly performed by this structure in mediating such behavior processes as arousal, attention to exteroceptive, or environmental, stimuli, voluntary movement, and memory. The desynchronized pattern, on the other hand, has been suggested as a correlate of the functions of the hippocampus that regulate "automatic" behaviors, that inhibit attention to environmental stimuli, and that process information derived from response-produced, or proprioceptive, feedback. For a more detailed presentation of these theories, the reader should consult Bennett (1971, 1975), Black (1975), Vanderwolf (1971), Vanderwolf, Kramis, Gillespie, & Bland (1975), and Winson (1975).

Hippocampal Theta and Memory

W. R. Adey and his colleagues have suggested that hippocampal theta activity reflects the role of the hippocampus in the processing, consolidation, and recall of information (Adey, Dunlop, & Hendrix, 1960; Adey & Walter, 1963; Adey, Walter, & Hendrix, 1961; Elazar & Adey, 1967a, 1967b; Holmes & Adey, 1960). Their conclusions were made on the basis of data collected in a number of studies that comprehensively examined the electrical activity of the hippocampal system—that is, the hippocampus and related structures, during acquisition and performance of a delayed-response task or a visual-discrimination problem. Their findings were similar regardless of which of these tasks was used. Since the majority of their experiments used the two-choice simultaneous-brightness-discrimination problem in a straight alley runway, I will confine my discussion to the results obtained with this task. You will recall from the last chapter that animals can learn a two-choice simultaneous-discrimination problem without an intact hippocampus. Unfortunately, this was learned well after Adey began his inquiries. Nevertheless, it is still possible that, when the hippocampus is intact, it participates in simultaneous-visual-discrimination performance. It is similarly plausible that its functions in this behavior process are reflected by specific rhythms. This relates to another drawback of the brain-lesion technique: it can at times obscure how the intact brain works.

In the Adey paradigm, each trial in the visual-discrimination task began when the cat was placed in the start box at one end of the alley. After a 500-Hz tone was presented, the door opened and the cat was able to view the opposite end of the apparatus, where there were two translucent plexiglass windows separated by a divider, with a metal dish under each. One of these windows was lit from behind throughout each trial. Approaching the lighted window directly was a correct response and was rewarded with food.

Adey and his associates (1960) found that, with every training trial, a very regular, rhythmic train of theta at 5–6 Hz appeared in the dorsal hippocampus and entorhinal cortex (an area of cortex below the ventral hippocampus; see Figure 11-2) as their cats approached the food reward. Computer analysis of the EEG data uncovered some interesting findings. Cross-correlation analyses, as described in Chapter 4, were computed between the electrical activities of the hippocampus and of the entorhinal cortex to determine the time relationship between these two regions at different levels of training. It was found that, in early training, the theta electrical pattern of the hippocampus led that of the entorhinal cortex by 20–35 msec. In contrast, this time relationship in the same animals was reversed once the correct approach response to the lighted window was well established. In this latter case, the EEG activity of the entorhinal cortex led that of the hippocampus by as much as 65 msec.

These observations led Adey and his associates to postulate that hippocampal theta may signal the active involvement of the hippocampus in the processing, consolidation, and recall of information. More specifically, Adey (1966) wrote that "deposition of a memory trace in extrahippocampal systems may depend on such wave trains (theta) and subsequent recall on the stochastic reestablishment of similar wave patterns" (p. 25). Substantiation of such a view would, of course, provide support for the more general theory that consolidation of information into memory results from alterations in the spatiotemporal firing pattern of brain cells. In the last chapter, I noted that Penfield and Milner (1958), on the basis of human clinical observations, proposed that the initial recording of memory traces is accomplished by hippocampal mechanisms. In their formulations, Adey and his colleagues suggested an electrophysiological correlate of this postulated consolidation function.

In later research, Elazar and Adey (1967a) examined subtle shifts in hippocampal electrical activity that took place as a function of trial segments and amount of training. A sample of their data is shown in Figure 11-3. As indicated in this figure, the trial segments analyzed were (a) the prestimulus epoch—before the tone was presented—(b) the stimulus epoch—between presentation of the tone and opening of the start-box door—(c) the approach epoch—when the animal approached the food and made its decision as to which side to approach—and (d) the postapproach epoch. These EEG data were spectrally analyzed—a process described in Chapter 4.

The computer analysis indicated that the dominant frequency (spectral peak) in the theta range was 4 Hz for the prestimulus epoch, 5 Hz for the stimulus epoch, 6 Hz during the approach epoch, and 4–5 Hz in the postapproach epoch. These shifts became more pronounced and regular as training progressed. In addition, these investigators reported that the peak of theta activity did not shift to 6 Hz during the approach segment of the trial if the cats made an incorrect choice. For this reason, Elazar and Adey proposed that the 6-Hz theta activity that accompanied correct approaches was the essential electrophysiological correlate of functions performed by the hippocampus in information processing and memory consolidation.

In their investigations, Elazar and Adey (1967b) also computed the spectral peaks from records obtained from extrahippocampal regions—specifically, the amygdala, subthalamus, midbrain reticular formation, and visual cortex. They found that spectral peaks in the theta range, particularly at 5 and 6 Hz, appeared in all of these regions during the approach epoch in the advanced stages of training, but the peaks were less distinct and more variable than in the hippocampus. Nevertheless, evidence for the occurrence of these theta waves in cortical and subcortical structures during learning and performance led these authors to conclude that "during consolidation of learning, neural circuits of interacting structures comprising hippocampus, subthalamus, midbrain reticular formation, and cerebral cortex are formed.

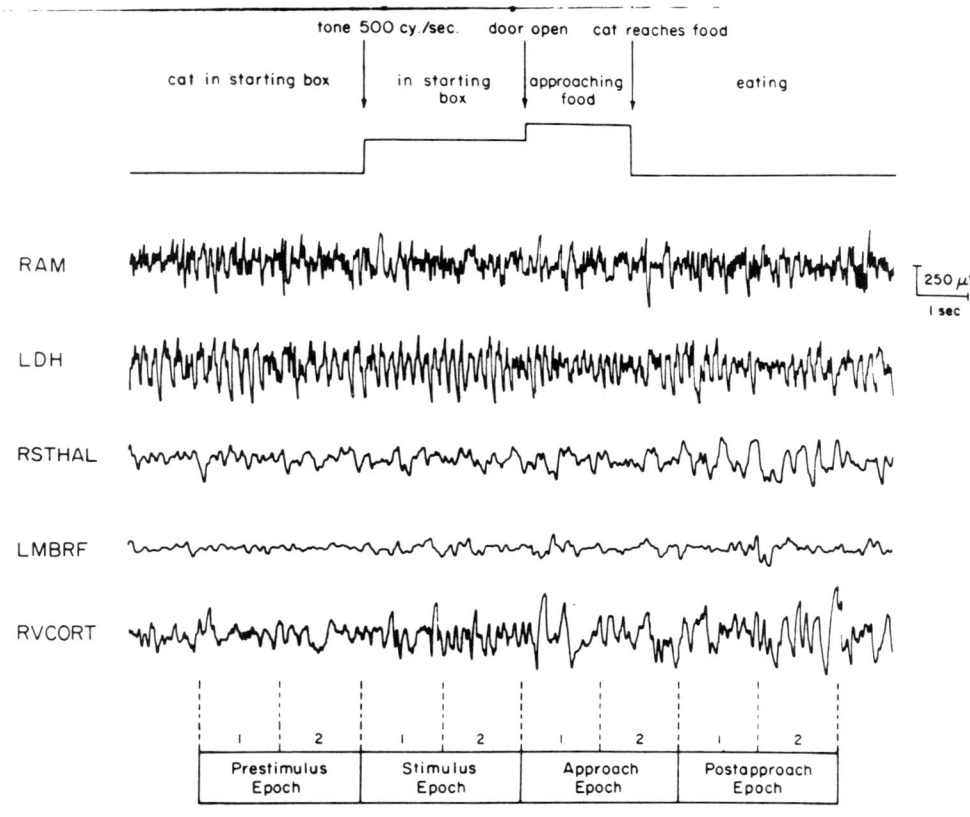

tone 500 cy./sec.   door open   cat reaches food

cat in starting box   in starting   approaching   eating
                       box   food

250 μV

1 sec

RAM

LDH

RSTHAL

LMBRF

RVCORT

	2		2		2		2
Prestimulus Epoch		Stimulus Epoch		Approach Epoch		Postapproach Epoch	

*Figure 11-3
A fragment of the EEG record of one of Elazar and Adey's cats. At the bottom of the figure, the segmentation of the record for spectral analysis is shown. For each behavioral epoch, two periods (marked 1 and 2), each of 1.6 sec in length, were analyzed. RAM = right amygdala; LDH = left dorsal hippocampus; RSTHAL = right subthalamus; LMBRF = left midbrain reticular formation; RVCORT = right visual cortex. From "Spectral Analysis of Low Frequency Components in the Electrical Activity of the Hippocampus During Learning, " by Z. Elazar and W. R. Adey,* Electroencephalography and Clinical Neurophysiology, *1967, 23, 225–240. Copyright © 1967 by ASP Biological and Medical Press. Reprinted by permission of ASP Biological and Medical Press,* Elsevier Division, Amsterdam.

In such neural circuits the hippocampus represents the constant link and probably has a leading role, while participation of other structures has a more subtle, facultative and protean character" (Elazar & Adey, 1967b, p. 317).

Hippocampal Electrical Activity and Processes of Attention

Adey and his associates have clearly demonstrated that changes in the electrical activity of the brain accompany the learning process. However, their data do not necessarily imply that the observed alterations in patterns of hippocampal electrical activity reflect hippocampal involvement in general learning and memory processes per se. Investigations of the electrical activity of the cat hippocampus by Grastyán and his co-workers (Grastyán, Karmos, Vereczkey, & Kellényi, 1966; Grastyán, Lissák, Madarász, & Donhoffer, 1959) and by my associates and me (Bennett, 1969, 1970, 1973, 1975; Bennett & Gottfried, 1970; Bennett, Hébert, & Moss, 1973;

Bennett, Nunn, & Inman, 1971) have led to an alternate view of the significance of hippocampal EEG patterns. We have proposed that theta in the cat reflects the role of the hippocampus in analyzing information derived from exteroceptive stimulation; that is, theta is a correlate of attention to environmental cues. This bioelectric rhythm does not reflect general or global processing/consolidation/recall functions of the hippocampus.

Quite early in their experiments, Grastyán and his colleagues showed that the theta response is elicited only by "meaningful" stimuli and occurs as a correlate of relatively long-duration attention or investigatory response directed toward the stimulus. This finding is illustrated in the hippocampal tracings shown in Figure 11-4.

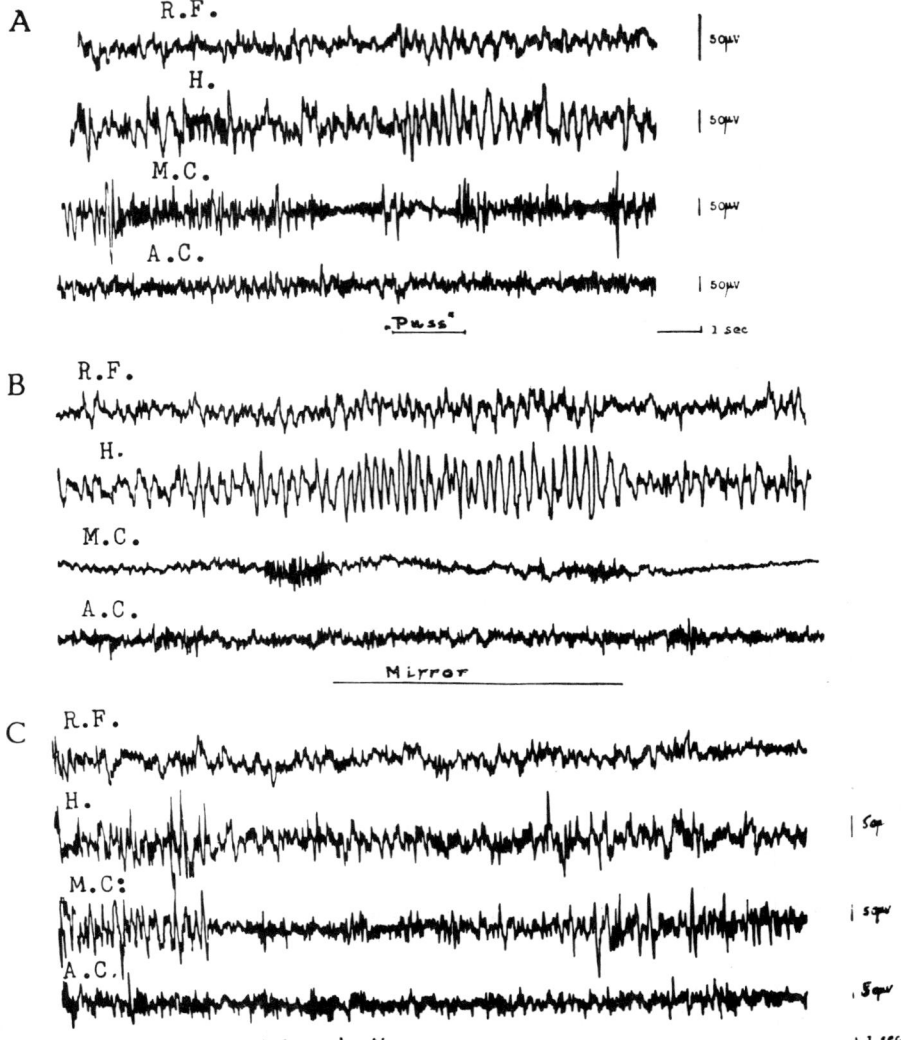

Figure 11-4
(A) The EEG pattern of a cat exposed to the stimulus "puss." The response is slow and rhythmic (5 Hz). (B) A similar marked change occurs when the cat looks in a mirror. (C) The first presentation of the neutral sound stimulus desynchronizes the activity of the hippocampus and the neocortex. R. F. = reticular formation; H. = hippocampus; M. C. = motor cortex; A. C. = auditory cortex. From "Hippocampal Electrical Activity during the Development of Conditioned Reflexes," by E. Grastyán, K. Lissák, L. Madarász, and H. Donhoffer, Electroencephalography and Clinical Neurophysiology, 1959, 11, 409–430. Copyright © 1959 by ASP Biological and Medical Press. Reprinted by permission of ASP Biological and Medical Press, Elsevier Division, Amsterdam.

The auditory stimulus "puss" and the sight of its own image in a mirror elicited from the cat a theta response of 5 Hz. In contrast, a neutral, 1000-Hz tone elicited neither a behavioral orienting response toward the source of the stimulus nor a theta pattern. However, following a few associations of this neutral stimulus with an electric shock, the stimulus acquired significance, in the sense that further presentations of the previously neutral stimulus elicited both a vigorous orienting response toward the source of the sound and hippocampal theta activity. This finding is illustrated in Figure 11-5.

219
Electro-
physiological
Correlates
of Learning
and Performance

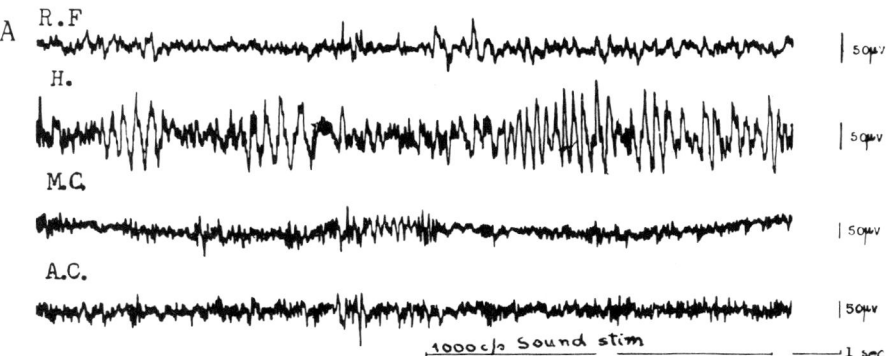

Figure 11-5
A few associations
of the formerly
indifferent sound
stimulus with an
electric shock
evokes a vigorous
orienting reaction
and slow potentials
(5 Hz) in the
hippocampus. From
"Hippocampal
Electrical Activity
during the
Development of
Conditioned
Reflexes," by
E. Grastyán,
K. Lissák,
L. Madarász, and
H. Donhoffer,
Electroencepha-
lography and
Clinical
Neurophysiology,
1959, 11, 409–430.
Copyright © 1959
by ASP Biological
and Medical Press.
Reprinted by
permission of ASP
Biological and
Medical Press,
Elsevier Division,
Amsterdam.

In his inquiries, Grastyán additionally recorded patterns of hippocampal electrical activity during conditioned-approach and -avoidance learning. In the conditioned-approach task, the animal learned to approach a food cup following presentation of a stimulus—a tone of a specific pitch. The avoidance task was a two-way active-avoidance problem. In this problem, the animal also learned to respond to an auditory signal. In the case of both of these tasks, the cats' hippocampal records were dominated by desynchronized activity, except when an animal made a long orienting response toward the speaker from which the signal came. This behavioral orienting response was invariably correlated with hippocampal theta activity. Hence, according to Grastyán and his fellow researchers, theta does not signal hippocampal involvement in memory processes. Instead, hippocampal theta signals hippocampal mediation of behavioral orienting or attention responses.

Results generally supportive of Grastyán's formulations have been obtained in my laboratory. In summarizing our findings, I have concluded (Bennett, 1973, 1975) that the most apparent factor determining whether learning and performance are accompanied by hippocampal theta or desynchronization is whether successful performance requires the cats to attend to environmental stimuli and process information derived from them. On the basis of data collected in a number of experiments in my laboratory, my colleagues and I have found that, in tasks that could be learned by attending to exteroceptive stimuli, both original learning and performance were accompanied by theta activity (for example, in successive or simultaneous auditory or brightness discriminations in an operant-conditioning chamber, in light-cued-DRL schedule in an operant chamber, and in simultaneous brightness discrimination in a straight alley runway). Learning and performance of tasks that could not be mastered by attending to environmental cues (for example, CRF schedule, noncued-DRL schedule in an operant chamber) and instead required attention to proprioceptive feedback (response-produced cues) for their solution were accompanied by hippocampal desynchronization.

The relation of hippocampal theta to processes of attention to exteroceptive stimuli can best be illustrated by our experiments that examined the electrical activity of the hippocampus while animals learned and were shifted from a continuous (CRF) to a differential-reinforcement-of-low-rates-of-responding (DRL) schedule that was either the normal, noncued variety (Bennett & Gottfried, 1970) or the cued type (Bennett, Hébert, & Moss, 1973). In both of these experiments, the animals were initially given 10 sessions of CRF practice and were then gradually shifted to DRL 20 second. The shaping procedure was necessary so that the cats would not cease responding altogether; it is very difficult to get cats to continue performing on a DRL schedule. To master the DRL schedules, the cats had to learn to wait a relatively long time between successive bar-presses and were therefore required to inhibit their tendency to respond at the fast rate acquired under the CRF condition.

Mastery of the noncued-DRL problem required attention to proprioceptive feedback; no other cues were available to the cats to guide their behavior. In contrast, in the cued-DRL condition, the onset of a light over the bar signaled the end of the time-out interval and the availability of reinforcement for the next bar-press. The EEG results obtained in these two experimental paradigms were contrasting. As shown in Figure 11-6, which is based on data obtained in the Bennett and Gottfried (1970) study, the electrical activity of the hippocampus was desynchronized during learning and performance of noncued DRL. In sharp contrast, as illustrated in Figure 11-7, the interresponse intervals were dominated by theta when animals learned and performed the cued-DRL schedule (Bennett, Hébert, & Moss, 1973).

Apparently, the appearance of theta in the cat is related not to general memory functions but rather to specific processes of attention. In support of the view that theta is not necessary for memory consolidation, researchers have shown, as reviewed in the last chapter, that the hippocampus is needed for mastery of the noncued-DRL task, which was correlated with hippocampal desynchronization in the cats. On the other hand, the integrity of the hippocampus was not required for animals to learn the cued DRL, which was accompanied by hippocampal theta (Pellegrino & Clapp, 1971; Rickert, Bennett, Anderson, Corbett, & Smith, 1973).

Why did Adey and his associates find extensive theta activity during approach performance in the simultaneous-discrimination problem? More than likely it was because this task required the animal to process exteroceptive stimulation as it made its approach response. Shifts in the characteristics of the theta response occurred during the course of learning, presumably because the nature of the task-oriented attention responses changed as the cats learned to attend only to those stimuli that would help guide their subsequent behavior.

Is Theta Necessary?

Even if theta does accompany and reflect learning and memory processes in general, a question remains regarding its significance. That is, is theta necessary for the occurrence of these processes? A perhaps more answerable question is the following: Is theta necessary for the occurrence of behaviors with which it is correlated? In two studies, we (Bennett, 1973; Bennett, Nunn, & Inman, 1971) examined this issue. Illustrative of our endeavors is my (1973) research. In this experiment, I investigated the effects of centrally blocking hippocampal theta on

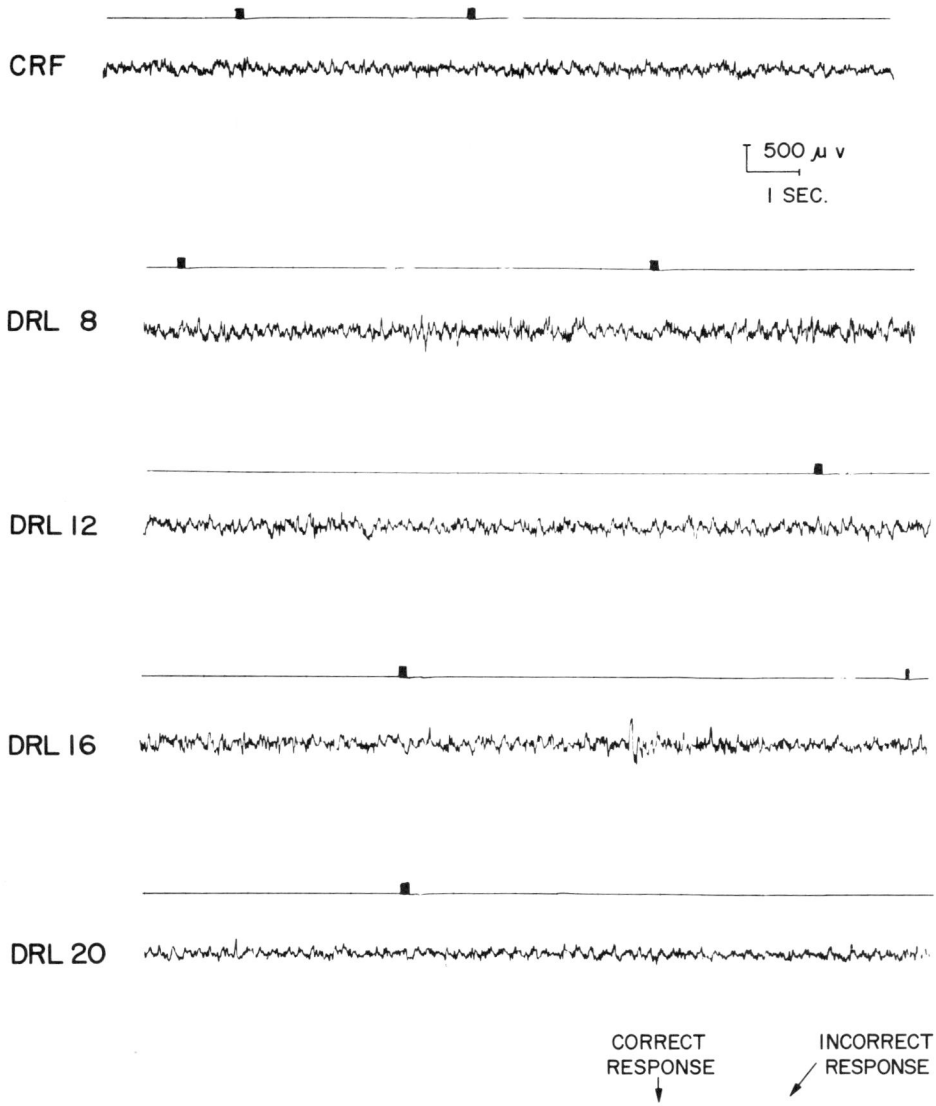

CRF

DRL 8

DRL 12

DRL 16

DRL 20

T 500 μ v
I SEC.

CORRECT
RESPONSE

INCORRECT
RESPONSE

Figure 11-6
Hippocampal electrical activity during performance on continuous-reinforcement (CRF) and differential-reinforcement-of-low rates-of-responding (DRL) schedules. Note that cat hippocampograms are dominated by desynchronized activity. Based on data published by Bennett and Gottfried (1970).

original learning and retention of Adey's simultaneous-brightness-discrimination problem, the performance of which is normally accompanied by theta on 90–95% of the approach trials. The major purpose of this inquiry was to determine whether theta was essential to consolidation and recall of information in the Adey paradigm, as Adey and his associates had proposed.

Theta blocking was accomplished by injecting 2 μl of the anticholinergic agent scopolamine hydrobromide into the medial septal nucleus of cats via a chronically

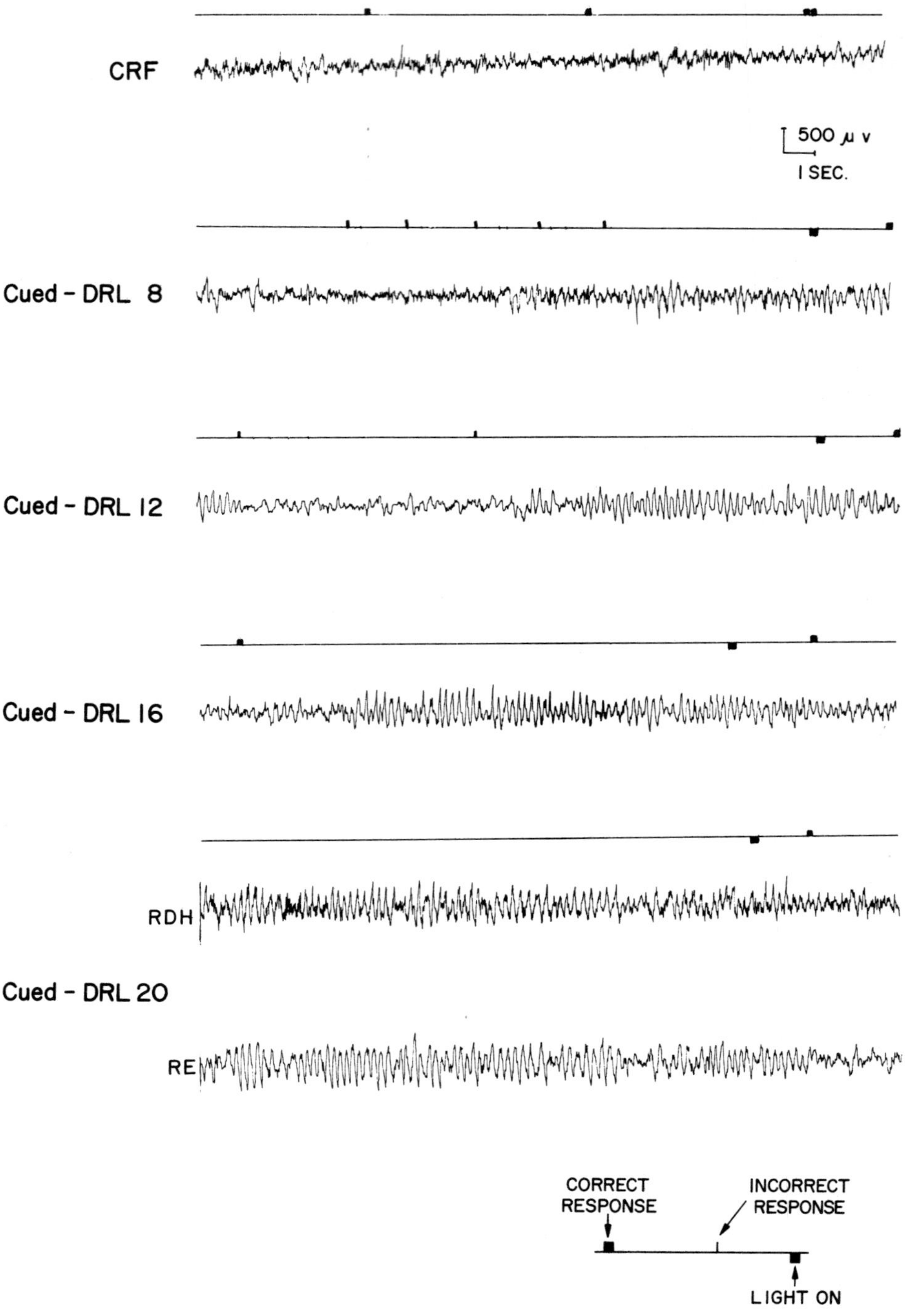

*Figure 11-7
Electrical activity of
the cat hippocampus
during CRF and
cued-DRL training.
Performance on the
cued-DRL
schedules was
accompanied by
theta. The tracing
from the entorhinal
cortex during cued
DRL 20 illustrates
that the electrical
activity of this
region closely
parallels that of the
hippocampus. Based
on data published
by Bennett, Hébert,
and Moss (1973).*

CRF

500 μv

1 SEC.

Cued – DRL 8

Cued – DRL 12

Cued – DRL 16

RDH

Cued – DRL 20

RE

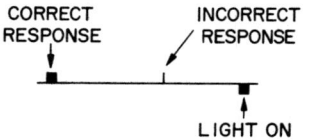

CORRECT
RESPONSE

INCORRECT
RESPONSE

LIGHT ON

implanted cannula. The septum was chosen for the site of injection because the activity of some of the cells in the medial nucleus of the septal region acts as a "pacemaker" for the hippocampal theta response. The blocking procedure resulted in theta accompanying only 6–8% of the approach responses during original learning and retention, as compared with 92–93% of the trials under the nondrugged condition. Electrical activity recorded from the hippocampus of the same cat during nondrugged and drugged approach performance is shown in Figure 11-8.

223

*Electro-
physiological
Correlates
of Learning
and Performance*

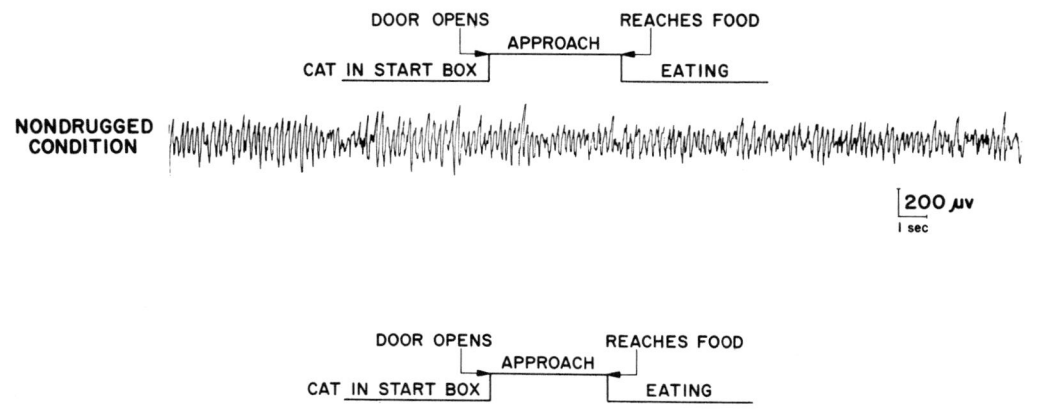

*Figure 11-8
The effect of a
central injection of
scopolamine
hydrobromide on
the electrical
activity of the dorsal
hippocampus during
correct approach
performance in the
cat. From "The
Effects of Centrally
Blocking
Hippocampal Theta
Activity on
Learning and
Retention," by T. L.
Bennett,* Behavioral
Biology, *1973, 9,
541–552. Copyright
1973 by Academic
Press, Inc. Reprinted
by permission.*

Independent groups of cats were administered scopolamine hydrobromide centrally either during original learning or during retention test sessions. The effects of theta blocking on the rate of original learning and the amount retained are graphically portrayed in Figure 11-9. Analysis of the results indicated that neither the rate of original task acquisition nor the amount retained were affected by theta blocking. At least for this experimental situation, it appeared that theta was not necessary for the occurrence of learning and performance behaviors with which this bioelectric rhythm is normally correlated. Further, it was apparent that the occurrence of theta during performance was required neither for the laying down of memory traces nor for the subsequent recall of information from memory. Clarification of the necessity of theta for its correlated behavior processes and the necessity of hippocampal desynchronization will require further research.

Species Differences in the Electrical Activity of the Hippocampus

There are distinct species differences in the electrical activity of the hippocampus. All species studied exhibit widespread theta in the hippocampus during Stage REM sleep, but here the similarities end. These differences in the electrical activity of the hippocampus probably indicate that the electrical correlates of this structure's functions vary across species (Douglas, 1967; Gray, 1970).

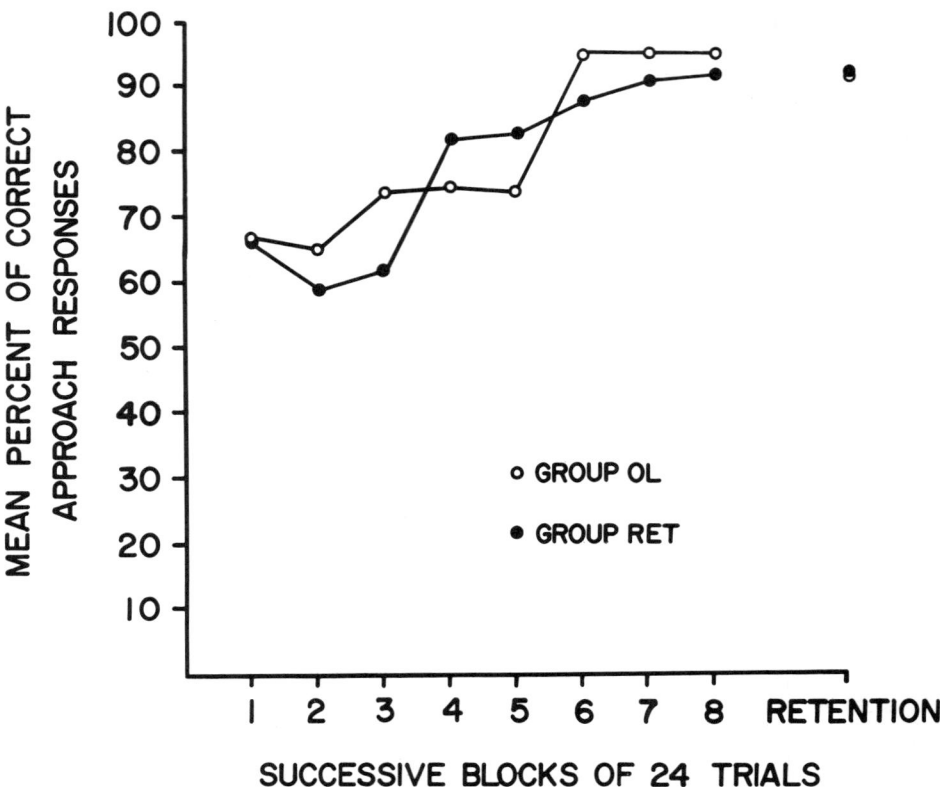

Figure 11-9 Discrimination-learning curves and retention scores for groups OL *and* RET. *Theta blocking occurred for group* OL *during original learning and for group* RET *during retention test sessions. From "The Effects of Centrally Blocking Hippocampal Theta Activity on Learning and Retention," by T. L. Bennett,* Behavioral Biology, *1973, 9, 541–552. Copyright 1973 by Academic Press, Inc. Reprinted by permission.*

Theta is very difficult to observe in the hippocampal EEG records of primates; the usual electrical activity of the primate hippocampus is desynchronized. However, through spectral-analysis techniques it is possible to demonstrate a dominant peak in the theta range for hippocampal records when monkeys perform a delayed-alternation problem (Crowne, Konow, Drake, & Pribram, 1972). The occurrence of activity in the hippocampal theta range under these circumstances is consistent with a view relating theta to the processing of information derived from exteroceptive stimulation.

In the cat, there seems to be a balance between the amount of theta and the amount of desynchronization occurring in the hippocampus. In contrast to theta in primates, as you've seen, theta in felines can easily be detected by visual analysis of hippocampal EEG records. The rat and rabbit reflect the other end of the continuum of ease of observing rhythmic slow-wave activity in hippocampal records. In these species, slow-wave activity is the dominant pattern, and relatively little desynchronized activity is observed.

In the rat and rabbit, there are two components of the synchronous slow-wave activity observed in the hippocampal EEG tracings (Vanderwolf, Kramis, Gillespie, & Bland, 1975). The patterns are apparently mediated by two distinct inputs from the brain stem that converge on the hippocampus. One input, whose activity is blocked by anticholinergic agents such as scopolamine hydrobromide or atropine sulfate, produces a rhythmic theta-wave pattern with a frequency of 5–7 Hz. The second system cannot be disrupted by administration of anticholinergic agents, and it produces a rhythmic slow-wave activity with a mean frequency greater than 7 Hz and as high as 12 Hz.

Thus, in rodents there are two patterns of slow-wave activity that appear, usually concurrently, in hippocampal EEG records. One of these is in the theta range, and one is not. My own analysis of the data published by Vanderwolf and his associates leads me to conclude that the slow-wave response in the theta range may be a correlate of attention to environmental stimuli. Vanderwolf has proposed that the faster rhythmic activity is a correlate of hippocampal mediation of patterns of voluntary movement such as walking, rearing, and head movements. Since these two patterns normally occur at the same time, it is hard to separate out their behavior correlates. Vanderwolf and others have indicated that hippocampal desynchronization in the rat accompanies the performance of relatively stereotyped, or automatic, response patterns, such as eating and grooming.

It is of interest to note that the fast-frequency component of rhythmic slow-wave activity is not observed in the cat. As was indicated earlier, I have published data clearly demonstrating a lack of correspondence between patterns of voluntary movement and theta activity in the cat (Bennett, 1969). Only the anticholinergic-sensitive theta pattern is observed in the feline hippocampus (Bennett, 1973; Bennett, Nunn, & Inman, 1971). It is also of interest to note that the region of the hippocampus from which the most distinct slow-wave activity can be recorded differs from the rat to the cat. In the rat, the most distinct slow-wave activity can be recorded from hippocampal region CA 1, while, in the cat, theta is most prominent from region CA 4 (see Figure 11-2). It would appear that, in broadest perspective, the most constant correlation of hippocampal theta activity in a number of species is their orienting toward and attending to stimuli in their environment (Isaacson, 1974). However, there is also an association of rhythmic activity of a higher frequency than the theta range with bodily movements in some species, such as the rat and the rabbit.

Fast, or High-Frequency, EEG Rhythms

An EEG pattern referred to as "fast" rhythmic activity has also generated a great deal of interest among neuroscientists. Fast rhythmic EEG patterns often have dominant frequencies, or spectral peaks, at 40 Hz. Bursts of fast rhythmic activity have been recorded from many regions of the cortex and subcortex during arousal, attention, and learning. As you will see, the occurrence of 40 Hz in the neocortex bears an interesting relation to learning and performance—a relation that has led Sheer (1970) to refer to this bioelectric pattern as the "consolidation rhythm."

In subcortical regions, the occurrence of fast rhythmic activity is most pronounced in certain rhinencephalic zones—particularly the olfactory bulb and the amygdala. Lesse (1960), using cats, was one of the first to study the 40-Hz burst activity of the basolateral amygdala. An example of **amygdala fast activity** is shown in Figure 11-10. The amygdala fast is evoked by meaningful or noxious stimuli, such as food, water, a mouse or dog, and loud noises. It appears before avoidance learning has become apparent and persists long after avoidance is well learned.

A number of researchers have provided evidence suggesting that the amygdala fast is an electrophysiological correlate of the olfactory orienting response (for example, Delgado, Johnston, Wallace, & Bradley, 1970; Sheer, 1970). Its occurrence

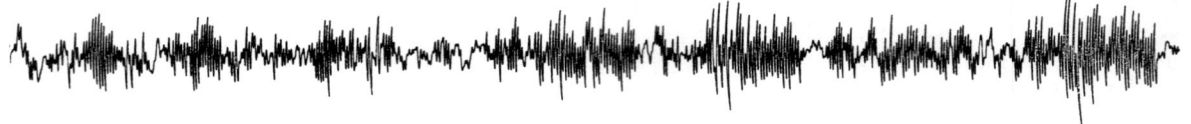

Figure 11-10
*A burst of fast,
40-Hz activity
against a
background of
desynchronized
activity. This
spindling was
recorded from the
basolateral
amygdala of a cat.*

500 μV

I SEC.

seems to be highly correlated with sniffing and the movement of air through the nasal passages (Gault & Leaton, 1963). Bilateral ablation of the olfactory bulb abolishes the amygdala fast, and ipsilateral nasal occlusion abolishes it ipsilaterally while potentiating it contralaterally (Sheer, 1970). As Sheer has indicated, the ecological significance of this rhythm is obvious. For quadruped animals in particular, the processing of olfactory information during attention or orienting behaviors is an essential component of exploratory, feeding, and sexual behaviors.

Bursts of fast rhythmic activity can also be recorded from the neocortex. Sheer and his associates have studied these patterns during learning and performance of a visual-discrimination problem (Sheer, 1970). In their research, cats learned an operant task in which bar-presses were reinforced with a milk reward if they were emitted in the presence of a 7/sec flickering light (positive stimulus). Bar-presses emitted when the negative stimulus—a 3/sec flashing light—was present were not reinforced. Recordings were obtained from various regions of the neocortex, and training was continued until the animals met a learning criterion of three times more bar-presses being made during periods when the positive stimulus was on than during intervals when the negative stimulus was presented, for three consecutive days.

Some interesting differences in the electrical activity of certain neocortical regions were correlated with different aspects of performance on this task when the criterion level of training had been reached. These patterns were restricted to the visual and motor neocortex. Specifically, there was a marked increase in the amount of electrical activity at a spectral peak of 40 Hz in the visual and motor cortex when the animals emitted reinforced bar-presses. Under the assumption that this rhythm is a correlate of consolidation processes, Sheer named this bioelectric response the "consolidation rhythm." This rhythm would also presumably reflect recall processes during performance. It is important to note that the occurrence of 40 Hz in the visual and motor cortex was found to be uncorrelated with the appearance of 40 Hz in amygdala records. Furthermore, olfactory-bulb ablations, which abolished the amygdala fast activity, had no effects on the EEG fast patterns of the neocortex during performance of this visual-discrimination problem.

Sheer also reported that he and his associates observed an EEG correlate of behavioral inhibition during periods of refraining from responding when the negative stimulus was presented. The interval during which a bar-press would not have been reinforced was dominated by 20-Hz activity in the visual and motor cortex. This EEG pattern was not simply a correlate of motor inhibition, since no shift to the 20-Hz peak

226

of electrical activity occurred during refraining from responding in the presence of the positive cue.

Sheer's findings are intriguing. More work on the behavior correlates of these neocortical EEG patterns is warranted. It would be interesting to know whether these patterns are correlates of general information processing, consolidation, and recall processes or rather are more closely related to the attention component of discrimination learning. Along these lines, it would be worthwhile to investigate the relationship of the neocortical 20-Hz and 40-Hz rhythms to the theta and desynchronized electrical activities of the hippocampus.

Microelectrode Investigations of the Electrophysiological Correlates of Learning and Performance

As indicated in Chapter 4, some neuroscientists have contended that, since macroelectrodes (such as those used in the experiments described previously in this chapter) record regional EEG patterns and because neurons that are functionally related are not necessarily located together, it is difficult, if not impossible, to obtain meaningful correlations between summed EEG patterns and possible brain functions. Such an argument is considerably weakened by microelectrode data such as those published by Ranck (1973a).

In an elegant series of experiments, Ranck has shown that there are cells in the septum and hippocampus of the rat whose individual firing patterns invariably correlate with the appearance of hippocampal theta activity. Ranck reports that these "theta cells" increase their firing rate if and only if a regular theta rhythm occurs in the hippocampus. In terms of behavior correlates, an increase in the rate of firing of the theta cells and the appearance of hippocampal theta activity accompany the same behavior patterns (see also Feder & Ranck, 1973).

Until the 1960s, microelectrode studies were confined to acute surgical preparations. With subsequent technological advances, it has become possible to record the firing pattern of a single cell in chronically implanted, unrestrained animals. The refinements in microelectrode methodology have continued, so that it is now possible to obtain records of firing from a single cell in unrestrained, vigorously moving subjects for several hours with almost no distortion of the record due to movement artifact (see Ranck, 1973b). Experimental investigations of alterations in the firing patterns of single cells in the mammalian nervous system may be divided into two categories: (1) attempts to alter the discharge rate of single units by applying reinforcement and (2) examinations of normal alterations in the discharge pattern of single cells during learning and performance.

Attempts to Alter the Discharge Rate of Single Units via Reinforcement

The first published account of conditioning of the firing rate of single cells was by Olds and Olds (1961). In this study, individual cells were located that were spontaneously active, and increases in their rate of discharge were reinforced by application of rewarding electrical brain stimulation. Particularly in the hippocampus, cells were found that responded to this treatment procedure. After only 1–20 reinforcements, cells that usually responded at a rate of only once or twice per second increased their firing rate to levels of up to 30 discharges per second. Unfortunately, it soon became evident that overt postural changes or receptor adjustments were being reinforced and what were being recorded were the central electrophysiological correlates of these behavior alterations. For example, a neuron would increase its firing rate if the rat sniffed or moved its limb. Reinforcement would then be delivered, and the subject would repeat the response that led to reinforcement.

Fetz (1969) demonstrated similar changes in the rate of firing of neurons when food was used as the reinforcer. In his research, the activity of single units in the precentral motor cortex of unanesthetized Rhesus monkeys was conditioned by selective reinforcement of high rates of neuronal discharge with a banana-flavored food pellet. In addition to food reinforcement, the monkeys usually received either visual or auditory feedback related to the unit's firing pattern. This sensory feedback probably served as a training aid. For example, two of the monkeys were exposed to a click sound for each firing of the single cell under observation. Thus, high rates of clicking could have signaled the animal that reinforcement would soon be delivered.

The average firing rate of a prefrontal-cortex cell as a function of training conditions is shown in Figure 11-11. As you can see, the rate of firing was low during

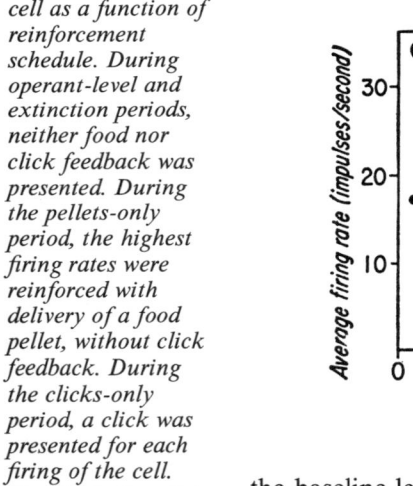

Figure 11-11
The firing rate of a precentral-cortex cell as a function of reinforcement schedule. During operant-level and extinction periods, neither food nor click feedback was presented. During the pellets-only period, the highest firing rates were reinforced with delivery of a food pellet, without click feedback. During the clicks-only period, a click was presented for each firing of the cell. Finally, both pellets and clicks were provided. From "Operant Conditioning of Cortical Unit Activity," by E. E. Fetz, Science, 1969, 163, 955–957. Copyright 1969 by the American Association for the Advancement of Science. Reprinted by permission.

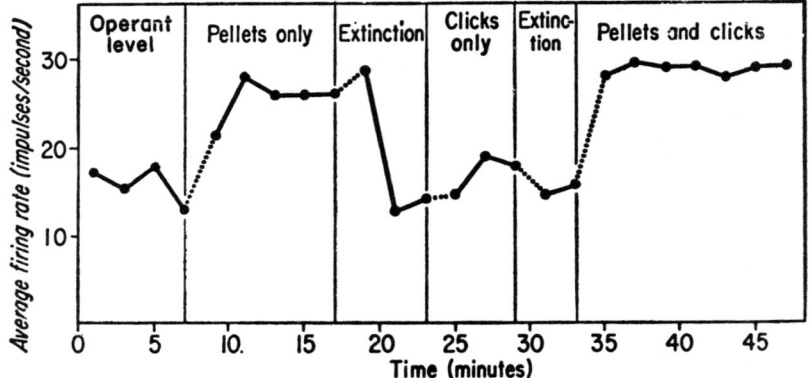

the baseline level. However, the firing rate significantly increased during reinforcement periods. The discharge rate subsequently returned to a baseline level of firing when reinforcement for high rates of responding was discontinued—that is, during extinction. Fetz reported that, after several reinforcement sessions, monkeys could increase the firing rate of some isolated cells by as much as 500% over baseline levels. These findings are quite impressive, but, although Fetz tries to rule out the possibility, it seems quite possible that his findings are best explained by the fact that the observed alterations in the firing rate of the individual neurons were correlated with alterations in patterns of gross movement, with postural changes, or with receptor adjustments.

In an attempt to circumvent this problem, Olds and his associates (Olds, 1965, 1967; Olds & Hirano, 1969) repeated their investigations. In these later experiments, cells were conditioned only during periods when the animals remained motionless. In these studies, hungry animals were rewarded with food pellets for altering the discharge rate of individual neurons. The operant-conditioning procedure required that the rat first stand quite motionless and then, while standing still, show a greatly increased firing rate of the particular neuron being studied. As in the earlier inquiries of these researchers, hippocampal units were most responsive to the training procedures and showed large increments in their rate of discharge following conditioning.

229

Electro-
physiological
Correlates
of Learning
and Performance

Olds and his associates have interpreted these alterations in firing rate as related to a temporary memory trace of a motivationally significant event—a view in accord with the notion that the hippocampus is involved in the transfer of new information to long-term memory. However, as was indicated in the last chapter, this view of the role of the hippocampus in learning must be seriously questioned in light of recent experimental findings. As was the case with the earlier data of Olds and his associates, these more recent findings are somewhat difficult to interpret. Although these investigators have attempted to rule out alternative interpretations of the alterations in firing rate, it is still possible that they were recording from units that increased their firing rate in direct correspondence with the degree of inhibition of movement. Another possibility is that they recorded from units that increased their firing rate in response to changes in heart rate, respiration, or some other relatively covert vegetative response.

Changes in the Firing Rate of Neurons during Learning and Performance

Other single-unit inquiries have observed changes in ongoing cellular activity during learning and performance behavior. One of the most comprehensive investigations of this sort was conducted by Ranck and his colleagues (Feder & Ranck, 1973; Ranck, 1973a). In the rat dorsal hippocampus, Ranck differentiated two types of neurons: theta cells, which were mentioned earlier, and "complex spike cells"—so named because of the complex spike burst they exhibited during discharge. As indicated, theta cells were found to increase their firing rate when theta EEG activity was recorded from macroelectrodes located in the dorsal hippocampus. Increases in the firing rate of theta cells were correlated with the appearance of voluntary motor responses (for example, walking, looking around, making postural adjustments, jumping, and exploring). In contrast, a decrease in their rate of firing accompanied the onset of hippocampal desynchronization and the performance of relatively automatic behavior patterns (for example, eating, drinking, grooming, teeth chattering, and performing a well-established bar-press response for a food reward, under either continuous or fixed-ratio 50—reinforcement for 50 bar-presses—reinforcement schedules).

Ranck further reported that the firing rate of complex spike cells also correlated with alterations in overt behavior but bore no relationship to hippocampal theta activity. Ranck identified several distinct types of complex spike cells according to their correlated overt behavior. For example, an *approach-consummate cell* fired most rapidly during successful completion of certain consummatory behaviors. A cell of this type would increase its firing rate during approach to, exploration of, and eating of a food pellet. An *approach-consummate-mismatch unit* fired when an approach-consummate cell fired, but it would additionally increase its rate of discharging if the rat's behavior was not consummated. Such a unit would not only fire at a higher rate during a rat's approach to water and during drinking but also during exploration of a water hole after the water bottle had been removed.

A number of researchers have observed changes in the rate of firing of single units during acquisition and performance of various classically or operantly conditioned responses (see the review by Leiman & Christian, 1973). For example, Woody, Vassilevsky, and Engle (1970) studied the firing rate of single units following presentation of a conditioned stimulus (CS, a click) during classical conditioning of an eye-blink response in cats. The neurons studied were in the coronal-precruciate area—one of the cortical regions regulating the eye-blink response. After conditioning, the CS was followed by more frequent and longer discharges of units in this area, and there was a decrease in the latency of firing after presentation of the CS.

Changes in the activity of single cells are also observed during operant conditioning. Travis and his associates (Travis, Hooten, & Sparks, 1968; Travis & Sparks, 1967; Travis, Sparks, & Hooten, 1968) investigated the responsiveness of units in the globus pallidus of the basal ganglia of monkeys trained to bar-press for a food reward. They found that, during a response sequence in which an animal obtained and consumed a familiar reward, approximately 30% of the cells sampled were inhibited. However, the firing of these units was not inhibited when the monkeys grasped unfamiliar or inedible objects or when the monkeys were consuming an unfamiliar food. These researchers suggested that these units mediated the chaining of stimulus-response sequences. Future research should clarify the nature of the behavior functions, if any, of these very intriguing units.

Some very interesting single-unit research has examined variation in the reactivity of individual neurons during learning and performance as a function of whether an appetitive or aversive stimulus was used to control behavior. A study by Fuster and Uyeda (1971) is illustrative of this approach. They demonstrated that individual neurons in the limbic system of the monkey brain react with changes in their rate of discharge to visual stimuli associated with food reward and electric shock.

Fuster and Uyeda's subjects were trained in a pattern discrimination in which a pattern of horizontal light bands served as a food signal and a pattern of vertical light bands as a shock signal. After six seconds of exposure to one of these signals, a screen in front of two levers was raised for four seconds so that the animal could press one of the levers. The animals were trained to respond to the food signal by pressing the lever on the right; doing so resulted in delivery of a banana-flavored food pellet. Pressing the left lever resulted in no reinforcement. If the shock signal was presented, then the monkey had to press the left-hand lever. Failure to press this bar during the four-second response period or pressing the food lever resulted in application of a mild, brief electric shock to the animal. Unit records were obtained after the animals had learned to respond at a level of 85% correct or better, and unit data were analyzed for the six-second period of signal presentation. A total of 469 units were studied in this very thorough inquiry.

The units examined were selected from the hippocampus, the amygdala, and the pyriform cortex adjacent to the amygdala. Because of the histological techniques used to assess the location of the units under examination, no reliable separation could be made between records derived from the two components of the hippocampus—Ammon's horn and the dentate gyrus. The majority of the amygdala units studied were from the basolateral nuclear complex. Units from the pyriform cortex included selections from the cortex of the medial and ventral surfaces of the temporal lobes.

Three categories of units were isolated. Some neurons responded with either excitation or inhibition to both the food and the shock signals. A record from a unit located in the hippocampus that responded to both signals with an increase in firing is shown in Figure 11-12. Note that presentation of a neutral stimulus, in the bottom tracing, did not affect this unit's discharge pattern. A second group of units was discovered that selectively responded to either the food signal or the shock signal. A unit from the hippocampus that was inhibited by the shock signal but whose firing pattern was unaffected by the food signal is shown in Figure 11-13. A third group of neurons was found to be excited by one of the signals and inhibited by the other. However, such reciprocally reacting cells were rare.

All three categories of units described above were found in each of the three large subdivisions of the rhinencephalon examined, although the proportions were different from region to region. Although the proportion of responsive units was found to be greater in the hippocampus and pyriform cortex, units that differentially responded to the signals were most common in the amygdala. The finding of a comparatively high incidence of units in the amygdala that differentially reacted to the two signals suggested to Fuster and Uyeda that neurons of the amygdala generally respond in a selective fashion to the appetitive and aversive properties of sensory stimuli. The investigators concluded that their results supported the theory that an essential function of the amygdala in mediating behavior is to identify reinforcing stimuli.

Later work by Olds and Segal was able to demonstrate a difference in the firing pattern between units in the dentate gyrus and in Ammon's horn (Segal & Olds, 1972, 1973; Segal, Disterhoft, & Olds, 1972). They found that units located in CA 1 and CA 3 of Ammon's horn did not differentially react to appetitive or aversive signals.

Figure 11-12
Records from a unit in the hippocampus: excitatory responses to both food and shock. From "Reactivity of Limbic Neurons of the Monkey to Appetitive and Aversive Signals," by J. M. Fuster and A. A. Uyeda, Electroencephalography and Clinical Neurophysiology, 1971, 30, 281–293. Copyright © 1971 by ASP Biological and Medical Press. Reprinted by permission of ASP Biological and Medical Press, Elsevier Division, Amsterdam.

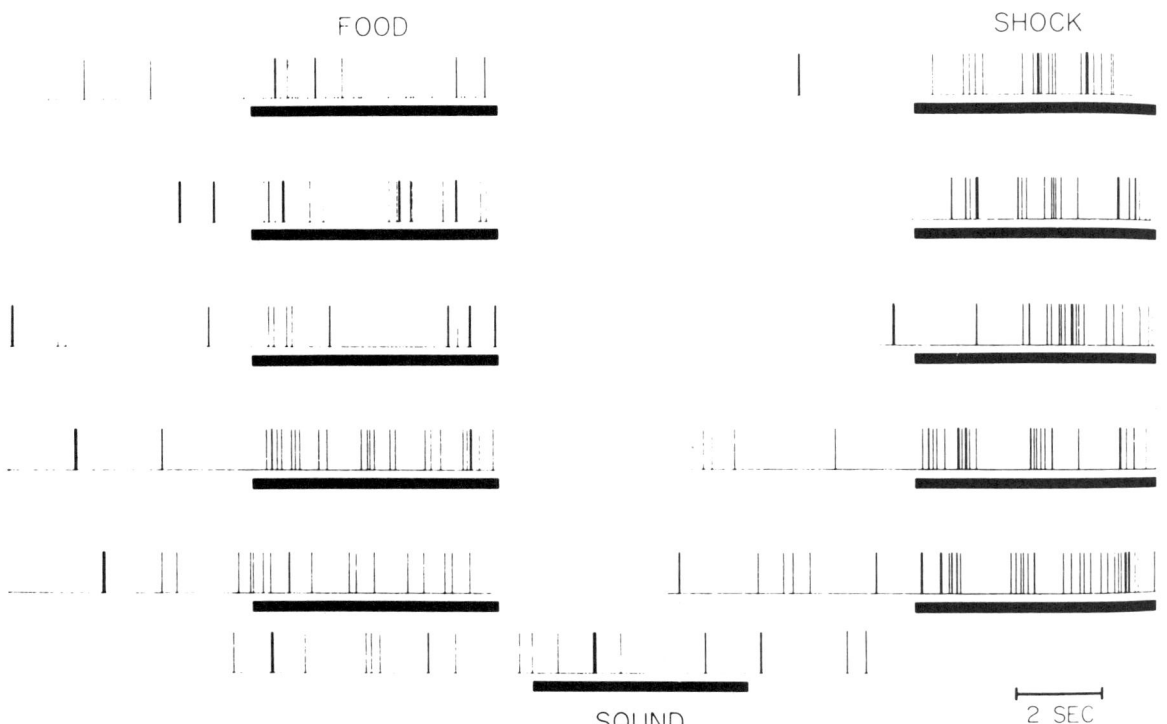

FOOD   SHOCK

SOUND   2 SEC

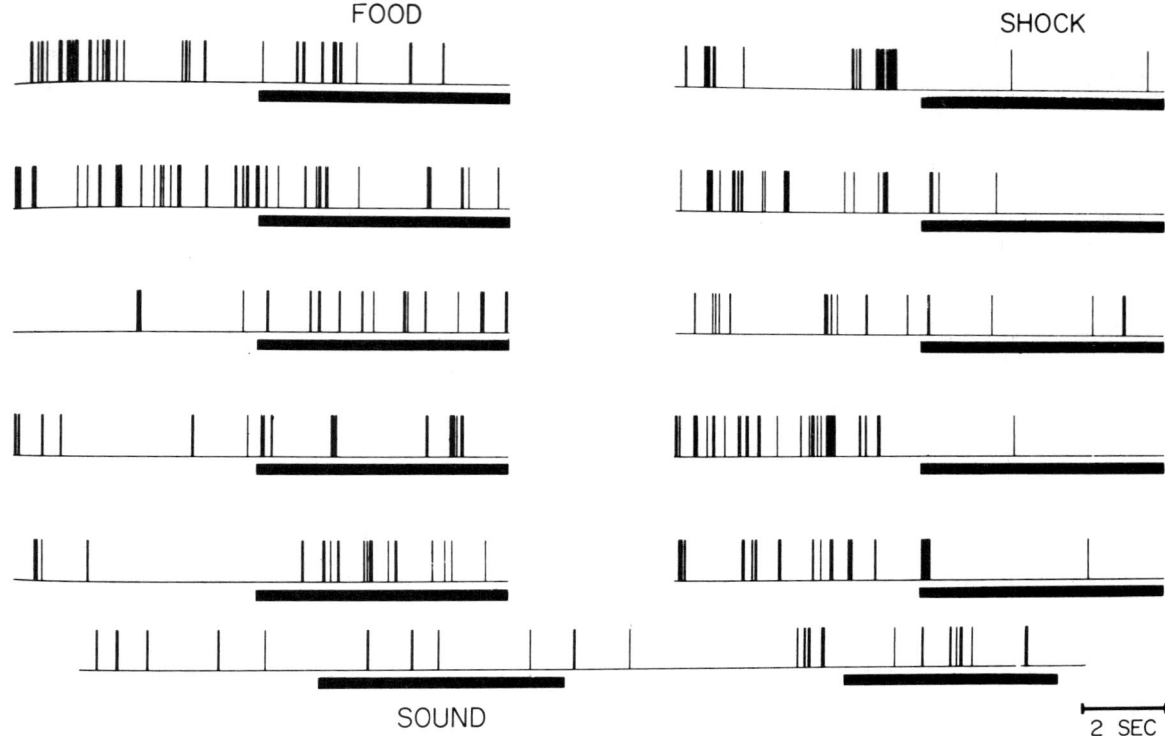

FOOD

SHOCK

SOUND

2 SEC

Figure 11-13
The record from a hippocampal unit inhibited by the shock signal. From "Reactivity of Limbic Neurons of the Monkey to Appetitive and Aversive Signals," by J. M. Fuster and A. A. Uyeda, Electroencephalography and Clinical Neurophysiology, *1971, 30, 281–293. Copyright © 1971 by ASP Biological and Medical Press. Reprinted by permission of ASP Biological and Medical Press, Elsevier Division, Amsterdam.*

Rather, these units increased their firing rate to both conditioned signals. In contrast, units in the dentate gyrus acted reciprocally to the two signals. That is, these units reacted to the food signal by increasing their rate of firing and to the aversive signal by inhibiting it.

With regard to appetitive signals alone, Olds and his associates (Olds, Mink, & Best, 1969; Phillips & Olds, 1969) reported that there are units, most frequently located in the hippocampus and hypothalamus, that seem to respond in anticipation only of food or only of water. In the Olds, Mink, and Best study, units were monitored in rats that were trained to depress a pedal and then, after 0.25 second, remain motionless for 1.75 seconds to obtain a reward. There were two pedals—one for food and one for water. The firing patterns of the units were analyzed during the 1.75 second waiting period. In the Phillips and Olds study, the rats were trained to depress a bar and remain motionless for two seconds. After the first second had elapsed, one of three tones was presented. The tone signaled that food, water, or nothing would be delivered for a subsequent bar-press.

Analysis of the results of these inquiries indicated that certain units would increase their discharge rate if the animal was hungry and the tone signaled the availability of food or if a deprived animal was waiting for food. This latter finding is illustrated in Figure 11-14. Units were also found that increased their firing rate only in anticipation of the delivery of a water reward. In the Phillips and Olds experiment, for example, certain units were isolated that increased their firing rate if the rat was thirsty and the tone signaled the availability of water. In the experiments by Olds and

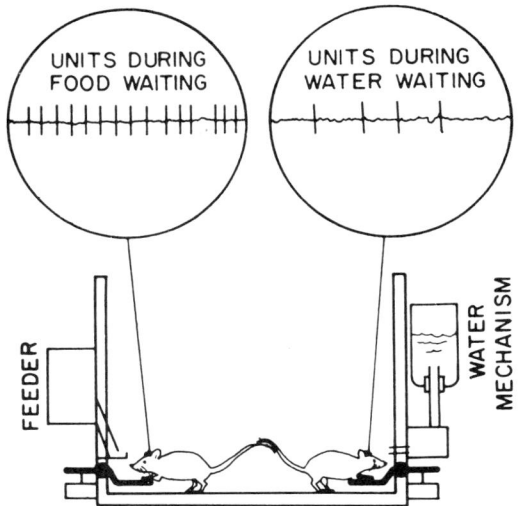

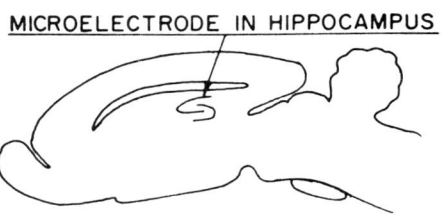

MICROELECTRODE IN HIPPOCAMPUS

his associates, the units responded if and only if the anticipated reward was relevant to the animal's current motivational state. While it seems very plausible that these results indicate the functions of units in controlling or mediating eating and drinking, Olds (1969) prefers to interpret them as indicating that short-term or immediate memories of eating and drinking behaviors related to this task are stored in the hippocampus.

The results obtained with unit recordings are certainly intriguing. They seem to indicate that changes in the firing patterns of cells are correlated with learning and performance. Unfortunately, it is still too soon to decide whether these alterations reflect memory consolidation and recall processes per se or whether they reflect ongoing sensory, motor, and motivational components of learned behavior sequences.

DC, or Steady Potentials

In contrast to EEG and unit records, in which changes in bioelectric patterns are often measured in terms of milliseconds, brain voltages that change slowly over time—over a period of seconds or minutes—have also been studied and related to learning and performance. As described in Chapter 4, these latter changes are called *DC*, or *steady-potential, shifts.* Some of the problems encountered in studying these phenomena, in terms of apparatus requirements, and the early history of research on steady-potential phenomena were summarized in Chapter 4.

The term *steady potential (SP),* as used with reference to the cortex, refers to "the maintained or nonrhythmic difference of potential between the surface of the cortex and the immediately subjacent white matter" (Rowland, 1968, p. 5). Steady potentials range in amplitude from 0.5 to 5 mv and exhibit a slow shift as a function of time, but they rarely change by more than approximately 0.5 mv over several hours if an animal is left undisturbed. Steady potentials apparently result from and reflect both the depolarization of glia cells and the massed activity of neurons (Castellucci &

Goldring, 1970; Sheafor & Rowland, 1974; Ransom & Goldring, 1973a, 1973b, 1973c).

Glia cells, which have not been mentioned previously, are actually by far the most common cells in the brain. Over 90% of the cells in the brain are glia cells. While there are approximately 12 billion neurons in the brain, there are 120 billion glia (Nurnberger, 1958). Glia cells, which surround nerve cells and their branches, have often been thought simply to make up a type of connective tissue. Recent evidence, however, has led to the conclusion that glia cells perform important nutritive and regulatory roles in nerve-cell function. Some theorists have proposed that activity in glia cells may, in addition, serve as the basis for temporary, or short-term, memory.

Current interest in steady-potential (SP) phenomena has followed Caton's 19th-century lead (see Chapter 4); researchers have attempted to determine meaningful relationships between SP shifts and behavior. Excellent reviews on SP phenomena are provided by Rowland (1968) and by Rowland and Anderson (1971). In the examples cited below, the SP shift appears as a shift in the baseline of the EEG record.

SP Shifts Correlated with Arousal, Attention, and Drive Level

All novel stimuli evoke SP shifts, which exhibit rapid decrement with repetitions of the stimulus. The SP shift appears most prominently in the cortical sensory projection area associated with the modality of the stimulus being presented (Gumnit, 1961; Köhler & Wegener, 1955; Lickey & Fox, 1966). This phenomenon is illustrated in Figure 11-15, which shows SP shifts in the rat cortex during repeated presentations of a moderately intense light in a darkened chamber (from Rowland, 1968). It is interesting that the SP shift under these conditions apparently was correlated with the behavioral orienting, or attention, response. Diminution of the orienting response as the animal habituated to the stimulus was reflected by a decrease in and finally a disappearance of the SP shift.

In contrast to SP shifts that follow neutral stimuli, SP shifts that accompany stimuli having biological significance for the animal do not show decrements in amplitude simply as a function of repeated presentations (Rowland, 1968). Rowland and his associates have demonstrated this with respect to the following stimuli: food, perineal stimulation in the estrus rat and cat, peripheral electric shock, and positively and negatively reinforcing electrical stimulation of the hypothalamus.

In the case of these biologically significant stimuli, decrements in the SP shift appear to be directly related to decreases in the relevant drive state. An example of this finding is shown in Figure 11-16. In this example, records of SP phenomena were obtained while a food-deprived cat lapped an evaporated milk/fishmeal homogenate. As illustrated by this figure, when hungry cats were presented with food, they exhibited an SP shift that sometimes reached 1–2 mv over the first 5–10 minutes of eating. The slope of this shift was the steepest at the onset of eating and gradually declined until the SP shift reached its maximum amplitude, when the cat approached satiety. After eating stopped, the SP reversed its direction and returned to the baseline level (Rowland, Bradley, School, & Deutschman, 1967). Taken together, the data discussed thus far in this section suggest that the occurrence and maintenance of SP shifts are related to the arousal, attention, and drive level of an organism. Thus, SP shifts may provide us with an additional physiological index of these processes.

235

*Electro-
physiological
Correlates
of Learning
and Performance*

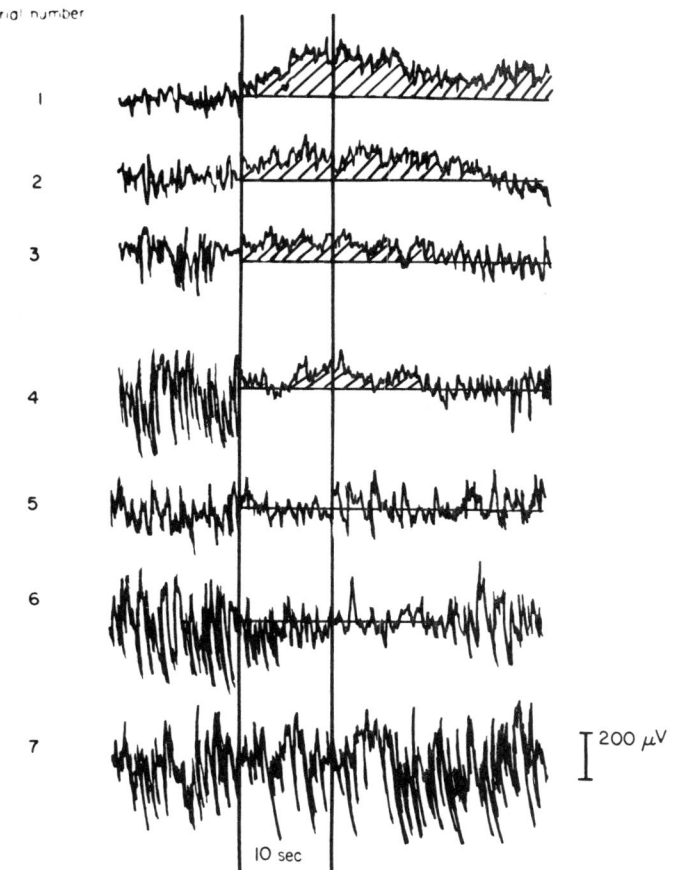

Trial number

10 sec

200 μV

Figure 11-15
*The progressive loss
of SP shift with
repeated
presentations of a
light. From
"Cortical Steady
Potential (Direct
Current Potential)
in Reinforcement
and Learning," by
V. Rowland. In E.
Stellar and J. M.
Sprague (Eds.),*
Progress in
Physiological
Psychology, *(Vol.
2). Copyright 1969
by Academic Press,
Inc. Reprinted by
permission.*

SP Shifts and Attention in Humans

Evidence that SP shifts are related to processes of attention is also provided by research conducted by Walter and his associates (for example, Walter, 1964). They have described an SP shift in humans that occurs during the interval between presentation of a meaningful stimulus and the reaction to this cue. Called the **expectancy wave** or **E-Wave,** this SP shift appears when stimuli are paired. According to Walter (1964), in the typical experimental paradigm of this sort, the subject learns that, if there is a click (conditional stimulus), there will be flashes of light (imperative stimulus), so press the button (imperative response). In this situation, an E-Wave is evoked in the frontal cortex immediately after the conditional stimulus is presented and endures until the imperative response is emitted. Thereafter, the response declines back to the baseline. This SP shift is elicited by attention to the conditional stimulus and occurs during sensory-motor associations.

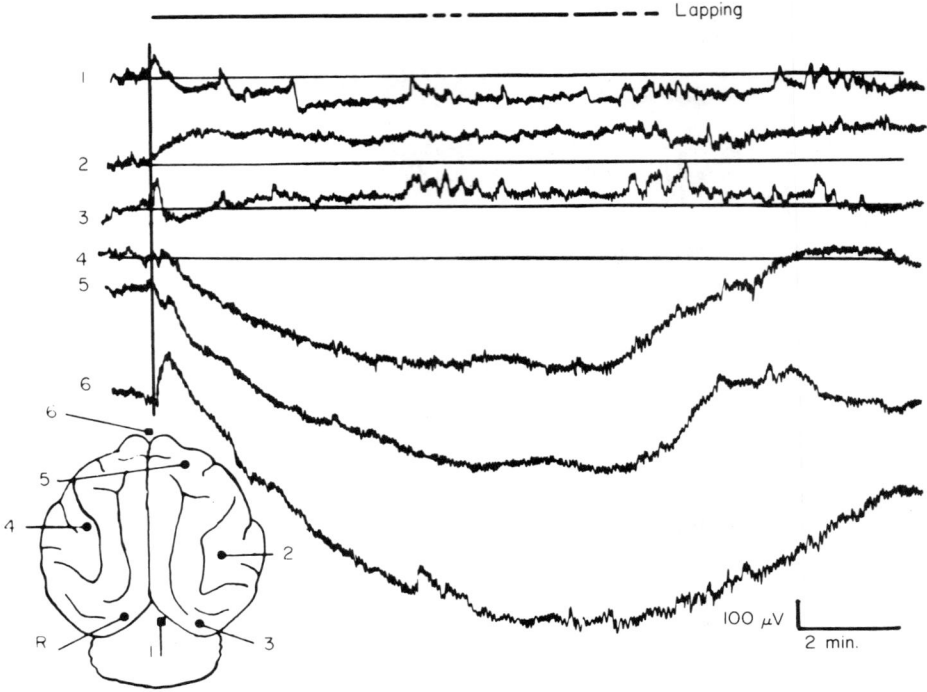

Figure 11-16
The shift in the
steady potential of a
cat that is lapping,
recorded
simultaneously from
six sites. From
"Cortical Steady
Potential (Direct
Current Potential)
in Reinforcement
and Learning," by
V. Rowland. In E.
Stellar and J. M.
Sprague (Eds.),
Progress in
Physiological
Psychology *(Vol. 2).*
Copyright 1968 by
Academic Press, Inc.
Reprinted by
permission.

SP Shifts during Operant Behavior in Infrahuman Species

Schedules of Reinforcement. Rowland and Anderson (1971) reported observations they had made of cortical SP shifts in rats on various schedules of reinforcement. They found that the development of stable patterns of responding on fixed-interval and fixed-ratio schedules of reinforcement was accompanied by the appearance of a systematic pattern of SP shifting. These SP shifts were recorded from visual, motor, and somatosensory cortical regions. Fixed-interval (FI) training involved reinforcing the first bar-press that was emitted one minute (FI 1-minute schedule) or two minutes (FI 2-minute schedule) after the last rewarded response. Failure of the subject to respond within an additional five seconds, for the FI-1 schedule, or 10 seconds, for the FI-2 schedule, resulted in the resetting of the time-out-from-reinforcement interval. As shown in Figure 11-17, an SP shift anticipated and accompanied bar-pressing. It increased in amplitude until the animal performed the rewarded bar-press, indicated by the arrow. Subsequent eating of the food pellet and absence of bar-pressing were correlated with a return of the SP to the baseline level or beyond (rebound).

Figure 11-18 illustrates SP shifts recorded during stable fixed-ratio (FR-50) performance. Under this schedule, every 50th bar-press was rewarded. This figure indicates that an SP shift developed prior to each reinforced bar-press, a larger shift accompanied food delivery, and a slow return to the baseline accompanied the cessation of eating the food pellet and the return to bar-pressing. Therefore, the

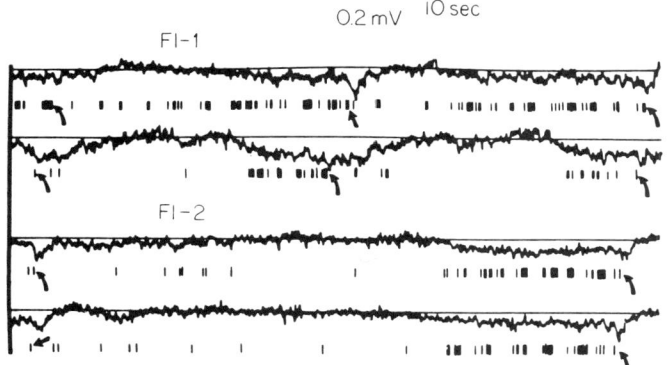

Figure 11-17
SP shifts recorded
in a rat during FI-1
and FI-2 schedules
of reinforcement.
The arrows indicate
reinforcement.
Adapted from
"Brain Steady
Potential Shifts," by
V. Rowland and R.
Anderson. In E.
Stellar and J. M.
Sprague (Eds.),
Progress in
Physiological
Psychology (Vol. 4).
Copyright 1971 by
Academic Press, Inc.
Reprinted by
permission.

pattern of shift during ratio performance was basically similar to that observed during interval performance. The fact that the direction of the SP shift was toward increased positivity (or decreased negativity) during the first half of the FR-50 cycle and then changed directions would argue that the observed SP shifting was not simply a motor-system correlate of bar-pressing. Rather, the direction and amplitude of the SP appeared to be a correlate of anticipatory arousal and drive level (Rowland & Anderson, 1971).

Maze Running. In research conducted in Rowland's laboratory, Wisenfeld (1969) recorded SP shifts from the cortical surface of the visual and motor cortex of rats performing a food-reinforced turning habit in a T-maze. The opening of the start-box door elicited a large SP shift, the amplitude of which decreased as the animal entered the goal box. Subsequent eating was accompanied by an SP shift in

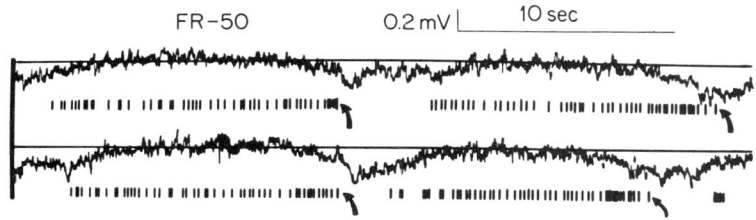

Figure 11-18
SP shifts recorded
during stable FR-50
performance. The
arrows indicate
reinforcement.
Adapted from
"Brain Steady
Potential Shifts," by
V. Rowland and R.
Anderson. In E.
Stellar and J. M.
Sprague (Eds.),
Progress in
Physiological
Psychology (Vol. 4).
Copyright 1971 by
Academic Press, Inc.
Reprinted by
permission.

the opposite direction. Partial extinction of this behavioral response (as defined by an increase in choices of the previously nonrewarded side to 50% of the trials) was correlated with marked reductions in the amplitude of all of these shifts.

An examination of SP shifts during performance of this learned pattern of responding thus provides additional support for the view that SP shifts, at least in part, reflect central processes related to arousal, attention, and motivation, or drive, level. Whether these electrophysiological responses also reflect memory mechanisms is still a question.

Because of the bewildering complexity of the mammalian nervous system and of behavior characteristic of mammalian species, some researchers, in their quest for an understanding of the neurophysiology of learning, have examined the simplest kinds of learning in animals with primitive nervous systems. Their model of the learning process has been the phenomenon of habituation, and the nervous systems examined have included such invertebrates as annelids, insects, crustacea, and mollusks. In this final section of the chapter, we will first examine the phenomenon of habituation as a model for the learning process and then review behavioral and electrophysiological studies of habituation in the marine mollusk *Aplysia. Aplysia* is a superb preparation to work with because a number of nerve cells in its primitive nervous system, or ganglion, are exceptionally large. The size of these brain cells allows the investigator to identify them visually, record from them for prolonged periods of time, and identify the same cell in different individuals of the species. The interconnections have been determined for a number of these identifiable single neurons (for example, Frazier, Kandel, Kupfermann, Waziri, & Coggeshall, 1967).

Habituation

Habituation refers to a decrease in the tendency to respond to a behaviorally irrelevant stimulus. One possible physiological correlate of the habituation process was described in the previous section. It was indicated that the magnitude of SP shifts shows a rapid decrement following repeated presentation of a neutral stimulus. Habituation is the opposite of **sensitization**—an increase in response tendency as a result of repeated stimulation. Habituation should be distinguished from other decremental processes that are not themselves habituation. For example, habituation, which is a behavioral response differs from adaptation, which involves a decrease of sensitivity in a sensory receptor cell. Adaptation was discussed in Chapter 5. Habituation also does not include decreases in responding due to fatigue or to decreases in motivation.

Thompson and Spencer (1966) have described the features of habituation. They include (1) a decrease in response with repeated stimulation, (2) recovery of response tendency if the stimulus is withheld, (3) generalization of habituation to stimuli that are similar to the stimulus being repeated, (4) greater habituation with more frequently presented stimuli, (5) more pronounced habituation to weaker stimuli, and (6) **dishabituation**—the recovery of a habituated response after a single presentation of a novel stimulus. It is important to note that habituation is produced by stimuli that have no consequences for the animal. Thompson and Spencer and others have argued that both habituation and dishabituation represent primitive examples of learning. Clarifying the nature of these processes may aid our understanding of more general learning phenomena and their physiological substrates.

Habituation in Aplysia

An excellent series of experiments that ties behavioral habituation to a defined nerve network has been conducted by Kandel in collaboration with Carew, Castellucci, Kupfermann, and Pinsker (for example, Carew & Kandel, 1973; Carew,

Pinsker, & Kandel, 1972; Castellucci, Pinsker, Kupfermann, & Kandel, 1970; Kupfermann, Castellucci, Pinsker, & Kandel, 1970; Kupfermann & Kandel, 1969; Pinsker, Kupfermann, Castellucci, & Kandel, 1970). These findings are reviewed by Kupfermann (1975).

239

*Electro-
physiological
Correlates
of Learning
and Performance*

In this research, the behavioral response measured in *Aplysia* was the gill-withdrawal reflex, which is a component of a larger defensive withdrawal response to potentially noxious tactile stimuli. Gill withdrawal in *Aplysia* can be reliably experimentally elicited by tactile stimuli. This latter response will generally habituate in five to ten trials. Besides showing a decrease in response with repeated presentations of the same stimulus, the gill-withdrawal reflex also exhibits several other features characteristic of the habituation process. After rest, the response recovers. Greater degrees of habituation are produced with shorter interstimulus intervals and less intense stimuli. Dishabituation can be reliably produced by a change in the locus of the tactile stimulus. Because habituation did not result in changes in the magnitude of spontaneous gill contractions observed by these researchers, the behavior alteration was true habituation rather than the product of generalized fatigue.

The neural circuit mediating the gill-withdrawal reflex has been defined by these investigators. It consists of four motor neurons within the abdominal ganglion—the primitive brain of *Aplysia*. These motor neurons have both monosynaptic and polysynaptic connections with mechanoreceptors in the skin. Electrophysiological inquiries using microelectrodes positioned in these motor neurons demonstrated that repetitive tactile stimulation that produced behavioral habituation was accompanied by a decrease in the number of action potentials generated and in the amplitude of EPSPs recorded from these motor neurons. Restoration of reflex responsiveness following either rest or application of a dishabituating stimulus was associated wtih an increase in the amplitude of the evoked EPSP and an increase in the number and frequency of action potentials in these same cells.

These researchers carried the analysis of the habituation phenomenon one step further by investigating the cellular mechanisms mediating both habituation and dishabituation. Their data indicated that these two processes involved changes in the functional effectiveness of synapses between sensory and motor neurons. Habituation was found to be correlated with a decrement in the excitability of these synapses. In contrast, dishabituation was found to be due to an excitatory input superimposed upon the decrement and perhaps resulting from an enhanced release of transmitter substance. Alterations in synaptic transmission have long been suspected of being important physiological substrates of learning and memory. This point will be elaborated on in Chapter 13. Let me emphasize at this point that the findings obtained by Kandel and his colleagues indicate that data obtained even from an organism as primitive as *Aplysia* can aid our search for the neural substrates of behavior.

Chapter Summary and Conclusions

In this chapter, research into electrophysiological correlates of learning and performance was surveyed. Interest in these phenomena has at least in part been generated by the theory that memory processes may be reflected by alterations in the spatial and temporal pattern of electrical activity in the brain. As you will remember, such a view was postulated because of the lack of good evidence for the existence of centers or regions of neural tissue that are crucially involved in basic learning and memory functions.

Several approaches to studying the electrophysiological correlates of learning and performance were presented. These included electroencephalography, single-unit recording, and studies of steady-potential shifts. The central problem for users of all of these approaches is to determine the basis for any electrophysiological changes that may be observed—a problem that was exemplified by the hippocampal theta controversy. It is often difficult, if not impossible, to determine whether the observed changes reflect information processing, memory consolidation, and recall rather than such things as arousal, receptor adjustments, attention, movement, and drive level, which are only correlated with—not synonymous with—acquisition, storage, and recall of information.

The chapter concluded with a discussion of behavioral and physiological studies of the habituation process in the marine mollusk *Aplysia. Habituation* means a decrease in response tendency to a behaviorally irrelevant stimulus. Habituation can be considered a simple model of learning. Studying the neural basis of habituation in an animal with a simple nervous system, such as *Aplysia,* may eventually clarify our understanding of the electrophysiological correlates and physiological substrates of complex learning processes in humans.

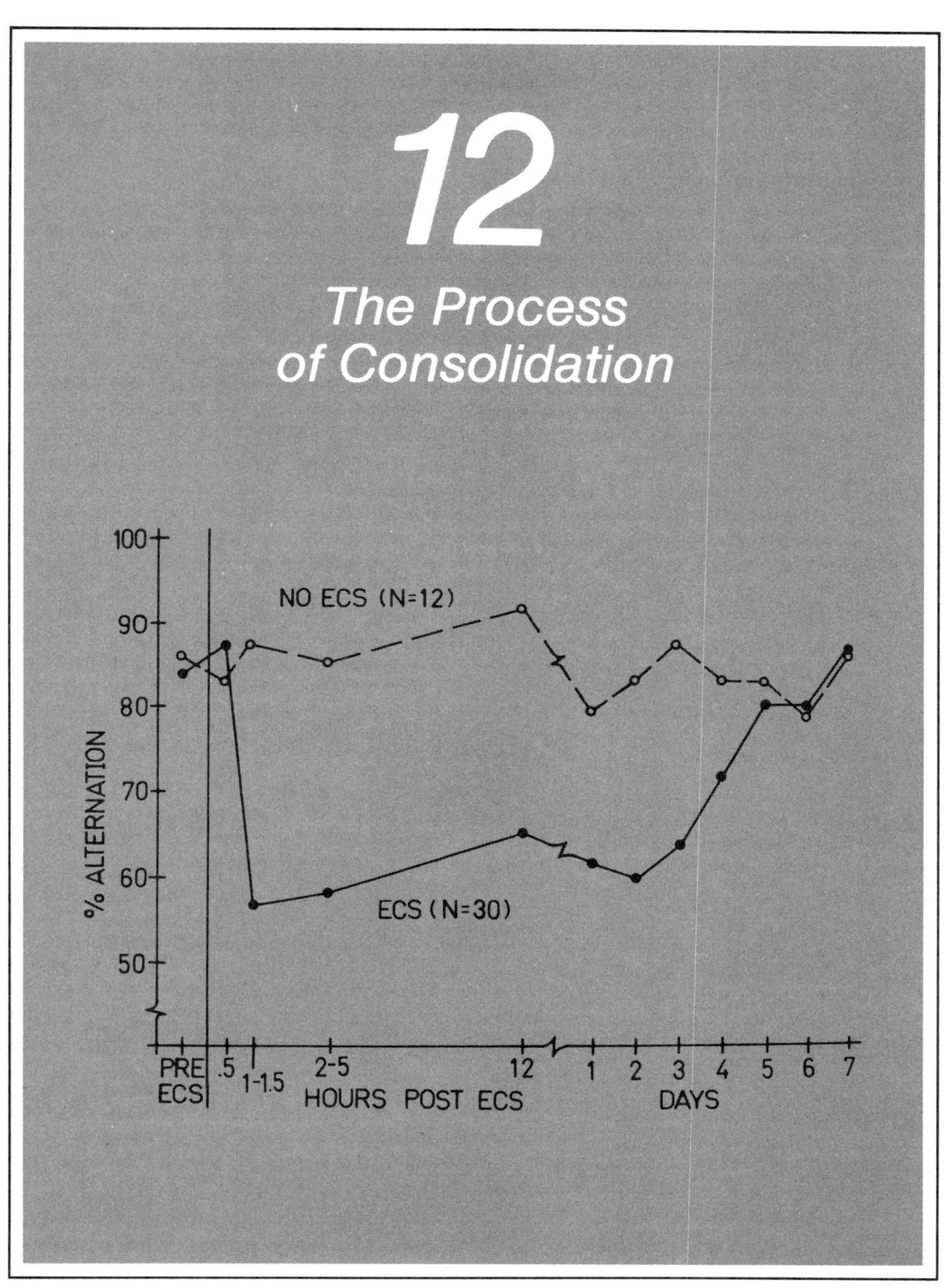

In 1900, Müller and Pilzecker proposed a theory designed to account for many of the phenomena of remembering. Basically, the theory stated that neural processes initiated during learning continued through time and that they became more firmly established because of this persisting activity. The process of firmly establishing or stabilizing long-term memory traces is called **consolidation.** Müller and Pilzecker's basic formulation has persisted, and, as an extension, most contemporary learning theorists assert that the consolidation of new information into long-term, more or less permanent memory takes place in two stages.

According to this view, memory traces are in a very labile form immediately after an experience has occurred. They become "permanent," "fixed," or consolidated after a period of time. Many present-day anatomical theories of memory also support a two-stage concept of memory consolidation—a concept that has its roots in the very influential two-factor learning theory of Hebb (1949). The anatomical theorists generally contend that memory traces are initially represented by **reverberatory circuits** that encompass neurons originally involved in processing the incoming information. Reverberatory circuits are circular nervous pathways that can reactivate themselves over and over. Short-term memories are postulated to be held by this reverberatory activity until permanent anatomical changes occur in the nervous system. There is evidence to support the existence of reverberatory circuits. For example, Burns (1958) reported that a single electrical stimulus applied through an electrode can initiate bursts of electrical activity in isolated slabs of cortex for periods of up to 30 minutes or longer. However, it is not clear whether such electrical activity performs a role in either short-term memory or memory-consolidation processes. It is also unclear whether reverberatory circuits could persist long enough and thereby maintain memories long enough for structural changes necessary for long-term memory to occur. Such anatomical changes are thought to constitute the substrate for the consolidation process.

Two anatomical changes that have been proposed as possible substrates for long-term, relatively permanent memory storage are the enlargement of existing presynaptic terminals between adjacent nerve cells (Eccles, 1953) and the development of new presynaptic terminals. As you'll remember from Chapter 2, the presynaptic terminals contain the transmitter substances that make synaptic transmission possible.

Experimental investigations of the process of memory consolidation became possible following the introduction of **electroconvulsive shock (ECS)** by Cerletti and Bini in 1938 as a treatment for psychiatric patients. This treatment is still in vogue. It consists of passing a brief but very intense electric current through a subject's head via electrodes placed on opposite sides of the head. ECS may produce brief periods of unconsciousness, convulsions, and EEG seizures similar to those observed during a grand mal epileptic episode.

242

The breakthrough regarding the use of ECS for studying memory-consolidation processes came when it was discovered (for example, Flescher, 1941) that human patients subjected to ECS treatments experienced **retrograde amnesia**—loss of memory for immediately preceding events. This observation has precipitated a flood of experimental inquiries over the years that have used ECS to study memory-consolidation processes. An excellent, comprehensive review of much of that work is provided by McGaugh and Herz (1972). Most of the work with infrahuman species has used either rats or mice. In the experiments I'll describe, the ECS treatment consisted of passing a brief current through the animal by means of electrodes attached to both ears or placed on both eyes. The current was usually of sufficient intensity to elicit convulsions.

The Initial Use of ECS to Study Consolidation Processes

In a classic study published in 1949, Duncan brought the ECS technique from the psychiatric setting into the animal experimental laboratory, where it could be systematically used in carefully controlled studies as an experimental tool to study the memory-consolidation process. His initial inquiry was to serve as the impetus for hundreds of subsequent laboratory investigations. In Duncan's experiment, rats were given one trial per day on an active-avoidance task. Subjects in different groups were administered ECS 20 seconds, 40 seconds, 60 seconds, 4 minutes, 15 minutes, 1 hour, 4 hours, or 14 hours after each daily trial. The results are shown in Figure 12-1. As

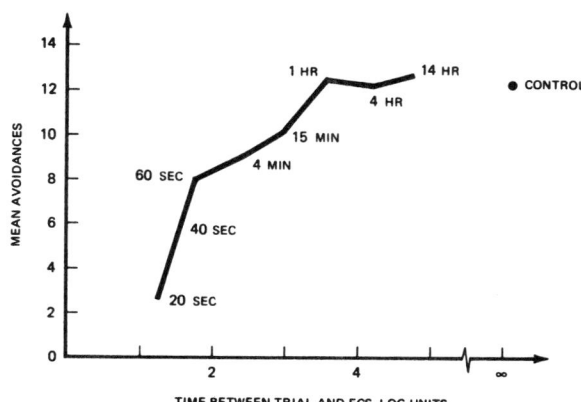

TIME BETWEEN TRIAL AND ECS, LOG UNITS

Figure 12-1
Mean avoidance responses by rats on 18 daily trials in an active-avoidance task as a function of the trial-ECS interval (expressed in log units). From "The Retroactive Effect of Electroshock on Learning," by C. P. Duncan, Journal of Comparative and Physiological Psychology, *1949, 42, 32–44. Copyright 1949 by the American Psychological Association. Reprinted by permission.*

indicated by this graph, learning was significantly retarded in those rats that received ECS shortly after each trial. In general, the longer the delay between training and ECS treatment, the smaller was the deficit produced.

Duncan's data appeared to support the general theory that memory traces need a period of undisturbed gestation before they can become permanently consolidated. Such an interpretation of these findings has not, however, been uncritically accepted.

Many subsequent investigations have sought to clarify the basis for the observed behavior deficits following ECS treatments, and several alternative interpretations have been proposed. These alternative views suggest that, instead of interrupting memory-consolidation processes per se, ECS treatments yield other behavior changes that are mistaken for evidence of a memory impairment. One theory is that ECS leads to the development of fear, and another is that it causes the conditioning of incompatible, or competing, responses.

Alternative Interpretations of the ECS Effect

ECS and the Development of Fear. Coons and Miller (1960) hypothesized that ECS may have aversive properties for the subject and that, therefore, an ECS-induced fear of the goal may develop. In the type of active-avoidance learning paradigm used by Duncan, the subject had a choice of not responding and receiving a shock to the feet or successfully avoiding and receiving a shock to the head—that is, an ECS treatment. If the rat chose the former over the latter, it does not necessarily mean that memory of the avoidance response was not consolidated. This is a very critical issue because, if the ECS effects simply reflect a punishment phenomenon, then data collected using this experimental methodology are irrelevant to the problem of memory storage. Along these lines, it is interesting to note that human patients undergoing a series of ECS treatments are often upset after a treatment and quite commonly develop an aversion to this sort of therapy. However, this may result partly from the fact that they do not recall the events leading up to the ECS treatment (Gallinek, 1956).

To test this interpretation, Coons and Miller had their rats learn active-avoidance responses. The first experiment was basically a replication of Duncan's research, and the findings generally confirmed his results. In addition, however, Coons and Miller discovered that rats that received ECS soon after each training trial exhibited increased emotion, as indexed by increased urination and defecation.

The second experiment described in the Coons and Miller paper was designed to separate the aversive from the amnesic effects of ECS treatments. In this experiment, the animals were first trained in the active-avoidance task. They were initially placed in the "dark" compartment of the apparatus. If they did not move to the lighted side within about 10 seconds, they were shocked until they did. After they had learned this response, the conditions were reversed, with shock introduced on the previously safe side. In this passive-avoidance phase, foot-shock was delivered in the lighted compartment whenever an avoidance response (moving from the dark side) was emitted; staying in the dark compartment was the new avoidance response. Animals were administered one passive-avoidance trial each day for twelve days, and ECS was administered 20 seconds, 60 seconds, or one hour after each training trial. Since the response to be learned was suppression of a previously acquired response, the longer the animal stayed in the dark compartment, the better it was at learning.

The results of this inquiry are shown in Figure 12-2. Under these conditions, the *sooner* ECS followed a training trial, the *faster* was the rate of learning. Statistical analysis of these data indicated that the 20-second group was significantly better than the 60-second group, which was in turn significantly faster at learning than the one-hour group. These results appeared to clearly support the view that ECS has aversive effects, at least when administered repeatedly. The findings therefore provided support for the "acquired fear" interpretation of the effects of ECS on learned behavior.

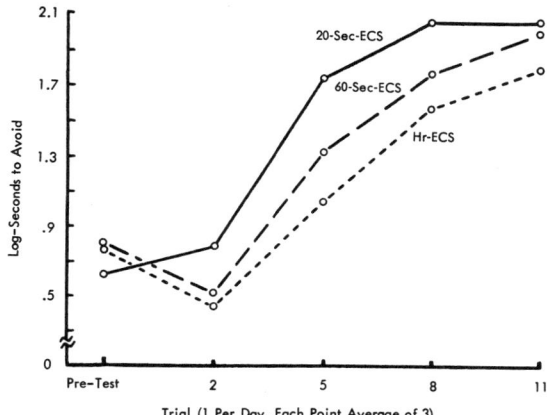

Figure 12-2
*The effects of ECS
on passive
avoidance. Rats
were given one
passive-avoidance
trial per day, and
ECS was
administered 20
seconds, 60 seconds,
or one hour after
each training trial.
Learning was better
(that is, the animal
stayed in the dark
compartment and
avoided the lighted
compartment
longer) the shorter
the training
trial-ECS interval.
From "Conflict vs.
Consolidation of
Memory Traces to
Explain 'Retrograde
Amnesia' Produced
by ECS," by E. E.
Coons and N. E.
Miller,* Journal of
Comparative and
Physiological
Psychology, *1960,
53, 524–531.
Copyright 1960 by
the American
Psychological
Association.
Reprinted by
permission.*

Subsequent research, however, has demonstrated that the acquired-fear hypothesis cannot totally account for the effects of ECS on learning and retention. For example, data published by McGaugh and Madsen (1964) suggested that only amnesic effects resulted from ECS treatments during early trials with repeated ECS treatments. In contrast, after a number of treatments, the animals tended to avoid the place in a maze where ECS was administered. Because of the potential fear-producing effects of ECS when applied over a series of daily learning trials, recent investigations have generally employed one-trial learning tasks and a single application of ECS.

Numerous researchers have demonstrated that a single application of ECS will disrupt subsequent behavior. For example, Bureš and Burešová (1963) found such effects in a passive-avoidance situation. If normal rats were placed in an apparatus that had two adjacent compartments, one of which was considerably smaller than the other, the animals spent most of their time in the small compartment. If they were then shocked in the small compartment and placed back into the apparatus on the next day, they avoided the small compartment. Bureš and Burešová reported that, if rats were administered a single ECS treatment up to 6 hours after they had received foot-shock in the small compartment, they would return to the small compartment on the next day more often than animals not administered ECS. In a one-trial/one ECS treatment such as that used by Bureš and Burešová, the possibility that the effects of ECS were due to learned fear responses was minimized.

Another way of controlling for the possibility that the ECS-treated subject is learning fear responses that interfere with performance is to administer ECS in a relatively nonaversive manner. This can be accomplished in several ways. In one of the early ECS studies, Friedman (1953) found that no aversion to ECS developed in rats subjected to ECS treatments twice a day for four successive days if the experimenter prevented the behavior convulsions that normally occur during this treatment by anesthetizing the rats with ether prior to applying the ECS. The animals still showed a memory deficit—a finding that has been replicated (for example, McGaugh & Alpern, 1966). Friedman's data are very interesting. They suggest that the aversive component of ECS treatment may be linked to the behavior seizures rather than to the passage of electricity through the brain.

Another way to control for the aversive effects of ECS is to vary the method of delivery. Kesner, Gibson, and LeClair (1970) reported that, if ECS was delivered through cortical electrodes rather than the usual ear clips, no aversion to ECS treatment developed. They suggested that the ears of the rat become sensitive to the ear clips following repeated treatments. A third way to separate the aversive and amnesic effects of ECS is to administer ECS in the home cage rather than in the test apparatus. This technique reduces the possibility that ECS will become associated with the response being measured. When this procedure is followed, a performance deficit will still occur in the convulsed subjects (Leonard & Zavala, 1964; Quartermain, Paolino, & Miller, 1965).

There are other data that are simply inconsistent with the notion that the observed effects on behavior result from the aversive properties of the ECS. For example, if ECS produces its effects because of its aversive attributes, then it should produce faster extinction of an operant response if administered after each extinction trial. This prediction has not been empirically supported. Several investigators have reported that ECS yields increased rather than decreased resistance to extinction of both aversively and appetitively motivated behaviors (for example, Madsen & Luttges, 1963; Gerbrandt & Thomson, 1964; Greenough & Schwitzgebel, 1966).

ECS and the Development of Competing Responses. A second alternative interpretation of the basis for the ECS effect is that ECS leads to the development of responses that are incompatible with performance of the previously learned response (Lewis & Maher, 1965; Black & Suboski, 1971). More specifically, this view contends that ECS interferes with performance by causing the animal to be less active in the testing chamber. Such an interpretation must be questioned, however, in light of the fact that ECS produces deficits in passive- as well as active-avoidance tasks. Since learning in a passive-avoidance situation is indexed by increases in the latency of approach to a previously rewarded goal, one would expect that ECS would facilitate learning of this type of task. However, the opposite has been found (for example, Bureš & Burešová,1963; McGaugh & Alpern, 1966).

Also inconsistent with the competing-responses interpretation is the fact, mentioned earlier, that subjects administered ECS in their home cages still show retrograde amnesia (Leonard & Zavala, 1964; Quartermain et al., 1965). The conditioned-inhibition view assumes that the behavioral inhibition becomes conditioned to the environmental cues of the training chamber in which the ECS was administered. Administering the ECS in the home cage controls for this possibility.

In light of the data reviewed thus far in this chapter, the most parsimonious explanation for the effects of ECS on memory is that the ECS treatment disrupts the memory-consolidation process. We will next examine experimental research that has attempted to clarify the nature of the ECS-induced retrograde amnesia by seeking to determine (1) the maximally effective training–ECS interval, (2) the factors affecting the extent of ECS-induced retrograde amnesia, and (3) the permanence of the ECS-produced retrograde amnesia.

Further Clarification of the ECS-Induced Amnesia

Duration of the Training-ECS Interval

Experimental investigations of ECS have generally agreed that the treatment must be administered fairly soon after training. Just how soon has been the subject of some disagreement. Some researchers have reported that significant amnesic effects will occur even if ECS treatment is delayed for periods of up to several hours after training (Kopp, Bohdanecky, & Jarvik, 1968; McGaugh, 1966; Paolino & Hine, 1973; Springer, Schoel, Klinger, & Agranoff, 1975). In contrast, other experimenters have reported that amnesia followed ECS only if the animals were treated within a few seconds after training (Chorover & Schiller, 1965; Lee-Teng & Sherman, 1966; Schiller & Chorover, 1967). Such contradictions about the nature of the retrograde-amnesia gradient following administration of ECS are quite common in the experimental literature, but, as McGaugh and Herz (1972) indicated, a simple explanation has not yet been offered to account for these divergent results.

In light of these discrepancies, some researchers have argued that the actual amnesic gradient is very short—in the order of a minute or less; impairments in performance observed with longer training-ECS intervals probably indicate effects on behavior other than a loss of memory (Chorover & Schiller, 1966; Spevack & Suboski, 1969). Others have proposed that the obtained effects on performance with long training-ECS intervals still represent deficits in memory-consolidation processes but that the effect is on other phases of the consolidation process than those affected by short-duration training-ECS intervals (Paolino, Quartermain, & Levy, 1969; Paolino & Levy, 1971).

Factors Affecting the ECS-Induced Retrograde-Amnesia Gradient

A number of experimenters have shown that certain features of the research methodology employed in ECS experiments may affect the ECS-induced retrograde-amnesia gradient. Some of these features are: (1) the parameters of the ECS treatment, (2) training variables, (3) the criterion used to assess retention, and (4) subject differences.

Parameters of the ECS Treatment. Characteristics of the ECS treatment have been found to affect the retrograde-amnesia gradient. In general, there is a direct relationship between the severity of the ECS treatment and the amount of retention impairment observed (Mah & Albert, 1973). Several experiments have shown that, with increases in the intensity of the ECS current, there is a corresponding increase in the amount of amnesia produced and that, further, with increases in ECS intensity, the length of time following training during which application of ECS can disrupt memory processes is lengthened (for example, Buckholz & Bowman, 1972; Haycock & McGaugh, 1973; Hughes, Barrett, & Ray, 1970a; Zornetzer & McGaugh, 1971a, 1971b). Apparently, the effects of ECS treatments on memory depend on the interaction of ECS intensity and the length of the training-ECS treatment interval (TTI). For a constant TTI, a higher intensity of ECS will produce greater amnesia, and, for a given ECS intensity, a shorter TTI will produce greater interference with memory processes (Haycock & McGaugh, 1973).

When the severity of the ECS treatment is increased by lengthening of its duration, the result is ambiguous. Some researchers have found that longer-duration ECS currents produce greater amnesia (Alpern & McGaugh, 1968; Buckholz & Bowman, 1972), but Paolino and his associates (1969) have not. The severity of the ECS treatment can also be increased by administering more than one ECS after training. For example, Mah, Albert, & Jamieson (1972) administered two rather than one ECS treatment after passive-avoidance training and found a much greater retention deficit than in the animals receiving one. Jamieson (1972) reported that the amnesic effect produced by a series of five ECSs spaced one minute apart was far greater than that produced by a single ECS. In summary, all of these results suggest that the degree of amnesia produced by ECS varies directly with ECS severity.

Characteristics of the Training Situation. The retrograde-amnesia gradient can also be influenced by characteristics of the training situation. For example, an early study by Thompson (1958) demonstrated that the degree of amnesia produced by ECS varied inversely with the amount of training prior to the ECS treatment (see also Keyes, 1973a) and directly as a function of task difficulty. Similarly, Lewis, Miller, and Misanin (1968) and Miller (1970) found that, in the case of one-trial passive-avoidance training, increasing the subject's familiarity with the testing apparatus prior to training significantly decreased the disruptive effects of ECS on memory. Miller also demonstrated that, as the complexity of the training environment was increased, more familiarity with the training apparatus was needed to attenuate the disruptive effects of ECS.

The strength of the positive or negative reinforcement used during training can also affect the characteristics of the retrograde-amnesia gradient. For example, increasing the duration of foot-shock in passive-avoidance training reduces significantly the disruptive effects of ECS treatment applied after training (Chorover & Schiller, 1965; Ray & Bivens, 1968). With regard to appetitively motivated behavior, Peeke, McCoy, and Herz (1969) reported that the degree of amnesia for an appetitively motivated problem produced by ECS depended directly upon the length of deprivation. The longer their rats were deprived of water, the more resistant to disruption by ECS was a learned operant to obtain a water reward.

The Criterion Used to Assess Retention. The characteristics of the ECS-produced retention gradient depend upon the criterion of retention (Schneider, Kapp, Aron, & Jarvik, 1969) as well as on the response measure being used (Adams & Calhoun, 1972; Hine & Paolino, 1970; Mendoza & Adams, 1969). In the Hine and Paolino experiment, ECS given to rats immediately after one-trial passive-avoidance training disrupted subsequent passive-avoidance behavior, but the rats still exhibited heightened arousal in the post-ECS testing. This finding suggested that the animals had retained the physiological concomitants of a fear response associated with the passive-avoidance paradigm. This result cannot be explained by suggesting that the cardiac alterations reflected the aversive properties of ECS treatment, because control animals given only the ECS treatment did not show heart-rate changes. Hine and Paolino postulated that their findings might indicate that consolidation was more rapid for the generalized fear response than for the overt behavioral index of retention. More recently, Caul and Barrett (1972) have shown that under certain conditions ECS will both attenuate the cardiac changes normally associated with passive-avoidance training and yield an amnesia of the learned avoidance response.

Subject Differences. A fourth factor that can affect the ECS-induced amnesia gradient is subject differences. For example, McGaugh, Landfield, and Dawson (1972) reported that the gradient may vary as a function of the strain of mice used. Heinze (1970) has similarly reported that the degree of amnesia produced by ECS varies with the strain of rats employed in an experiment.

Recovery from Retrograde Amnesia. It was once generally assumed that ECS treatments interfere with memory consolidation by upsetting biologically constant neural processes and thereby exert permanent effects on recall. For this reason, few experimenters investigated the permanence of the ECS-induced retrograde amnesia. It has now been well established that the effect of ECS on memory processes is quite variable. In the material just presented, you saw some of the factors that can affect the degree of amnesia produced. The number of possible interactions among all of these variables indicates the complexity of the ECS phenomenon.

Experiments conducted to examine the permanence of the ECS-induced amnesia have produced somewhat divergent results. A number of experiments have demonstrated instances of recovery from ECS-produced retrograde amnesia. Typically, in these studies, there is an initial amnesia, resulting from the ECS treatment, that lasts for about 24 hours. This amnesia is then followed by a recovery of the "lost" memory (for example, Adams & Calhoun, 1972; Kohlenberg & Trabasso, 1968; Koppenall, Jagoda, & Cruce, 1967; Miller, 1968; Zinkin & Miller, 1967). This finding—that recovery of memory can sometimes occur after ECS treatment—has been taken by some researchers as evidence that ECS affects recall, or retrieval, rather than consolidation processes. This interpretation is certainly plausible, but it leads to a controversy that's hard to resolve. It is difficult to know whether a certain procedure has interrupted consolidation or recall processes, since consolidation is always indexed by some measure of recall.

It should be pointed out that this recovery phenomenon is not the most common finding. Surveys of the available literature by Mah and Albert (1973) and by McGaugh and Dawson (1971) indicate that usually little or no recovery from ECS-induced retrograde amnesia is observed. Some researchers have reported that the amnesic effect did not abate after a month or more (for example, Luttges & McGaugh, 1967).

The data on the permanence of the ECS-induced retrograde amnesia found by Luttges and McGaugh are graphed in Figure 12-3. In this study, mice were given one trial in a step-through passive-avoidance problem, similar to that used by Bureš and Burešová (1963), and were treated with foot-shock and ECS as indicated in the graph. Independent groups were tested for retention of the passive-avoidance habit 14 hours, 1 week, or 1 month after their original treatment. This graph indicates virtually no recovery of passive avoidance in the animals receiving passive-avoidance training followed by ECS treatment (foot-shock/ECS group), even a month after training. Similar findings regarding the permanence of the ECS effect were obtained by Chevalier (1965), Geller, Jarvik, and Robustelli (1970), Jamieson (1972), King and Glasser (1970), Ray and Barrett (1969), and others. Hughes and his associates (Hughes et al., 1970a, 1970b) reported that the degree of amnesia in ECS-treated rats may actually increase with the passage of time.

McGaugh and Herz (1972) state that these conflicting results regarding the permanence of retrograde amnesia following ECS have not yet been accounted for satisfactorily. However, they suggest that incomplete amnesia may result when the ECS treatment used is not sufficient to totally stop the consolidation process. According to this reasoning, incomplete interference with memory storage may provide a basis for at least some recovery. Consistent with this proposal are data

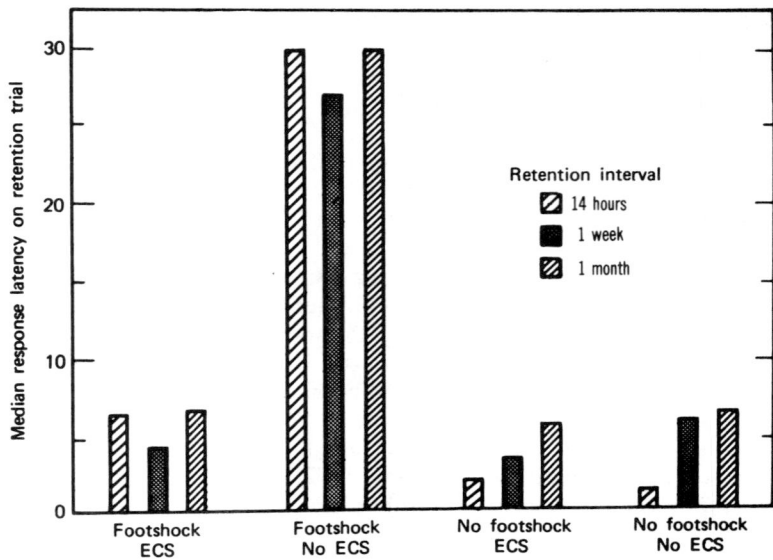

reported by Miller (1968) and by Pagano, Bush, Martin, and Hunt (1969). They found that no recovery of memory on several test trials occurred when a high-intensity ECS was given following passive-avoidance training but that, with a low-intensity ECS, there was a partial recovery of the learned avoidance habit.

The Reminder Effect. Several researchers have reported an interesting phenomenon with respect to recovery from ECS-induced retrograde amnesia called the **reminder effect** (DeVietti & Bucy, 1975; DeVietti & Hopfer, 1974; Galluscio, 1971; Koppenall et al., 1967; Lewis et al., 1968; Miller, Ott, Berk, & Springer, 1974; Miller & Springer, 1972; Quartermain, McEwen, & Azmitia, 1970, 1972). The reminder effect is the fact that memory, suppressed by an ECS treatment after training, can be partially recovered by exposure of animals to elements of the training situation during the interval between training/ECS and later testing. The reminder effect has been demonstrated for both aversively and appetitively motivated tasks, although almost all inquiries have used aversively motivated tasks.

The general procedure used to produce the reminder effect under aversively motivated conditions can be summarized as follows. The animal is given training on a one-trial passive-avoidance task and then given an ECS treatment. Twenty-four hours later, the rat is given a retention test. The subject is administered a foot-shock (reminder stimulus) outside of the testing chamber at some interval after this first retention test. A second retention test is given 24 hours after the first, and the animal's retention score typically improves significantly. The finding that there is a recovery of the memory thought not to have been consolidated has led a number of researchers to conclude that ECS treatments influence recall but not consolidation of information.

At face value, the reminder-effect data appear to strongly argue that memory-retrieval rather than memory-storage processes have been disrupted by ECS treatments. However, proponents of the view that ECS disrupts consolidation processes have been quick to propose alternative explanations of these data. As I've indicated, it is often difficult to decide whether an experimental manipulation has disrupted consolidation or recall processes, because consolidation deficits can only be indexed by a later retrieval impairment. Perhaps it would be appropriate to describe an ECS-induced learning impairment as reflecting a disruption along a consolidation/recall continuum.

Researchers supporting the view that ECS disrupts memory storage have pointed out that ECS rarely yields a total retrieval deficit when ECS-treated animals are compared with appropriate control subjects—that is, subjects treated exactly as the experimental animals except for the ECS treatment. Additionally, they have stressed that reminder treatment, while certainly increasing retention, often falls far short of yielding complete recovery of the lost memory (for example, Galluscio, 1971; Miller & Springer, 1972). As a result of these observations, Cherkin (1972) has reinterpreted the reminder-effect data in terms of the memory-storage view. Cherkin argues that the reminder stimulus serves as a weak training trial that generalizes to and summates with any residual memory that survived ECS. The increased retention that is observed after reminder treatment thus results from a summation of these two rather weak memory traces rather than the release of an already-stored memory.

There are data available that tend to support Cherkin's interpretation of the reminder effect (Cherkin, 1972; Gold, Haycock, Macri, & McGaugh, 1973; Haycock, Gold, Macri, & McGaugh, 1973; Kesner & Conner, 1974). In general, these studies have shown that animals that are partially amnesic following initial ECS treatments are able to profit from a reminder stimulus but that totally amnesic subjects do not show the reminder effect. Presumably, the partially amnesic animals were able to generalize and add the experience of the foot-shock administered outside of the testing chamber to the partial memory trace for the passive-avoidance habit (Haycock et al., 1973).

Whether the ECS-induced performance deficit reflects consolidation or retrieval impairments may, as previously indicated, be a very difficult issue to satisfactorily resolve. It is also entirely possible that ECS yields both retroactive and proactive inhibitory influences. That is, ECS may both interfere with the ability to store, or consolidate, information and disrupt the ability to recall whatever information is already stored.

The Biological Basis of the ECS Effect

Similarities between the Effects of ECS and Hippocampal Lesions

Several researchers have pointed out some interesting similarities between the effects of ECS and of hippocampal lesions on behavior. Whether these findings indicate that ECS produces hippocampal malfunction, which in turn accounts for the ECS effect, is uncertain. Some of the parallel behavior alterations produced by ECS and hippocampectomy are as follows.

Aversively Motivated Behavior. As you've seen, most ECS studies employ tests of passive avoidance to assess a memory deficit, and, as was reviewed in the last chapter, animals with hippocampal lesions are severely deficient on this task (for example, Isaacson & Wickelgren, 1962; Kimble, 1963). Rats given ECS reach criterion *faster* than control animals in a two-way shuttle-box active-avoidance task (Pirch, 1969; Vanderwolf, 1963). This is very interesting for two reasons. First, one would predict that, if ECS yields retrograde amnesia, ECS-treated animals should be impaired, not facilitated, in their ability to learn this task. Second, this finding is of interest because hippocampectomized animals are similarly superior to normal animals in their ability to learn this type of avoidance problem (for example, Isaacson, Douglas, & Moore, 1961).

Food-Motivated Tasks. Regarding appetitively motivated tasks, Keyes and Young (1973) and Keyes (1973a) have demonstrated that ECS produces an increase in responding during extinction of a lever-press operant task. Keyes and Dempsey (1973) found, similarly, that ECS administered immediately after acquisition of a runway task yielded increased resistance to extinction. These findings are identical to the effects produced by hippocampal lesions, as you saw in the last chapter. Hippocampectomized rats show increased resistance to extinction of both a bar-press (for example, Jarrard, 1965) and a runway response (for example, Jarrard, Isaacson, & Wickelgren, 1964). Keyes (1973b) has also reported that rats were deficient in their ability to master a discrimination reversal when trained four hours after receiving ECS. Deficiency in the ability to learn a discrimination reversal is another well-established effect of hippocampal lesions (Kimble & Kimble, 1965; Thompson & Langer, 1963).

Spontaneous Alternation. **Spontaneous alternation** is the tendency for normal animals to alternate between the two goal boxes of a T-maze on consecutive trials when no reward is provided for responses to either side. A normal rat alternates—that is, visits the alley of a T-maze opposite to that entered on the previous trial—approximately 85% of the time. In contrast, hippocampectomized rats alternate only about 50% of the time. Their spontaneous-alternation behavior has been abolished, since alternation has fallen to a chance level (Roberts, Dember, & Brodwick, 1962).

Spontaneous alternation appears to be highly and specifically related to hippocampal function. A variety of brain lesions to extrahippocampal structures have no effect whatsoever on this behavior (Douglas, 1972; Douglas, Peterson, & Douglas, 1973). For this reason, Douglas, Pagano, Lovely, and Peterson (1973) argued that, if the similarity between the effect of ECS and the effect of hippocampectomy is more than just coincidental, a single ECS treatment should dramatically attenuate spontaneous-alternation behavior.

To test this possibility, Douglas and his associates examined T-maze spontaneous-alternation behavior in rats. An alternation test consisted of a pair of trials; an alternation response was said to occur if the subject entered opposite arms of the maze on those two trials. Prior to ECS treatment, the rats were given one or two alternation tests per day until they had received a total of 25. At that point, each subject was removed from the apparatus and taken to another room, where ECS was administered. The ECS electrodes were attached to the control animals, but no current was passed through them. All animals were awake and responsive by 20 minutes after ECS, and the first test was given 30 minutes post-ECS. Two tests were then administered between 1 and 1½ hours after the ECS treatment, four tests between 2 and 5 hours after ECS, and two tests at each of the following intervals after ECS: 12, 24, 48, 72, 96, 120, 144, and 196 hours. The control subjects were similarly tested.

The results of this inquiry are graphed in Figure 12-4. It can be seen that ECS greatly reduced spontaneous alternation for an extended period. Alternation was significantly depressed in the experimental subjects for the first 72 hours (3 days) following ECS treatment, as compared with both their own pretest scores and the alternation rates of control subjects during the posttreatment test sessions. During this period, the alternation behavior of the ECS-treated subjects was not significantly above a chance level of 50%. It was not until the seventh day after ECS that spontaneous alternation returned to pretest levels, but recovery was almost complete by the fifth day. Keyes (1973b) has also demonstrated that ECS temporarily abolished spontaneous alternation.

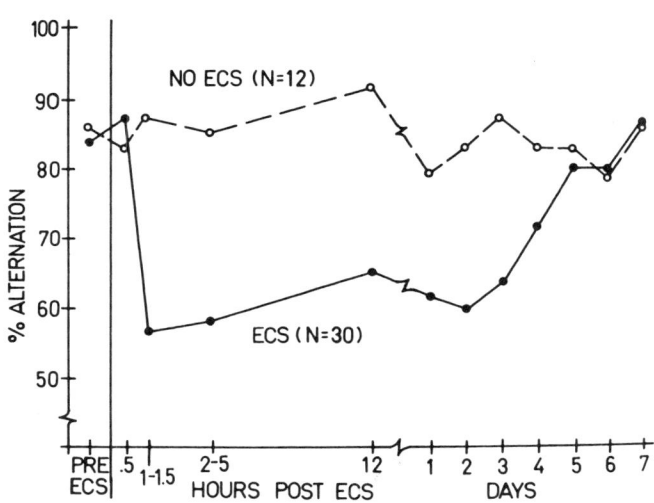

*Figure 12-4
Spontaneous
alternation before
and after ECS.
From "The
Prolonged Effects of
a Single ECS on
Behavior Related to
Hippocampal
Function," by R. J.
Douglas, R. R.
Pagano, R. H.
Lovely, and J. J.
Peterson,*
Behavioral Biology,
*1973, 8, 611–617.
Copyright 1973 by
Academic Press, Inc.
Reprinted by
permission.*

Figure 12-4 also indicates that spontaneous alternation did not attenuate until the tests administered between 1 and 1½ hours after ECS treatment. Douglas and his associates suggest that this finding indicates that the effects of ECS on alternation behavior are not immediate but rather require an incubation period of somewhere between 0.5 and 1 hour. These findings, regarding the effects of ECS on spontaneous alternation, provide the most striking similarity between the effects of ECS and of hippocampal ablations. As Douglas and his associates indicate, although these findings suggest that ECS yields hippocampal malfunction, they do not prove it. The similarities between the effects of ECS and of hippocampectomy are intriguing, but they may simply indicate that the two experimental methods are disrupting parallel, not identical, processes.

Other Neurological Issues Regarding the ECS Effect

Other questions regarding the effects of ECS on memory consolidation and recall processes need to be answered. Not the least of these is: What neurobiological mechanisms are affected by the ECS treatment to produce the amnesic effect? ECS may produce its effects on memory by altering the electrical activity of the brain, which, as you've seen, some researchers contend serves as a basis for memory storage. Many investigators have supposed that brain seizures produced by ECS are the basis for the retrograde-amnesia effect. However, data reviewed by McGaugh, Zornetzer, Gold, and Landfield (1972) suggest that the relationship between brain seizures and amnesia is not causal; rather, both the amnesia and the seizures are consequences of the neural disturbances produced by the electrical stimulation. Sometimes the thresholds for producing brain seizures and amnesia are comparable, but at other times they are not. Under some conditions, the intensity of the current needed to yield retrograde amnesia greatly exceeds the threshold required to produce brain seizures. Under different experimental conditions, the current level required to produce amnesia is less than that needed to produce brain seizures.

Another possibility is that ECS produces its effects on memory by disrupting the production of macromolecules, which many investigators contend constitute a template for permanent memory. Protein synthesis has been implicated in memory-consolidation processes. Several experiments have shown that brain protein synthesis is partially inhibited for a short period following ECS treatment (Agranoff, 1972; Dunn, 1971; MacInnes, McConkey, & Schlesinger, 1970). However, as McGaugh, Zornetzer, Gold, and Landfield (1972) indicate, it is unclear whether the observed inhibition of brain protein synthesis following ECS is an essential correlate of either the brain seizures or the retrograde amnesia. They point out that studies using antibiotics to block protein synthesis obtain significant amnesic effects only if the degree of protein-synthesis inhibition is at least 80–90% (for example, Agranoff, 1968; Barondes, 1968). In contrast, the inhibition of protein synthesis produced by ECS is only around 20%. Therefore, it is unlikely that the amnesia produced by ECS results from an interference with brain protein synthesis. A great deal of attention has been directed in recent years toward the possible role of macromolecules in memory processes. This research will be reviewed in the next chapter.

Chapter Summary and Conclusions

In this chapter, I reviewed experiments that have investigated the nature of the consolidation process. *Consolidation* refers to the process of encoding long-term or permanent memory traces. Experimental investigations of the consolidation process became possible following the discovery that application of electroconvulsive shock can disrupt memory processes. Evidence bearing on the theory that ECS disrupts consolidation processes and alternative interpretations of the ECS-induced retention deficit were presented. Some of the parameters affecting the ECS-induced retrograde amnesia were explored.

It was concluded that, although the weight of the evidence supports the view that ECS disrupts memory processes, it is unclear whether ECS disrupts consolidation of information or rather blocks the expression of previously stored memory. It was suggested that ECS may disrupt both of the processes. Similarities between the effects of ECS and hippocampal lesions were reviewed. It was indicated that, although the effects of these two procedures are strikingly similar, it is unclear whether they result from the disruption of identical or parallel processes. Findings regarding the neurobiological mechanisms that may be affected by ECS to yield the amnesic effect were discussed. The possibilities were evaluated that ECS produces amnesia by severely disrupting the electrical activity of the brain or by interfering with the production of macromolecules, which may constitute a template for memory. It was indicated that neither of these factors could presently be directly related to the ECS effect.

13

The Biochemistry of Learning and Memory

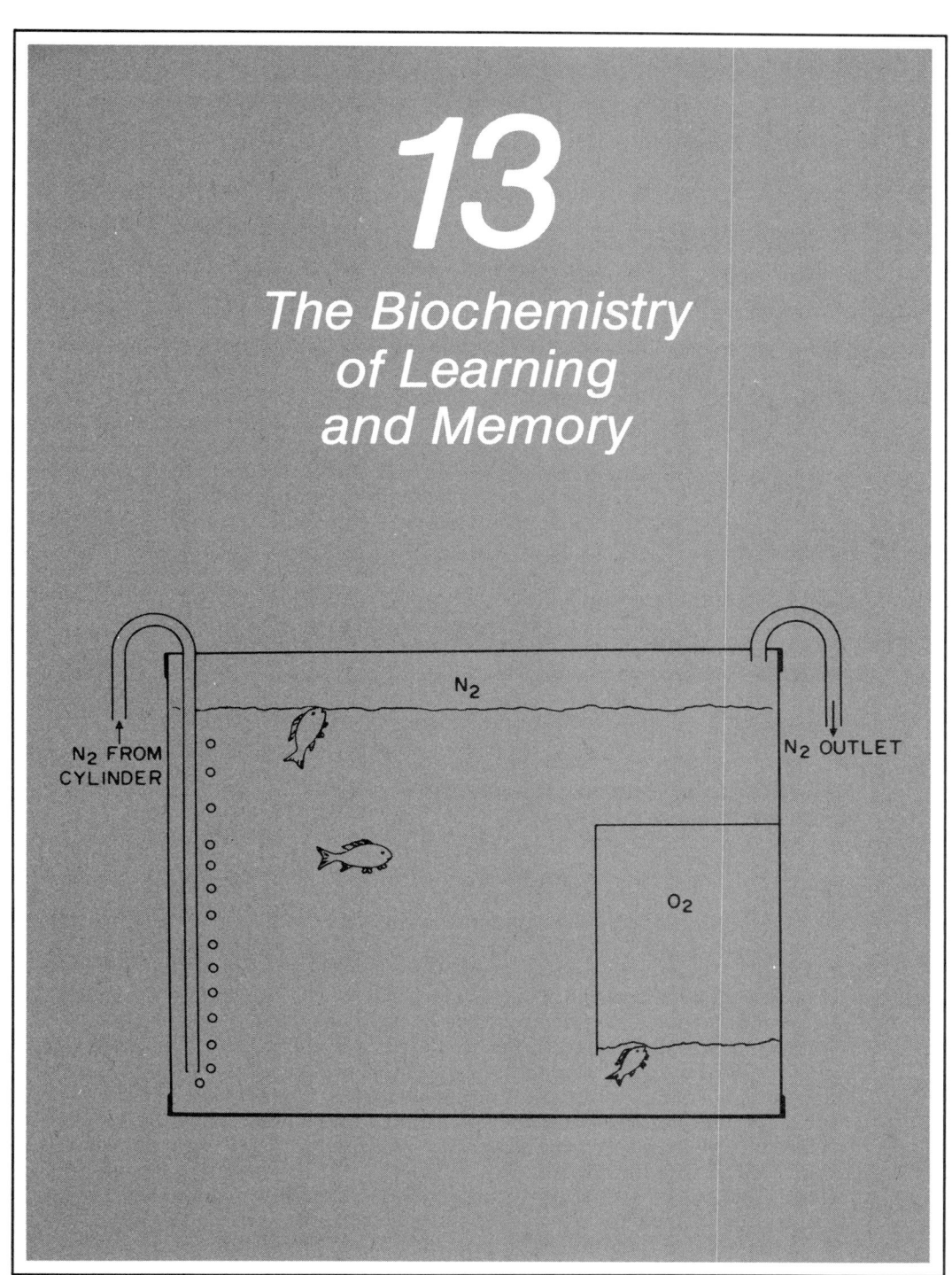

The search for the engram, or memory trace, in the brain must end at the cellular level since alterations in cellular activities undoubtedly mediate both the memory-consolidation process and changes in the spatiotemporal firing patterns of neurons that reflect this process. When discussing cellular functions and activities, we have to relate them to protein molecules. This is because the metabolic functions and structural features of cells are determined by the nature and quantity of proteins that the cells manufacture. In view of the crucial role performed by protein molecules in cellular physiology, it is appropriate to assume that the protein-synthesis mechanism performs a major role in the activities of the neurophysiological substrates of memory consolidation.

Several distinct methodological approaches have been employed by neuroscientists attempting to clarify the biochemical basis of learning and memory. Among these are investigations of (1) the effects of environmental enrichment on brain indexes, (2) changes in brain chemistry following learning and performance, (3) the transfer of memory by brain extracts, and (4) the effects of antimetabolite drugs on acquisition and recall. In this chapter, I will review representative studies that have used these various approaches to study the molecular basis of memory.

The Effects of Environmental Enrichment on Brain Indexes

One of the first major attempts to relate protein synthesis and other neural indexes to either experience or learning was a series of experiments initiated in the early 1960s by E. L. Bennett, Diamond, Krech, and Rosenzweig at the University of California, Berkeley. Excellent reviews of their comprehensive endeavors are provided by Bennett, Rosenzweig, and Diamond (1969), Rosenzweig (1971), and Rosenzweig, Bennett, and Diamond (1972).

In most of the experiments conducted by this research group, littermate rats were assigned to either an enriched condition (EC) or a nonenriched environment. An animal reared under the EC conditions was housed with a group of 10–12 others in a large cage containing a variety of stimulus objects, or "toys," such as ladders, wheels, boxes, and platforms. It should be noted that social stimulation is unnecessary to produce the results detailed below; the results appear in rats exposed individually to an enriched environment (Rosenzweig & Bennett, 1972). Nonenriched environments were of two types, which produced similar outcomes, as indexed by cerebral measures. Under the standard-colony condition (SC), rats were reared three to a cage, and, in the isolated condition (IC), the subjects were raised individually in cages.

After the rats were maintained in the different conditions for the experimental rearing period of 30 to 80 days, they were sacrificed, and various anatomical and biochemical measures were made of their brains. The results reported below were produced not only by rearing weanling rats in an enriched environment but also by exposing young-adult (105 days old) or year-old rats to the enriched environment (Rosenzweig et al., 1972).

Upon analysis of their data, these researchers discovered a number of differences in the cerebral cortex of animals reared in the EC, as opposed to the SC and IC, conditions. These differences included variations in tissue weight, in the amounts of certain enzymes, and in a number of anatomical indexes. In general, the effects of differential rearing conditions were especially prominent in the occipital, or visual, cortex. However, several experiments have indicated that visual experience per se is unnecessary for the observed effects. These differences are observed in blind rats reared in an enriched environment (for example, Krech, Rosenzweig, & Bennett, 1963).

The most consistent finding, and one that has been replicated sixteen times (Rosenzweig et al., 1972), is that rats reared in the EC condition had a heavier cerebral cortex than did their littermates reared under either the SC or IC conditions. This difference is not due simply to variations in fluid content of the brains of animals reared under the various conditions (Bennett, Rosenzweig, & Diamond, 1968). Animals reared in the enriched environment also had thicker cerebral cortices, and there was more protein in their brains.

At the cellular level, occipital-cortex measures indicated that the number of neurons was not greater for the EC-reared subjects but that the cross-section area of their neuronal cell bodies was greater by about 13% (Diamond, 1967). Further, the occipital cortex of the EC-raised rats showed increases in the glia/neuron ratio (Altman & Das, 1964; Diamond, Law, Rhodes, Lindner, Rosenzweig, Krech, & Bennett, 1966), in the size of synaptic junctions (Møllgaard, Diamond, Bennett, Rosenzweig, & Lindner, 1971), and in the density of dendritic endings of pyramidal cells (Globus, Rosenzweig, Bennett, & Diamond, 1973; Volkmar & Greenough, 1972).

Differences in the concentration of certain brain enzymes were also noted following differential rearing conditions. In the EC rats, as compared with the SC and IC animals, there were larger amounts of acetylcholinesterase and cholinesterase present. As you saw in Chapter 2, these two substances are concerned with transmission of nerve impulses at many brain synapses in that they inactivate the synaptic transmitter acetylcholine. The EC subjects also showed greater amounts of hexokinase—an enzyme important in energy transformation.

Because of the posited functions of the hippocampus in learning and memory, Diamond, Rosenzweig, and Bennett (1971) undertook an examination of hippocampal thickness in littermates reared under different conditions. It was found that the hippocampi of the EC rats were thicker than those of their IC littermates. However, the observed differences were of smaller magnitude and less reliability than the EC/IC differences in cortical thickness. Other subcortical measures have been taken (see Bennett et al., 1969), but, in general, the effects in the subcortex have been small.

Relating the Environment-Enrichment Effect to Behavior

Several researchers—for example, Hymovich (1952) and Forgays and Read (1962)—have shown that rearing animals in an enriched environment such as that used by the Berkeley group leads to superior problem-solving ability in adults. It would be nice, then, if one could directly relate differences in cerebral measures to problem-solving scores. Unfortunately, attempts to do this have been unsuccessful. Rosenzweig (1971) writes that "while we have been able to demonstrate both significant cerebral effects and significant behavioral effects of prior environmental manipulations, we have not found any simple way of relating these two sets of observations" (p. 327). Thus, the significance of these neural changes following environmental enrichment remains unclear (Rosenzweig et al., 1972).

This failure may have arisen because these researchers attempted to measure transfer effects from a generally enriched environment to quite different task situations. A more fruitful approach might be to examine cerebral changes arising from exposure to certain stimuli in the early environment. More specifically, research could be conducted using a transfer-of-perceptual-learning paradigm, such as that used by my associates and me and by Gibson and Walk and their colleagues (see Chapter 10).

As discussed in Chapter 10, the transfer-of-perceptual-learning paradigm involves preexposing animals to specific stimuli (such as circles and triangles) during rearing. As adults, the animals learn to discriminate between these stimuli as a test of whether they have learned something about these shapes. As I indicated in that chapter, studies of this type have generally shown that animals—usually rats—preexposed to specific stimuli can later learn to discriminate between them much more rapidly than can animals that didn't have this early experience.

It would be interesting to determine whether preexposure to specific shapes produces changes in cerebral indexes, and, if such changes do occur, whether they are directly related to, or highly correlated with, learning ability. If such a relationship did occur, it might suggest a neural substrate for the early-experience effect observed in the transfer-of-perceptual-learning paradigm.

The research of the Berkeley group has uncovered some very interesting phenomena regarding the effects of general environmental enrichment on neural indexes, including brain chemistry. A different approach, which has been applied by several neuroscientists, is to seek changes in brain chemistry following learning and performance of specific responses.

Changes in Brain Chemistry Accompanying Learning and Performance

Researchers using this approach have often attempted to relate their findings to changes in the genetic materials of brain cells—**RNA (ribonucleic acid)** and **DNA (deoxyribonucleic acid)**. DNA regulates cellular processes since it directs protein synthesis via its management of messenger RNA. One of the many important functions of RNA is the synthesis of synaptic transmitter substances, such as acetylcholine. It has long been established that increased activity of brain cells is correlated with an increase in the amount of RNA in their cytoplasm (for example, Brattgård, 1952). For this reason, a number of researchers have postulated that learning results in the formation of novel RNA or protein molecules, which then serve as a template for permanent memory. One of the first to suggest this possibility was Monné (1948), but most of the current interest in biochemical models of memory can be traced directly to the work of Holger Hydén (1959).

The basic methodology for assessing the role of nucleic acids and protein in learning and memory—one that has been used by Hydén and his associates—is to examine quantitative and/or qualitative changes in these substances in the nervous system following training. In principle this is a simple procedure, but in practice it is not always easy. Chapouthier (1973) indicates that a major difficulty in interpreting the results of such experiments is that it is not always possible to distinguish between chemical changes occurring in the brain after learning and changes occurring in brain chemistry after stimulation without learning. Increases in RNA and protein synthesis occur in the nervous system after various types of stimulation without learning (for example, Debold, Firshein, Carrier, & Leaf, 1967; Rappoport & Daginawala, 1968; Ungar, 1970a).

Another problem for molecular theories of learning occurs at the conceptual level. This problem concerns the mechanisms involved in the formation of novel RNA and ultimately the protein molecules that presumably serve as a template for the memory trace. The type of protein produced by any cell is dictated by the DNA found in the genes of the cell. The RNA manufactured and, in turn, the protein synthesized, are faithful replicas of the DNA template of the gene. This is a necessary condition for survival of the cell and of the organism. In his writings, Hydén has emphasized that the RNA produced during learning is different from that synthesized by the same cells during nonlearning. This supposition requires that the neurons manufacture RNA that is different from that dictated by their DNA—a notion that runs contrary to all of our understanding of cell processes.

Bonner (1966, 1972) has proposed a molecular model of memory that circumvents this problem. He hypothesized that electrical input to a cell during learning may *derepress* parts of a gene or genes that were previously repressed or not maximally active. Therefore, while learning may not change the basic structure of the DNA, it may yield a derepression or activation of parts of the genes as they already exist. Derepression of such a previously repressed gene would yield an increase in RNA synthesis following learning—a finding reported by several investigators. Ultimately, this process would allow for the manufacture of substances that render a particular synapse or synapses more sensitive (or less sensitive) to transmission of nerve impulses. The gene sites, once derepressed, could maintain this state forever, thereby causing a permanent change in the protein-synthesis characteristics of the brain cells and presumably allowing for the encoding or consolidation of a unit of permanent memory.

Experimental Findings

In the late 1950s, Hydén developed the methodology necessary to measure the composition of minute quantities of RNA. These techniques provided a tool by which experimenters could directly evaluate whether learning indeed resulted in the formation of a unique RNA. In the initial investigations conducted by Hydén and his colleagues (Hydén & Egyházi, 1962, 1963), rats learned to obtain food by balancing on and climbing up a long narrow wire that was set at an angle of 45 degrees. The composition of the RNA extracted from neurons in the vestibular nucleus of the medulla—a nucleus important in balance (see Figure 6-7)—was then compared to that of RNA obtained from control rats. The controls did not learn the task; instead, they were swung for an equivalent amount of time to stimulate their vestibular nuclei.

The results of this study were clear cut. The RNA content was different in that part of the brain concerned with balance when learning to balance had been acquired. Thus, the results apparently supported Hydén's theory. However, these findings have been criticized on several grounds. The most serious criticism has to do with the appropriateness of the control group. It is plausible that the different treatments—balancing and swinging—stimulated different aspects of the vestibular system. Therefore, the differences in RNA observed may have reflected these procedural differences rather than memory in the trained animals.

In other investigations, Hydén and his associates (Hydén & Egyházi, 1964; Hydén & Lange, 1965) have assessed changes in the composition of RNA extracted from the motor cortex of rats that had been forced to reach with their nonpreferred paw for food at the end of a tube. Rats, like people, have distinct "handedness" preferences. The change in handedness resulting fom using the nonpreferred paw was regarded as learning. Upon analysis of their results, the investigators discovered that the RNA extracted from the two sides of the motor cortex differed both in composition and in concentration. No interhemispheric differences were noted in the quantity or composition of RNA in rats allowed to use their preferred paw to obtain food.

Using similar behavior-assessment techniques, Hydén and Lange (1971a, 1971b, 1972) have shown that differences in the concentration of the brain-specific protein S-100 may be obtained from pyramidal nerve cells in the hippocampus of rats forced to use their nonpreferred paw to obtain food. Again, these measures were compared with measures from control subjects allowed to continue using their preferred paw. The researchers reported that the amount of S-100 increased during learning. Further, they reported that intraventricular injection of antiserum against the S-100 protein during the course of training prevented the rats from further learning but did not affect their general motor functions. The site of action of the antiserum was found to be the hippocampus. In contrast, control subjects injected with inactivated antiserum showed no loss in their ability to learn to use their nonpreferred paw. These findings are graphically portrayed in Figure 13-1.

On the basis of these observations, Hydén and Lange (1972) concluded that the brain-specific protein S-100 is linked to the transfer-of-handedness learning process. In spite of the elegance of these experiments, it is difficult to conclude that the observed changes in brain chemistry reflected memory encoding. Rather, the observed changes in both RNA and protein may have resulted from massive activation of previously relatively inactive regions of the motor system. Thus, the changes in brain chemistry may have been reflective of and necessary for performance of the new motor response rather than related to the encoding of a memory of this response.

Some very interesting changes in RNA composition in nerve cells of monkeys subjected to more conventional training paradigms have been reported by Hydén, Lange, Mihailović, and Petrović-Minić (1974) and by Mihailović, Krzalić, Petrović, and Čupić (1971). In these experiments, rhesus monkeys were given visual-discrimination and delayed-alternation training. The amount of RNA per nerve cell and the composition of this extracted RNA were determined for pyramidal nerve cells from region CA 3 of the hippocampus, from the fifth cellular level of the inferotemporal neocortex, and from the gyrus principalis of the frontal association cortex. Why did these researchers sample RNA composition from these specific regions? It was because, as reviewed in Chapter 10, the inferotemporal cortex has

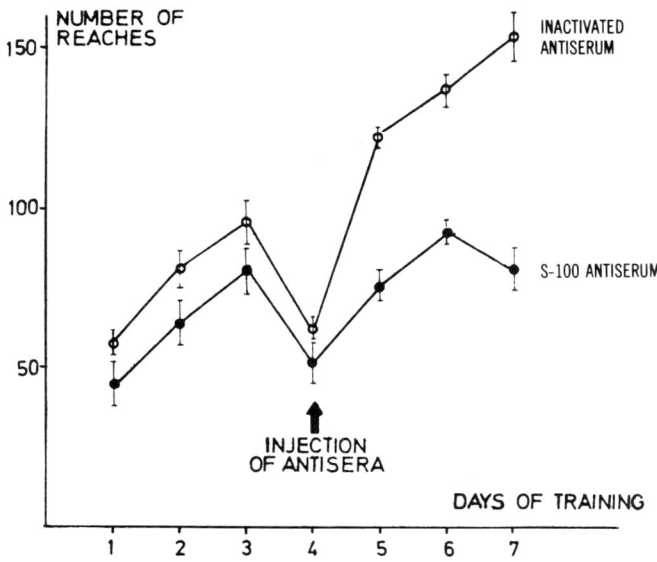

Figure 13-1
The number of reaches with the nonpreferred paw by rats injected with S-100 antiserum and by control animals injected with inactivated antiserum. From "Correlation of the S-100 Brain Protein with Behavior," by H. Hydén and P. W. Lange. In J. Gaito (Ed.), Macromolecules and Behavior, *(2nd ed.).* Copyright 1972 by Plenum Publishing Corporation. Reprinted by permission.

been implicated in visual-discrimination learning (for example, Mishkin, 1954; Mishkin & Pribram, 1954). The gyrus principalis has been specifically related to delayed-alternation performance (Butters & Pandya, 1969; Butters, Pandya, Sanders, & Dye, 1971; Weiskranz, 1964; Weiskranz, Mihailović, & Gross, 1962). Finally, the hippocampus was examined because of its postulated role in the establishment of new behavior (see Chapter 10).

Behavioral testing was conducted in a modified Wisconsin General Testing Apparatus (WGTA). Prior to the beginning of training, the monkeys were pretrained to displace the covers from two food wells situated in front of them to obtain a piece of apple. When they had learned to do this consistently, training on the test problems began. Visual-discrimination training required the animals to discriminate between two different shapes to obtain the reward. The food was always hidden in the food well under the positive stimulus, which was randomly alternated from side to side as trials progressed. The stimulus panels were a yellow hexagon and a yellow hourglass on black backgrounds.

Delayed-alternation training involves components of two functions that are related to frontal-lobe function: the ability to alternate from side to side and the ability to learn a delayed response. Training on the delayed-alternation problem involved teaching the animal to lift the cover off the food well opposite to that from which the cover was removed during the previous trial (alternation component). Between successive trials, an opaque screen was lowered in front of the food wells for seven seconds (delay component).

For both of these tasks, monkeys were administered 30 reinforced trials per day until they achieved a performance criterion of 80–100% correct choices for a session, and they were then sacrificed. The composition of RNA extracted from the regions of interest was then assessed. The RNA from these experimental animals was compared to that obtained from trained control animals. This control group is one of the many excellent features of these researchers' work. Animals in the trained control group allowed these researchers to control for changes in RNA composition due to nonspecific motor, sensory, and other behavior components of the learning process. These control subjects—one group for each behavior task—were exposed to the same training conditions and were presented with the same number of trials as the experimental subjects. However, the rewards were presented randomly—that is, independently of the response emitted by the monkey.

The most interesting results of this study emerged upon analysis of the samples obtained from experimental and control animals subjected to visual-discrimination training. The greatest changes in RNA composition were noted in the inferotemporal cortex, which is the cortical region that has been directly implicated in this type of learning. Lesser but still significant changes were noted in the composition of RNA samples extracted from the hippocampus of these monkeys. No changes whatsoever were noted in RNA samples from the gyrus principalis of the frontal lobe—a region that has been shown to be unnecessary for visual-discrimination learning (Weiskrantz, 1964; Weiskrantz et al., 1962).

In contrast, delayed-alternation training did induce significant changes in the RNA composition of cells from the gyrus principalis. Hydén and his associates concluded that the lack of change in RNA from this region following visual-discrimination learning, along with the alterations noted following delayed-alternation performance, emphasize the specific involvement of the gyrus principalis in delayed-alternation performance. Interestingly enough, significant changes in RNA composition were also noted in the inferotemporal cortex and the hippocampus following delayed-alternation learning, and they were similar to those induced by visual-discrimination learning. Possibly, these changes indicated that some common functions are required for these two problems. Even though the critical cues for delayed performance are not visual, the animal is attending to cues in its visual field while performing this problem. Hence, it would be of interest to determine whether similar changes would occur in the inferotemporal cortex—a region unnecessary for this type of learning—if animals learned a delayed-alternation problem in the dark.

We have now seen that changes in RNA content occur in hippocampal pyramidal cells during transfer of handedness, delayed-alternation learning, and visual-discrimination behavior. The integrity of the hippocampus is necessary for alternation learning; it may also be necessary for handedness transfer, but it is certainly not absolutely essential for visual-pattern-discrimination learning. Therefore, as I have suggested before, the hippocampal changes may be correlates of performance rather than of memory-consolidation processes.

It is very difficult to isolate the exact processes that resulted in the observed changes in neural RNA and protein that have been reviewed in the last few pages. However, some excellent strides have been made in this direction. The model employed in these last experiments by Hydén and Mihailović and their associates is an excellent one for answering these questions; the controls used in these studies were very good. The further development and use of antisera to inactivate specific proteins associated with specific learning processes will also produce some very exciting and provocative findings in the years to come.

Transfer of Memory by Brain Extracts

Since its introduction in research conducted by McConnell and his associates (McConnell, 1962), the concept of chemical transfer of learned information has been the most controversial area of research in neuropsychology. The *memory transfer* proponents claim to have demonstrated that learned behavior may be transferred to naïve recipient animals by the injection of certain types of brain extracts from trained donor animals. In the pages that follow, we will examine McConnell's early planarian work and some of the criticisms that have been leveled against it. We will then look at a variety of more recent research that has examined both the phylogenetic and the behavioral generality of this phenomenon. Many excellent reviews of this topic are available (for example, Chapouthier, 1973; Fjerdingstad, 1973; McConnell & Jacobson, 1973; Smith, 1974). Fjerdingstad (1971) has edited an entire text devoted to this subject, entitled *Chemical Transfer of Learned Information.*

Experiments on Planarians

The storm of controversy began in the early 1960s when McConnell suggested that memories could be transferred from one planarian to another. The planarian is a flatworm found in both fresh and salt water throughout the world. It rarely attains a length of over 2.5 cm. Phylogenetically speaking, it is the most primitive species to have bilateral symmetry, true synapses, and a brain. Further, the planarian possesses remarkable abilities of regeneration. As McConnell and Jacobson (1973) indicate, one can cut a planarian into 50 to 100 pieces, and, within weeks, each part will grow an entire organism that is as large as the one from which the pieces were taken!

McConnell's memory-transfer work dates back to his and Thompson's discovery that planarians can be classically conditioned (Thompson & McConnell, 1955). In their classical-conditioning paradigm, the conditioned stimulus was light and the unconditioned stimulus was electric shock. The animal showed an unconditioned response to the shock: contracting and turning. The training procedure involved giving the animals 150 trials during which light preceded the shock onset. Successive trials were separated by 20–30 seconds. Over the course of training, the experimental animals showed a statistically significant increase in their rate of responding to the onset of the conditioned stimulus, as compared with control subjects given only 150 presentations of the light alone or 150 trials of the shock alone. These results were interpreted by Thompson and McConnell as having demonstrated classical conditioning in this very primitive invertebrate species.

This experiment was justly criticized on a number of points, the most important of which was the appropriateness of the control groups. Thompson and McConnell failed to control adequately for pseudoconditioning effects. *Pseudoconditioning* refers to the fact that the animals' behavior may have changed not because they had learned to associate light onset with impending shock but rather because the planarians had been stimulated (and hence were possibly sensitized) by the occurrence of so much shock and light. However, when proper controls were used to control for the possibility of pseudoconditioning, planarians still appeared to demonstrate true classical conditioning (Jacobson, Horowitz, & Fried, 1967). Other researchers have shown that planarians can learn elementary operant tasks that require left/right discriminations (for example, Best & Rubenstein, 1962; Chapouthier, Pallaud, & Ungerer, 1968; Corning, 1964; Griffard & Pierce, 1964; McConnell & Shelby, 1970). Thus, the weight of the evidence appears to indicate that, under ideal conditions, planarians are capable of learning simple associations.

In light of the planarian's incredible regenerative capacities, McConnell and his associates wondered how well regenerated planarians would retain a classically conditioned response learned by the original intact animal. They trained planarians in the Thompson/McConnell classical-conditioning paradigm, cut them in half, let them rest for a month (during which the head sections grew new tails and the tail sections grew new heads), and then retrained them on the task. As shown in Table 13-1, the original planarians took an average of 134 trials to begin responding to the onset of the light alone at least 92% of the time. This same criterion was attained by the animals regenerated from the head in only 40 training trials, while the planarians regenerated from the tail sections reattained criterion in an average of approximately 43 trials. Since the conditions of testing were such that the minimum number of trials the regenerates could reach criterion in was 23, these scores reflected a high degree of savings. Two of the tail sections—E-2 and E-5 in Table 13-1—showed almost perfect retention of training.

Table 13-1. The Number of Responses Required by Original and Regenerated Planarians to Reach a Behavioral Criterion

S	*Original Training*	*Retest Head*	*Retest Tail*
E-1	99	50	51
E-2	191	37	24
E-3	97	48	72
E-4	83	35	44
E-5	200	30	25
M	134	40	43.2

From "The Effects of Regeneration upon Retention of a Conditioned Response in the Planarian," by J. V. McConnell, A. L. Jacobson, and D. P. Kimble, *Journal of Comparative and Physiological Psychology,* 1959, *52,* 1–5. Copyright 1959 by the American Psychological Association. Reprinted by permission.

These findings were incredible; they precipitated another storm of controversy. That the tail end of the trained planarians had to regenerate an entire new brain with new synapses, yet apparently retained learned information, was an idea that many neuroscientists simply could not accept. It was just too inconsistent with established theories on how the brain processes information. Primarily for this reason, these observations of McConnell and his associates have been criticized. For example, Brown, Dustman, and Beck (1966a, 1966b) have argued that the greater responsiveness to light noted in the regenerated subjects resulted from the fact that the regenerated planarians were smaller than the original ones and that, in general, smaller planarians are more responsive to light than larger ones (Van Deventer & Ratner, 1964). This is an important criticism because it suggests that the regenerated animals differed from the original planarians with regard to sensitivity to the testing paradigm. As you'll see, this criticism has repeatedly surfaced in the experimental memory-transfer literature.

McConnell and his co-workers' findings, which at the time appeared to suggest that memory could survive regeneration, were followed by the even more spectacular and disquieting finding that memory could be transferred by feeding trained planarians to untrained subjects (John, 1964; McConnell, 1962). In his demonstration of this phenomenon, McConnell took advantage of the fact that, when certain species of planarians are starved, they become cannibalistic. He trained planarians using the standard Thompson/McConnell light/shock classical-conditioning paradigm. Once the "donors" had attained a criterion response rate of 92%, he chopped them into small pieces and fed them to hungry, untrained planarians. Other cannibals were fed untrained worms, and both groups were administered the classical-conditioning training. The results of this experiment were positive; that is, the animals that had consumed the trained planarians conditioned more rapidly than the subjects that had consumed the naïve donors. McConnell (1962) claimed to have obtained a "transfer of memory through cannibalism."

A rather devastating critique of the memory-transfer-through-cannibalism notion was leveled by Hartry, Keith-Lee, and Morton (l964). These investigators replicated McConnell's training paradigm and found that planarians that had cannibalized previously conditioned subjects required significantly fewer trials to acquire the conditioned reflex than did naïve planarians. However, the same finding was also observed in planarians that had cannibalized untrained planarians exposed only to photic stimuli or only handled. Hence, it appeared that it was not learning that was being transferred during the cannibalism but rather an increased activity level or sensitization.

The possible confounding effects of increased activity or sensitization in the recipient animals were partially controlled for in an experiment by McConnell and Shelby (1970). In this experiment, planarians were trained in a T-maze, one arm of which was light gray and the other dark gray. The worms showed no initial preference for either arm, and half of the donors were trained to go to the light arm and half to the dark arm. Criterion performance required that they make 9 out of 10 correct choices for two days in a row. The donor planarians required an average of 200 trials to achieve this criterion. They were then cut into pieces and fed to untrained cannibals. Other subjects ate untrained animals.

Four groups of recipients were used. Group I cannibals were trained to go to the same arm of the maze as their donor (positive-transfer group). Group II subjects learned to go to the side the opposite of the one their donors had learned to approach (negative-transfer group). Group III was fed two donors, one of which had been trained to go to the dark side and the other to the light side (conflicting-instructions or ± group). Finally, the animals in group IV were fed nontrained worms (0 group). The results of this study are given in Table 13-2. Group I subjects attained criterion significantly sooner than the remaining groups, and Group II was significantly superior in its rate of task acquisition to Groups III and IV. The difference between Groups III and IV was not significant. It is hard to explain the results of this experiment except as demonstrating transfer of information. The finding that Group I is superior to the other groups makes an alternative interpretation hard to support. However, the superiority of Group II to Group IV tends to suggest that both an

Table 13-2. Mean Trials to Criterion in a T-Maze for Four Groups of Planarians Fed Different Types of Donor Animals

	Group I (+ Group)	Group II (− Group)	Group III (± Group)	Group IV (0 Group)
mean trials to criterion	113.8	166.3	263.8	228.8

From "Memory Transfer Experiments in Invertebrates," by J. V. McConnell and J. M. Shelby. In G. Ungar (Ed.), *Molecular Mechanisms in Memory and Learning.* Copyright 1970 by Plenum Publishing Corporation. Reprinted by permission.

increase in arousal or sensitization and a transfer of information may have contributed to the obtained findings. In view of the implications of these findings, the McConnell and Shelby study needs to be replicated in a number of independent laboratories.

Another question the planarian researchers attempted to answer was: What is the chemical basis of the transfer effect? Under the supposition that RNA may mediate the effect, RNA was extracted from donor animals trained on the Thompson/McConnell light/shock classical-conditioning paradigm. This extracted RNA was then injected into untrained planarians. Control animals were injected with RNA extract from untrained animals. It was found that the planarians injected with RNA from trained subjects conditioned significantly faster than did the animals injected with the control substance (Fried & Horowitz, 1964; Jacobson, Fried & Horowitz, 1966a, 1966b; Zelman, Kabat, Jacobson, & McConnell, 1963). Thus, regardless of whether the transfer effect in this paradigm reflects the transfer of learned information or sensitization, it appears that these effects can be duplicated by simply injecting RNA extract from trained donors into naïve recipients.

Experiments with Vertebrates

In 1965, four independent research groups located around the world applied the planarian memory-transfer paradigm to rodents and concluded that they had found an interanimal transfer of a learned response. The procedures used in these studies involved the extraction of brain material from trained rodents and the injection of this material into untrained animals. The recipients then reportedly showed a tendency to respond similarly to the way the donors had in a training situation. The route of administration of the transfer agent in these and subsequent inquiries was intraperitoneal, intravenous, or intracranial, and the materials injected included brain homogenates and extracts from brain homogenates composed mainly of RNA or water-soluble protein fractions.

The behavior tendencies reported to have been transferred in these initial studies published in 1965 included approaching a food cup (Babich, Jacobson, Bubash, & Jacobson, 1965), approaching one of the arms of a T-maze on the basis of brightness cues (Fjerdingstad, Nissen, & Røigaard-Petersen, 1965), pushing a translucent door open to obtain food in response to the onset of a light (Reinis, 1965), and habituation of a startle response to a sound stimulus (Ungar & Oceguera-Navarro, 1965). These initial reports of apparently successful transfer were soon followed by a series of negative results from other laboratories (Byrne et al., 1966; Gross & Carey, 1965; Luttges, Johnston, Buck, Holland, & McGaugh, 1966). Although additional positive results were published, many other researchers also reported an inability to replicate the basic observations.

Both the difficulties in replicating the interanimal transfer effect and the controversy regarding the meaning of this effect have continued. One loud objection has been that the physiological or neurological mechanisms by which a transfer could be accomplished are either nonexistent or unknown (for example, Barondes, 1972). Another problem is the adequacy of the behavioral data to support a learning interpretation of the transfer effect. The lack of many good replication studies, inadequate control in many of the studies, and improper statistical analysis of the data have prevented many of the experiments from demonstrating in a definitive fashion that learned information has been transferred. Nevertheless, as will be seen, the transfer effect has been reported in a variety of tasks. Hence, whatever the true explanation is for this phenomenon, the transfer effect seems to show a high degree of generality.

As indicated, much of the resistance to the possibility of interanimal transfer of learned information has been generated by the fact that the biological mechanisms required to produce the effect are unknown (Davis, 1970; Smith, 1974). The interanimal transfer phenomenon requires that, during the interval between injection and testing in the recipient subjects, the active ingredient be transported to the site of action in the brain. During its transport, the material must escape degradation. Next, the active material must be selectively absorbed by cells performing functions identical to those performed by the cells that produced the material in the donor animals. Finally, the material must interact with the biochemistry of the recipient cells in such a way as to create that state that existed in the cells of the donor prior to extraction. There is simply no direct evidence to support the existence of such mechanisms.

Furthermore, the fact that intraperitoneal administrations of the transfer agent yield transfer effects calls into question the existence of such biological mechanisms or, at the very least, casts doubt on their importance in producing the observed behavior alterations. Fjerdingstad (1973) and Luttges & his associates (1966) report that at least 99% of the material administered intraperitoneally never reaches the brain but rather is excreted in the feces and urine. These findings suggest that much of the action of at least intraperitoneally administered transfer agents is peripheral; that is, it acts outside of the brain. Hence, it is probably more parsimonious to suggest that many of the transfer effects reflect changes in such variables as arousal, which in turn affects the sensitivity of the animal to cues associated with the training situation. As you'll see, however, some results—particularly those using appetitively motivated tasks—are difficult to account for by resorting to a simple arousal interpretation of the obtained results.

The transfer shows wide phylogenetic and behavioral generality. It has been demonstrated in a wide variety of species, including goldfish (Fjerdingstad, 1973) and mice (for example, Essman & Lehrer, 1967). However, the rat has been the species chosen by most investigators. Interspecific transfers have also been reported. Babich, Jacobson, and Bubash (1965) used hamsters as donors and rats as recipients, and Benner and Radcliffe (1970) used rats as donors and mice as recipients.

A large variety of aversively and appetitively motivated tasks have been used to demonstrate the transfer phenomenon. Detailed reviews of these experimental paradigms are provided by Chapouthier (1973) and Smith (1974). Only a few examples will be cited here. With regard to aversively motivated tasks, Gay and Raphelson (1967, 1970) have reported the interanimal transfer effect for passive avoidance of one chamber of a three-chambered apparatus. Trained donors were given foot-shock in the dark chamber and permitted to escape to the light chamber at the other end. Recipients of brain extracts from these donors were found to spend less time in the dark chamber of the apparatus than did recipients of extracts from untrained control donors. Although these results tended to suggest that something learned about the apparatus had been transferred, the validity of a learning interpretation of these results is open to question because of the absence of an important control group. Specifically, there should have been a group of donors that had received shock not contingent upon performance, so that it could be determined whether sensitization or arousal was being transferred. In the absence of this control, we are unable to draw any conclusions regarding what was transferred.

A study by Frank, Stein, and Rosen (1970) provided evidence to support a "transfer of arousal" interpretation of the Gay and Raphelson results. They replicated the Gay and Raphelson research, except that a group of stressed control donors was also used. The stressed control donors were rolled back and forth in a glass jar. Recipient mice were then injected with RNA extract from the brains of trained, naïve control, or stressed control animals. In confirmation of Gay and Raphelson's results, Frank and his associates found that recipients of extracts from the donors who were shocked in the test chamber remained outside of the black compartment longer than did recipients of the brain extracts from naïve donors. However, the recipients of RNA extract from the stressed controls—that is, the mice that were rolled around in the jar—avoided the dark compartment even more than did the recipients of trained-donor extract! Needless to say, these findings argue that something different from learned information was probably contributing to the effects observed by Gay and Raphelson. Frank and his associates suggest that the most likely factor transferred was a general stress factor.

Gay and Raphelson failed to clarify the basis for the transfer effect, but Ungar, in a series of experiments, has gone on to isolate a protein he named *scotophobin.* He has argued that scotophobin is the active neurochemical ingredient mediating the interanimal transfer effect in this paradigm (Ungar, 1967, 1968, 1969, 1970b; Ungar, Desiderio, & Parr, 1972). He has even reported success in producing a synthetic scotophobin that produced the same effects as the biological material when injected into recipients. Other researchers have reported difficulty in replicating the results with the synthetic (Goldstein, Sheehan, & Goldstein, 1971), and the validity of the chemistry involved in both the identification and synthesis of scotophobin by Ungar and his associates has been criticized by Stewart (1972). Stewart argues that the chemical evidence for the composition of the biological material scotophobin is largely invalidated by the probable presence of impurities resulting from Ungar's analytical methods. Further, Stewart contends that Ungar's comparison of the synthetic material with the isolated biological material is "cursory and inconclusive" (p. 209).

Interanimal transfer of learning on appetitively motivated tasks have also been reported by a number of researchers. In a very clever paradigm, Cheney (1970) trained some donors on a DRL schedule in which they had to wait at least 30 seconds between successive bar-presses to obtain a food reward. Another group of donors received practice on a fixed-ratio (FR) schedule in which they received one reinforcement for each 20 bar-presses. This schedule typically produces high rates of responding. The recipients, which had been performing on a DRL 10-second schedule, were given brain homogenate from different donor groups every eight days. The effects were very interesting: recipient response rates were reduced by half following injections of brain homogenates from the DRL-30 trained donors but increased by 40% after injections of homogenates obtained from the FR-20 subjects! It is unclear whether these effects were mediated by transfer of learned information, transfer of arousal level, or a combination of the two. However, there are some data obtained with appetitively motivated tasks that cannot be accounted for by a transfer-of-arousal explanation (Braud & Braud, 1972; Fjerdingstad, 1973).

Fjerdingstad (1973) reported transfer effects using what he referred to as "oxygen reinforced approach training." In this paradigm, Fjerdingstad took advantage of the tendency of goldfish to surface to take in air when the oxygen content of the water is decreased. He found that, by providing an oxygen-free environment on the surface of the water, as shown in Figure 13-2, while making oxygen available from a small area near the bottom of the aquarium, this surfacing behavior could be reversed. The fish would now go to the bottom when oxygen deprived. This task was learned very rapidly by the donors. When naïve recipients were injected intracerebrally with RNA extracts from the donors, they were found to surface significantly less often in response to oxygen deprivation than control recipients injected with RNA extracts from naïve fish. These results appear to demonstrate the transfer of a learned behavior tendency.

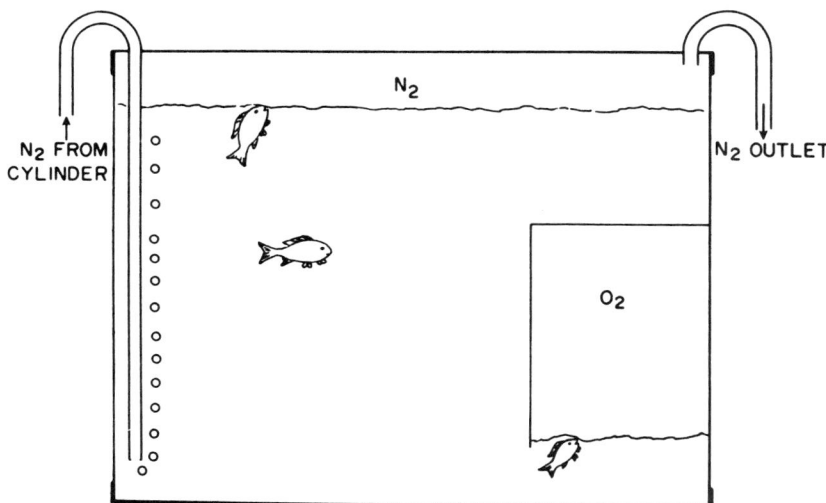

Figure 13-2
Apparatus for
oxygen-reinforced
training of goldfish.
Oxygen is washed
out of the water by
a stream of
nitrogen, and a
nitrogen atmosphere
is left over the
surface. From
"Transfer of
Learning in
Rodents and Fish,"
by E. J.
Fjerdingstad. In W.
B. Essman and S.
Nakajima (Eds.),
Current
Biochemical
Approaches to
Learning and
Memory. Copyright
1973 by Spectrum
Publications.
Reprinted by
permission of
Spectrum
Publications, New
York.

Another study that appeared to demonstrate the transfer of a learned behavior tendency in a relatively unambiguous fashion was an inquiry by Braud and Braud (1972). In this experiment, donors were trained in a Y-maze to choose the larger of two circles (3.2 versus 7 cm in diameter) to obtain a food reward. The rats received 10 trials per day for 12 days. At the end of this training regimen, all animals had performed at a level of 90% correct or better for the last two days. The donor brains were then homogenized and injected intraperitoneally into recipients. Control subjects received intraperitoneal injections of brain homogenates from untrained animals.

Testing involved a transposition task. *Transposition* refers to the fact that, if an animal is trained to go to the larger of two stimuli and then presented with the old positive stimulus and a new, larger cue, it will approach the larger stimulus. The subject is said to have transposed—that is, to have responded to the relative aspects of the cues. Braud and Braud tested the recipients for transposition by presenting them on nonrewarded trials with a 7-cm circle (the old positive stimulus for the donors) and a 12-cm stimulus. The rats that had received homogenates from naïve animals did not show a preference for either of the two stimuli. In contrast, the recipients of trained-donor extract preferred the larger of the test stimuli and made significantly more approaches to the large circle than did the control subjects. Not only was there evidence that the extract from the trained donors produced a transfer of transposition, but there was also evidence that it facilitated learning of the original discrimination task, as compared with the performance of both the control recipients and the original donors (see Figure 13-3).

The results published by both Fjerdingstad (1973) and Braud and Braud (1972) provide some of the strongest evidence for interanimal transfer of learned information. The question remains as to what has actually been transferred. For example, in the Braud and Braud inquiry some general activation effect may have been produced by the trained extracts. This factor would account for the more rapid discrimination learning of the animals that had received extracts from the trained donors.

Figure 13-3
Comparison of correct responses (mean percent) on daily reinforced training sessions of the original discrimination problem, for donors, experimental recipients, and control recipients. From "Biochemical Transfer of Relational Responding (Transposition)," by L. W. Braud, and W. G. Braud, Science, 1972, 176, 942–943. Copyright 1972 by the American Association for the Advancement of Science. Reprinted by permission.

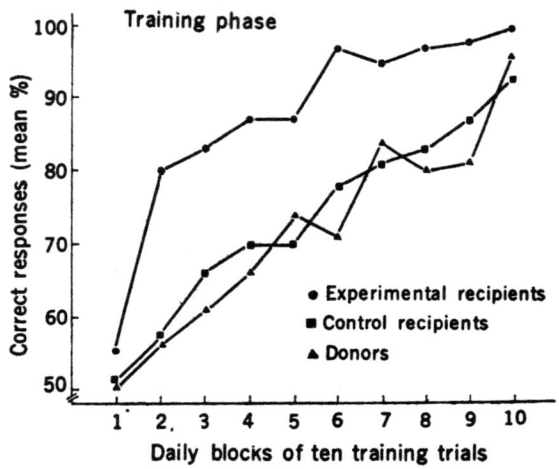

Unfortunately, these investigators used the intraperitoneal route for administering brain homogenates. As I noted, it appears unlikely that significant amounts of transfer substance administered in this fashion ever reach the brain. The Fjerdingstad data may also reflect the influence of some as yet unidentified arousal factor. It is also possible that the transfer effect represents an interaction between a transferred sensitivity or stress factor and some actual learned behavior tendency.

In evaluating the memory-transfer experiments, scepticism is warranted because, as was discussed earlier in this chapter, there is simply no evidence to support the existence of the biological mechanisms that would be required to produce such a transfer of information. Also, the memory-transfer hypothesis would require that a new macromolecule be synthesized for each response an organism learns to make. This proposition runs counter to all of our understanding of neural functions (Barondes, 1972). Of course, we cannot rule out such a possibility, and so future research will have to decide the fate of the memory-transfer hypothesis.

The Effects of Antimetabolite Drugs on Acquisition and Recall

Earlier in this chapter, I indicated that it is commonly assumed that the consolidation of long-term memory is mediated by RNA and protein-synthesis mechanisms. To assess the validity of this view, many neuroscientists have investigated the effects on learning and memory of certain drugs that interfere with the metabolic processes involved in RNA and protein synthesis. The results of these studies will be summarized below.

Inhibition of RNA Synthesis

The two principal antimetabolite drugs that have been used to examine the effects of RNA-synthesis inhibition are 8-azaguanine and actinomycin-D. These agents inhibit the processes by which DNA produces RNA. The first researchers to examine the effects of RNA-synthesis inhibition on learning and memory were Dingman and Sporn (1961). In their study, 8-azaguanine was injected into rats either before or after the subjects learned to escape from a water-filled maze. The rats that had been injected before training showed a significant acquisition impairment. However, the animals injected after training showed no loss of retention.

At face value, these findings appeared to indicate that RNA synthesis was important for the original consolidation of information but not for its subsequent recall. However, in a later paper, Dingman and Sporn (1964) indicated that their initial findings were not conclusive because of severe side effects of the drug. Basically, the rats were made sick by 8-azaguanine, and it is well known that almost any treatment that makes an animal ill will have more disruptive effects on original learning than on retention and performance. In spite of the fact that their findings were confounded and therefore not clearly interpretable, their research was important. It was the first attempt to study consolidation and recall processes by using an antimetabolite agent that inhibited the synthesis of the proposed substrates of these processes. Their research thus provided great impetus to later, similar inquiries. The problem of whether observed changes in behavior following administration of certain RNA- and protein-synthesis inhibitors arise from altered brain metabolism or merely from side effects of the drugs is still central to many of the experiments in this area of research.

Another popular RNA-synthesis inhibitor that has been used in studies of learning and memory is actinomycin-D. This drug is a more potent RNA-synthesis inhibitor than 8-azaguanine. It is possible to achieve up to 95% inhibition of cerebral RNA synthesis in mice by intracranial injections of this agent (Cohen & Barondes, 1966; Barondes & Jarvik, 1964). Nevertheless, researchers have not consistently demonstrated that memory deficits follow its administration. For example, administration of actinomycin-D was found to affect neither original learning nor retention of either a passive-avoidance (Barondes & Jarvik, 1964) or a simple maze-learning problem (Cohen & Barondes, 1966). Long-term studies were prevented because of the extremely high toxicity of this drug.

More recently, Oshima, Gorbman, and Shimada (1969) injected homing salmon with actinomycin-D. Homing salmon, when ready to spawn, have a legendary ability to find their way back to the small fresh-water stream from which they emerged as small fish. It is assumed by many students of fish behavior that the salmon become imprinted to the olfactory cues present in their aqueous nursery. When they go to sea, they "remember" these stimuli. After remaining in the ocean for about five years, they swim back to the small stream to spawn and die. As detailed by Hasler (1956), the fish find their way back from the ocean to the mouth of the river, where it enters the ocean, by using the sun as a compass. Once at the mouth of the river, the completion of their homeward journey is guided by their sense of smell. Like any other animal, they can follow an odor to its source. The salmon detect the cues from their original stream and then follow the concentration gradient upstream, choosing the correct turn at each tributary, until they arrive at the stream in which they were hatched.

In the study by Oshima and his associates, actinomycin-D administration was found to inhibit the ability of homing salmon to learn an olfactory discrimination between their home water and other types of natural stream water. This is a task that normally is performed very efficiently by these animals. On the basis of their findings, Oshima and his colleagues postulated that the RNA-synthesis inhibition had disrupted their long-term memory of their home water's olfactory attributes. This is an interesting possibility, but, in light of the severe side effects and high toxicity of actinomycin-D, the basis for the altered performance is unclear. The altered discrimination may simply have reflected side effects of this antimetabolite such as we saw in the experiments using 8-azaguanine as the RNA-synthesis inhibitor.

The Effects of Protein-Synthesis Inhibition on Memory

The Puromycin Effect. Antimetabolite drugs that interfere with the RNA-directed synthesis of protein molecules have also been used to study the biochemical substrates of memory. The principal drugs that have been used in these investigations are puromycin, cyclohexamide, acetoxycyclohexamide, and anisomycin. Intracerebral injections of puromycin following training have been shown to interfere with the retention of an acquired response in a variety of species and testing situations. Intracranial injections of this drug result in amnesia for a previously learned avoidance response in mice (for example, Barondes & Cohen, 1966, 1967; Flexner, Flexner, & Stellar, 1963; Flexner, Flexner, Roberts, & De la Haba, 1964) and in goldfish (for example, Agranoff, 1972; Agranoff, Davis, & Brink, 1965, 1966; Agranoff & Klinger, 1964; Davis & Agranoff, 1965; Davis, Bright, & Agranoff, 1965; Springer, Schoel, Klinger, & Agranoff, 1975). Puromycin administrations also disrupt retention of a learned position reversal in mice (Flexner et al., 1963) and rats (Moss, 1973), retention of a color discrimination in Japanese quail (Mayor, 1969), and memory for shuttle-box extinction in goldfish and bar-press extinction in rats (Braud & Broussard, 1973).

The first examination of the effects of puromycin on retention was conducted in the Flexner laboratory using mice (Flexner, Flexner, & Stellar, 1963). Adult white mice were trained in a right/left position discrimination in a Y-maze under shock-avoidance motivation. The mouse was placed in the stem of the Y, and, to avoid shock, it had to move into the correct arm within five seconds. If it entered the incorrect arm, it received foot-shock until it moved into the correct arm. Training was continued in a single session until the animal reached a criterion of nine out of ten correct responses. Retention testing involved the same procedures, and the mice were retrained to criterion. Flexner and his associates report that normal subjects retain excellent memory of this problem for at least five weeks after training.

To test for the effects of intracerebral injections of puromycin on retention of this task, the Flexner group injected puromycin into the temporal lobes one to six days after acquisition of the task. The effect of these administrations was to inhibit protein synthesis by approximately 80% for a duration of 8 to 10 hours in both the temporal-lobe neocortex and the hippocampus. Retention tests were given three days after the puromycin injections to allow the animals the opportunity to recover from the side effects of this drug. It was found that puromycin injections given one or two days after original training yielded a total loss of memory for the task. However, if temporal injections were given three to six days after original training, they were often ineffective in abolishing memory. To affect memory at these intervals, it was necessary to inject puromycin in several loci of the brain, including the temporal region, the frontal region, and the ventricles. More recently, Nakajima (1973) has been able to demonstrate that temporal injections alone can block memory even if administered as long as seven days after training if the puromycin is injected at a very slow rate.

The data obtained by the Flexners and their associates are supportive of the view that protein synthesis serves as the basis for memory consolidation. Block the manufacture of protein, their data suggest, and you will disrupt memory processes. Their differential findings regarding the efficiency of temporal applications of puromycin in blocking memory following different training-injection intervals were used to infer that different anatomical regions may participate in short-term and long-term memory. They interpreted these data as suggesting that short-term, or immediate, memory of an event may be located in the temporal-lobe neocortex and hippocampus. In contrast, long-term, or consolidated, information is more diffusely organized and has no precise cortical location. However, such a view may be unwarranted, since Nakajima (1973) was unable to replicate the finding of differential effects of temporal puromycin injections at different training-injection intervals. Also, Deutsch (1969) has suggested that the Flexner data may simply indicate that a larger dose of puromycin was required to suppress memory processes when given several days, as opposed to a day, after training. Hence, the small dose present after temporal injections may be sufficient to interfere with recently acquired information, but a higher dose, as was present after the multiple-loci administrations, may be needed to abolish more firmly established memories.

Agranoff and his associates have studied the effects of intracerebral injections of puromycin on memory of a shuttle-box active-avoidance response in goldfish. In these experiments, goldfish were individually trained in tanks divided in half by an underwater barrier, as shown in Figure 13-4. At the beginning of a trial, a light was turned on at the end of the tank in which the fish was placed. Twenty seconds later, an intermittent shock was applied to the illuminated side of the apparatus, and it

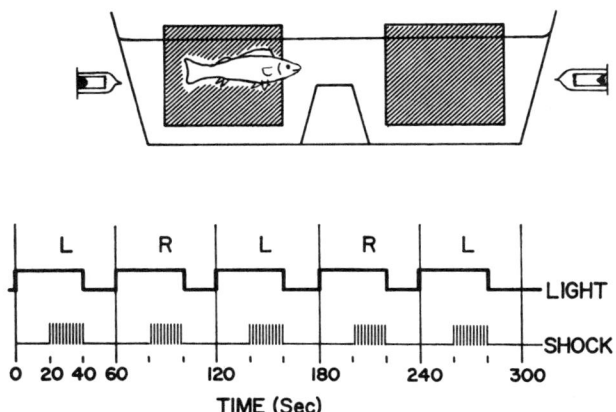

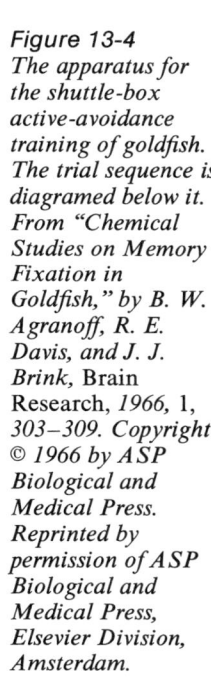

Figure 13-4
The apparatus for the shuttle-box active-avoidance training of goldfish. The trial sequence is diagrammed below it. From "Chemical Studies on Memory Fixation in Goldfish," by B. W. Agranoff, R. E. Davis, and J. J. Brink, Brain Research, 1966, 1, 303–309. Copyright © 1966 by ASP Biological and Medical Press. Reprinted by permission of ASP Biological and Medical Press, Elsevier Division, Amsterdam.

continued for 20 seconds. Fish that had not already swum to the dark, or safe, side did so quickly when the shock was applied. Forty seconds after the start of the trial, both the light and the shock were ended. After a 20-second intertrial interval, the previously safe side was illuminated, and the procedure was repeated. The fish received five trials in five minutes and then were given five minutes rest in the dark. A block of five trials is outlined in Figure 13-4. Agranoff and his colleagues gave their subjects 20 trials during the first day of training. The fish usually successfully avoided the shock on about three of the first block of 10 trials and improved during the next block of 10 trials. If they were then given another 10 trials, they improved even more.

An interesting aspect of this training procedure is that, if up to a month was allowed to pass between trial 20 and trial 21, the goldfish performed just as well on the third block of trials as they would have if only the five-minute rest interval had elapsed. Hence, they appeared to retain a good memory of this training experience. In Agranoff's puromycin studies, three days were allowed to elapse between trials 20 and 21. On the fourth day, the researchers compared the performance of goldfish that had received intracerebral puromycin injections with that of goldfish that had received control saline injections. All the injections had been given on the first day, following the 20 trials. Using this procedure, Agranoff and his associates found that 90 to 210 μg of puromycin administered up to 30 minutes after initial training impaired retention but that there was no effect if it was injected 60 minutes or longer after the first session (Agranoff, Davis, & Brink, 1966). If puromycin was injected before training began, on the first day, it did not affect the rate of original learning, but retention on the fourth day of testing was still disrupted. Agranoff concluded that puromycin does not affect short-term memory but does interrupt the processes by which short-term memory is consolidated into permanent memory.

Interpretations of the Puromycin Effect. On the basis of findings such as those reported by the Flexner group and by Agranoff and his colleagues, many neuroscientists concluded that puromycin causes amnesia by temporarily reducing protein synthesis in the central nervous system. For this reason, these findings have been taken as evidence that protein metabolism serves as a template for long-term memory storage. As you've seen, the theory that protein molecules serve as a template for permanent memory is certainly a reasonable one in light of our current knowledge about cellular processes. However, as Agranoff and his associates (Agranoff & Klinger, 1964) and the Flexner group (Flexner, Flexner, & Stellar, 1963) emphasized early in their investigations, it is not clear whether the puromycin-induced amnesia resulted from a disruption of protein synthesis or rather from other effects of this drug on the physiology of the organism. Further, it is unclear, on the basis of retention test sessions, whether the drug administrations blocked original consolidation processes or blocked recall of information. The research to be reviewed next suggests that (1) puromycin disrupts recall rather than consolidation processes and (2) the effects of puromycin on memory processes result from factors other than a disruption of protein synthesis.

A basic corollary of the theory that puromycin blocks consolidation of information into permanent memory is that the observed performance deficits should be irreversible. If memory was not stored, it should not later recover. However, this is not the case. Flexner and Flexner (1967, 1968a) reported that intracerebral injections of isotonic saline solution brought about a recovery of an aversively conditioned position habit when applied as long as 60 days after the response had been eliminated by puromycin. Flexner and Flexner (1970) later reported that not only isotonic saline solution but also other salt solutions, an ultrafiltrate of blood, and water alone produced the same recovery phenomenon. A possible explanation of this recovery phenomenon will be presented below, but, for now, let me emphasize that these findings indicate that the puromycin effect apparently reflects an inability to recall previously stored information rather than a disruption of consolidation processes.

The idea that puromycin may produce its effects through processes other than the interruption of protein synthesis has arisen as a result of several studies. For example, it has been demonstrated that intracerebral administrations of other protein-synthesis inhibitors, such as acetoxycyclohexamide and cyclohexamide, do not always yield amnesia for a previously learned habit, even for those tasks on which puromycin usually has a very potent effect (Flexner & Flexner, 1966). Cyclohexamide and acetoxycyclohexamide are at least as potent as, if not more potent than, puromycin as protein-synthesis inhibitors. Further, the disruptive effects of puromycin can be circumvented by the addition of acetoxycyclohexamide or cyclohexamide to the puromycin injections (Barondes & Cohen, 1967; Flexner & Flexner, 1966). When these additions were made, there was no disruption of memory, even though the mixture of these agents yielded profound protein-synthesis inhibition and remained in the brain as long as the drugs would have if injected separately (Flexner & Flexner, 1966). These results indicated that puromycin's effects were not due to its suppression of protein synthesis. Why, then, does puromycin yield a retention deficit? Two of the hypotheses that have been offered to account for this finding are as follows.

Cohen, Ervin, and Barondes (1966) attempted to find a basis for Barondes and Cohen's (1967) observation that cyclohexamide did not disrupt retention of an aversively motivated position habit, as did puromycin. They investigated the electrical activity of the mouse hippocampus five hours after intracerebral injections of saline, cyclohexamide, or puromycin. The recordings were obtained from unanesthetized animals. As shown in Figure 13-5, puromycin markedly suppressed the electrical activity of the hippocampus five hours after its application, while cyclohexamide did not. Additionally, it was found that frequent seizure activity appeared in

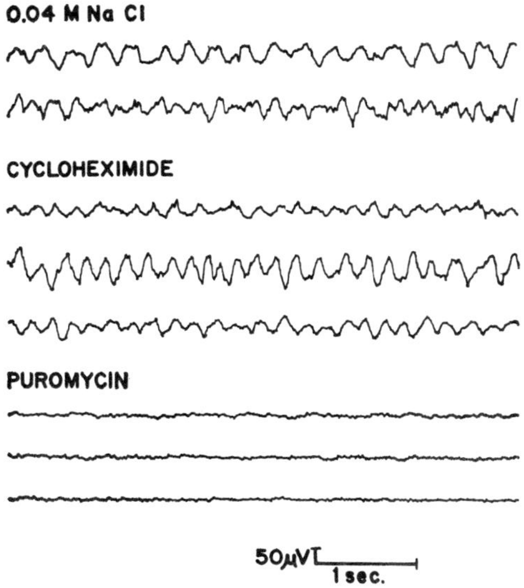
0.04 M Na Cl
CYCLOHEXIMIDE
PUROMYCIN
50μV
1 sec.

Figure 13-5
The electrical activity recorded from the hippocampus of mice that have undergone intracerebral injections of saline solution, cyclohexamide, or puromycin. The recordings were made five hours after the injections. From "Puromycin and Cyclohexamide: Different Effects on Hippocampal Electrical Activity," by H. D. Cohen, F. Ervin, and S. H. Barondes, Science, *1966,* 154, *1557–1558. Copyright 1966 by the American Association for the Advancement of Science. Reprinted by permission.*

the records of the puromycin-injected animals shortly after the drug was given. Finally, if the anticonvulsant drug diphenylhydantoin was given at the time of the puromycin injections, it attenuated puromycin's amnesic effect.

Cohen and his associates interpreted these results as suggesting that the effect of puromycin on memory is due, at least in part, to disturbances of cerebral electrical activity. Because of puromycin's effect on cerebral activity, which is independent of its suppression of cerebral protein synthesis, Barondes (1970) has concluded that "puromycin is not a useful drug for studying the hypothesis that memory storage is mediated by the synthesis of protein" (p. 29). Research by Flexner and Flexner (1967, 1968b) and by Roberts, Flexner, and Flexner (1970) has suggested another hypothesis to account for the effect of puromycin on memory processes.

In view of the finding that potent protein-synthesis inhibitors do not necessarily produce memory deficits in those situations in which puromycin does and the finding that the memory blockage can be reversed by intracerebral injections of several solutions, these researchers have postulated that puromycin does not interrupt memory-consolidation processes but rather interferes with the recall of information. Specifically, the Flexner group has suggested that the injected puromycin causes the synthesis of abnormal peptides, which intefere with normal synaptic functions involved in recall. A peptide is made up of amino acids bonded together. Proteins are also composed of amino acids, linked together by peptide bonds; therefore, all proteins are peptides. Whether the abnormal peptide that these researchers postulate represents a protein or a protein fraction is unclear. However, it is referred to as *peptidal puromycin.*

The hypothesis advanced by these researchers is that the injected puromycin is converted to peptidal puromycin, which then becomes bonded to synaptic membranes and thereby blocks transmission necessary for recall of previously consolidated information. By using radioactively labeled puromycin, these investigators have demonstrated that peptidal puromycin remains in the brains of puromycin-treated mice for at least 58 days. Hence, the possibility that such abnormal peptides block recall is a real one (Flexner & Flexner, 1968b). The "protection" of memory from the action of puromycin afforded by acetoxycyclohexamide and cyclohexamide may occur because these latter agents suppress the formation of the abnormal peptides. The recovery of memory produced by injections of inorganic solutions into previously puromycin-injected subjects may result from a displacement of peptidal puromycin from the blocked synaptic sites. When the blockage is thereby removed, normal transmission and recall of information can proceed.

Further work on this problem by Roberts, Flexner, and Flexner (1970) suggested that the blocked postsynaptic sites may be adrenergic receptors—that is, receptors for impulses transmitted across synapses by norepinephrine. They further suggest that "a stable modification of adrenergic sites may be involved in the formation and persistence of the memory trace" (p. 312). This proposition is not necessarily in conflict with Deutsch's (1969, 1973) view that the cholinergic system is involved in memory. Roberts and his associates suggest that the two systems may be involved in memory in an interactive fashion. For example, it is possible that the adrenergic system acts to increase the sensitivity of the cholinergic system, or, as Burn (1965) suggests, acetylcholine may mediate the release of norepinephrine.

The puromycin data underscore two problems inherent in neuropsychological research. First, they point out the pitfalls involved in assuming that a retention deficit necessarily reflects a loss of consolidation skills. Second, the puromycin data demonstrate the danger of assuming that a drug's effects on learning and memory processes are due to the action—for example, inhibition of protein synthesis—for which the drug was administered.

The Effects of Induced Electrical Silence in the Hippocampus on Later Retention. Earlier, I indicated that one of the effects of puromycin is to produce abnormalities in hippocampal EEG patterns. In light of this observation, an interesting series of experiments suggested itself to Carlton and his associates. They wondered if it would be possible to produce retention deficits, in the absence of significant protein-synthesis inhibition, by inducing "electrical silence" in the hippocampus. For a review of their work, the reader should refer to a chapter by Carlton and Markiewicz (1973).

A simple conditioned emotional response (CER) paradigm was used in these investigations. During the first session, thirsty rats were allowed to lap water from a drinking tube in the test chamber. During training on the next day, a tone was presented several times, and the termination of this auditory signal was accompanied by brief, inescapable, painful electric shock. Twenty-four hours after the tone/shock conditioning trials were presented, intrahippocampal injections of 25% potassium chloride (KCl) were given to the rats. KCl solutions of this strength have been employed in a number of studies to effect temporary, reversible lesions of neural tissue (see Schneider, 1973, for a review). In the studies by Carlton and his colleagues, the behavior of KCl-injected rats was compared with that of similarly trained control animals that had had isotonic saline injected into their hippocampi.

Three days after the intracerebral injections, the animals were returned to the chamber and tested for their retention of the tone/shock association. It should be noted that the intervals used by Carlton between original training and injection (24 hours) and between injection and retention tests (3 days) were the same as those successfully used by the Flexner group to demonstrate the puromycin effect. In Carlton's research, retention testing involved the following procedure.

The animals were returned to the testing chamber in a water-deprived state. After a rat had emitted 100 licks at the drinking tube, the tone that had previously been associated with shock was sounded. The auditory signal remained on until the subject made an additional 10 licks or for a maximum of 300 seconds. The behavior exhibited by the saline-injected control rats and the KCl-injected experimental animals was found to be quite different. While the saline-administered rats showed complete suppression of licking during presentation of the tone (CER), the animals that had received intrahippocampal injections of 25% KCl solution showed almost no suppression of licking. In addition, and as shown in Figure 13-6, these researchers found that the magnitude of the retention deficit bore a direct relationship to the duration of the electrical silence induced by the KCl injections. That is, the longer the electrical silence induced by KCl administrations, the shorter the duration of suppression of licking suppressed during retention testing three days later.

The retention deficits produced by electrical silence in the hippocampus are thus similar to those yielded by puromycin administrations. Similar effects of intrahippocampal injections of KCl solutions on conditioned suppression (CER) have been reported by Hughes (1969) and by Kapp and Schneider (1971). Henderson, Henderson, and Greene (1973) have also shown that intrahippocampal KCl administrations disrupt passive-avoidance and alternation performance. The similarity between the effects of KCl and of puromycin injections does not necessarily imply, however, that the two disrupt identical physiological processes. The EEG abnormalities occurring after administration of these two agents may arise from two

Figure 13-6
Suppression time
(the amount of time
that elapsed before
the animal emitted
10 licks following
presentation of the
tone associated with
shock), plotted as a
function of minutes
of electrical silence
in the hippocampus.
From "Studies on
the Physiological
Bases of Memory,"
by P. L. Carlton
and B. Markiewicz.
In E. Stellar and J.
M. Sprague (Eds.),
Progress in
Physiological
Psychology *(Vol. 5).*
Copyright 1973 by
Academic Press, Inc.
Reprinted by
permission.

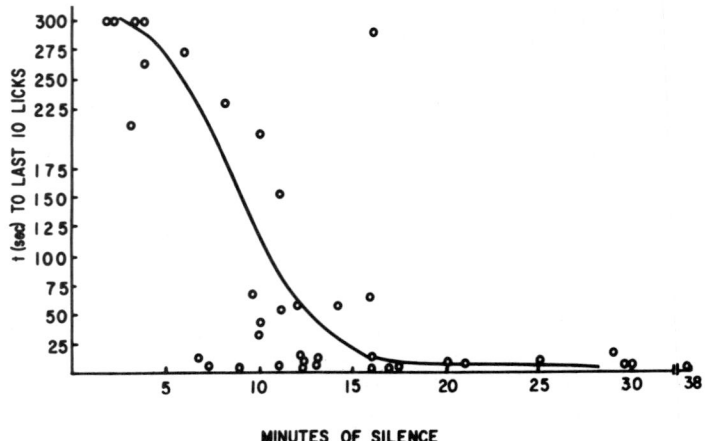

MINUTES OF SILENCE

different causes. Further, the nature of the KCl-induced retention deficit is unclear. It could reflect a disruption of either consolidation or recall processes. If the KCl effect results from the same physiological factors as does the puromycin effect, it is likely that the KCl-induced retention deficits reflect an inability to recall stored information rather than a disruption of consolidation processes.

The Effects of Anisomycin on Memory Processes. The puromycin data cannot be used to substantiate the theory that protein macromolecules form a template for permanent memory, but there are data from investigations that used other protein-synthesis inhibitors that provide strong support for this view. For example, in research into the effects of inhibition of protein synthesis on retention of a passive-avoidance task, Flood, Rosenzweig, E. L. Bennett, and Orme (1973, 1974) used anisomycin as their amnesic agent. Anisomycin is an effective blocker of cerebral protein synthesis, but its side effects are not as severe as those of the other protein-synthesis inhibitors I've discussed. Its effects on the EEG, as compared with those of puromycin and cyclohexamide, have not yet been reported. The chief advantage of anisomycin over other protein-synthesis inhibitors is that it doesn't have severe toxic effects. Therefore, successive doses of anisomycin can be applied to vary the length of time after training during which protein synthesis is suppressed.

In the research conducted by Flood and his associates, a one-trial step-through passive-avoidance training paradigm was used. The apparatus consisted of two adjacent compartments—one black and one white—separated by a small hole. Fifteen minutes after receiving a subcutaneous injection of anisomycin, the mice were placed in the black compartment. Twenty seconds later, the light was turned on in the white compartment, and a door covering the hole between the two compartments was opened. Foot-shock was delivered to the animal five seconds after it entered the white compartment and continued until it returned to the black side. Retention testing procedures were the same as those used during original training except that no shock was given. Latencies, to a maximum of 300 seconds, to enter the white compartment were recorded. Amnesia was defined as a latency of 20 seconds or less.

The most important results of the inquiries by Flood and his associates concerned the effects of varying the length of protein-synthesis inhibition on retention of this previously acquired habit. If protein synthesis does indeed serve as the basis for the formation of permanent memory traces, then it would be predicted that, the longer protein synthesis is inhibited, up to some maximally effective length of time, the greater will be the memory loss. Flood's experiments confirmed this prediction. For example, in one experiment it was found that a single pretraining injection inhibited cerebral protein synthesis 80% or more for two hours; a second injection given two hours after the first maintained this degree of suppression for a total of four hours. It was found that the two successive injections caused significantly more amnesia than did the single injection when animals were given a retention test a week after original training. Hence, increasing the duration of inhibition of protein synthesis yielded greater amnesia for the passive-avoidance problem.

Similarly, Squire and Barondes (1974) and Squire and Davis (1975) have shown that administration of anisomycin prior to training yields impaired memory for an object discrimination in mice tested for retention 5, 7, or 14 days after original training. Control mice were injected with saline solution. It is interesting to note that they found no effects of anisomycin on the rate of original learning despite the fact that protein synthesis was inhibited by over 90% during this period. In contrast to Flood and his associates, however, they reported that the degree of amnesia produced by the drug did not differ as a function of the duration of inhibition of protein synthesis after training. Rather, they found that the extent of amnesia was directly related to the degree of protein-synthesis inhibition occurring during training. This latter conclusion was based on the finding that lower doses of anisomycin administered before training produced less protein-synthesis inhibition and less amnesia. These results are also supportive of the theory that protein molecules serve as a template for memory. The divergence of these findings from those reported by Flood and his associates probably resulted from differences in the tasks used in their experiments.

The anisomycin data provide some of the strongest support to date for the theory that protein synthesis is required for and provides the substrate underlying permanent memory. More research is needed with this drug, and other actions of anisomycin, besides its suppression of protein synthesis, need clarification. For example, the effects of anisomycin on cerebral EEG patterns have not yet been reported. Further, it is uncertain whether anisomycin interferes with the formation of memory traces as information is consolidated or whether, on the other hand, this agent blocks the recall of stored information. Because of anisomycin's low toxicity and mild side effects, this drug will provide a valuable tool for experimental investigations of memory.

Cyclohexamide and the Reminder Effect. Amnesia for a previously acquired step-through passive avoidance also results from either subcutaneous (Flood, Rosenzweig, Bennett, & Orme, 1972) or intrahippocampal (Eichenbaum, 1975) administrations of the protein-synthesis inhibitor cyclohexamide. Examination of the nature of the cyclohexamide-induced amnesia in this experimental situation has led some researchers to conclude that the cyclohexamide interfered with recall rather than with original information storage (Quartermain, McEwen, & Azmitia, 1970, 1972). Quartermain and his associates drew this conclusion on the basis of their finding that a reminder effect similar to that seen after ECS could be demonstrated in cyclohexamide-treated rats. As discussed in Chapter 12, the *reminder effect* refers to the finding that recovery from amnesia can be produced by exposing the animals to elements of the training situation. This recovery phenomenon argues for the view that the effect of the amnesia-inducing agent is to make previously stored information inaccessible rather than to disrupt the initial consolidation of this information.

As indicated, Quartermain and his associates demonstrated the reminder effect in cyclohexamide-induced amnesic subjects. Furthermore, the reminder effect could even be demonstrated when cyclohexamide doses far in excess of those normally needed to produce total amnesia were administered to the rats. Hence, in these studies it does not appear as if the recovery can be explained by saying that the original amnesia produced was only partial—an explanation that has been offered for the reminder effect following ECS-induced amnesia.

The issue of whether protein-synthesis inhibitors produce consolidation or retrieval impairments cannot be satisfactorily resolved at present. The evidence reviewed suggests that at least some of the retention losses result from recall deficits. As I suggested in my review of the ECS phenomenon, it is certainly possible that amnesic agents exert both retroactive and proactive influences over memory processes. Protein-synthesis inhibitors may interfere with both the process of initial memory storage and the ability to recall or retrieve previously consolidated information.

For a number of years, investigators of the memory-consolidation process have contended that changes at the molecular level serve as a template for the memory trace, but only in the past 15 years has evidence to support this supposition emerged. We have examined some of these findings in this chapter. Unfortunately, this field of inquiry is so young that in some instances more questions than answers have emerged from the experiments. Nevertheless, in its infancy, research examining the molecular basis of memory has already established itself as a most promising approach to unraveling the mystery of the brain's operations.

Chapter Summary and Conclusions

Attempts to discover the biochemical substrates of the memory trace were reviewed in this chapter. The four broad areas of inquiry examined were (1) the effects of environmental enrichment on brain indexes, (2) changes in brain chemistry following learning and performance, (3) the transfer of memory by brain extracts, and (4) the effects of antimetabolite drugs—that is, RNA- or protein-synthesis inhibitors—on acquisition and recall. The substrates of memory must ultimately be traced to the cellular level since some changes in the characteristics of synaptic transmission between brain cells must serve as the basis for alterations in the electrical activity of neurons as they convey information into or out of memory.

It was shown that the brain does indeed react differently as a function of varied environmental or training experiences. The chief problem with studies using this approach is determining whether the observed changes in neural indexes were specifically related to the encoding of information. Great promise for research efforts of this type is held out by investigations by Hydén and his colleagues, which have demonstrated the synthesis of unique, brain-specific protein in regions of the brain specifically involved in the task being mastered. Whether the synthesis of this protein is related to consolidation processes or to performance variables is not clear at this time.

Since its beginning, experimentation on transfer of learned information by brain extracts has been the most controversial area of research in neuropsychology. Unfortunately, this field of inquiry has been plagued by a lack of replicated observations, inadequate controls, and improper statistical analyses of the data. Nevertheless, the transfer effect appears to be a real phenomenon. Whether actual stored information or general activation is transferred from the donor to the recipient has been hotly debated. It was suggested that, in evaluating the memory-transfer experiments, scepticism is warranted. This is because the biological mechanisms that would be required to produce such a transfer of information have simply not been shown to exist. In addition, the memory-transfer hypothesis requires that a unique macromolecule be synthesized for each response that an organism learns to make. This proposition runs counter to all of our understanding of neural processes.

In the final section of this chapter, the effects of antimetabolite drugs on memory processes were examined. It was shown that administration of these agents does indeed yield retention deficits. However, several interpretative problems regarding these findings were noted. First, it was shown that the amnesic effects were not necessarily related to the effects the drug was administered for. For example, the puromycin-induced amnesia was shown not to be related to the fact that puromycin produces a high degree of cerebral protein-synthesis inhibition. Rather, the effects of puromycin on retention seem to be related to the formation of abnormal peptides in the presence of this drug or to the disruptive effects of this agent on cerebral EEG patterns. A further question regarding the effects of antimetabolite drugs on memory processes concerns the nature of the amnesic deficit. Research from several studies suggests that the effect of chemically induced amnesia may be to interfere with the expression of memory rather than with the ability to store, or consolidate, recently acquired information.

The question of the nature of the protein-synthesis-inhibition-induced amnesia has not been resolved. It is possible that all amnesic agents, ECS, RNA-synthesis inhibitors, protein-synthesis inhibitors, and others—influence memory by interfering with both the consolidation of new information and the retrieval of information from memory. Since a consolidation impairment is always indexed by a retention deficit in these experiments, this issue may be difficult to resolve. Nevertheless, the data currently available are at least consistent with the theory that protein macromolecules serve as the basis for the encoding or consolidation of memory.

Glossary

ablation: The damaging or surgical removal of brain tissue. Also called *lesion* or *extirpation.* It is the oldest and still most widely used technique for studying brain functions.

absolute refractory period: A period corresponding to the spike potential, which signals membrane depolarization. It is a period during which additional neuronal activity cannot be induced by a stimulus of any strength.

accessory arcuate nucleus (of the thalamus): See cortical relay nuclei.

acetoxycyclohexamide: See antimetabolite drugs.

acetylcholine (ACh): An excitatory synaptic transmitter at the neuromuscular junction—the junction between a muscle and the nerve fiber that activates it. It is also thought to act as an excitatory transmitter in the brain. Neurons that release ACh are called *cholinergic* neurons.

acetylcholinesterase (AChE): An enzyme, found in the synaptic cleft of cholinergic synapses, that inactivates acetylcholine and allows the permeability of the postsynaptic membrane to sodium ions to return to its resting level.

actinomycin-D: See antimetabolite drugs.

action potential: The all-or-none spike discharge that travels down the axon of a neuron. It is also called a *nerve impulse.*

action tremor: See intention tremor.

acute preparation: A surgical preparation in which an animal is experimented on during surgery and then sacrificed at the end of the session.

adaptation: A reduction in the sensitivity or responsiveness of a sensory receptor during prolonged stimulation.

adenohypophysis: See pituitary.

adenosine triphosphate (ATP): A compound made up of adenosine diphosphate (ADP) and a high-energy phosphate bond. The breakdown of ATP and the resultant release of energy provide the energy for cellular processes.

adequate stimulus: The type of stimulus (for example, mechanical, thermal, or electromagnetic) to which a given receptor cell is maximally sensitive.

adipsia: Cessation of drinking.

adrenal cortex: The outer region of the adrenal glands, where adrenocorticosteroids are produced.

adrenalin: A common term for epinephrine.

adrenal medulla: The inner part of the adrenal glands, where epinephrine and norepinephrine are produced.

adrenergic: Neurons that release the excitatory transmitters epinephrine or norepinephrine are called *adrenergic.*

affective: Pertaining to the emotions. *Affective behavior* is synonymous with *emotional behavior.*

affective attack: A pattern of attack behavior, elicited by electrical stimulation of the hypothalamus, in which the animal shows full-blown rage and attacks its prey.

afferent: In a direction toward the center. In neurons, *afferent* means toward the cell body. In the nervous system, *afferent* describes information or pathways arriving at a structure in the central nervous system from the peripheral nervous system. Compare with efferent.

all-or-none law: The law that an action potential will either take place at a certain amplitude or not at all. This property contrasts with the graded potentials of the postsynaptic membrane.

alpha motor neuron: A neuron the cell body of which is located in one of the ventral horns of the spinal cord. Also called *ventral-horn cells,* these neurons are involved in transmitting motor information. The axons of alpha motor neurons synapse with skeletal muscle fibers, whose contractions they control. Since alpha motor neurons ultimately mediate all movements—both reflexive and voluntary—they are often called the *final common pathway.*

alpha waves: See synchronous activity.

amacrine cells: Cells that collect and conduct neural activity within the retina.

Ammon's horn: See hippocampus.

amygdala: See rhinencephalon. A rhinencephalic structure consisting of several nuclei, which are grouped into two nuclear complexes: the basolateral complex and the corticomedial complex. The basolateral nuclear complex includes the lateral nucleus, the basal lateral nucleus, and the basal medial nucleus. The corticomedial complex includes the central, cortical, and medial nuclei.

amygdala fast activity: A synchronous, 40-Hz brain-wave pattern that occurs in the basolateral amygdala complex in response to biologically significant exteroceptive stimuli.

amygdalotemporal fasciculus: A pathway connecting the amygdala with the temporal-lobe neocortex.

androgen: A male sex hormone.

androstenedione: One of the principal male sex hormones.

anestrus: The opposite of estrus. A period during which the sexual receptivity of a female is low or totally suppressed.

angiotensin: A substance produced in the blood, through the action of the enzyme renin, in response to hypovolemia. It has two effects on thirst regulation. First, it results in increased water retention by the kidneys. Second, it has a direct excitatory effect on the hypothalamic regions controlling drinking, so that drinking is initiated.

angstrom (Å): A unit of measure equal to one billionth of a meter.

anion: See ion.

anisomycin: See antimetabolite drugs.

anorexia: A hypersensitivity to the taste quality of food so that only very tasty foods are consumed.

anterior: A directional term indicating toward the front. *Anterior* is used interchangeably with *cephalic* and *rostral.* It is the opposite of posterior.

anterior nucleus (of the thalamus): See association nuclei.

antidiuretic hormone (ADH): A hormone that is released into the blood from the pituitary and that produces increased water reabsorption by the kidneys. Its release is mediated by osmoreceptor cells in the hypothalamus.

antimetabolite drugs: Chemical agents that interfere with cellular metabolic processes involved in RNA and protein synthesis. Two inhibitors of RNA synthesis are 8-azaguanine and actinomycin-D. Protein-synthesis inhibitors include puromycin, cyclohexamide, acetoxycyclohexamide, and anisomycin.

aphagia: Cessation of eating.

aqueous humor: A thin, watery fluid that is an ultrafiltrate of blood and that fills the space between the cornea and the lens of the eye.

arachnoid: See meninges.

archicerebellum: See cerebellum.

ascending reticular activating system (ARAS): See reticular formation.

associated movements: Unconscious, involuntary movements of muscles that accompany the movements of other muscles—for example, the swinging of the arms during walking.

association cortex: Neocortex that is neither sensory nor motor in function and that is assumed to be involved in complex behavior processes such as emotion, learning, and memory.

association nuclei (of the thalamus): Nuclei of the thalamus that receive few, if any, direct projections from ascending sensory fibers; they project to association areas of the neocortex. They have been implicated in complex behavior functions, including learning and memory. They are the anterior nucleus, dorsomedial nucleus, submedial nucleus, lateral dorsal nucleus, lateral posterior nucleus, and pulvinar.

athetosis: See hyperkinetic disorders.

atropine sulfate: A cholinergic blocking agent.

audition: The sense of hearing.

auditory radiations: The fiber pathways between the medial geniculate body of the thalamus and the auditory cortex (superior gyrus of the temporal lobe—areas 41 and 42).

autonomic nervous system: The portion of the nervous system made up of the autonomic nerves and ganglia. The autonomic nervous system controls visceral functions such as heart rate, blood pressure, respiration, gastrointestinal functions, and sweating.

axon: The single extension of a neuron that conducts nerve impulses away from the cell body to other neurons.

axo-axonic synapse: See synapse.

axo-dendritic synapse: See synapse.

axon hillock: A slight elevation in the neuron where the cell body connects to the axon. It is the point at which postsynaptic potentials in the cell body are converted into an action potential.

axo-somatic synapse: See synapse.

ballism: See hyperkinetic disorders.

basal ganglia: The collective term for the nuclei overlying the thalamus that are involved in the control of movement. The basal ganglia include the caudate nucleus, putamen, and globus pallidus. The putamen and globus pallidus together form the lenticular nucleus. The basal ganglia taken together are sometimes called the *corpus striatum.*

basic cutaneous senses: The senses of pain, touch or pressure, cold, and warmth that arise from the skin.

basilar membrane: See inner ear. The organ of Corti, which contains the auditory receptor cells, rests upon and runs the length of the basilar membrane.

basolateral nuclear complex (of the amygdala): See amygdala.

beta waves: See synchronous activity.

bipolar cells: Cells in the retina that relay neural activity from the retina to the brain.

bipolar electrode: See electrode.

brachium of the inferior colliculus: A fiber pathway between the inferior colliculi of the midbrain and medial geniculate body of the thalamus.

brachium of the superior colliculus: A fiber pathway between the superior colliculi of the midbrain and the lateral geniculate body of the thalamus.

bradykinin: A possible chemical mediator of pain sensations arising in the skin.

brain: A collection of nervous tissue and supporting tissue within the skull. The brain and spinal cord together compose the central nervous system.

brain atlas: See stereotaxic method.

brain stem: The combined hindbrain and midbrain upon which the forebrain rests. Sometimes the diencephalon and even the basal ganglia are considered part of the brain stem. When the diencephalon and basal ganglia are included, *brain stem* is being used to refer to everything between the spinal cord and the cerebral hemispheres.

brain wave: An undulation in the electroencephalogram or in the electrical activity of the brain.

broad-band cell: A type of cell in the lateral geniculate body of the thalamus that is either excited or inhibited by all visual stimuli.

bulboreticular facilitatory area: The portion of the descending reticular formation that produces an increase in muscle tone either in specific muscles or throughout the body.

bulboreticular inhibitory area: The portion of the descending reticular formation that produces a decrease in muscle tone.

carbachol: A synthetic cholinergic transmitter.

cardiac muscle: The heart muscle.

cation: See ion.

caudal: See posterior.

caudate nucleus: See basal ganglia.

cellular membrane: The outer boundary of the cell. It is composed of lipids and proteins and controls the flow of substances into and out of the cell.

central canal: A canal that extends the length of the spinal cord and contains cerebrospinal fluid.

central nervous system: The portion of the nervous system that is made up of the brain and spinal cord.

central sulcus: The sulcus dividing the frontal lobe from the parietal lobe.

central summation: The process of algebraic summation of excitatory postsynaptic potentials (EPSPs) and inhibitory postsynaptic potentials (IPSPs). If their sum is above the threshold for firing the neuron, an action potential will be generated.

cephalic: See anterior.

cerebellar peduncles (superior, middle, and inferior): Bilateral fiber bundles that connect the cerebellum to the rest of the brain.

cerebellum: A structure of the metencephalon. It is involved in sensory-motor coordination. It is functionally divided into three regions: archicerebellum, paleocerebellum, and neocerebellum.

cerebrospinal fluid: A clear liquid, similar to blood plasma in composition. It circulates in the sub- arachnoid space—between the pia mater and the arachnoid layers of the meninges. Cerebrospinal fluid is also found in four interconnected spaces, or ventricles, within the brain and in the central canal that extends down the spinal cord. It performs important functions in nutrition of the brain and spinal cord.

chemical stimulation: See intracranial chemical stimulation.

chemoreceptors: Receptors for the senses of smell and taste.

cholinergic: Neurons that release the excitatory transmitter acetylcholine are called *cholinergic.*

chorea: See hyperkinetic disorders.

choroid coat: The middle layer of the eyeball. It is darkly pigmented and serves to darken the interior of the eye.

chronic preparation: a surgical preparation in which an animal has stimulating or recording electrodes permanently implanted in its brain. The experiment is conducted after the animal recovers from surgery.

ciliary muscles: The muscles of the eye that control the shape of the lens so that objects at different distances from the eye can be brought into focus.

cingulate gyrus: See rhinencephalon.

cingulum bundle: A pathway connecting the cingulate gyrus with the hippocampus and the amygdala.

cochlea: A bony, tubular structure in the inner ear that consists of three canals: the scala vestibuli, the scala media, and the scala tympani. The scala vestibuli is separated from the scala media by Reissner's membrane, and the basilar membrane separates the scala media from the scala tympani. The scala media contains the auditory receptor cells and a viscous fluid called *endolymph* or *cochlear fluid,* which is set into motion by movements of the stapes against the oval window.

cochlear fluid: Endolymph. *See* cochlea.

cochlear nuclei (dorsal and ventral): The first relay nuclei in the auditory pathway. They are located in the medulla.

complex cell of the visual cortex: A cell that responds to line stimuli, such as bars of light, of a specific orientation anywhere in the field of vision. A complex cell will fire continuously if the line stimulus is moved across the visual field.

concentration gradient: The relative concentration of a substance on two sides of a membrane—for example, the difference between the concentration of a substance in the extracellular fluid and the concentration of it in the intracellular fluid.

cones: Visual receptor cells of the retina. They allow an organism to distinguish color and fine details of stimuli. They will not function under low levels of illumination, as the rods do.

conjugate eye movements: Movement of both eyes simultaneously in the same direction.

consolidation: The process of firmly establishing or stabilizing long-term memory traces.

consolidation rhythm: A synchronous neocortical brain-wave pattern with a frequency of 40 Hz, which has been related by some investigators to processes of memory consolidation and recall.

contralateral: A directional term meaning on the opposite side. The opposite of ipsilateral.

cornea: The frontal portion of the sclera of the eye. It is transparent and allows light to enter. With the lens, it focuses light on the receptive surface of the eye (the retina).

corner detectors: See higher-order hypercomplex cell of the visual cortex.

coronal plane: A flat section perpendicular to the anterior/posterior axis. It is also called a *frontal plane.* It divides the brain into front and back sections.

corpus callosum: A prominent, sickle-shaped band of nerve fibers that crosses between and interconnects the cerebral hemispheres.

corpus luteum: A follicle that has undergone a series of changes following expulsion of the ovum. It secretes large amounts of estrogens, which modify the tissues of the uterus in preparation for implantation of a fertilized egg.

corpus striatum (striate body): See basal ganglia.

cortical relay nuclei (of the thalamus): Nuclei of the thalamus that receive projections from sensory systems and in turn send information to specific sensory projection areas of the neocortex. They include the lateral geniculate body (relay for vision), the medial geniculate body (relay for hearing), the posterior ventral nuclear complex (relay for somesthesis and proprioception), the accessory arcuate nucleus (relay for taste), and the lateral ventral nucleus (relay for cerebellar feedback).

corticomedial nuclear complex (of amygdala): See amygdala.

corticospinal tracts (lateral and anterior): Fiber tracts of the pyramidal motor system that descend from the medulla. *See* pyramidal decussation.

cranial nerves: The 12 pairs of nerves that enter the brain directly along the brain stem and connect the brain to the receptors and effectors of the head.

cribiform plate: The bony plate in the nasal cavity through which axonal fibers of the olfactory receptors exit.

cross adaptation: The process by which adaptation to one taste quality significantly affects the taste sensation for a subsequently ingested substance.

cross correlation: A technique of computer analysis of the electroencephalogram that allows a determination of the similarity between two simultaneously recorded patterns of electrical activity. It also allows the experimenter to determine whether the electrical activity is traveling from one structure to another.

cutaneous: Of or pertaining to the skin.

cutaneous senses: See basic cutaneous senses and somesthesis.

cyclohexamide: See antimetabolite drugs.

cytoplasm: The protoplasmic material inside a cell, excluding the cell's nucleus. It consists of proteins, other organic materials and ions in water. The cytoplasm is separated from the extracellular space by the cell membrane.

dark adaptation: A gradual increase in visual sensitivity, under low levels of illumination, that is related to the resynthesis of rhodopsin.

DC potential: See steady potential.

decerebrate rigidity: A condition of extreme muscular and postural rigidity that occurs following transection of the brain stem between the superior and inferior colliculi of the midbrain. It occurs because the normal inhibitory influences exerted by the cortex and basal ganglia over the bulboreticular facilitatory area have been removed.

delta waves: See synchronous activity.

dendrites: The branched extensions of a neuron that receive input from other neurons and conduct this information, in the form of postsynaptic potentials, toward the cell body.

dentate gyrus: See hippocampus.

deoxyribonucleic acid (DNA): Nucleic acid, found in the nucleus of cells, that forms the genetic material—the genes—which make up the chromosomes. DNA controls cellular processes through its direction of protein synthesis.

depolarization: What happens to a neuron when an action potential occurs. Membrane potential is reversed due to a rapid influx of sodium ions.

dermis: The inner layer of the skin. It contains a rich supply of free nerve endings, cutaneous somatosensory receptors, cutaneous glands, and blood vessels. The dermis merges into the subcutaneous tissue without any distinct border.

desynchronized activity: An irregular, low-amplitude brain-wave response.

diencephalon: See forebrain.

disarthria: An inability to perform motor patterns involving a succession or progression of movements due to damage of the cerebellum. In a person suffering this disability, complex skill patterns, such as running, writing, and talking, become almost totally uncoordinated.

dishabituation: The recovery of a habituated response after a single presentation of a novel stimulus.

doctrine of specific nerve energies: A law formulated by Johannes Müller (1838). It states that, regardless of the nature of the initiating stimulus, a given receptor always gives rise to the same psychological experience.

dopamine: See excitatory synaptic transmitter.

dorsal: A directional term indicating toward the top of the brain or the back of an animal. The opposite of ventral.

dorsal horns: The dorsal gray region of the spinal cord, which contains the cell bodies of neurons involved in transmitting sensory information. Contrast with ventral horns.

dorsal root ganglion: A ganglion (grouping of cell bodies) that lies outside the spinal cord and that is formed by the cell bodies of sensory neurons.

dorsomedial nucleus (of the thalamus): See association nuclei.

double-cannula system: A technique used for intracranial chemical stimulation. An outer cannula, which is permanently attached to the skull, serves as a guide through which an injection cannula is introduced. Chemicals are injected through the injection cannula into the brain.

duplicity theory of vision: The theory that the rods and cones of the retina compose two functional systems. The rod system functions at low levels of illumination but is insensitive to color and fine detail. The cones are sensitive to color and fine details but will not operate under low levels of illumination.

dura mater: See meninges.

ECS: See electroconvulsive shock.

efferent: In a direction away from the center. In neurons, *efferent* means away from the cell body. In the nervous system, efferent can refer to impulses arising in one brain region and being sent to another. Compare with *afferent.*

8-azaguanine: See antimetabolite drugs.

electrical gradient: In cell biology, a difference in the concentration of ions on the two sides of a cell membrane, which produces a net electrical change.

electroconvulsive shock (ECS): A procedure in which brief but very intense electric current is passed through a subject's head via electrodes placed on opposite sides of the head. ECS may produce brief periods of unconsciousness, EEG seizures, and convulsions. It is used both clinically, as a psychiatric tool, and experimentally, to produce retrograde amnesia.

electrode: a conductor (usually very thin wire) that is used either to apply electrical current to tissue or to record ongoing electrical responses from the tissue. Electrodes can be either monopolar (single) or bipolar (double). A monopolar electrode is a single wire inserted into the brain. Since current must flow in a closed circuit, an indifferent, or reference, electrode attached to the skull or imbedded in the skin must be used to complete the circuit. Bipolar electrodes consist of two wires placed close together. The current flows through or is recorded between the two tips. Macroelectrodes record the electrical activity of large populations of neurons, while microelectrodes record the firing pattern of individual neurons.

electroencephalogram (EEG): The record of an electroencephalograph.

electroencephalograph: A machine that records the electrical activity of the brain through electrodes attached to the scalp of the subject or implanted in the subject's brain. Its record is called an *electroencephalogram (EEG).*

electromagnetic receptors: Receptors that detect light on the receptive surface of the eye (the retina).

encephalization of function: The process by which the neocortex assumed some of the functions of more primitive brain regions during evolution.

end bulbs of Krause: A type of cutaneous receptor once thought to detect sensations of cold. This theory was never verified.

endocrine glands (system): Internal organs, including the pituitary, thyroid, adrenal, ovary, and testis, that secrete hormones into the blood.

endolymph: Cochlear fluid. *See* cochlea.

end-plate potential: The partial depolarization of a muscle fiber, produced by acetylcholine. It is similar to an excitatory postsynaptic potential.

engram: A memory trace, or a structural change that takes place during learning and serves as the physiological substrate of memory.

entorhinal cortex: Cortex surrounding the ventral hippocampus that is medial to the rhinal sulcus on the ventral surface of the brain.

enzyme: A protein that controls chemical reactions in living tissue.

epidermis: The outer layer of the skin. The epidermis can be subdivided into an outer, dead layer and an inner, living layer. The outer layer contains neither nerve fibers nor blood vessels. The inner layer also has no blood vessels, but it does contain some free nerve endings.

epilepsy: A disorder characterized by abnormal brain-wave patterns. In extreme cases, it may be accompanied by brain-wave seizure activity, loss of consciousness, and convulsions.

epinephrine: A hormone, produced by the adrenal medulla, that arouses the body in emergencies by increasing heart rate, respiration, oxygen uptake, blood flow, and so on. *See also* excitatory synaptic transmitter.

equilibrium potential: The potential or voltage difference across a cell membrane that exists when electrical and concentration gradients are in balance and no other forces are tending to move a type of ion either into or out of the cell.

equipotentiality: The principle developed by Lashley to describe the finding that all regions of a specific sensory area of the neocortex were equally capable of maintaining a discrimination habit based on the sensory modality being investigated. For example, any part of the visual cortex was capable of maintaining a visual pattern discrimination.

ESB: Electrical stimulation of the brain. It can be either pleasurable or aversive, depending upon the locus and parameters of stimulation. *See* pleasure center, reward system, and self-stimulation.

estrogen: One of the principal female sex hormones.

estrus: A period of heightened female sexual receptivity found in infrahuman mammals.

ethomoxane: An adrenergic blocking agent.

eustachian tube: A canal between the middle ear and the back of the mouth that allows air pressure to be equalized on the two sides of the tympanic membrane.

excitation: Electrical impulses (postsynaptic potentials and action potentials) that are conducted by neurons.

excitatory postsynaptic potential (EPSP): A brief (15 msec) depolarization evoked in a neuron (usually in the dendrites or soma) by the action of excitatory synapses between adjacent neurons. If the EPSP surpasses the threshold for the neuron, an action potential will be generated at the axon hillock.

excitatory synaptic transmitter: A chemical that is released from a presynaptic terminal button and initiates an excitatory postsynaptic potential (EPSP) on the postsynaptic membrane. Some proposed excitatory transmitters are acetylcholine, dopamine, serotonin (5-hydroxytryptamine), histamine, substance P, epinephrine, and norepinephrine.

expectancy wave (E-wave): A steady-potential shift that occurs in humans between presentation of a meaningful stimulus and the reaction to it.

external auditory meatus: See outer ear.

exteroceptive stimulation: Stimulation arising from the environment—that is, outside the body—as in the sensations of vision, audition, taste, and olfaction.

extirpation: See ablation.

extracellular fluid: The liquid found outside of the cells. The extracellular fluid is separated from the intracellular fluid by the cell membrane.

extrapyramidal motor system: The motor system involved in the process of facilitating or "smoothing out" patterns of movement that are initiated by the pyramidal motor system. It originates in diffuse areas of the cortex and synapses with a number of areas (the basal ganglia, several brain stem nuclei, the cerebellum, and the reticular formation) on its descent to the spinal cord.

Factor I: See inhibitory synaptic transmitter.

fasciculus cuneatus: A fiber pathway of the medial lemniscal system that conducts somesthetic sensory impulses from the arms and upper trunk to the nucleus cuneatus in the medulla.

fasciculus gracilis: A fiber pathway of the medial lemniscal system that conducts somesthetic sensory impulses from the legs and lower trunk to the nucleus gracilis in the medulla.

feeding center: See lateral hypothalamic feeding mechanism.

final common pathway: See alpha motor neuron.

fissure: See neocortex.

follicles: Tissue formations in the ovary that produce ova (egg cells).

follicle-stimulating hormone (FSH): A pituitary gonadotrophic hormone that stimulates the growth of follicles in the ovaries of females. In males, it interacts with interstitial cell-stimulating hormone (ICSH) to bring about the complete maturation of spermatozoa.

footplate (of stapes): See middle ear.

forebrain. The portion of the brain composed of the diencephalon and telencephalon. The major structures of the diencephalon are the hypothalamus, the pituitary, the subthalamus, and the thalamus. The telencephalon is made up of the basal ganglia, the rhinencephalon, and the cerebral hemispheres.

fornix: A fiber pathway connecting the septal region with the hippocampus and the hypothalamus.

fovea: The point of the retina on which an image is focused by the lens of the eye. It is densely packed with and occupied only by cones.

free nerve endings: Somesthetic receptors involved in detecting light cutaneous pressure, or touch sensations, and pain.

frequency theory (of auditory pitch perception): The theory that pitch is coded by the vibrating of the basilar membrane at a frequency corresponding to the frequency of the tone. Fibers in the auditory system that then carry impulses from the inner ear also fire at the frequency of the tone being presented, according to this theory.

frontal eye field: Area 6 of the premotor cortex, which controls discrete movements of the head and eyes.

frontal lobe: See neocortex.

frontal lobotomy: A technique of psychosurgery that involves severing the connections of portions of the frontal lobes with the rest of the brain.

frontal plane: See coronal plane.

gamma aminobutyric acid (GABA): See inhibitory synaptic transmitter.

ganglion: A group of nerve-cell bodies outside of the brain and spinal cord. Plural: ganglia.

ganglion cells: Cells in the retina that relay neural activity from the retina to the brain.

glia cells: Cells in the central nervous system that perform important nutritive and regulatory roles in nerve-cell function. Some theorists have proposed that they are involved in short-term memory storage.

globus pallidus: See basal ganglia.

glomerulus: Groups of dendrites and cell bodies of mitral cells in the olfactory bulbs that synapse with fibers from the olfactory receptors.

glucostatic theory (of hunger regulation): The theory that hunger reflects an attempt on the part of an animal to keep glucose levels constant in the body.

glycine: See inhibitory synaptic transmitter.

gonadotrophic hormones: Hormones released by the

anterior pituitary (adenohypophysis) that control the hormonal secretory activities of the gonads (testes and ovaries).

gonads: Ovaries of the female and testes of the male.

graded potential: The size of a postsynaptic potential is graded, in that it depends directly on the size of the stimulus initiating it. This contrasts directly with the all-or-none activity of axons.

gray matter: Regions of the central nervous system containing cell bodies; they look gray. Areas made up of nerve fibers appear white.

gyrus: Plural: gyri. *See* neocortex.

gyrus principalis: A gyrus of the frontal association cortex that appears to be crucially involved in delayed-alternation performance.

habituation: A decrease in the tendency to respond to a behaviorally irrelevant stimulus. The opposite of sensitization.

hair cells: Receptors in the organ of Corti whose mechanical displacement produces neural impulses that provide the basis for auditory sensations.

hair nerve ending: A touch receptor that is coiled around the base of a body hair and is stimulated by any movement of the hair around which it is entwined. These receptors adapt quickly and probably detect information about an object moving across the surface of the skin.

hedonic system: That system in the brain that mediates experiences of pleasure.

hedonistic: To act in such a way that pleasant things are approached and unpleasant things are avoided.

Hering's opponent-process theory of vision: A theory of color vision, according to which there are three visual pigments in the cones of the retina. One of these mediates white/black vision—that is, white, black, and gray sensations. A second pigment mediates red/green vision, and a third pigment is involved in yellow/blue vision. Contrast with the Young-Helmholtz trichromatic theory of vision.

hertz: Cycles per second. Abbreviation: Hz.

higher-order hypercomplex cell of the visual cortex: A cell that responds to an edge stimulus moving across the visual field as long as the edge is of a specific width. Some of these cells respond specifically to two edges that form a 90° angle and are called *corner detectors.*

hindbrain: The portion of the brain composed of the myelencephalon and the metencephalon. The medulla is the major structure of the myelencephalon. The major structures of the metencephalon are the pons and cerebellum.

hippocampal desynchronization: A fast, irregular, low-amplitude brain-wave response that can be recorded from the hippocampus under certain conditions. Its appearance has been linked to several possible functions of the hippocampus, including inhibition of attention responses to

environmental stimuli, processing of information derived from response-produced, or proprioceptive, stimulation, and regulation of "automatic" motor patterns.

hippocampal theta activity. A synchronous brain-wave pattern with a frequency of 4–7 Hz that can be recorded from the hippocampus under certain conditions. Its appearance has been correlated by different theorists with possible functions performed by the hippocampus in regulating arousal, attention to environmental, or exteroceptive, stimuli, voluntary movement, and memory.

hippocampus (hippocampal formation): See rhinencephalon. The hippocampus is paleocortex and is made up of two interlocking gyri: the dentate gyrus and Ammon's horn.

histamine: A possible chemical mediator of pain sensations arising in the skin. It has also been suggested as an excitatory synaptic transmitter.

histology: A technique for preparing cell tissue for microscopic analysis. The tissue is first hardened or fixed, then sliced into thin sections using a microtome, and finally stained before examination.

horizontal cells: Cells that collect and conduct neural activity within the retina.

horizontal section: A section perpendicular to the sagittal plane. The horizontal plane divides the brain into dorsal and ventral portions.

hormones: Chemical substances secreted by the endocrine glands into the bloodstream and carried to various target organs.

human growth hormone: A growth hormone secreted by the pituitary of individuals of all ages. It promotes growth of tissue throughout the body.

hydrocephalus: A clinical condition due to interference with the absorption of cerebrospinal fluid. It involves the accumulation of excess cerebrospinal fluid in the brain. As a result, the bones of infants afflicted with this disorder are forced apart, until the head reaches an enormous size. The brain is usually severely compressed, and extreme mental retardation results.

hypercomplex cell of the visual cortex: A cell that responds to line stimuli of a specific orientation that do not exceed a certain length.

hyperkinetic disorders: Motor disorders resulting from damage to the basal ganglia; they are characterized by excessive and abnormal movement. Examples are chorea, athetosis, and ballism. Parkinson's disease has both hyperkinetic and hypokinetic (lacking some movement capabilities) components.

hypermetamorphosis. Part of the Klüver-Bucy syndrome. A tendency to be dominated by a compulsive impulse to attend and react immediately to every object.

hypertonia: A significantly increased level of muscle tone that tends to restrict body movement and facial expression. Hypertonia may result from damage to the basal ganglia.

hypervolemia: A condition of higher-than-normal volume of intravascular (inside the circulatory system) fluids. It results from drinking large amounts of water.

hypokinetic disorders: Motor disorders resulting from damage to the basal ganglia and characterized by a loss of some movement capabilities. Parkinson's disease has some hypokinetic as well as hyperkinetic components.

hypothalamic hyperphagia: A condition of extreme overeating leading to gross obesity. It results from bilateral lesions of the ventromedial hypothalamic nuclei.

hypothalamic-hypophyseal portal vessels: Vessels that allow hypothalamic releasing factors to travel from the hypothalamus to the pituitary.

hypothalamic neurosecretory hormones: See hypothalamic releasing factors.

hypothalamicohypophyseal fibers: Fibers arising primarily in the supraoptic and periventricular nuclei of the hypothalamus. They convey impulses to the posterior pituitary (neurohypophysis).

hypothalamic releasing factors: Hormones, synthesized in the hypothalamus, that travel through the hypothalamic-hypophyseal portal vessels to the adenohypophysis, where they cause pituitary hormones to be released into the blood.

hypothalamus: A group of small nuclei, lying ventral to the thalamus, that forms a junction between the midbrain and the thalamus. It helps to regulate the behavioral expression and physiological concomitants of basic drive states. Through its interactions with the pituitary it regulates endocrine-gland functions.

hypovolemia: Condition of less-than-normal volume of intravascular (inside the circulatory system) fluids from prolonged water deprivation.

immediate memory: See short-term memory.

incus (anvil): See middle ear.

indifferent electrode: See electrode.

inferior colliculus: Primitive midbrain center for hearing. Plural: colliculi.

inferotemporal cortex: Association cortex of the monkey ventrolateral temporal lobe, which is a higher-processing area for learned responses involving vision. Destruction of this region has been shown to produce psychic blindness—a component of the Klüver-Bucy syndrome.

infundibulum: The stalk joining the pituitary to the hypothalamus.

inhibitory interneuron: See reciprocal inhibition.

inhibitory postsynaptic potential (IPSP): A brief (15 msec) hyperpolarization evoked in a neuron (usually in the dendrites or soma) by the action of inhibitory synapses between adjacent neurons. The IPSP makes the neuron less likely than normal to be excited by subsequent excitatory impulses.

inhibitory synaptic transmitter. A chemical that is released from a presynaptic terminal button and that initiates an inhibitory postsynaptic potential (IPSP) on the postsynaptic membrane. Some proposed inhibitory transmitters are glycine, gamma aminobutyric acid (GABA), factor I, and serotonin (5-hydroxytryptamine).

injection cannula: See double-cannula system.

inner ear: The innermost division of the ear. It contains the cochlea, which in turn contains the auditory receptor cells. The inner ear also contains the vestibular system, which is involved in the maintenance of posture and balance.

intention tremor: A disorder resulting from damage to the cerebellum. When the afflicted individual moves a limb to a new position, the limb overshoots the mark. Due to the overshoot, movement is initiated in the opposite direction. The corrective movements occur repeatedly as each pass overshoots the intended destination. As a result, the limb will oscillate several times before it finally arrives at its intended destination.

interneuron: A neuron that lies between and synapses with two other neurons. Also called an *internuncial neuron.*

internuncial neuron: See interneuron.

interstitial cell-stimulating hormone (ICSH): A pituitary gonadotrophic hormone that regulates secretion of testosterone by the male testes.

intracellular fluid: The liquid found inside the cell. The intracellular fluid is separated from the extracellular fluid by the cell membrane.

intracranial chemical stimulation: The process of injecting chemicals directly into brain tissue to either stimulate or temporarily ablate the tissue.

intralaminar nuclei (of the thalamus): See intrinsic nuclei.

intrinsic nuclei (of the thalamus): Nuclei of the thalamus that interconnect nuclei within the thalamus and connect the thalamus with other subcortical structures. They have no projections to the neocortex. Functionally, these nuclei are probably involved in attention shifts and in integration of visceral impulses that mediate pain. They are also called the *subcortical, intralaminar,* or *midline nuclei* of the thalamus.

ion: An atom that has lost or gained one or more electrons and thereby obtained a net electrical charge. A cation is a positively charged ion, and an anion is a negatively charged ion.

ipsilateral: A directional term meaning on the same side. The opposite of contralateral.

iris: The colored part of the eye at the front of the eye. It contains muscle fibers that control the size of the pupil and thereby regulate the amount of light falling on the receptive surface of the eye (the retina).

K-complexes: See Stage 2 sleep.

Klüver-Bucy Syndrome: An abnormal pattern of behavior in monkeys resulting from bilateral removal of the temporal lobes. It is characterized by hypersexuality, a loss of aggressiveness, and dramatic alterations in reactions to objects in the environment. *See* psychic blindness, oral tendencies, hypermetamorphosis.

Korsakoff's psychosis: An extreme memory deficit involving an inability to add recently acquired information to long-term memory. It is associated with brain damage resulting from chronic alcoholism.

lateral: A directional term indicating toward the side. Contrast with medial.

lateral dorsal nucleus (of the thalamus): See association nuclei.

lateral fissure: The sulcus that separates the temporal lobe from the parietal lobe.

lateral geniculate body (of the thalamus): See cortical relay nuclei.

lateral hypothalamic feeding mechanism: The process whereby the lateral hypothalamic area, when stimulated, causes a well-fed animal to start eating and, when lesioned, causes aphagia (cessation of eating) and adipsia (cessation of drinking) leading to death unless the animal is maintained by tube feeding. If the animal is tube fed, it goes through a series of four stages of recovery of eating and drinking called the *lateral hypothalamic syndrome.*

lateral hypothalamic syndrome: A series of four stages in the recovery of eating and drinking behavior following lateral hypothalamic lesions.

lateral lemniscus: A fiber path carrying auditory impulses from the dorsal cochlear nucleus and the superior olivary complex to the inferior colliculi.

lateral posterior nucleus (of the thalamus): See association nuclei.

lateral ventral nucleus of the thalamus: A thalamic nucleus that operates in conjunction with the basal ganglia to regulate movement. *See* cortical relay nuclei.

lens: A transparent structure behind the pupil of the eye that focuses light waves on the receptive surface of the eye (the retina).

lenticular nucleus: See basal ganglia.

lesion: See ablation.

limbic system: See rhinencephalon.

lipostatic theory (of hunger regulation): The theory that animals are sensitive to the overall amount of fat stored in their bodies and alter their food intake to maintain an optimal fat level.

longitudinal plane: See sagittal plane.

long-term memory: Information that has been relatively permanently stored in the brain. Long-term memory is thought to be due to some structural or physiological alteration at the synaptic level.

lordosis: A response shown by a quadruped female when she is mounted from the rear by a male. It consists of arching the back and raising and exposing the genitalia.

luteinizing hormone (LH): A pituitary gonadotrophic hormone that acts together with follicle-stimulating hormone (FSH) to accelerate growth of follicles in the ovaries.

macroelectrode: See electrode.

macula: The central region of the retina, it is occupied predominantly by cones. It contains the fovea—the point of the retina on which the lens of the eye focuses an image.

malleus (hammer): See middle ear.

mammilotegmental tract: A fiber pathway joining many regions of the hypothalamus to the brain stem reticular formation.

mammilothalamic tract: A fiber pathway joining the mammillary region of the hypothalamus with the anterior nucleus of the thalamus—an association nucleus.

mass action: Principle developed by Lashley to account for the effects of cortical lesions on maze learning. He found that the severity of the performance deficit was directly related to the amount of bilateral damage to the cortex, regardless of its locus. The principle of mass action was also found to be applicable to complex learning in monkeys.

massa intermedia: A bridge between the two halves of the thalamus.

mechanoreceptors: Receptors that detect bending, or displacement, of either the receptor or cells adjacent to it.

medial: A directional term indicating toward the midline, or middle. Contrast with lateral.

medial forebrain bundle: A fiber pathway joining the anterior and lateral hypothalamus to rhinencephalic regions.

medial geniculate body (of the thalamus): See cortical relay nuclei.

medial lemniscal system: One of the neural systems involved in conducting somesthetic sensory impulses in the brain. The other is the spinothalamic system.

medial lemniscus: A fiber tract carrying taste sensations from the nucleus solitarius in the medulla to the accessory arcuate nucleus of the thalamus and somatosensory sensations from the medulla to the posteroventral nuclear complex of the thalamus.

medial thalamocortical radiations: Fiber pathways between the anterior nucleus of the thalamus and the cingulate gyrus.

medulla oblongata: The major structure of the myelencephalon, it contains vital nuclei involved in the regulation of such autonomic processes as respiration, heart action, and gastrointestinal function.

Meissner's corpuscle: A touch or pressure receptor of the skin that detects the texture of objects. This receptor is very abundant in the fingertips, lips, and other areas of the skin where the touch modality is particularly sensitive. These receptors adapt very rapidly and so are probably very sensitive to objects moved across the skin.

memory retrieval: The process of retrieving information stored in long-term memory.

meninges: Protective membranes (dura mater, pia mater, and arachnoid) that surround the brain and spinal cord.

mesencephalon: See midbrain.

metencephalon: See hindbrain.

microelectrode: See electrode.

micron: A unit of measure equal to a hundred thousandth of a meter.

microtome: See histology.

microvilli: Fine, finger-like extensions of taste receptors that increase the receptive surface of the taste cells.

midbrain: The most recently evolved portion of the brain that still retains the basic tubular structure of the spinal cord. It contains the superior and inferior colliculi. Also called the *mesencephalon.*

middle ear: A small air-filled cavity between the tympanic membrane and the inner ear. Suspended in the middle-ear space are three small bones, or ossicles, called the *malleus, incus,* and *stapes.* Vibrations in this chain of ossicles transmit sound waves from the tympanic membrane to the inner ear. The footplate of the stapes fits up against the oval window of the inner ear.

midline nuclei (of the thalamus): See intrinsic nuclei.

mitochondrion: Plural: mitochondria. The so-called power plants of cells. It is possible that the mitochondria synthesize synaptic transmitters.

mitral cells: Neurons whose cell bodies are in the glomerulus of the olfactory bulbs. They receive inputs from olfactory receptor cells, and their axons form the olfactory nerve.

monopolar electrode: See electrode.

motor end plate: See neuromuscular junction.

motor unit: A motor neuron and the muscle fibers that it activates.

myasthenia gravis: A disease characterized by severe muscle fatigue and paralysis. It occurs either because the sole feet in the neuromuscular junction are unable to secrete adequate amounts of acetylcholine or because the postsynaptic membrane (muscle fiber) has lost its normal sensitivity to this transmitter.

myelencephalon: See hindbrain.

myelinated: See myelin sheath.

myelin sheath: A fatty covering around the axon that is formed by Schwann cells in the peripheral nervous system and by neuroglia in the central nervous system. Axons with a well-developed myelin sheath are called *myelinated fibers,* while axons with a rudimentary myelin covering are called *unmyelinated fibers.*

myoclonic twitches: Small twitches or jerks in the body muscles that occur during Stage REM sleep. *See* Stage REM sleep.

negative afterpotential: An interval following the relative refractory period of an action potential during which the axon is partially depolarized and can therefore be fired by a subthreshold stimulus.

neocerebellum: See cerebellum.

neocortex: The most recently evolved portion of the brain. It is greatly enlarged in primates, especially humans, and it forms the cerebral hemispheres. The cerebral hemispheres can, for convenience, be divided into four lobes: frontal, parietal, occipital, and temporal. The surface of the cerebral hemispheres of humans is convoluted. The ridges are called *gyri* (singular: *gyrus*); the grooves are called fissures or sulci (singular: sulcus).

nerve cell: See neuron.

nerve impulse: See action potential.

nervous system: The system of cells in the body that is specialized to transmit electrochemical information. It is commonly divided into the central nervous system, the peripheral nervous system, and the autonomic nervous system.

neural tube: The initial stage in the embryological development of the brain.

neuroglia: See myelin.

neurohypophysis: See pituitary.

neuromuscular junction: The synapse-like structure between a motor neuron and the muscle it activates.

neuromuscular synapse: The junctional region between a sole foot of a motor neuron and a muscle-fiber membrane.

neuron: The basic functional cellular unit of the nervous system. It is a cell that is specialized to conduct electrochemical signals, which form the basis for information transmission.

night blindness: A condition in which the rods do not operate, due to a long-term vitamin-A deficiency. Vitamin A is required for the synthesis of rhodopsin, which in turn mediates the sensitivity of the rods to visual processes under low levels of illumination.

nodes of Ranvier: Periodic interruptions (approximately 1 mm apart) in the myelin sheath, at which the axon comes into direct contact with the extracellular fluid.

non-REM sleep: Stages 1–4 of sleep. Sometimes referred to as Slow-Wave Sleep (SWS).

norepinephrine: A hormone produced by the adrenal medulla that arouses the body in emergencies by increasing heart rate, respiration, oxygen uptake, blood flow, and so on. *See also* excitatory synaptic transmitter.

nuclei of raphe: A brain-stem group of nuclei thought to be involved in the onset of Slow-Wave Sleep.

nucleus: In cellular biology, *nucleus* refers to the central dense region of the cell, which is the master control for cellular activities. In neuroanatomy, *nucleus* refers to a collection of nerve-cell bodies, such as the ventromedial nucleus of the hypothalamus.

nucleus cuneatus: A nucleus of the medial lemniscal system that is a somesthetic sensory relay. It is located in the medulla and receives inputs from the fasciculus cuneatus.

nucleus gracilis: A nucleus of the medial lemniscal system that is a somesthetic sensory relay. It is located in the medulla and receives inputs from the fasciculus gracilis.

nucleus locus coeruleus: A nucleus of the caudal pons that is responsible for triggering the inhibition of muscle tone that accompanies the onset of Stage REM sleep.

nucleus solitarius: A nucleus in the medulla that is the first relay for taste sensations arising from the taste receptors. Fibers from this nucleus carry impulses to the accessory arcuate nucleus of the thalamus via a tract called the *medial lemniscus.*

nystagmus: Rapid side-to-side movements of the eyes.

obstinate progression: A disorder resulting from damage to the caudate nucleus of the basal ganglia or to the subthalamus. The animal with this disorder will walk in an almost normal fashion until a barrier is placed in its path. If this happens, the animal will simply butt its head against the barrier and try to keep walking.

occipital lobe: See neocortex.

olfaction: The sense of smell.

olfactory bulb: The area at the base of each cerebral hemisphere where axons from the olfactory receptors synapse.

opponent-process theory of vision: See Hering's opponent-process theory of vision.

opsin: See rhodopsin.

optic chiasm: An area at the base of the brain in front of the pituitary where half of the optic nerve fibers cross to the opposite side of the brain.

optic disc: The blind spot of each eye, where fibers from the ganglion cells collect and exit from the retina. There are no rods and cones in the optic disc.

optic nerve: A nerve composed of axons from the ganglion cells that travel to the optic chiasm.

optic radiations: The fiber pathways of the visual system that transmit signals from the lateral geniculate body of the thalamus to the visual cortex of the occipital lobe.

optic tract: The visual pathway posterior to the optic chiasm. Each pathway has fibers from both eyes.

oral tendencies: Part of the Klüver-Bucy syndrome. A strong and compulsive tendency to examine all objects by mouth.

organ of Corti: A structure resting upon and running the length of the basilar membrane. It contains auditory receptor cells (hair cells) that bend in response to vibrations of the cochlear fluid. This bending produces neural impulses in the auditory nervous system.

osmolality: A measure of the concentration of solutes on either side of a membrane.

osmoreceptors: Neurons that change their firing rate as their volume is changed in response to changes in the osmolality (concentration of solutes) of the extracellular fluid.

osmosis: The movement of water through a membrane in response to an unequal distribution of solutes on the two sides of the membrane.

ossicles: Bones in the middle ear (the malleus, incus, and stapes) that transmit sound waves from the tympanic membrane to the inner ear.

outer cannula: See double-cannula system.

outer ear: The part of the ear that collects sound stimuli. It consists of the pinna (the cartilaginous flappy structure we normally call the ear), the external auditory meatus (ear canal), and the tympanic membrane (eardrum).

oval window: A membrane-covered opening in the outer wall of the inner ear. Vibration of the stapes against the oval window sets the cochlear fluid of the inner ear in motion.

ovulation: The release of an ovum by the ovaries.

ovum: An egg cell.

pacinian corpuscles: A type of pressure or touch receptor that is located deep in the dermis and underlying tissue. They adapt very rapidly and are only excited by very rapid movement of the tissues. They are important for detecting rapid, deep touch or pressure sensations and vibrating stimuli.

paleocerebellum: See cerebellum.

pallium: See neocortex.

Papez circuit: A neuroanatomical system, which Papez (1937) proposed, that regulates emotion. It consists of the hypothalamus, the anterior nucleus of the thalamus, the cingulate gyrus, the hippocampus, and their interconnections. Papez's effort was the first attempt to define a neuroanatomical system mediating behavior.

papillae: Small elevations or ridges of tissue on the tongue, soft palate, hard palate, pharynx, larynx, and other areas of the oral cavity that contain the taste buds.

parabiotic animals: A pair of highly inbred laboratory animals that have been surgically joined together at the intestines so that part of the food ingested by one animal crosses over to and is absorbed by its partner.

parietal lobe: See neocortex.

Parkinson's disease (paralysis agitans): See hyperkinetic disorders.

peripheral nervous system: The portion of the nervous system composed of the spinal and cranial nerves.

periventricular fibers: Fibers making up a pathway joining the hypothalamus and the dorsomedial and midline nuclei of the thalamus.

permeability: The property of a cell membrane that allows substances to pass through it. *Permeability* is often used to describe a cell membrane in terms of the ease with which a substance can pass through it.

phasic phenomena (of Stage REM sleep): See Stage REM sleep.

phrenology: The view that the brain can be separated into different centers or organs, each controlling a separate behavior process.

pia mater: See meninges.

pinna: See outer ear.

pitch: The sensation of sound that is related to the sound-wave frequency. The greater the frequency of a sound, the higher the perceived pitch.

pituitary (hypophysis): A small gland attached to the base of the brain, below the hypothalamus, by a stalk called the *infundibulum.* It is often called the *master gland* because, together with the hypothalamus, it regulates other endocrine glands. It is divided into two lobes: anterior (adenohypophysis) and posterior (neurohypophysis). The functions of the posterior lobe are regulated by nerve fibers arising in the hypothalamus, while the activities of the anterior lobe are regulated by neurosecretions from the hypothalamus.

place theory (of auditory pitch perception): The theory that the essential cues for pitch perception are provided first by the place of stimulation on the basilar membrane and later by the locus of activation of fibers in the auditory pathways.

pleasure center: A region of the brain that an animal will work to have electrically stimulated. Humans report pleasurable experiences following stimulation of such a region.

pons: A structure of the metencephalon. It contains fibers that connect the two hemispheres of the cerebellum and fibers that carry ascending and descending information within the central nervous system. Regions of the pons are involved in certain sleep phenomena.

ponto-geniculo-occipital (PGO) waves: Sharp spikes in the EEG record that originate in the pons, travel to the lateral geniculate body of the thalamus, and arrive at the occipital cortex during Stage REM sleep. *See* Stage REM sleep.

positive afterpotential: A period of decreased excitability or hyperpolarization that immediately follows the negative afterpotential of an action potential. A stimulus must be of greater-than-normal strength to fire an axon during this period. The positive afterpotential results from potassium overshoot; that is, more potassium ions move to the extracellular fluid than are required for electrical recovery.

postcentral gyrus: The cortical receiving area of the somatosensory system (areas 3, 2, and 1).

posterior: A directional term indicating toward the back. *Posterior* is used interchangeably with *caudal.* It is the opposite of anterior.

posterior ventral nuclear complex (of thalamus): See cortical relay nuclei.

postsynaptic inhibition: See inhibitory postsynaptic potential.

prandial drinking: Drinking that is only secondary to eating. The animal will drink only to wet its mouth and thereby make it easier to consume food.

precentral gyrus: See primary motor area.

prefrontal association cortex: The neocortical region anterior to the motor and premotor areas, which is classified as association cortex.

premotor area: The region of the neocortex concerned with gross movement of the limbs (area 6) and discrete movements of the head and/or eyes (area 8).

presynaptic inhibition: A process, involving an axo-axonic synapse, that results in a decrease in the amount of transmitter released at an excitatory synaptic terminal so that the excitatory postsynaptic potential is in turn diminished in size.

primary auditory projection area: The region of the temporal lobe of the neocortex that receives projections from the auditory system (areas 41 and 42). Also called the *superior gyrus of the temporal lobe.*

primary motor area: The neocortical region (precentral gyrus, area 4) concerned with the control of discrete movements. *See also* pyramidal motor system.

primary odors: The odoriferous qualities whose mixture forms the basis of the olfactory sensations we experience. Likely candidates for primary odors are camphoraceous (mothballs), musky, floral, pepperminty, putrid (rotten eggs), ethereal (dry cleaning fluid), and pungent (vinegar).

primary tastes: The taste qualities whose mixture accounts for the broad spectrum of taste sensations we experience. The primary tastes are sweet, sour, bitter, and salt.

primary visual projection area: The region of the occipital lobe of the neocortex that receives projections from the visual system (area 17).

proactive interference: A deficit in the ability to learn new information due to interference from previously learned information. Response perseveration is an example of proactive interference.

progesterone: One of the principal female sex hormones.

propagation of an action potential: The processes involved in conduction of a nerve impulse down an axon.

proprioceptive: Pertaining to sensations arising from movement or body position.

prosencephalon: In embryological development, the portion of the neural tube that later develops into the forebrain.

protein: A large molecule that is composed of chains of amino acids. Proteins are the essential building blocks of living tissue.

psychic blindness: Part of the Klüver-Bucy syndrome. A loss of memory for the significance of objects. *See* inferotemporal cortex.

psychosurgery: The use of brain surgery to treat

disorders that are primarily behavioral in nature.

pulvinar (of the thalamus): See association nuclei.

pupil: The adjustable opening in the iris of the eye that controls the amount of light falling on the receptive surface of the eye (the retina).

puromycin: See antimetabolite drugs.

push-pull cannula system: An intracranial chemical-stimulation technique in which a precision infusion/withdrawal pump is used to inject a small amount of a substance through one tube implanted in the brain and withdraw it through an adjacent one. The technique allows the investigator to apply a much smaller amount of the injected substance than is possible with more traditional methods.

putamen: See basal ganglia.

pyramidal decussation: The location in the medulla where 80% of the descending fibers of the pyramidal motor system cross the midline to control muscle fibers on the opposite side of the body from that in which they originated. They then descend as the lateral corticospinal tract. The remaining 20% of the fibers descend as the anterior corticospinal tract and cross the midline just prior to their termination.

pyramidal motor system: The system of motor pathways in the central nervous system that controls precise, voluntary movements such as those involved in writing, using a typewriter, playing a piano, fielding a baseball, and talking. Most of the cell bodies in this system originate in the precentral gyrus of the neocortex (area 4) and descend directly down the spinal cord to synapse with alpha motor neurons that control muscle contractions or with interneurons that in turn synapse with alpha motor neurons.

quadrigeminal bodies: See inferior colliculus and superior colliculus.

quiet biting attack: A pattern of attack behavior, elicited by electrical stimulation of the hypothalamus, in which the animal quietly stalks its prey, pounces, and kills.

radiation theory (of olfaction): The theory that particles stimulating olfactory receptors differentially absorb and radiate heat and light energy, depending upon their molecular structure. It contended that these processes are responsible for different olfactory sensations.

rapid eye movements (REMs): Movements of the eyes that occur during Stage REM sleep. *See* Stage REM sleep.

recent memory: See short-term memory.

receptor potential: A potential change produced by a stimulus applied to a receptor cell. It is a graded potential, in that its size is directly proportional to the intensity of the stimulus producing it.

reciprocal inhibition: The process by which two sets of neurons controlling antagonistic muscles relate so that one muscle will relax while the other contracts during movement. Also called *Sherington's inhibition.* The relaxation of one of the antagonistic muscle groups is mediated by inhibitory interneurons.

red nucleus: A brain-stem nucleus that operates in conjunction with the basal ganglia in the regulation of movement.

reference electrode: See electrode.

reflex: An automatic, involuntary response to a stimulus, such as the knee jerk.

reflex arc: The neural circuit of a reflex. It extends from the sensory receptor through the spinal cord to the muscle that is activated.

Reissner's membrane: See cochlea.

relative refractory period: The phase of an action potential following the absolute refractory period. During this interval, a new action potential can be triggered only by a stronger stimulus than is normally required.

relaxed wakefulness: A condition of drowsiness characterized by 8–13 Hz alpha activity.

reminder effect: The finding that recovery from an ECS-induced retrograde amnesia may occur if the animals are exposed to some elements of the training situation during the interval between training/ECS treatment and later testing. A similar phenomenon has been shown to occur after cyclohexamide-induced amnesia.

REM-rebound effect: The tendency to make up for lost Stage REM sleep time when deprived of this stage of sleep for several successive sleep periods.

renin: A substance secreted by the kidneys in response to hypovolemia. It is an enzyme that enables one of the plasma proteins to be converted into angiotensin.

repolarization: Electrical recovery of the resting membrane potential following an action potential. Repolarization is accomplished by the movement of potassium ions to the extracellular fluid and is necessary before a neuron can fire again.

response-inhibition deficit: See response perseveration.

response perseveration: The tendency of an animal to persist with a previously rewarded pattern of responding that is no longer appropriate. Also called a *response-inhibition deficit.*

resting membrane potential: The voltage or potential difference that occurs across a cell membrane. In neurons, it is equal to -70 mv. It corresponds to the period when the nerve cell is not firing and is electrically recovered.

reticular formation: A mixture of nerve cells and fibers in the ventral brain stem. It extends from the myelencephalon into the posterior hypothalamus. Descending fibers of the reticular formation influence movement. The ascending reticular formation plays a crucial role in behavior arousal. Hence it is often called the *ascending reticular activating system.*

retina: The receptive surface of the eye. It is densely packed with visual receptor cells—the rods and cones.

retinal receptive field: The region of the retina that influences the firing rate of a cell in the visual cortex.

retinene: See rhodopsin.

retrograde amnesia: Loss of memory for events that immediately preceded brain trauma due to injury or surgery. Long-term memory remains intact.

reverberatory circuit: A circular nervous pathway that can reactivate itself over and over again. In the occipital lobe, nerve fibers from area 17 project to area 18 and through it to area 19. Both area 18 and area 19 send fibers back to area 17, thus establishing potential reverberatory circuits. Some theorists have proposed that short-term memory is mediated by neural activity in reverberatory circuits.

reversible lesion: A temporary ablation of neural tissue, which can be created by cooling the tissue or applying a chemical to it.

reward system: The anatomical areas of the brain electrical excitation of which will sustain self-stimulation.

rhinencephalon: Historically, *rhinencephalon* designated a group of structures thought to process olfactory information. These included the olfactory bulbs and tracts, the septal area, the hippocampus, the amygdala, and the cingulate gyrus. It has now been shown that only the olfactory bulbs and tracts are directly concerned with olfaction. The other structures are concerned with higher behavior processes, including emotion, motivation, learning, performance of learned responses, and memory. The rhinencephalon along with the hypothalamus and certain portions of the thalamus make up the limbic system.

rhodopsin: Also called *visual purple,* it is a visual pigment that mediates the low-illumination sensitivity of the rods. It is a combination of an opsin, or protein material, called *scotopsin* and the yellow pigment retinene.

rhombencephalon: In embryological development, the portion of the neural tube that later develops into the hindbrain.

ribonucleic acid (RNA): A type of nucleic acid found chiefly in the cytoplasm of cells. It is involved in protein synthesis.

rods: Visual receptor cells of the retina. Rods are sensitive to levels of illumination but are insensitive to color and do not allow for the fine-detail vision that the cones provide.

rostral: See anterior.

Ruffini endings: A type of pressure or touch receptor located deep in the dermis and underlying tissue. They adapt very slowly and probably provide information regarding continuous displacement of deep tissue and heavy, continuous pressure. Ruffini endings were at one time thought to transmit sensations of warmth, but that theory was never verified.

sagittal plane: A vertical section extending from the front to the back. It is also called a *longitudinal section.* A medial sagittal section divides the brain into its two hemispheres.

saltatory conduction: The process by which an action potential is conducted along a heavily myelinated axon, appearing to jump from one node of Ranvier to the next.

satiety center: See ventromedial hypothalamic satiety mechanism.

scala media: See cochlea.

scala tympani: See cochlea.

scala vestibuli: See cochlea.

Schwann cells: See myelin.

sclera (sclerotic coat): The "white" of the eye. It forms the outermost layer of the eyeball. The frontal portion of the sclerotic coat is the *cornea.*

scopolamine hydrobromide: A cholinergic blocking agent.

scotopsin: See rhodopsin.

self-stimulation: When an animal works or performs a required response in order to deliver electrical stimulation to its brain.

sensitization: An increase in response tendency as a result of repeated stimulation. The opposite of habituation.

septal area (septum): See rhinencephalon.

septal rage syndrome: The tendency, in some species, to exhibit hyperemotionality and indiscriminate attack behavior following bilateral septal lesions.

serotonin (5-hydroxytryptamine): See excitatory synaptic transmitter and inhibitory synaptic transmitter. Increases in serotonin, thought to be produced by the nuclei of raphe, may suppress the arousal effects of the ascending reticular activating system and lead to Slow-Wave Sleep.

shearing: See tectorial membrane.

Sherington's inhibition: See reciprocal inhibition.

short-term memory: Recently acquired information that has not yet been stored in permanent or long-term memory. Also called immediate or recent memory.

simple cell of the visual cortex: A cell that responds to line stimuli, such as bars of light, of a specific orientation and in a fixed part of the retinal receptive field. It will cease firing if the position of the line stimulus is changed, even though the orientation of the line is maintained.

skeletal muscle: Muscle attached to the skeleton that controls movements and postural reflexes.

sleep spindles: See Stage 2 sleep.

Slow-Wave Sleep (SWS): Used by animal researchers to refer collectively to the non-REM sleep stages 1–4. *Slow-Wave Sleep* is a term used by researchers of human sleep phenomena to denote Stages 3 and 4 combined.

smooth muscle: Muscle that regulates all visceral activity except heart action.

sodium-potassium pump: The mechanism that enables a cell membrane to achieve a balance of sodium and potassium ions between the extracellular fluid and the intracellular fluid—a distribution that is not equal to that which would result from the equilibrium potential. During the resting state, the sodium-potassium pump in neurons moves sodium out of the cell and potassium into the cell.

sole feet: The endings of a motor neuron at a neuromuscular synapse, or junction.

solitary tract (tractus solitarius): A fiber tract that carries impulses arising from the taste buds to the nucleus solitarius in the medulla.

solutes: Particles in solution.

soma: The neuron cell body.

somesthesis: The sensations of pain, touch or pressure, cold, and warmth that arise from the skin (cutaneous senses), muscles, and organs of the body.

spatial summation: The process by which simultaneous excitation of progressively greater numbers of excitatory presynaptic terminals yields increases in the size of an excitatory postsynaptic potential. Inhibitory postsynaptic potentials also exhibit summation.

spatiotemporal: Existing in both space and time.

spectral analysis: A technique of computer analysis of the electroencephalogram that allows a determination of the most common frequency.

spectrally opponent cell: A type of cell in the lateral geniculate body of the thalamus that fires in a manner consistent with Hering's opponent-process theory of vision. For example, some of these cells are excited by red light but inhibited by green. Others react in the opposite way. Additional spectrally opponent cells show an increase in their firing rate to blue light while decreasing their rate of firing to yellow light or vice versa.

sperm: Male reproductive cells.

spike potential: See absolute refractory period.

spinal cord: The bundle of nerve cells and fibers that runs through the spinal column. The spinal cord and the brain together compose the central nervous system.

spinothalamic system: One of the neural systems involved in conducting somesthetic sensory impulses in the brain. The other is the medial lemniscal system.

spinothalamic tracts (ventral and lateral): Fiber pathways carrying somesthetic information from the spinal cord to the posteroventral nuclear complex of the thalamus.

spontaneous alternation: The tendency of normal rats to alternate between the two goal boxes of a T-maze on consecutive trials when no reward is given for responses to either side.

spreading depression: The application of a solution of 25% potassium chloride to brain tissue to yield a reversible lesion.

Stage 1 sleep: A stage of light sleep in which the EEG is desynchronized, as it is during behavior arousal.

Stage 2 sleep: A stage of sleep characterized by sleep spindles (brief bursts of 12–15 Hz activity) and wave patterns called K-complexes.

Stage 3 sleep: A stage of deep sleep defined by an EEG record in which at least 20% but not more than 50% of the record consists of delta waves with a frequency of 2 Hz or less.

Stage 4 sleep: A stage of deep sleep defined by an EEG record in which more than 50% of the record consists of delta waves of 2 Hz or slower.

Stage REM sleep: A stage of sleep characterized by a desynchronized EEG record similar to that observed during Stage 1 sleep. The physiological indexes of Stage REM are divided into tonic and phasic phenomena. The tonic phenomena are the Stage 1 EEG pattern, the theta waves present throughout the hippocampus, and a loss of muscle tone. The phasic phenomena are rapid eye movements (REMs), myoclonic twitches, ponto-geniculo-occipital (PGO) waves, and short-term fluctuations of autonomic activity. Stage REM is correlated with vivid dreaming in humans.

stapes (stirrup): See middle ear.

steady potential (SP): The maintained or nonrhythmic difference of voltage between the surface of the neocortex and the immediately underlying white matter. Steady-potential shifts have been correlated with behavior processes and appear to be related to arousal, attention, and drive level of an animal.

stereochemical theory (of olfaction): The theory that there are differently shaped receptor cells for the primary odors. Molecules of odoriferous substances are also differently shaped, and they produce their effects by fitting into the correct receptor "slots."

stereotaxic instrument: See stereotaxic method.

stereotaxic method: The process of making ablations or implanting electrodes using a stereotaxic instrument. A stereotaxic instrument holds an animal in a fixed position while electrode carriers are adjusted, to allow for precise implantation of lesioning or recording electrodes. The site of implantation is often determined from a brain atlas—a book that indicates where an electrode should be placed in the three principal axes (anterior/posterior, lateral, and vertical) to reach a given brain locus.

stomach distension: Stretching of the stomach due to ingestion of large amounts of solid food and/or liquid.

striated muscle: See skeletal muscle.

stria terminalis: A fiber tract connecting the anterior hypothalamus with the amygdala and the amygdala with the septal area.

subarachnoid space: A space between the pia mater and arachnoid layers of the meninges that contains cerebrospinal fluid.

subcortical nuclei (of thalamus): See intrinsic nuclei.

submedial nucleus (of thalamus): See association nuclei.

substance P: See excitatory synaptic transmitter.

substantia nigra: A brain-stem nucleus that operates in conjunction with the basal ganglia in the regulation of movement.

subthalamus: A transitional zone between the dorsal thalamus and the midbrain tegmentum. It contains nuclei that form part of the extrapyramidal motor system and operate in conjunction with the basal ganglia in the regulation of movement.

sulcus: Plural: sulci. *See* neocortex.

superior colliculus: Primitive midbrain center for vision. Plural: colliculi.

superior gyrus of the temporal lobe: Location of the auditory cortex (areas 41 and 42).

superior olivary complex: A relay in the auditory system, it is located in the pons. It is the first place in the auditory pathway where binaural interactions occur.

synapse: The microscopic junction (100–500Å) between a terminal button of one neuron and a dendrite (axo-dendritic synapse), soma (axo-somatic synapse), or axon (axo-axonic synapse) of another neuron. Neurotransmitters mediate the transmission of information across a synapse.

synaptic vesicles: Small spherical structures found in the terminal buttons of axons; they contain synaptic transmitter substances.

synchronous activity: A very regular pattern of brain-wave activity, in which the waves are of approximately the same height or amplitude and occur at about the same frequency. Synchronous patterns have been given Greek-letter names corresponding to their average frequency—that is, to the number of waves or cycles per second (Hz). Alpha waves = 8–12 Hz, beta waves = 18 Hz and above, delta waves = 0.5–3 Hz, and theta waves = 4–7 Hz.

tactile discs: Touch or pressure receptors of the skin that are very abundant in areas of the body, such as the fingertips, where touch sensitivity is acute. They adapt relatively slowly and are probably involved in our ability to be cognizant of continuous contact of objects with the body.

taste bud: A cluster of cells on the base of the papillae of the tongue, soft palate, hard palate, pharynx, larynx, and other areas of the oral cavity that contains the taste receptors.

tectorial membrane: A membrane suspended immediately above the basilar membrane in the organ of Corti of the middle ear. Differences in the movements of the tectorial and basilar membranes that occur when the cochlear fluid vibrates cause the tectorial membrane to slide

across the basilar membrane. This brushing, which is called *shearing,* produces a generator potential in the auditory receptor cells (hair cells).

tectum: The dorsal surface of the midbrain, which contains the superior and inferior colliculi.

tegmentum: The ventral portion of the midbrain. It contains ascending and descending fiber tracts.

telencephalon: See forebrain.

temporal lobe: See neocortex.

temporal summation: The process by which a new excitatory postsynaptic potential adds to what is left of a preceding excitatory postsynaptic potential. Inhibitory postsynaptic potentials also exhibit temporal summation.

terminal arborizations: The branching of an axon near its end.

terminal button: The end of a terminal arborization. It contains transmitter substance, which is necessary for the transmission of information across the synaptic junction.

testosterone: One of the principal male sex hormones.

thalamus: A structure in the diencephalon that serves to relay information to the cortex.

thermoreceptors: Receptors that are sensitive to changes in temperature.

thermostatic theory (of hunger regulation): The theory that hunger arises in response to a decrease in body temperature and that animals eat in order to keep their body temperature from decreasing. According to this theory, animals stop eating when they become warm.

theta waves: See synchronous activity.

threshold: The lowest level of stimulation or the least amount of depolarization necessary to produce an action potential.

tonic phenomena (of Stage REM sleep): See Stage REM sleep.

tonotopic organization: The view that neurons originating from adjacent parts of the basilar membrane of the organ of Corti are maximally sensitive to specific different tones and remain arranged in a systematic order throughout the different levels of the auditory system.

transorbital leucotome: A device used in a psychosurgical procedure called *transorbital leucotomy.*

transorbital leucotomy: A technique of psychosurgery in which a transorbital leucotome (surgical ice pick) is driven through the bony cavity above the eye and into the base of the frontal lobes. The handle of the leucotome is then swung to sever the fibers in the frontal lobes.

trichromatic theory of vision: See Young-Helmholtz trichromatic theory of vision.

tympanic membrane: See outer ear.

unit recording: Recording the electrical activity of single cells. Records may be made extracellularly or intracellularly.

unmyelinated: See myelin sheath.

ventral: A directional term indicating toward the

base of the brain and the belly side of an animal. The opposite of dorsal.

ventral-horn cell: See alpha motor neuron.

ventral horns: The ventral gray region of the spinal cord, which contains the cell bodies of neurons involved in transmitting motor information. Contrast with dorsal horns.

ventral noradrenergic bundle: A fiber pathway ascending from midbrain nuclei to several limbic system structures. It passes close to the ventromedial hypothalamic nuclei. It has been suggested that damage to this pathway, rather than to the ventromedial nuclei, produces the syndrome of hypothalamic hyperphagia.

ventricles: A system of four interconnected spaces in the brain that contain cerebrospinal fluid.

ventromedial hypothalamic satiety mechanism: The mechanism postulated to account for the fact that stimulation of the ventromedial hypothalamic nucleus will cause a hungry animal to stop eating, and lesioning of it will cause an animal to overeat until it is grossly obese.

visual accommodation: The process of self-adjustment of the lenses of the eyes so that objects at different distances from the eye can be brought into focus.

visual purple: See rhodopsin.

vitreous humor: A clear, viscous, gelatinous substance that fills the space between the back of the lens and the retina of the eye.

white matter: Regions of the central nervous system that are made up of nerve fibers and therefore appear white. Areas comprised of cell bodies appear gray.

Young-Helmoholtz trichromatic theory of vision: A theory of color vision that states that the retina contains three different types of cones, which contain different photosensitive pigments. The different pigments make each cone sensitive to one of the three primary colors (red, green, or blue). Combinations of output from these receptors determine the colors or hues that we see. If the influence of all of these outputs is equal, we will see white. Contrast with Hering's opponent-process theory of vision.

References

Abramov, I., & Gordon, J. Vision. In E. C. Carterette & M. P. Friedman (Eds.), *Handbook of perception* (Vol. 3): *Biology of perceptual systems.* New York: Academic Press, 1973, 327–357.

Adams, H. E., & Calhoun, K. S. Indices of memory recovery following electroconvulsive shock. *Physiology and Behavior,* 1972, *9,* 783–787.

Adams, R. D., & Sidman, R. L. *Introduction to neuropathology.* New York: Blakiston, 1968.

Adey, W. R. Neurophysiological correlates of information transaction and storage in brain tissue. In E. Stellar & J. M. Sprague (Eds.), *Progress in physiological psychology* (Vol. 1). New York: Academic Press, 1966.

Adey, W. R., Dunlop, C. W., & Hendrix, C. E. Hippocampal slow waves: Distribution and phase relationships in the course of approach learning. *Archives of Neurology,* 1960, *3,* 74–90.

Adey, W. R., & Walter, D. O. Application of phase detection and averaging techniques in computer analysis of EEG records in the cat. *Experimental Neurology,* 1963, *7,* 186–209.

Adey, W. R., Walter, D. O., & Hendrix, C. E. Computer techniques in correlation and spectral analyses of cerebral slow waves during discrimination behavior. *Experimental Neurology,* 1961, *3,* 501–524.

Adolph, E. F. Urges to eat and drink in rats. *American Journal of Physiology,* 1947, *151,* 110–125.

Agnew, H. W., Webb, W. B., & Williams, R. L. The effects of stage 4 sleep deprivation. *Electroencephalography and Clinical Neurophysiology,* 1964, *17,* 68–70.

Agranoff, B. W. Biological effects of antimetabolites used in behavioral studies. In D. H. Efron et al. (Eds.), *Psychopharmacology: A review of progress, 1957–1967,* (U. S. Public Health Service Publication No. 1836). Washington, D. C.: U. S. Government Printing Office, 1968, 909–917.

Agranoff, B. W. Further studies on memory formation in the goldfish. In J. L. McGaugh (Ed.), *Chemistry of mood motivation and memory.* New York: Plenum Press, 1972, 175–185.

Agranoff, B. W., Davis, R. E., & Brink, J. J. Memory fixation in goldfish. *Proceedings of the National Academy of Sciences,* 1965, *54,* 788–793.

Agranoff, B. W., Davis, R. E., & Brink, J. J. Chemical studies on memory fixation in goldfish. *Brain Research,* 1966, *1,* 303–309.

Agranoff, B. W., & Klinger, P. D. Puromycin effect on memory fixation in the goldfish. *Science,* 1964, *146,* 952–953.

Ahmad, S. S., & Harvey, J. A. Long-term effects of septal lesions and social experience on shock-elicited fighting in rats. *Journal of Comparative and Physiological Psychology,* 1968, *66,* 596–602.

Aitkin, L. M., Anderson, D. J., & Brugge, J. F. Tonotopic organization and discharge characteristics of single neurons in nuclei of the lateral lemniscus of the cat. *Journal of Neurophysiology,* 1970, *33,* 421–440.

Albert, D. J., & Mah, C. J. Passive avoidance deficit with septal lesions: Disturbance of response inhibition or response acquisition? *Physiology and Behavior,* 1973, *11,* 205–213.

Albert, D. J., & Storlien, L. H. Hyperphagia in rats with cuts between the ventromedial and lateral hypothalamus. *Science,* 1969, *165,* 599–600.

Allen, W. F. Effects of destroying three localized cerebral cortical areas for sound on correct conditioned differential responses of the dog's foreleg. *American Journal of Physiology,* 1945, *144,* 415–428.

Allen, W. F. Fiber degeneration in Ammon's horn resulting from extirpations of pyriform and other cortical areas and from transections of horn at various levels. *Journal of Comparative Neurology,* 1948, *88,* 425–438.

Alpern, H. P., & McGaugh, J. L. Retrograde amnesia as a function of duration of electroshock stimulation. *Journal of Comparative and Physiological Psychology,* 1968, *65,* 265–269.

Alpers, B. J., & Mancall, E. L. *Clinical neurology* (6th ed.). Philadelphia: F. A. Davis, 1971.

Altman, J., & Das, G. D. Autoradiographic examination of the effects of enriched environments on the rate of glial multiplication in the adult rat brain. *Nature,* 1964, *204,* 1161–1163.

Amoore, J. E., Johnston, J. W., Jr., & Rubin, M. The stereochemical theory of odor. *Scientific American,* 1964, *210,* 42–49.

Amsel, A., Glazer, H., Lakey, J. R., McCuller, T., &

Wong, P. T. P. Introduction of acoustic stimulation during acquisition and resistance to extinction in the normal and hippocampally damaged rat. *Journal of Comparative and Physiological Psychology,* 1973, *84,* 176–186.

Anand, B. K., & Brobeck, J. R. Hypothalamic control of food intake in rats and cats. *Yale Journal of Biology and Medicine,* 1951, *24,* 123–140.

Anand, B. K., & Brobeck, J. R. Food intake and spontaneous activity of rats with lesions in the amygdaloid nuclei. *Journal of Neurophysiology,* 1952, *15,* 421–430.

Anand, B. K., & Dua, S. Feeding responses induced by electrical stimulation of the hypothalamus in cats. *Indian Journal of Medical Research,* 1955, *43,* 113–122.

Anand, B. K., Dua, S., & Schoenberg, K. Hypothalamic control of food intake in cats and monkeys. *Journal of Physiology,* 1955, *127,* 143–152.

Anchel, H., & Lindsley, D. B. Differentiation of two reticulohypothalamic systems regulating hippocampal activity. *Electroencephalography and Clinical Neurophysiology,* 1972, *32,* 209–226.

Andersen, P., Bliss, T. V. P., & Skrede, K. K. Unit analysis of hippocampal population spikes. *Experimental Brain Research,* 1971, *13,* 208–221.

Anderson, R. Differences in the course of learning as measured by various memory tasks after amygalotomy in man. In E. Hitchcock, L. Laitinen, & K. Vaernet (Eds.), *Psychosurgery.* Springfield, Ill.: Charles C Thomas, 1972.

Andersson, B. The effect and localization of electrical stimulation of certain parts of the brain stem in sheep and goats. *Acta Physiologica Scandinavica,* 1951, *23,* 8–24.

Andersson, B. Polydipsia caused by intrahypothalamic injections of hypertonic NaCl-solutions. *Experientia,* 1952, *8,* 157–158.

Antelman, S. M., & Brown, T. S. Hippocampal lesions and shuttlebox avoidance behavior: A fear hypothesis. *Physiology and Behavior,* 1972, *9,* 15–20.

Anton, B. S., & Bennett, T. L. Hippocampal lesions during rearing and transfer of perceptual learning in rats. *Physiological Psychology,* 1974, *2,* 523–528.

Artemenko, D. P. Role of hippocampal neurons in theta-wave generation. *Nierofiziologiya,* 1972, *4,* 531–539.

Aserinsky, E., & Kleitman, N. Regularly occurring periods of eye motility and concomitant phenomena during sleep. *Science,* 1953, *118,* 273–274.

Avery, D. D. Intracranial electrical stimulation. In D. Singh & D. D. Avery (Eds.), *Physiological techniques in behavioral research.* Monterey, Calif.: Brooks/Cole, 1975.

Babich, F. R., Jacobson, A. L., & Bubash, S. Cross-species transfer of learning: Effect of ribonucleic acid from hamsters on rat behavior. *Proceedings of the National Academy of Sciences,* 1965, *54,* 1299–1302.

Babich, F. R., Jacobson, A. L., Bubash, S., & Jacobson, A. Transfer of a response to naïve rats by injection of ribonucleic acid extracted from trained rats. *Science,* 1965, *149,* 656–657.

Bandler, R. J., Jr. Facilitation of aggressive behavior in the rat by direct cholinergic stimulation of the hypothalamus. *Nature,* 1969, *221,* 1035–1036.

Bandler, R. J., Jr. Cholinergic synapses in the lateral hypothalamus for the control of predatory aggression in the rat. *Brain Research,* 1970, *20,* 409–424.

Bandler, R. J., Jr. Direct chemical stimulation of the thalamus: Effects on aggressive behavior in the rat. *Brain Research,* 1971, *26,* 81–93. (a)

Bandler, R. J., Jr. Chemical stimulation of the rat midbrain and aggressive behavior. *New Biology,* 1971, *229,* 222–223. (b)

Bard, P. A diencephalic mechanism for the expression of rage with special reference to the sympathetic nervous system. *American Journal of Physiology,* 1928, *84,* 490–515.

Bard, P. On emotional expression after decortication with some remarks on certain theoretical views, Parts I and II. *Psychological Review,* 1934, *41,* 309–329, 424–429.

Bard, P., & Mountcastle, V. B. Some forebrain mechanisms involved in expression of rage with special reference to suppression of angry behavior. *Research Publications of the Association for Research in Nervous and Mental Disease,* 1948, *27,* 362–404.

Barondes, S. H. Effects of inhibitors of cerebral protein synthesis on "long term" memory in mice. In D. H. Efron et al. (Eds.), *Psychopharmacology: A review of progress, 1957-1967* (U. S. Public Health Service Publication No. 1836). Washington, D. C.: U. S. Government Printing Office, 1968, 905–908.

Barondes, S. H. Some critical variables in studies of the effect of inhibitors of protein synthesis on memory. In W. L. Byrne (Ed.), *Molecular approaches to learning and memory.* New York: Academic Press, 1970, 27–34.

Barondes, S. H. Memory transfer. *Science,* 1972, *176,* 631–632.

Barondes, S. H., & Cohen, H. D. Puromycin effects on successive phases of memory storage. *Science,* 1966, *151,* 594–595.

Barondes, S. H., & Cohen, H. D. Comparative effects of cyclohexamide and puromycin on cerebral protein synthesis and consolidation of memory in mice. *Brain Research,* 1967, *4,* 44–51.

Barondes, S. H., & Jarvik, M. E. The influence of actinomycin-D on brain RNA synthesis and on memory. *Journal of Neurochemistry,* 1964, *11,* 187–195.

Beach, F. A. Effects of cortical lesions upon the copulatory behavior of male rats. *Journal of*

Comparative Psychology, 1940, *29,* 193–239.

Beach, F. A. Hormonal factors controlling the differentiation, development, and display of copulatory behavior in the ramstergig and related species. In E. Tobach, L. R. Aronson, & E. Shaw (Eds.), *The biopsychology of development.* New York: Academic Press, 1971, 249–296.

Beach, F. A. Behavioral endocrinology: An emerging discipline. *American Scientist,* 1975, *63,* 178–187.

Beatty, W. W., Beatty, P. A., O'Briant, D., Gregoire, K. C., & Dahl, B. L. Factors underlying deficient passive-avoidance behavior by rats with septal lesions. *Journal of Comparative and Physiological Psychology,* 1973, *85,* 502–514.

Beatty, W. W., & Schwartzbaum, J. S. Enhanced reactivity to quinine and saccharin solutions following septal lesions in the rat. *Psychonomic Science,* 1968, *8,* 483–484.

Beck, L. H., & Miles, W. R. Some theoretical and experimental relationships between infrared absorption and olfaction. *Science,* 1947, *106,* 511.

Beidler, L. M. Dynamics of taste cells. In Y. Zotterman (Ed.), *Olfaction and taste.* New York: Macmillan, 1963.

Békésy, G. von. Zur Theorie des Hörens; Die Schwingungsform der Basilmembran. *Physik Zeits.,* 1928, *29,* 793–810.

Békésy, G. von. *Experiments in Hearing.* New York: McGraw-Hill, 1960.

Benner, R. G., & Radcliffe, G. Induction of conditioned avoidance in unreinforced recipient rats treated with brain extracts from conditioned donors. *Journal of Biological Psychology,* 1970, *12,* 17–20.

Bennett, E. L., Rosenzweig, M. R., & Diamond, M. C. Rat brain: Effects of environmental enrichment on wet and dry weights. *Science,* 1968, *163,* 825–826.

Bennett, E. L., Rosenzweig, M. R., & Diamond, M. C. Time courses of effects of differential experience on brain measures and behavior of rats. In W. L. Byrne (Ed.), *Molecular approaches to learning and memory.* New York: Academic Press, 1969, 55–89.

Bennett, T. L. Evidence against the theory that hippocampal theta is a correlate of voluntary movement. *Communications in Behavioral Biology,* 1969, *4,* 165–169.

Bennett, T. L. Hippocampal EEG correlates of behavior. *Electroencephalography and Clinical Neurophysiology,* 1970, *28,* 17–23.

Bennett, T. L. Hippocampal theta activity and behavior: A review. *Communications in Behavioral Biology,* 1971, *6,* 37–48.

Bennett, T. L. The effects of centrally blocking hippocampal theta activity on learning and retention. *Behavioral Biology,* 1973, *9,* 541–552.

Bennett, T. L. The electrical activity of the hippocampus and processes of attention. In R. L. Isaacson & K. H. Pribram (Eds.), *The hippocampus (Vol. 2): Neurophysiology and behavior.* New York: Plenum Press, 1975, 71–99.

Bennett, T. L., Anton, B. S., & Levitt, L. Stimulus relevancy and transfer of perceptual learning. *Psychonomic Science,* 1971, *25,* 159–160.

Bennett, T. L., & Ellis, H. C. Tactual-kinesthetic feedback from manipulation of visual forms and nondifferential reinforcement in transfer of perceptual learning. *Journal of Experimental Psychology,* 1968, *77,* 495–500.

Bennett, T. L., & Gottfried, J. Hippocampal theta and response inhibition. *Electroencephalography and Clinical Neurophysiology,* 1970, *29,* 196–200.

Bennett, T. L., Hébert, P. N., & Moss, D. E. Hippocampal theta activity and the attention component of discrimination learning. *Behavioral Biology,* 1973, *8,* 173–181.

Bennett, T. L., Nunn, P. J., & Inman, D. P. Effects of scopolamine on hippocampal theta and correlated discrimination performance. *Physiology and Behavior,* 1971, *7,* 451–454.

Berger, H. Über das Elektrenkephalogramm des Menschen. *Archiv für Psychiatrie und Nervenkrankheiten,* 1929, *87,* 527–570.

Berger, R., & Meier, G. The effects of selective deprivation of states of sleep in the developing monkey. *Psychophysiology,* 1966, *2,* 354–371.

Best, J. B., & Rubenstein, I. Maze learning and associated behavior in planaria. *Journal of Comparative and Physiological Psychology,* 1962, *55,* 560–566.

Bianchi, L. The functions of frontal lobes. *Brain,* 1895, *18.*

Black, A. Hippocampal electrical activity and behavior. In R. L. Isaacson & K. H. Pribram (Eds.), *The hippocampus* (Vol. 2): *Neurophysiology and Behavior.* New York: Plenum, 1975.

Black, M., & Suboski, M. D. Incubation and ECS-produced gradients in one-trial and multitrial discriminated-avoidance conditioning in rats. *Journal of Comparative and Physiological Psychology,* 1971, *74,* 325–330.

Blass, E. M., & Epstein, A. N. A lateral preoptic osmosensitive zone for thirst in the rat. *Journal of Comparative and Physiological Psychology,* 1971, *76,* 378–394.

Blum, J. S. Cortical organization in somesthesis. Effects of lesions in posterior associative cortex on somato-sensory function in *Macaca mulatta. Comparative and Physiological Monograph,* 1951, *20,* 219–249.

Blum, J. S., Chow, K. L., & Pribram, K. H. A behavioral analysis of the organization of the parieto-temporo-preoccipital cortex. *Journal of Comparative Neurology,* 1950, *93,* 53–100.

Boitano, J., Lubar, J., Auer, J., & Furnald, M. Effects of hippocampectomy on consummatory behavior and movement-inhibition in rats. *Physiology and Behavior,* 1968, *3,* 901–906.

Bond, D., Randt, C. T., Bidder, T. G., & Rowland, V. Posterior septal fornical and anterior thalamic lesions in the cat. *Archives of Neurology and Psychiatry*, 1957, *78*, 143–162.

Bonner, J. Molecular biological approaches to the study of memory. In J. Gaito (Ed.), *Macromolecules and behavior*, New York: Appleton-Century-Crofts, 1966, 158–164.

Bonner, J. Molecular biological approaches to the study of memory. In J. Gaito (Ed.), *Macromolecules and behavior* (2nd ed.). New York: Appleton-Century-Crofts, 1972, 361–366.

Booth, D. A. Localization of the adrenergic feeding system in the rat diencephalon. *Science*, 1967, *158*, 515–517.

Booth, D. A. Mechanism of action of norepinephrine in eliciting an eating response on injection into the rat hypothalamus. *Journal of Pharmacology and Experimental Therapeutics*, 1968, *160*, 336–348.

Boring, E. G. *A history of experimental psychology* (2nd ed.). New York: Appleton-Century-Crofts, 1950.

Bower, G. H., & Miller, N. E. Rewarding and punishing effects from stimulating the same place in the rat's brain. *Journal of Comparative and Physiological Psychology*, 1958, *51*, 669–674.

Brady, J. V. The paleocortex and behavioral motivation. In H. F. Harlow & C. N. Woolsey (Eds.), *Biological and biochemical bases of behavior*. Madison: University of Wisconsin Press, 1958, 193–235.

Brady, J. V. Temporal and emotional effects related to intracranial electrical self-stimulation. In E. R. Ramey & D. S. O'Doherty (Eds.), *Electrical studies on the unanesthetized brain*. New York: Hoeber, 1960, 52–77.

Brady, J. V. Motivational-emotional factors and intracranial self-stimulation. In D. E. Sheer (Ed.), *Electrical stimulation of the brain*. Austin, Texas: University of Texas Press and Hogg Foundation for Mental Health, 1961, 413–430.

Brady, J. V., & Nauta, W. J. H. Subcortical mechanisms in emotional behavior: Effective changes following septal forebrain lesions in the albino rat. *Journal of Comparative and Physiological Psychology*, 1953, *46*, 339–346.

Brady, J. V., & Nauta, W. J. H. Subcortical changes in emotional behavior: The duration of affective changes following septal and habenular lesions in the albino rat. *Journal of Comparative and Physiological Psychology*, 1955, *48*, 412–420.

Brain, W. R., & Walton, J. N. *Brain's diseases of the nervous system* (7th ed.). London: Oxford University Press, 1969.

Brattgård, S. O. The importance of adequate stimulation for the chemical composition of retinal ganglion cells during early postnatal development. *Acta Radiologica*, 1952, *Suppl. 96*, 1–80.

Braud, L. W., & Braud, W. G. Biochemical transfer of relational responding (transposition). *Science*, 1972, *176*, 942–943.

Braud, W. G., & Broussard, W. J. Effects of puromycin on memory for shuttle box extinction in goldfish and barpress extinction in rats. *Pharmacology, Biochemistry and Behavior*, 1973, *1*, 651–656.

Brazier, M. A. B. *A history of the electrical activity of the brain: The first half century*. London: Pitmar Medical Publishers, 1961.

Brierley, J. B., & Beck, E. The effects upon behavior of lesions in the dorsomedial and anterior thalamic nuclei of cat and monkey. In G. E. W. Wolstenholme & C. M. O'Conner (Eds.), *Neurological basis of behavior*. Boston: Little, Brown, 1958.

Brobeck, J. R. Food intake as a mechanism of temperature regulation in rats. *Federation Proceedings of the American Physiological Society*, 1948, *7*, 13.

Brobeck, J. R., Tepperman, J., & Long, C. N. H. Experimental hypothalamic hyperphagia in the albino rat. *Yale Journal of Biology and Medicine*, 1943, *15*, 831–853.

Broca, P. Remarques sur le siège de la faculté du language articulé. *Bulletin de la Société Anatomique de Paris*, 1861, *6*, 330–357.

Brody, E. B., & Rosvold, H. E. Influence of prefrontal lobotomy on social interaction in a monkey group. *Psychosomatic Medicine*, 1952, *14*, 406–415.

Brown, H. M., Dustman, R. E., & Beck, E. C. Experimental procedures that modify light response frequency of regenerated planaria. *Physiology and Behavior*, 1966, *1*, 245–249. (a)

Brown, H. M., Dustman, R. E., & Beck, E. C. Sensitization in planarian. *Physiology and Behavior*, 1966, *1*, 305–308. (b)

Brown, P. K., & Wald, G. Visual pigments in single rods and cones of the human retina. *Science*, 1964, *144*, 45–52.

Brown, S., & Schaefer, E. A. An investigation into the functions of the occipital and temporal lobe of the monkey's brain. *Philosophical Transactions of the Royal Society of London*, 1888, *179B*, 303–327.

Brown, T. S. General biology of sensory systems. In B. Scharf (Ed.), *Experimental sensory psychology*. Glenview, Ill.: Scott, Foresman, 1975, 69–111.

Brown, T. S., Gedvilas, G., & Marco, L. A. Effects of auditory cortical lesions on a test of frequency discrimination in the cat. *Proceedings of the 75th Annual Convention of the American Psychological Association*, 1967, *2*, 101–102.

Brown, T. S., Rosvold, H. E., & Mishkin, M. Olfactory discrimination after temporal lobe lesions in monkeys. *Journal of Comparative and Physiological Psychology*, 1963, *56*, 190–195.

Bruce, R. H. The effect of lessening the drive upon performance by white rats in a maze. *Journal of Comparative and Physiological Psychology*, 1938, *25*, 225–248.

Brücke, F., Petsche, H., Pillat, B., & Deisenhammer, E. Über veränderungen des hippocampus—elektrencephalogrammes beim kaninchen nach novocaininjektion in die septumregion. *Naunyn-Schmiedeberg's Arch. Exp. Pathol. Pharmakol.,* 1959, *237,* 276–284.

Brügger, M. Fesstrieb als hypothalamisches symptom. *Helvetica Physiologica et Pharmacologica Acta,* 1943, *1,* 183–198.

Brush, E. S., Mishkin, M., & Rosvold, H. E. Effects of object preferences and aversions on discrimination learning in monkeys with frontal lesions. *Journal of Comparative and Physiological Psychology,* 1961, *54,* 319–325.

Brutkowski, S. Functions of prefrontal cortex in animals. *Physiological Review,* 1965, *45,* 721–746.

Buckholtz, N. S., & Bowman, R. E. Incubation and retrograde amnesia studied with various ECS intensities and durations. *Physiology and Behavior,* 1972, *8,* 113–117.

Buddington, R. W., King, F. A., & Roberts, L. Emotionality and conditioned avoidance responding in the squirrel monkey following septal injury. *Psychonomic Science,* 1967, *8,* 195–196.

Bureš, J., & Burešová, O. Cortical spreading depression as a memory disturbing factor. *Journal of Comparative and Physiological Psychology,* 1963, *56,* 268–272.

Bureš, J., Petráň, M., & Zachar, J. *Electrophysiological methods in biological research,* (2nd ed.). New York: Academic Press, 1962.

Burkett, E. E., & Bunnell, B. N. Septal lesions and retention of DRL performance in the rat. *Journal of Comparative and Physiological Psychology,* 1966, *62,* 468–471.

Burn, J. H. *The autonomic nervous system* (2nd ed.). Oxford: Blackwell, 1965.

Burns, B. D. *The mammalian cerebral cortex.* London: Arnold, 1958.

Butter, C. M. Perseveration in extinction and in discrimination reversal tasks following selective frontal ablations in *Macaca mulatta. Physiology and Behavior,* 1969, *4,* 163–171.

Butters, N., & Pandya, D. Retention of delayed alternation: Effect of selective lesions of sulcus principalis. *Science,* 1969, *165,* 1271–1273.

Butters, N., Pandya, D., Sanders, K., & Dye, P. Behavioral deficits in monkeys after selective lesions within the middle third of the sulcus principalis. *Journal of Comparative and Physiological Psychology,* 1971, *76,* 8–14.

Byrne, W. L., Samuel, D., Bennett, E. L., Rosenzweig, M. R., Wasserman, E., Wagner, A. R., Gardner, R., Galambos, R., Berger, B. D., Margules, D. L., Fenichel, R. L., Stein, L., Corson, J. A., Enesco, H. E., Chorover, S. L., Holt, C. E., III, Schiller, P. H., Chiapetta, L., Jarvik, M. E., Leaf, R. C., Dutcher, J. D., Horowitz, Z. P., & Carlson, P. L. Memory transfer. *Science,* 1966, *153,* 658–659.

Cannon, W. B. The physiological basis of thirst.

Proceedings of the Royal Society, 1918, *B90,* 283–301.

Cannon, W. B. *Bodily changes in pain, hunger, fear and rage.* New York: Harper & Row, 1963.

Cannon, W. B., & Washburn, A. L. An explanation of hunger. *American Journal of Physiology,* 1912 *29,* 441–454.

Carew, T. J., & Kandel, E. R. Acquisition and retention of long-term habituation in *Aplysia:* Correlation of behavioral and cellular processes. *Science,* 1973, *182,* 1158–1160.

Carew, T. J., Pinsker, H. M., & Kandel, E. R. Long-term habituation of a defensive withdrawal reflex in *Aplysia. Science,* 1972, *175,* 451–454.

Carey, R. J. Quinine and saccharin preference—aversion threshold determinations in rats with septal ablations. *Journal of Comparative and Physiological Psychology,* 1971, *76,* 316–326.

Carlton, P. L., & Markiewicz, B. Studies on the physiological bases of memory. In E. Stellar & J. M. Sprague (Eds.), *Progress in Physiological Psychology* (Vol. 5). New York: Academic Press, 1973, 125–153.

Carter, C. S., Clemens, L. G., & Hoekema, D. J. Neonatal androgen and adult sexual behavior in the golden hamster. *Physiology and Behavior,* 1972, *9,* 89–96.

Castellucci, V., & Goldring, S. Contribution to steady potential shifts of slow depolarization in cells presumed to be glia. *Electroencephalography and Clinical Neurophysiology,* 1970, *28,* 109–118.

Castellucci, V., Pinsker, H., Kupfermann, I., & Kandel, E. Neuronal mechanisms of habituation and dishabituation of the gill withdrawal reflex in *Aplysia. Science,* 1970, *167,* 1745–1748.

Caton, R. The electrical current of the brain. *British Medical Journal,* 1875, *2,* 278–296.

Caul, W. F., & Barrett, R. J. Electroconvulsive shock effects on conditioned heart rate and suppression of drinking. *Physiology and Behavior,* 1972, *8,* 287–290.

Cerletti, V., & Bini, L. Electric shock treatment. *Bollettino Accademia Medica. Roma,* 1938, *64,* 36.

Chapouthier, G. Behavioral studies of the molecular basis of memory. In J. A. Deutsch (Ed.), *The physiological basis of memory.* New York: Academic Press, 1973, 1–17.

Chapouthier, G., Pallaud, B., & Ungerer, A. Relations entre deux reactions des planaires face à une discrimination droite-gauche. *Comptes Rendus Academie Sciences Serie D.,* 1968, *266,* 905–907.

Cheney, C. D. Transfer of a response rate bias in rats by injection of brain homogenate. *Journal of Biological Psychology,* 1970, *12,* 13.

Cherkin, A. Retrograde amnesia in the chick: Resistance to the reminder effect. *Physiology and Behavior,* 1972, *8,* 949–955.

Chevalier, J. A. Permanence of amnesia after a

single posttrial electroconvulsive seizure. *Journal of Comparative and Physiological Psychology,* 1965, *59,* 125–127.

Chi, C. C., & Flynn, J. P. Neural pathways associated with hypothalamically elicited attack behavior in cats. *Science,* 1971, *171,* 703–705.

Chorover, S. L., & Schiller, P. H. Short-term retrograde amnesia in rats. *Journal of Comparative and Physiological Psychology,* 1965, *59,* 73–78.

Chorover, S. L., & Schiller, P. H. Reexamination of prolonged retrograde amnesia in one-trial learning. *Journal of Comparative and Physiological Psychology,* 1966, *61,* 34–41.

Christman, R. J. *Sensory experience.* Scranton, Pa.: Intext Educational Publishers, 1971.

Clark, C. V. H., & Isaacson, R. L. Effect of bilateral hippocampal ablation on DRL performance. *Journal of Comparative and Physiological Psychology,* 1965, *59,* 137–140.

Clemes, S., & Dement, W. C. Effects of REM sleep deprivation on psychological functioning. *Journal of Nervous and Mental Disease,* 1967, *144,* 485–491.

Cohen, H., & Dement, W. C. Electrically induced convulsions in REM deprived mice: Prolongation of the tonic phase. *Psychophysiology,* 1968, *4,* 381.

Cohen, H. D., & Barondes, S. H. Further studies of learning and memory after intracerebral actinomycin-D. *Journal of Neurochemistry,* 1966, *13,* 207–211.

Cohen, H. D., Ervin, F., & Barondes, S. H. Puromycin and cyclohexamide: Different effects on hippocampal electrical activity. *Science,* 1966, *154,* 1557–1558.

Coons, E. E., & Miller, N. E. Conflict vs. consolidation of memory traces to explain "retrograde amnesia" produced by ECS. *Journal of Comparative and Physiological Psychology,* 1960, *53,* 524–531.

Coons, E. E., & Quartermain, D. Motivational depression associated with norepinephrine-induced eating from the hypothalamus: Resemblance to the ventromedial hyperphagic syndrome. *Physiology and Behavior,* 1970, *5,* 687–692.

Cooper, R. M., & Taylor, L. H. Thalamic reticular system and central grey: Self-stimulation. *Science,* 1967, *156,* 102–103.

Corbit, J. D., & Stellar, E. Palatability, food intake, and obesity in normal and hyperphagic rats. *Journal of Comparative and Physiological Psychology,* 1964, *58,* 63–67.

Corning, W. C. Evidence of a right-left discrimination in planarians. *Journal of Psychology,* 1964, *58,* 131–139.

Critchlow, V., & Bar-Sela, M. E. Control of the onset of puberty. In L. Martini & W. F. Ganong (Eds.), *Neuroendocrinology* (Vol. 2). London: Oxford University Press, 1967, 343–388.

Crowne, D. P., Konow, A., Drake, K. J., & Pribram, K. H. Hippocampal electrical activity in the monkey during delayed alternation problems. *Electroencephalography and Clinical Neurophysiology,* 1972, *33,* 567–577.

Cushing, H. A note upon the faradic stimulation of the postcentral gyrus in conscious patients. *Brain,* 1909, *32,* 44–53.

Davis, G. Intercellular transfer of information by RNA extracts. *Journal of Biological Psychology,* 1970, *11,* 10–17.

Davis, J. R., & Keesey, R. E. Norepinephrine-induced eating: Its hypothalamic locus and an alternate interpretation of action. *Journal of Comparative and Physiological Psychology,* 1971, *77,* 394–402.

Davis, R. C., Garafalo, L., & Kveim, K. Conditions associated with gastrointestinal activity. *Journal of Comparative and Physiological Psychology,* 1959, *52,* 466–475.

Davis, R. E., & Agranoff, B. W. Effects of electroconvulsive shock and of puromycin on memory in goldfish. *Federation Proceedings,* 1965, *24,* 329.

Davis, R. E., Bright, P. J., & Agranoff, B. W. Effects of ECS and puromycin on memory in fish. *Journal of Comparative and Physiological Psychology,* 1965, *60,* 162–166.

Deagle, J. H., & Lubar, J. F. Effects of septal lesions in two strains of rats on one-way and shuttle avoidance acquisition. *Journal of Comparative and Physiological Psychology,* 1971, *77,* 277–281.

DeArmond, S. J., Fusco, M. M., & Dewey, M. M. *Structure of the human brain: A photographic atlas.* New York: Oxford University Press, 1974.

Debold, R. C., Firshein, W., Carrier, S. C., III, & Leaf, R. C. Changes in RNA in the occipital cortex of rats as a function of light and dark during rearing. *Psychonomic Science,* 1967, *7,* 379–380.

Delacour, J. Effects of medial thalamic lesions in the rat: A review and an interpretation. *Neuropsychologia,* 1971, *9,* 157–174.

Delgado, J. M. R., Johnston, V. S., Wallace, J. D., & Bradley, R. J. Operant conditioning of amygdala spindling in the free chimpanzee. *Brain Research,* 1970, *23,* 347–362.

Delgado, J. M. R., Roberts, W. W., & Miller, N. E. Learning motivated by electrical stimulation of the brain. *American Journal of Physiology,* 1954, *179,* 587–593.

Dement, W. C. The effect of dream deprivation. *Science,* 1960, *135,* 1705–1707.

Dement, W. C. Recent studies on the biological role of rapid-eye-movement sleep. *American Journal of Psychiatry,* 1965, *122,* 404–408.

Dement, W. C. The biological role of REM sleep (circa 1968). In A. Kales (Ed.), *Sleep: Physiology and pathology.* Philadelphia: J. B. Lippincott Co., 1969, 245–265.

Dement, W. C., Greenberg, S., & Klein, R. The effect of partial REM-sleep deprivation and delayed recovery. *Journal of Psychiatric Research,* 1966, *4,* 141–152.

Dement, W. C., Henry, P., Cohen, H., & Ferguson, J. Studies on the effect of REM deprivation of humans and in animals. In S. Kety, E. Evarts, & H. Williams (Eds.), *Sleep and altered states of consciousness.* Baltimore: Williams & Wilkins, 1967, 456–468.

Dement, W. C., & Kleitman, N. Cyclic variations in EEG during sleep and their relation to eye movement, body motility, and dreaming. *Electroencephalography and Clinical Neurophysiology, 1957, 9,* 673–690. (a)

Dement, W. C., & Kleitman, N. The relation of eye movement during sleep to dream activity: An objective method for the study of dreaming. *Journal of Experimental Psychology,* 1957, *53,* 339–346.(b)

de Molina, F. A., & Hunsperger, R. W. Central representation of effective reactions in forebrain and brain stem: Electrical stimulation of amygdala, stria terminalis and adjacent structures. *Journal of Physiology,* 1959, *145,* 251–265.

de Molina, F. A., & Hunsperger, R. W. Organization of subcortical system governing defense and flight reactions in the cat. *Journal of Physiology,* 1962, *160,* 200–213.

Deutsch, J. A. The physiological basis of memory. *Annual Review of Psychology,* 1969, *20,* 85–104.

Deutsch, J. A. The cholinergic synapse and the site of memory. In J.A. Deutsch (Ed.), *The physiological basis of memory.* New York: Academic Press, 1973, 59–76.

Deutsch, J. A., & Deutsch, D. *Physiological psychology* (2nd ed.). Homewood, Ill.: Dorsey Press, 1973.

De Valois, R. L. Behavioral and electrophysiological studies of primate vision. In W. D. Neff (Ed.), *Contributions to sensory physiology* (Vol. 1). New York: Academic Press, 1965, 137–178.

De Valois, R. L., Abramov, I., & Mead, W. R. Single cell analysis of wave-length discrimination at the lateral geniculate nucleus in the macaque. *Journal of Neurophysiology,* 1967, *30,* 415–433.

De Valois, R. L., & Jacobs, G. H. Primate color vision. *Science,* 1968, *162,* 533–540.

De Valois, R. L., Jacobs, G. H., & Jones, A. E. Responses of single cells in primate red-green color vision system. *Optik,* 1963, *20,* 87–98.

DeVietti, T., & Bucy, C. E. Recovery of memory after reminder: Evidence for two forms of retrieval deficit induced by ECS. *Physiological Psychology,* 1975, *3,* 19–25.

DeVietti, T., & Hopfer, T. M. Reinstatement of memory in rats: Dependence upon two forms of retrieval deficit following electroconvulsive shock. *Journal of Comparative and Physiological Psychology,* 1974, *86,* 1090–1099.

Dewson, J. H., III, Cowey, A., & Weiskrantz, L. Disruptions of auditory sequence discrimination by unilateral and bilateral cortical ablations of superior temporal gyrus in monkey. *Experimental Neurology,* 1970, *28,* 529–548.

Diamond, I. T., Goldberg, J. M., & Neff, W. D. Tonal discrimination after ablation of auditory cortex. *Journal of Neurophysiology,* 1962, *25,* 223–235.

Diamond, I. T., & Neff, W. D. Ablation of temporal cortex and discrimination of auditory patterns. *Journal of Neurophysiology,* 1957, *20,* 300–315.

Diamond, M. C. Extensive cortical depth measurements and neuron size increases in the cortex of environmentally enriched rats. *Journal of Comparative Neurology,* 1967, *131,* 357–364.

Diamond, M. C., Law, F., Rhodes, H., Lindner, B., Rosenzweig, M. R., Krech, D., & Bennett, E. L. Increases in cortical depth and glia numbers in rats subjected to enriched environment. *Journal of Comparative Neurology,* 1966, *128,* 117–125.

Diamond, M. C., Rosenzweig, M. R., & Bennett, E. L. Unpublished data cited by Rosenzweig, M. R., in Effects of environment on development of brain and behavior. In E. Tobach, L. R. Aronson, & E. Shaw (Eds.), *The Biopsychology of Development.* New York: Academic Press, 1971, 303–342.

Dingman, W., & Sporn, M. B. The incorporation of 8-azaguanine into rat brain RNA and its effect on maze learning by the rat: An inquiry into the biochemical bases of memory. *Journal of Psychiatric Research,* 1961, *1,* 1–11.

Dingman, W., & Sporn, M. B. Molecular theories of memory. *Science,* 1964, *144,* 26–29.

Donovick, P. J., & Burright, R. G. Water consumption in rats with septal lesions following two days of water deprivation. *Physiology and Behavior,* 1968, *3,* 285–288.

Donovick, P. J., Burright, R. G., & Gittleson, P. L. Body weight and food and water consumption in septal lesioned and operated control rats. *Psychological Reports,* 1969, *25,* 303–310.

Dörner, G., Döcke, F., & Hinz, G. Homo- and hypersexuality in rats with hypothalamic lesions. *Neuroendocrinology,* 1969, *4,* 20–24.

Doty, R. L., Carter, C. S., & Clemens, L. G. Olfactory control of sexual behavior in the male and early-androgenized female hamster.*Hormones and Behavior,* 1971, *2,* 325–335.

Douglas, R. J. The hippocampus and behavior. *Psychological Bulletin,* 1967, *67,* 416–442.

Douglas, R. J. Pavlovian conditioning and the brain. In R. A. Boakes & M. S. Halliday (Eds.), *Inhibition and learning.* London: Academic Press, 1972, 529–533.

Douglas, R. J., Pagano, R. R., Lovely, R. H., & Peterson, J. J. The prolonged effects of a single ECS on behavior related to hippocampal function. *Behavioral Biology,* 1973, *8,* 611–617.

Douglas, R. J., Peterson, J., & Douglas, D. The ontogeny of a hippocampus-dependent response in two rodent species. *Behavioral Biology,* 1973, *8,* 27–37.

Douglas, R. J., & Pribram, K. H. Learning and limbic lesions. *Neuropsychologia,* 1966, *4,* 197–220.

Duncan, C. P. The retroactive effect of electroshock on learning. *Journal of Comparative and Physiological Psychology,* 1949, *42,* 32–44.

Dunn, A. Brain protein synthesis after electroshock. *Brain Research, Osaka,* 1971, *35,* 254–259.

Eaton, G. Effects of a single prepubertal injection of testosterone proprionate on adult bisexual behavior of male hamsters castrated at birth. *Endocrinology,* 1970, *87,* 934–940.

Eccles, J. C, *The neurophysiological basis of mind.* Oxford: Clarendon Press, 1953.

Eccles, J. C. *The physiology of nerve cells.* Baltimore: Johns Hopkins Press, 1957.

Eccles, J. C. *The physiology of synapses.* New York: Academic Press, 1964.

Edwards, D. A. Neonatal administration of androstenedione, testosterone, or testosterone proprionate: Effects on ovulation, sexual receptivity, and aggressive behavior in female mice. *Physiology and Behavior,* 1971, *6,* 223–228.

Edwards, D. A., & Burge, K. G. Early androgen treatment and male and female sexual behavior in mice. *Hormones and Behavior,* 1971, *2,* 49–58.

Egger, M. D., & Flynn, J. P. Amygdaloid suppression of hypothalamically elicited attack behavior. *Science,* 1962, *136,* 43–44.

Egger, M. D., & Flynn, J. P. Effects of electrical stimulation of the amygdala on hypothalamically elicited attack behavior in cats. *Journal of Neurophysiology,* 1963, *26,* 705–720.

Egger, M. D. & Flynn, J. P. Further studies on the effects of amygdaloid stimulation and ablation of hypothalamically elicited attack behavior in cats. In W. R. Adey & T. Tokizane (Eds.), *Progress in brain research* (Vol. 27): *Structure and function of the limbic system.* Amsterdam: Elsevier Publishing Co., 1967, 165–182.

Eichelman, B. S., Jr. Effect of subcortical lesions on shock-induced aggression in the rat. *Journal of Comparative and Physiological Psychology,* 1971, *74,* 331–339.

Eichenbaum, H. B. *Localization of memory by regional brain protein inhibition.* Unpublished doctoral dissertation, University of Michigan, 1975.

Elazar, Z., & Adey, W. R. Spectral analysis of low frequency components in the electrical activity of the hippocampus during learning. *Electroencephalography and Clinical Neurophysiology,* 1967, *23,* 225–240. (a)

Elazar, Z, & Adey, W. R. Electroencephalographic correlates of learning in subcortical and cortical structures. *Electroencephalography and Clinical Neurophysiology,* 1967, *23,* 306–319. (b)

Ellen, P., & Aitken, W. C., Jr. Analysis of DRL responding by rats with septal damage. *Physiological Psychology,* 1973, *1,* 16–20.

Ellen, P., Aitken, W. C., Jr., & Stahl, J. M. Pretraining effects on the DRL performance of rats with septal lesions. *Physiological Psychology,* 1973, *4,* 380–384.

Ellen, P., & Braggio, J. T. Reactions to DRL schedule change in rats with septal damage. *Physiological Psychology* 1973, *1,* 267–272.

Ellen, P., & Butter, J. External cue control of DRL performance in rats with septal lesions. *Physiology and Behavior,* 1969, *4,* 1–6.

Ellen, P., & Powell, E. W. Temporal discrimination in rats with rhinencephalic lesions. *Experimental Neurology,* 1962, *6,* 538–547.

Ellen, P., Wilson, A. S., & Powell, E. W. Septal inhibition and timing behavior in the rat. *Experimental Neurology,* 1964. *10.* 120–132.

Ellison, G. D., & Flynn, J. P. Organized aggressive behavior in cats after surgical isolation of the hypothalamus. *Archives Italiennes de Biologie,* 1968, *106,* 1–20.

Entingh, D. Perseverative responding and hyperphagia following entorhinal lesions in cats. *Journal of Comparative and Physiological Psychology,* 1971, *75,* 50–58.

Epstein, A. N., Fitzsimons, J. T., & Rolls (née Simons), B. J. Drinking induced by injection of angiotensin into the brain of the rat. *Journal of Physiology* (London), 1970, *210,* 457–474.

Epstein, A. N., & Teitelbaum, P. Regulation of food intake in the absence of taste, smell, and other oropharyngeal sensations. *Journal of Comparative and Physiological Psychology,* 1962, *55,* 753–759.

Essman, W. B., & Lehrer, G. M. Facilitation of maze performance by "RNA extracts" from maze trained mice. *Federation Proceedings,* 1967, *26,* 263.

Evans, E. F., Ross, H. F., & Whitfield, I. C. The spatial distribution of unit characteristic frequency in the primary auditory cortex of the cat. *Journal of Physiology,* 1965, *179,* 238–247.

Feder, R., & Ranck, J. B., Jr. Studies on single neurons in dorsal hippocampal formation and septum in unrestrained rats. II. Hippocampal slow waves and theta cell firing during bar pressing and other behaviors. *Experimental Neurology,* 1973, *41,* 532–555.

Feldberg, W., & Sherwood, S. L. Injection of drugs into the lateral ventricles of the cat. *Journal of Physiology,* 1954, *123,* 148–167.

Ferrier, D. *The functions of the brain.* London: Smith Elder, 1876.

Fetz, E. E. Operant conditioning of cortical unit activity. *Science,* 1969, *163,* 955–957.

Finan, J. L. Delayed response with pre-delay reinforcement in monkeys after removal of the frontal lobes. *American Journal of Psychology,* 1942, *55,* 204–214.

Fisher, A. E. Maternal and sexual behavior induced by intracranial chemical stimulation. *Science,* 1956, *124,* 228–229.

Fisher, A. E. Behavior as a function of certain neurobiochemical events. In R. Patton (Ed.), *Current trends in psychological theory: A bicentennial program.* Pittsburgh: University of Pittsburgh Press, 1961, 70–86.

Fisher, A. E. Chemical stimulation of the brain. *Scientific American,* 1964, *210,* 61–68.

Fitzsimons, J. T. Hypovolaemic drinking and renin. *Journal of Physiology* (London), 1966, *186,* 130P–131P.

Fitzsimons, J. T. The kidney as a thirst receptor. *Journal of Physiology* (London), 1967, *191,* 128P–129P.

Fitzsimons, J. T. The role of renal thirst factor in drinking induced by extracellular stimuli. *Journal of Physiology,* (London), 1969, *201,* 349–368.

Fitzsimons, J. T. The physiology of thirst: A review of the extraneural aspects of the mechanisms of drinking. In E. Stellar & J. M. Sprague (Eds.), *Progress in physiological psychology,* 1971, *4,* 119–201.

Fjerdingstad, E. J. (Ed.), *Chemical transfer of learned information.* Amsterdam: North-Holland Publishing Co., 1971.

Fjerdingstad, E. J. Transfer of learning in rodents and fish. In W. B. Essman & S. Nakajima (Eds.), *Current biochemical approaches to learning and memory.* Flushing, New York: Spectrum Publications, 1973, 73–98.

Fjerdingstad, E. J., Nissen, T., & Røigaard-Petersen, H. H. Effect of ribonucleic acid (RNA) extracted from the brain of trained animals on learning in rats. *Scandinavian Journal of Psychology,* 1965, *6,* 1–5.

Flescher, G. I. L'amnesia retrograde dopo l'elettroshock: Contributo allo studio della patogenesi delle amnesie in genere. *Schweizer Archiv fur Neurologie, Neurothirurgie und Psychiatrie,* 1941, *48,* 1–28.

Flexner, J. B., & Flexner, L. B. Restoration of memory lost after treatment with puromycin. *Proceedings of the National Academy of Sciences,* 1967, *57,* 1651–1654.

Flexner, J. B., & Flexner, L. B. Further observations on restoration of memory lost after treatment with puromycin. *Yale Journal of Biology and Medicine,* 1970, *42,* 235–240.

Flexner, J. B., Flexner, L. B., & Stellar, E. Memory in mice as affected by intracerebral puromycin. *Science,* 1963, *141,* 57–59.

Flexner, L. B., & Flexner, J. B. Effects of acetoxycyclohexamide and of an acetoxycyclohexamide-puromycin mixture on cerebral protein synthesis and memory in mice. *Proceedings of the National Academy of Sciences,* 1966, *55,* 369–374.

Flexner, L. B., & Flexner, J. B. Intracerebral saline: Effect on memory of trained mice treated with puromycin. *Science,* 1968, *159,* 330–331. (a)

Flexner, L. B., & Flexner, J. B. Studies on memory: The long survival of peptidyl-puromycin in mouse brain. *Proceedings of the National Academy of Sciences,* 1968, *60,* 923–927. (b)

Flexner, L. B. Flexner, J. B., Roberts, R. B., & De la Haba, G. Loss of recent memory in mice as related to regional inhibition of cerebral protein synthesis. *Proceedings of the National Academy of Sciences,* 1964, *52,* 1165–1169.

Flood, J. F., Rosenzweig, M. R., Bennett, E. L., & Orme, A. E. Influence of training strength on amnesia induced by pretraining injections of cyclohexamide. *Physiology and Behavior,* 1972, *9,* 589–600.

Flood, J. F., Rosenzweig, M. R., Bennett, E. L., & Orme, A. E. The influence of duration of protein synthesis inhibition on memory. *Physiology and Behavior,* 1973, *10,* 555–562.

Flood, J. F., Rosenzweig, M. R., Bennett, E. L., & Orme, A. E. Comparison of the effects of anisomycin on memory across six strains of mice. *Behavioral Biology,* 1974, *10,* 147–160.

Flourens, P. Recherches physiques sur les propriétés et fonctions du système nerveux dans les animaux vertébrés, *Archives Générales de Médecine,* 1823, *2,* 321–374.

Flynn, J. P. The neural basis of aggression in cats. In D. C. Glass (Ed.), *Neurophysiology and emotion,* New York: Rockefeller University Press and Russell Sage Foundation, 1967, 40–69.

Flynn, J. P., Vanegas, H., Foote, W., & Edwards, S. Neural mechanisms involved in a cat's attack on a rat. In R. E. Whalen, R. F. Thompson, M. Verzeano, & N. M. Weinberger (Eds.), *The neural control of behavior.* New York: Academic Press, 1970.

Fonberg, E. Aphagia produced by destruction of the dorsomedial amygdala in dogs. *Bulletin de L'Academie Polonaise des Sciences,* 1966, *14,* 719–722.

Forgays, D. G., & Read, J. M. Crucial periods for free-environmental experience on the rat. *Journal of Comparative and Physiological Psychology,* 1962, *55,* 816–818.

Foulkes, D. *The psychology of sleep.* New York: Scribner's 1966.

Fox, S. S., Kimble, D. P., & Lickey, M. E. Comparison of caudate nucleus and septal area lesions on two types of avoidance behavior. *Journal of Comparative and Physiological Psychology,* 1964, *58,* 380–386.

Frank, B., Stein, D. G., & Rosen, J. Interanimal "memory" transfer: Results from brain and liver homogenates. *Science,* 1970, *169,* 399–402.

Frazier, W. T., Kandel, E. R., Kupfermann, I., Waziri, R., & Coggeshall, R. E. Morphological and functional properties of identifiable cells in the abdominal ganglion of *Aplysia californica. Journal of Neurophysics,* 1967, *30,* 1288–1335.

Freeman, W., & Watts, J. W. *Psychosurgery in the treatment of mental disorders and intractable pain* (2nd ed.). Springfield, Ill.: Charles C Thomas, 1950.

French, G. M., & Harlow, H. F. Variability of delayed reaction performance in normal and brain-damaged rhesus monkeys. *Journal of Neurophysiology,* 1962, *25,* 585–599.

French, J. D. The reticular formation. *Scientific American*, 1957, *196*, 54–60.

Frey, M. von. Beitrage zur Sinnesphysiologie des Haut, *Ber Sächs Ges Wiss Leipzig Math-Phys Cl.*, 1895, *47*, 166–184.

Fried, C., & Horowitz, S. Contraction—a learnable response? *Worm Runner's Digest*, 1964, *6*, 3–6.

Fried, P. A. Effects of septal lesions on conflict resolution in rats. *Journal of Comparative and Physiological Psychology*, 1969, *69*, 375–380.

Fried, P. A. Limbic system lesions in rats: Differential effects in an approach-avoidance task. *Journal of Comparative and Physiological Psychology*, 1971, *74*, 349–353.

Friedman, M. H. Electroconvulsive shock as a traumatic (fear-producing) experience in the albino rat. *Journal of Abnormal and Social Psychology*, 1953, *48*, 555–562.

Fritsch, G., & Hitzig, E. Über die elektrische Erregbarkeit des Grosshirns. *Archiv für Anatomie Physiologie und Wissenschaftliche Medicin*, 1870, *37*, 300–332.

Fujita, Y, & Sato, T. Intracellular records from hippocampal pyramidal cells in the rabbit during theta rhythm. *Journal of Neurophysiology*, 1964, *27*, 1011–1025.

Fuller, J. L., Rosvold, H. E., & Pribram, K. H. The effect on affective and cognitive behavior in the dog of lesions of the pyriform-amygdala hippocampal complex. *Journal of Comparative and Physiological Psychology*, 1957, *50*, 89–96.

Fulton, J. F., & Jacobsen, C. F. The functions of the frontal lobes, a comparative study in monkeys, chimpanzees and man. *Abstract from the Second International Neurology Congress* (London), 1935, 70–71. Also in *Advances in Modern Biology* (Moscow), 1935, 113–123.

Fuster, J. M., & Uyeda, A. A. Reactivity of limbic neurons of the monkey to appetitive and aversive signals. *Electroencephalography and Clinical Neurophysiology*, 1971, *30*, 182–293.

Gallinek, A. Fear and anxiety in the course of electroshock therapy. *American Journal of Psychiatry*, 1956, *113*, 428–434.

Gallistel, C. R. Self-stimulation: The neurophysiology of reward and motivation. In J. A. Deutsch (Ed.), *The physiological basis of memory*. New York: Academic Press, 1973, 175–267.

Galluscio, E. H. Retrograde amnesia induced by electroconvulsive shock and carbon dioxide anesthesia in rats: An attempt to stimulate recovery. *Journal of Comparative and Physiological Psychology*, 1971, *75*, 136–140.

Ganong, W. F. *Review of medical physiology* (7th ed.). Los Altos, Calif.: Lange Medical Publications, 1975.

Gardner, D., & Kandel, E. R. Diphasic postsynaptic potential: A chemical synapse capable of mediating conjoint excitation and inhibition. *Science*, 1972, *176*, 675–678.

Gardner, E. *Fundamentals of neurology* (5th ed.). Philadelphia: W. B. Saunders, 1968.

Gault, F. P., & Leaton, R. N. Electrical activity of the olfactory system. *Electroencephalography and Clinical Neurophysiology*, 1963, *15*, 299–304.

Gay, R., & Raphelson, A. C. "Transfer of learning" by injection of brain RNA: A replication. *Psychonomic Science*, 1967, *8*, 369–370.

Gay, R., & Raphelson, A. C. A simplified behavior test of brain extractate transfer effects in rats. In W. L. Byrne (Ed.), *Molecular approaches to learning and memory*. New York: Academic Press, 1970, 171–178.

Geller, A., Jarvik, M. E., & Robustelli, F. Permanence of a long temporal gradient of retrograde amnesia induced by electroconvulsive shock. *Psychonomic Science*, 1970, *19*, 257–259.

Gerall, A. A. Hormonal factors influencing masculine behavior of female guinea pigs. *Journal of Comparative and Physiological Psychology*, 1966, *62*, 365–369.

Gerall, H. D., Ward, I. L., & Gerall, A. A. Disruption of the male rat's sexual behavior induced by social isolation. *Animal Behaviour*, 1967, *15*, 54–58.

Gerbrandt, L. K., & Thomson, C. W. Competing response and amnesic effects of electroconvulsive shock under extinction and incentive shifts. *Journal of Comparative and Physiological Psychology*, 1964, *58*, 208–211.

Giantonio, G. W., Lund, N. L., & Gerall, A. A. Effect of diencephalic and rhinencephalic lesions on the male rat's sexual behavior. *Journal of Comparative and Physiological Psychology*, 1970, *73*, 38–46.

Gibbs, F. A., Davis, H., & Lennox, W. G. The electroencephalogram in epilepsy and in conditions of impaired consciousness. *Archives of Neurology and Psychiatry*, 1935, *34*, 1133–1148.

Gibson, E. J., & Walk, R. D. The effect of prolonged exposure to visually presented patterns on learning to discriminate them. *Journal of Comparative and Physiological Psychology*, 1956, *49*, 239–242.

Gibson, W. E., Reid, L. D., Sakai, M., & Porter, P. B. Intracranial reinforcement compared with sugar water reinforcement. *Science*, 1965, *148*, 1357–1359.

Gittleson, P. L., & Donovick, P. J. The effect of septal lesions on learning and reversal of a kinesthetic discrimination. *Psychonomic Science*, 1968, *13*, 137–138.

Glees, P., Cole, J., Whitty, C. W. M., & Cairns, H. The effects of lesions in the cingular gyrus and adjacent areas in monkeys. *Journal of Neurology, Neurosurgery, and Psychiatry*, 1950, *13*, 178–190.

Glick, S. D., & Greenstein, S. Comparative learning and memory deficits following hippocampal and caudate lesions in mice. *Journal of Comparative and Physiological Psychology*, 1973, *82*, 188–194.

Globus, A., Rosenzweig, M. R., Bennett, E. L., &

Diamond, M. C. Effects of differential experience on dendritic spine counts in rat cerebral cortex. *Journal of Comparative and Physiological Psychology,* 1973, *82,* 175–181.

Gloor, P. Amygdala. In J. Field (Ed.) *Handbook of physiology; Section I: Neurophysiology* (Vol. 2). Washington, D. C.: American Physiological Society, 1960, 1395–1420.

Gold, P. E., Haycock, J. W., Macri, J., & McGaugh, J. L. Retrograde amnesia and the "reminder effect": An alternative interpretation. *Science,* 1973, *180,* 1199–1201.

Gold, R. M. Hypothalamic obesity: The myth of the ventromedial nucleus. *Science,* 1973, *182,* 488–489.

Goldberg, J. M., & Neff, W. D. Frequency discrimination after bilateral ablation of the cortical auditory areas. *Journal of Neurophysiology,* 1961, *24,* 119–128.

Goldstein, A., Sheehan, P., & Goldstein, J. Unsuccessful attempts to transfer morphine tolerance and passive avoidance by brain extracts. *Nature,* 1971, *223,* 126–129.

Goldstein, A. C. In H. Hoagland (Ed.), *Hormones, brain function, and behavior.* New York: Academic Press, 1957, 99.

Gotsick, J. E., & Marshall, R. C. Time course of the septal rage syndrome. *Physiology and Behavior,* 1972, *9,* 685–687.

Goy, R. W., Bridson, W. E., & Young, W. C. Period of maximal susceptibility of the prenatal female guinea pig to masculinizing actions of testosterone proprionate. *Journal of Comparative and Physiological Psychology,* 1964, *57,* 166–174.

Grady, K. L., Phoenix, C. H., & Young, W. C. Role of the developing rat testis in differentiation of the neural tissues mediating mating behavior. *Journal of Comparative and Physiological Psychology,* 1965, *59,* 176–182.

Grastyán, E., and Angyán, L. The organization of motivation at the thalamic level of the cat. *Physiology and Behavior,* 1967, *2,* 5–13.

Grastyán, E., Karmos, G., Vereczkey, L., & Kellényi, L. The hippocampal electrical correlates of the homeostatic regulation of motivation. *Electroencephalography and Clinical Neurophysiology,* 1966, *21,* 34–53.

Grastyán, E., Lissák, K., Madarász, L., & Donhoffer, H. Hippocampal electrical activity during the development of conditioned reflexes. *Electroencephalography and Clinical Neurophysiology,* 1959, *11,* 409–430.

Gray, J. A. Sodium amobarbital, the hippocampal theta rhythm, the partial reinforcement extinction effect and the psychophysiological nature of introversion. *Psychological Review,* 1970, *77,* 465–480.

Gray, J. A., Quintao, L., & Araujo-Silva, M. T. The partial reinforcement extinction effect in rats with medial septal lesions. *Physiology and Behavior,* 1972, *8,* 491–496.

Green, J. D. The hippocampus. In J. Field (Ed.), *Handbook of physiology; Section I: Neurophysiology* (Vol. 2). Washington, D. C.: American Physiological Society, 1960, 1373–1389.

Green, J. D., & Arduini, A. A. Hippocampal electrical activity and arousal. *Journal of Neurophysiology,* 1954, *17,* 533–557.

Green, J. D., Clemente, C. D., & de Groot, J. Rhinencephalic lesions and behavior in cats: An analysis of the Klüver-Bucy Syndrome with particular reference to normal and abnormal sexual behavior. *Journal of Comparative Neurology,* 1957, *108,* 505–545. (a)

Green, J. D., Clemente, C. D., & de Groot, J. Experimentally induced epilepsy in the cat with injury of Cornu Ammonis (hippocampus). *Archives of Neurology and Psychiatry,* 1957, *78,* 259–263. (b)

Greenblatt, M., & Solomon, H. C. *Frontal lobes and schizophrenia.* New York: Springer, 1953.

Greenough, W. T., & Schwitzgebel, R. L. Effect of a single ECS on extinction of a bar-press. *Psychological Reports,* 1966, *19,* 1227–1230.

Griffard, C. D., & Pierce, J. T. Conditioned discrimination in the planarian. *Science,* 1964, *144,* 1472–1473.

Gross, C. G., & Carey, F. M. Transfer of learned response by RNA injection: Failure of attempts to replicate. *Science,* 1965, *150,* 1749.

Gross, J., Feldman, M., & Fisher, C. *Eye movements during emergent stage 1 EEG in subjects with lifelong blindness.* Report to the Association for the Psychophysiological Study of Sleep: Washington, D. C., 1965.

Grosser, G. S., & Siegal, A. W. Emergence of a tonic-phasic model for sleep and dreaming. *Psychological Bulletin,* 1971, *75,* 60–72.

Grossman, S. P. Eating or drinking elicited by direct adrenergic or cholinergic stimulation of hypothalamus. *Science,* 1960, *132,* 301–302.

Grossman, S. P. Direct adrenergic and cholinergic stimulation of hypothalamic mechanisms. *American Journal of Physiology,* 1962, *202,* 872–882. (a)

Grossman, S. P. Effects of adrenergic and cholinergic blocking agents on hypothalamic mechanisms. *American Journal of Physiology,* 1962, *202,* 1230–1236. (b)

Grossman, S. P. Changes in food and water intake associated with an interruption of the anterior or posterior fiber connections of the hypothalamus. *Journal of Comparative and Physiological Psychology,* 1971, *75,* 23–31.

Grossman, S. P., & Grossman, L. Food and water intake following lesions of electrical stimulation of the amygdala. *American Journal of Physiology,* 1963, *205,* 761–765.

Grossman, S. P., & Grossman, L. Food and water intake in rats with parasagittal knife cuts medial or lateral to the lateral hypothalamus. *Journal of Comparative and Physiological Psychology,* 1971, *74,* 148–156.

Grossman, S. P., & Grossman, L. Persisting deficits

in rats "recovered" from transections of fibers which enter or leave hypothalamus laterally. *Journal of Comparative and Physiological Psychology,* 1973, *85,* 515–527.

Gulick, W. L. *Hearing: physiology and psychophysics.* New York: Oxford University Press, 1971.

Gumnit, R. J. The distribution of direct current responses evoked by sounds in the auditory cortex of the cat. *Electroencephalography and Clinical Neurophysiology,* 1961, *13,* 889–895.

Guyton, A. C. *Textbook of medical physiology* (4th ed.). Philadelphia: W. B. Saunders, 1971.

Haagen-Smith, A. J. Smell and taste. *Scientific American,* 1952, *186,* 28–32.

Hamilton, L. W. Intrabox and extrabox cues in avoidance responding: Effect of septal lesions. *Journal of Comparative and Physiological Psychology,* 1972, *78,* 268–273.

Han, P. W. Hypothalamic obesity in rats without hyperphagia. *Transactions of the New York Academy of Sciences,* 1967, *30,* 229–243.

Hara, K. Visual defects resulting from prestriate cortical lesions in cats. *Journal of Comparative and Physiological Psychology,* 1962, *55,* 293–298.

Hara, K., Cornwell, P. R., Warren, J. M., & Webster, I. H. Posterior extramarginal cortex and visual learning by cats. *Journal of Comparative and Physiological Psychology,* 1974, *87,* 884–904.

Harlow, H. F., & Dagnon, J. Problem solution by monkeys following bilateral removal of the prefrontal areas. I. The discrimination and discrimination-reversal problems. *Journal of Experimental Psychology,* 1943, *32,* 351–356.

Harris, G. W., & Levine, S. Sexual differentiation of the brain and its experimental control. *Journal of Physiology* (London), 1965, *181,* 379–400.

Harris, V. S., & Sachs, B. D. Copulatory behavior in male rats following amygdaloid lesions. *Brain Research,* 1975, *86,* 514–518.

Hart, B. L. *Experimental neuropsychology—a laboratory manual.* San Francisco: W. H. Freeman, 1969.

Hartry, A. L., Keith-Lee, P., & Morton, W. D. Planaria: Memory transfer through cannibalism reexamined. *Science,* 1964, *146,* 274–275.

Harvey, J. A., & Hunt, H. F. Effect of septal lesions on thirst in the rat as indicated by water consumption and operant responding for food reward. *Journal of Comparative and Physiological Psychology,* 1965, *59,* 49–56.

Hasler, A. D. Perception of pathways by fishes in migration. *Quarterly Review of Biology,* 1956, *31,* 200–209.

Haycock, J. W., Gold, P. E., Macri, J., & McGaugh, J. L. Noncontingent footshock attenuation of retrograde amnesia: A generalization effect. *Physiology and Behavior,* 1973, *11,* 99–102.

Haycock, J. W., & McGaugh, J. L. Retrograde amnesia gradients as a function of ECS-intensity. *Behavioral Biology,* 1973, *9,* 123–127.

Heath, R. G. Electrical self-stimulation of the brain in man. *American Journal of Psychiatry,* 1963, *129,* 511–577.

Hebb, D. O. *The organization of behavior: A neuropsychological theory.* New York: Wiley, 1949.

Heimberger, R. F., Whitlock, C. C., & Kalsbeck, J. E. Stereotaxic amygdalectomy for epilepsy with aggressive behavior. *Journal of the American Medical Association,* 1966, *198,* 741–745.

Heimer, L., & Larsson, K. Impairment of mating behavior in male rats following lesions in the preoptic-anterior hypothalamic continuum. *Brain Research,* 1967, *3,* 248–263.

Heinze, W. J. *Quantitative genetic analysis of learning and induced retrograde amnesia in the rodent Rattus norvedicus.* Unpublished doctoral dissertation, University of California, Berkeley, 1970.

Helmholtz, H. L. F. von. *Die Lehre von den Tonempfindugen als physiologische Grundlage für die Theorie der Musik.* Braunschweig: Viewig v. Sohn, 1863.

Henderson, J., Henderson, R., & Greene, E. Impairment of memory with administration of KCl to the hippocampus. *Behavioral Biology,* 1973, *9,* 655–670.

Hendricks, S. E. Influence of neonatally administered hormones and early gonadectomy on rats' sexual behavior. *Journal of Comparative and Physiological Psychology,* 1969, *69,* 408–413.

Henke, P. G. Persistence of runway performance after septal lesions in rats. *Journal of Comparative and Physiological Psychology,* 1974, *86,* 760–767.

Herberg, L. J. Hunger reduction produced by injecting glucose into the lateral ventricle of the rat. *Nature,* 1960, *187,* 245–246.

Herberg, L. J., & Franklin, K. B. J. Adrenergic feeding: Its blockade or reversal by posterior VMH lesions; and a new hypothesis. *Physiology and Behavior,* 1972, *8,* 1029–1034.

Hess, W. R. Stammganglein—Reizversuche, 10. Tagung der Deutschen Physiologischen Gesellschaft, Frankfurt am Main. *Berichten über die Gesamte Physiologie,* 1928, *42,* 554–555.

Hess, W. R. *Das zwischenhirn: Syndrome, lokalisationen, funktionen* (2nd ed.). Basel: Schwabe, 1954.

Hetherington, A. W., & Ranson, S. W. Hypothalamic lesions and adiposity in the rat. *Anatomical Record,* 1940, *78,* 149–172.

Hetherington, A. W., & Ranson, S. W. The spontaneous activity and food intake of rats with hypothalamic lesions. *American Journal of Physiology,* 1942, *136,* 609–617.

Hine, B., & Paolino, R. M. Retrograde amnesia: Production of skeletal but not cardiac response gradients by electroconvulsive shock. *Science,* 1970, *169,* 1224–1226.

Hitt, J. C., Bryon, D. M., & Modianos, D. T. Effects of rostral medial forebrain bundle and olfactory tubercle lesions upon sexual behavior of male rats. *Journal of Comparative and Physiological Psychology,* 1973, *82,* 30–36.

Hitzig, E. *Untersuchungen Über des Gehirns.* Berlin: Unger, 1874.

Hodgkin, A. L. Ionic movements and electrical activity in giant nerve fibers. *Proceedings of the Royal Society of London, Series B,* 1958, *148,* 1–37.

Hodos, W. H. Motivational properties of long durations of rewarding brain stimulation. *Journal of Comparative and Physiological Psychology,* 1965, *59,* 219–224.

Holmes, J. E., & Adey, W. R. Electrical activity of the entorhinal cortex during conditioned behavior. *American Journal of Physiology,* 1960, *199,* 741–744.

Horsley, V., & Clarke, R. H. The structure and functions of the cerebellum examined by a new method. *Brain,* 1908, *31,* 45–124.

Horvath, F. E. Effects of basolateral amygdalectomy on three types of avoidance behavior in cats. *Journal of Comparative and Physiological Psychology,* 1963, *56,* 380–389.

House, E. L., & Pansky, B. *A functional approach to neuroanatomy* (2nd ed.). New York: McGraw-Hill, 1967.

Howarth, C. I., & Deutsch, J. A. Drive decay: The cause of fast "extinction" of habits learned for brain stimulation. *Science,* 1962, *137,* 35–36.

Hubel, D. H. The visual cortex of the brain. *Scientific American,* 1963, *209,* 54–62.

Hubel, D. H., & Wiesel, T. N. Receptive fields, binocular interaction and functional architecture in the cat's visual cortex. *Journal of Physiology,* 1962, *160,* 106–154.

Hubel, D. H., & Wiesel, T. N. Shape and arrangement of columns in the cat's striate cortex. *Journal of Physiology,* 1963, *165,* 559–568.

Hubel, D. H., & Wiesel, T. N. Receptive fields and functional architecture in two nonstriate visual areas (18 and 19) of the cat. *Journal of Neurophysiology,* 1965, *28,* 229–289.

Hubel, D. H., & Wiesel, T. N. Receptive fields and functional architecture of the monkey striate cortex. *Journal of Physiology,* 1968, *195,* 215–243.

Hughes, K. R. Dorsal and ventral hippocampus lesions and maze learning: Influence of preoperative environment. *Canadian Journal of Physiology,* 1965, *19,* 325–332.

Hughes, R. A. Retrograde amnesia in rats produced by hippocampal injections of potassium chloride: Gradient of effect and recovery. *Journal of Comparative and Physiological Psychology,* 1969, *68,* 637–644.

Hughes, R. A., Barrett, R. J., & Ray, O. S. Retrograde amnesia in rats increases as a function of ECS-test interval and ECS intensity. *Physiology and Behavior,* 1970, *5,* 27–30. (a)

Hughes, R. A., Barrett, R. J., & Ray, O. S. Training to test interval as a determinant of a temporally graded ECS-produced response decrement in rats. *Journal of Comparative and Physiological Psychology,* 1970, *71,* 318–324. (b)

Hunsperger, R. W. Affektreaktionen auf elektrische Reizung im Hirnstamm der Katze. *Helvetica Physiologica et Pharmacologica Acta,* 1956, *14,* 70–92.

Hydén, H. Quantitative assay of compounds in isolated, fresh nerve cells and glial cells from control and stimulated animals. *Nature,* 1959, *184,* 433–435.

Hydén, H., & Egyházi, E. Nuclear RNA changes of nerve cells during a learning experiment in rats. *Proceedings of the National Academy of Sciences,* 1962, *48,* 1366–1373.

Hydén, H., & Egyházi, E. Glial RNA changes during a learning experiment with rats. *Proceedings of the National Academy of Sciences,* 1963, *49,* 618–624.

Hydén, H., & Egyházi, E. Changes in RNA content and base composition in cortical neurons of rats in a learning experiment involving transfer of handedness. *Proceedings of the National Academy of Sciences,* 1964, *52,* 1030–1035.

Hydén, H., & Lange, P. W. A differentiation in RNA response in neurons early and late in learning. *Proceedings of the National Academy of Sciences,* 1965, *53,* 946–952.

Hydén, H., & Lange, P. W. Brain-cell protein synthesis specifically related to learning. *Proceedings of the National Academy of Sciences,* 1971, *65,* 898–904. (a)

Hydén, H., & Lange, P. W. S-100 brain protein: Correlations with behavior. *Proceedings National Academy of Sciences,* 1971, *67,* 1959–1966. (b)

Hydén, H., & Lange, P. W. Correlation of the S-100 brain protein with behavior. In J. Gaito (Ed.), *Macromolecules and behavior* (2nd ed.). New York: Appleton-Century-Crofts, 1972, 131–143.

Hydén, H., Lange, P. W., Mihailović, L., & Petrović-Minić, B. Changes of RNA base ratio composition in nerve cells of monkeys subjected to visual discrimination and delayed alternation performance. *Brain Research,* 1974, *65,* 215–230.

Hymovich, B. The effects of experimental variations on problem-solving in the rat. *Journal of Comparative and Physiological Psychology,* 1952, *45,* 313–321.

Ingram, W. R., Barris, R. W., & Ranson, S. W. Catalepsy: An experimental study. *Archives of Neurology and Psychiatry,* 1936, *35,* 1175–1197.

Ireland, L. C., Hayes, W. N., & Schaub, R. E. The effects of bilateral hippocampal lesions on two-way active avoidance in the guinea pig. *Psychonomic Science,* 1969, *14,* 249–250.

Isaacson, R. L. *The limbic system.* New York: Plenum, 1974.

Isaacson, R. L., Douglas, R. J., & Moore, R. J. The effect of radical hippocampal ablation on acquisition of avoidance response. *Journal of Comparative and Physiological Psychology,* 1961, *54,* 625–628.

Isaacson, R. L., Olton, D. S., Bauer, B., & Swart, P. The effect of training trials on passive avoidance deficits in the hippocampectomized rats. *Psychonomic Science,* 1966, *5,* 419–420.

Isaacson, R. L., & Wickelgren, W. O. Hippocampal ablation and passive avoidance. *Science,* 1962, *138,* 1104–1106.

Iversen, S. D. Tactile learning and memory in baboons after temporal and frontal lesions. *Experimental Neurology,* 1967, *18,* 228–238.

Iversen, S. D. Brain lesions and memory in animals. In J. A. Deutsch (Ed.), *The physiological basis of memory.* New York: Academic Press, 1973, 305–364.

Jackson, W. J., & Strong, P. N. Differential effects of hippocampal lesions upon sequential tasks and maze learning by the rat. *Journal of Comparative and Physiological Psychology,* 1969, *68,* 442–450.

Jacobsen, C. F. The functions of the frontal association areas in monkeys. *Comparative Psychological Monographs,* 1936, *13,* 1–60.

Jacobson, A. L., Fried, C., & Horowitz, S. D. Planarians and memory: I. Transfer of learning by injection of ribonucleic acid. *Nature,* 1966, *209,* 599–601. (a)

Jacobson, A. L., Fried, C., & Horowitz, S. D. Planarians and memory: II. The influence of prior extinction on the RNA transfer effect. *Nature,* 1966, *209,* 601. (b)

Jacobson, A. L., Horowitz, S. D., & Fried, C. Classical conditioning, pseudoconditioning, or sensitization in the planarian. *Journal of Comparative and Physiological Psychology,* 1967, *64,* 73–79.

Jamieson, J. L. *Temporal patterning of electroshock and retrograde amnesia.* Unpublished doctoral dissertation, University of British Columbia, 1972.

Jansen, G. R., & Hutchison, C. F. Production of hypothalamic obesity by microsurgery. *American Journal of Physiology,* 1969, *217,* 487–493.

Jarrard, L. E. Hippocampal ablation and operant behavior in the rat. *Psychonomic Science,* 1965, *2,* 115–116.

Jarrard, L. E., & Isaacson, R. L. Hippocampal ablation in rats: Effects of intertrial interval. *Nature,* 1965, *207,* 109–110.

Jarrard, L. E., Isaacson, R. L., & Wickelgren, W. O. Effects of hippocampal ablation and intertrial interval on runway acquisition and extinction. *Journal of Comparative and Physiological Psychology,* 1964, *57,* 442–444.

Jarrard, L. E., & Lewis, T. C. Effects of hippocampal ablation and intertrial interval on acquisition and extinction in a complex maze. *American Journal of Psychology,* 1967, *80,* 66–72.

John, E. R. Studies in learning and retention in planaria. In M. A. Brazier (Ed.), *Brain function* (Vol. 2). Berkeley: University of California Press, 1964, 161.

John, E. R. *Mechanisms of memory.* New York: Academic Press, 1967.

John, E. R. Brain mechanisms of memory. In J. L. McGaugh (Ed.), *Psychobiology: Behavior from a biological perspective.* New York: Academic Press, 1971, 199–283.

John, E. R. Switchboard versus statistical theories of learning and memory. *Science,* 1972, *177,* 850–864.

Johnson, D. A. Developmental aspects of recovery of function following septal lesions in the infant rat. *Journal of Comparative and Physiological Psychology,* 1972, *78,* 331–348.

Johnson, D. A., Beliauskas, L. A., and Lancaster, J. DRL training and performance following anterior, posterior or complete septal lesions in infant and adult rats. *Physiology and Behavior,* 1973, *11,* 661–669.

Johnson, L. C. Are stages of sleep related to waking behavior? *American Scientist,* 1973, *61,* 326–338.

Johnson, L. C., Slye, E., & Dement, W. C. EEG and autonomic activity during and after prolonged sleep deprivation. *Psychonomic Medicine,* 1965, *27,* 415–423.

Johnson, W. A., & Tiefer, L. Sexual preferences in neonatally castrated male golden hamsters. *Physiology and Behavior,* 1972, *9,* 213–217.

Johnston, J. W., & Sandoval, A. Organoleptic quality and the stereochemical theory of olfaction. *Proceedings of the Scientific Section of the Toilet Goods Association,* 1960, *33,* 3–9.

Jouvet, M. Paradoxical sleep—a study of its nature and mechanisms. In K. Akert, C. Bally, & J. P. Schadé (Eds.), *Sleep mechanisms, progress in brain research,* 1965, *18,* 20–62.

Jouvet, M. Neurophysiology of the states of sleep. *Physiology Review,* 1967, *47,* 117–177. (a)

Jouvet, M. The states of sleep. *Scientific American,* 1967, *216,* 62–72. (b)

Jouvet, M. Neurohumoral basis of sleep. In L. Madow & L. H. Snow (Eds.), *The psychodynamic implications of the physiological studies on dreams.* Springfield, Ill.: Charles C Thomas, 1970, 3–23.

Judd, D. B., & Wyszecki, G. *Color in business, science and industry* (2nd ed.). New York: Wiley, 1963.

Jung, R., & Hassler, R. The extrapyramidal motor system. In J. Field (Ed.), *Handbook of physiology; Section 1: Neurophysiology* (Vol. 2). Washington, D. C.: American Physiological Society, 1960, 863–927.

Jung, R., & Kornmüller, A. E. Eine Methodik der Abkitung lokalisierter Potentialschwankungen aus subcorticalen Hirngebieten. *Archiv für Psychiatrie und Nervenkrankheiten,* 1938, *109,* 1–30.

Justesen, D. R., Sharp, J. C., & Porter, P. B. Self-stimulation of the caudate nucleus by instrumentally naïve cats. *Journal of Comparative and Physiological Psychology,* 1963, *56,* 371–374.

Kaada, B. R. Somato-motor, autonomic and electrocorticographic responses to electrical stimulation of "rhinencephalic" and other structures in primates, cat and dog. *Acta Physiologica Scandinavica,* 1951, *24,* Suppl. 83, 1–258.

Kaada, B. R., Rasmussen, E. W., & Kveim, O. Effects of hippocampal lesions on maze learning and retention in rats. *Experimental Neurology,* 1961, *3,* 333–355.

Kaada, B., Rasmussen, E., & Kveim, O. Impaired acquisition of passive avoidance behavior by subcallosal, septal, hypothalamic, and insular lesions in rats. *Journal of Comparative and Physiological Psychology,* 1962, *55,* 661–670.

Kales, A., Hodemaker, F. S., & Jacobson, A. *Reportable mental activity during sleep.* Report to the Association for the Psychophysiological Study of Sleep: New York, 1963.

Kales, A., Hodemaker, F. S., Jacobson, A., & Lichtenstein, E. L. Dream deprivation: An experimental reappraisal. *Nature,* 1964, *204,* 1337–1338.

Kapatos, G., & Gold, R. M. Evidence for ascending noradrenergic mediation of hypothalamic hyperphagia. *Pharmacology, Biochemistry, and Behavior,* 1973, *1,* 81–87.

Kapp, B. S., & Schneider, A. M. Selective recovery from retrograde amnesia produced by hippocampal spreading depression. *Science,* 1971, *173,* 1149–1151.

Keesey, R. E., & Powley, T. L. Hypothalamic, regulation of body weight. *American Scientist,* 1975, *63,* 558–565.

Kemble, E. D., & Tapp, J. T. Passive and active avoidance performance following small amygdaloid lesions in rats. *Physiology and Behavior,* 1968, *3,* 713–718.

Kennedy, G. C. The role of depot fat in the hypothalamic control of food intake in the rat. *Proceedings of the Royal Society, Series B,* 1953, *140,* 578–592.

Kent, E., & Grossman, S. P. Evidence for a conflict interpretation of anomalous effects of rewarding brain stimulation. *Journal of Comparative and Physiological Psychology,* 1969, *69,* 381–390.

Kent, M. A., & Peters, R. H. Effects of ventromedial hypothalamic lesions on hunger-motivated behavior in rats. *Journal of Comparative and Physiological Psychology,* 1973, *83,* 92–97.

Kerpelman, L. C. Preexposure to visually presented forms and nondifferential reinforcement in perceptual learning. *Journal of Experimental Psychology,* 1965, *69,* 257–262.

Kesner, R. P., & Conner, H. S. Cue-dependent recovery from ECS-induced amnesia: Evidence for time dependence. *Physiological Psychology,* 1974, *2,* 123–125.

Kesner, R. P., Gibson, W. E., & LeClair, M. J. ECS as a punishing stimulus: Dependency on route of administration. *Physiology and Behavior,* 1970, *5,* 683–686.

Keyes, J. B. ECS perseveration effect following varying amounts of training. *Physiological Psychology,* 1973, *1,* 2–4. (a)

Keyes, J. B. The effect of ECS on the hippocampus. *Physiological Psychology,* 1973, *1,* 357–360. (b)

Keyes, J. B., & Dempsey, G. L. The effect of motivational state on ECS-induced perseveration. *Physiological Psychology,* 1973, *1,* 133–135.

Keyes, J. B., & Young, A. ECS effects: The PRE. *Bulletin of the Psychonomic Society,* 1973, *1,* 39–40.

Khazan, N., & Sawyer, C. "Rebound" recovery from deprivation of paradoxical sleep in the rabbit. *Proceedings of the Society of Experimental Biology and Medicine,* 1963, *114,* 536–539.

Kierniesky, N. C., & Gerall, A. A. Effects of testosterone proprionate implants in the brain on the sexual behavior and peripheral tissue of the male rat. *Physiology and Behavior,* 1973, *11,* 633–640.

Kim, C., Kim, C. C., Kim, J. K., Kim, M. S., Chang, H. K., Kim, J. Y., & Lee, I. G. Fear response and aggressive behavior of hippocampectomized house rats. *Brain Research,* 1971, *29,* 237–251.

Kimble, D. P. The effects of hippocampal lesions in rats. *Journal of Comparative and Physiological Psychology,* 1963, *56,* 273–283.

Kimble, D. P. The hippocampus and internal inhibition. *Psychological Bulletin,* 1968, *70,* 285–295.

Kimble, D. P., & Coover, G. D. Effects of hippocampal lesions on food and water consumption in rats. *Psychonomic Science,* 1966, *4,* 91–92.

Kimble, D. P., & Gostnell, D. Role of cingulate cortex in shock avoidance behavior of rats. *Journal of Comparative and Physiological Psychology,* 1968, *65,* 290–294,

Kimble, D. P., & Kimble, R. J. Hippocampectomy and response perseveration in the rat. *Journal of Comparative and Physiological Psychology,* 1965, *60,* 474–476.

Kimble, D. P., & Kimble, R. J. The effect of hippocampal lesions on extinction and "hypothesis" behavior in rats. *Physiology and Behavior,* 1970, *5,* 735–738.

Kimble, D. P., Kirkby, R. J., & Stein, D. G. Response perseveration interpretation of passive avoidance deficits in hippocampectomized rats. *Journal of Comparative and Physiological Psychology,* 1966, *61,* 141–143.

Kimble, D. P., & Pribram, K. H. Hippocampectomy and behavior sequences. *Science,* 1963, *139,* 824–825.

King, F. A. Effects of septal and amygdaloid lesions on emotional behavior and conditioned avoidance responses in the rat. *Journal of Nervous and Mental Disease,* 1958, *126,* 57–63.

King, M. B., & Hoebel, B. G. Killing elicited by brain stimulation in rats. *Communications in Behavioral Biology,* 1968, *4,* 173–177.

King, R. H., & Glasser, R. L. Duration of electro-convulsive shock-induced retrograde amnesia in rats. *Physiology and Behavior,* 1970, *5,* 335–339.

Kirkby, R. J., Stein, D. G., Kimble, R. J., & Kimble, D. P. Effects of hippocampal lesions and duration of sensory input on spontaneous alternation. *Journal of Comparative and Physiological Psychology,* 1967, *64,* 342–345.

Kleitman, N. Patterns of dreaming. *Scientific American,* 1960, *203,* 82–88.

Kleitman, N. *Sleep and wakefulness.* Chicago: University of Chicago Press, 1963.

Kling, A. Effects of amygdalectomy and testosterone on sexual behavior of male juvenile macaques. *Journal of Comparative and Physiological Psychology,* 1968, *65,* 466–471.

Klüver, H., & Bucy, P. C. "Psychic blindness" and other symptoms following bilateral temporal lobectomy in rhesus monkeys. *American Journal of Physiology,* 1937, *119,* 352–353.

Klüver, H., & Bucy, P. C. Preliminary analysis of the functions of the temporal lobes in monkeys. *Archives of Neurology and Psychiatry,* 1939, *42,* 979–1000.

Kohlenberg, R., & Trabasso, T. Recovery of a conditioned emotional response after one or two electroconvulsive shocks. *Journal of Comparative and Physiological Psychology,* 1968, *65,* 270–273.

Köhler, W., & Wegener, J. Currents of the human auditory cortex. *Journal of Cellular and Comparative Physiology,* 1955, *Suppl. 1,* 25–54.

Konorski, J. *Conditioned reflexes and neuron organization.* London and New York: Cambridge University Press, 1948.

Kopp, R., Bohdanecky, Z., & Jarvik, M. E. Proactive effect of a single electro-convulsive shock (ECS) on one-trial learning in mice. *Journal of Comparative and Physiological Psychology,* 1968, *65,* 514–517.

Koppenall, R. J., Jagoda, E., & Cruce, J. A. F. Recovery from ECS-produced amnesia following a reminder. *Psychonomic Science,* 1967, *9,* 293–294.

Korner, A. F. REM organization in neonates: Theoretical implications for development and the biological function of REM. *Archives of General Psychiatry,* 1968, *19,* 330–340.

Korsakoff, S. S. Etudé médico-psychologique sur une forme des maladies de la mémoire. *Revue de Philosophie,* 1889, *28,* 501–530.

Krech, D., Rosenzweig, M. R., & Bennett, E. L. Effects of complex environment and blindness on rat brain. *Archives of Neurology,* 1963, *8,* 403–412.

Kriekhaus, E. E. Decrements in avoidance behavior following mammillothalamic tractotomy in cats. *Journal of Neurophysiology,* 1964, *27,* 753–767.

Kriekhaus, E. E., Coons, E. E., Greenspon, T.,

Weiss, J., & Lorenz, R. L. Retention of choice behavior in rats following mammillothalamic tractotomy. *Physiology and Behavior,* 1968, *3,* 125–131.

Kriekhaus, E. E., & Lorenz, R. L. Retention and relearning of lever-press avoidance following mammillothalamic tractotomy. *Physiology and Behavior,* 1968, *3,* 433–438.

Kriekhaus, E. E., & Randall, D. Lesions of mammillothalamic tract in rat produce no decrements in recent memory. *Brain,* 1968, *91,* 369–378.

Kriekhaus, E. E., Simmons, H. J., Thomas, G. J., & Kenyon, J. Septal lesions enhance shock avoidance behavior in the rat. *Experimental Neurology,* 1964, *9,* 107–113.

Kupfermann, I. Neurophysiology of learning. *Annual Review of Psychology,* 1975, *26,* 367–391.

Kupfermann, I., Castellucci, V., Pinsker, H., & Kandel, E. Neuronal correlates of habituation and dishabituation of the gill-withdrawal reflex in *Aplysia. Science,* 1970, *167,* 1743–1745.

Kupfermann, I., & Kandel, E. R. Neuronal correlates of a behavioral response mediated by the abdominal ganglion of *Aplysia. Science,* 1969, *164,* 847–850.

Kveim, O., Setekleiv, J., & Kaada, B. R. Differential effects of hippocampal lesions on maze and passive-avoidance learning in rats. *Experimental Neurology,* 1964, *9,* 59–72.

Larsson, K., & Heimer, L. Mating behavior of male rats after lesions in the preoptic area. *Nature,* 1964, *202,* 413–414.

Larsson, S. On the hypothalamic organization of the nervous mechanism regulating food intake. Part I. Hyperphagia from stimulation of the hypothalamus and medulla in sheep and goats. *Acta Physiologica Scandinavica,* 1954, *32, Suppl. 115,* 1–40.

Lashley, K. S. In search of the engram. *Society for Experimental Biology,* 1950, Symposium No. 4, 454–482.

Lashley, K. S. Cerebral organization and behavior. *Research Publications of the Association for Research in Nervous and Mental Disease,* 1958, *36,* 1–18.

Lawicka, W. The effect of the prefrontal lobectomy on the vocal conditioned reflexes in dogs. *Acta Biologiae Experimentalis* (Warsaw), 1957, *17,* 317–325.

Lawicka, W., & Konorski, J. The physiological mechanisms of delayed reactions. II. Delayed reactions in dogs and cats to directional stimuli. *Acta Biologiae Experimentalis* (Warsaw), 1959, *19,* 199–219.

Lawicka, W., & Konorski, J. The effects of prefrontal lobectomies on the delayed responses in cats. *Acta Biologiae Experimentalis* (Warsaw), 1961, *21,* 141–156.

Le Beau, J. Anterior cingulectomy in man. *Journal of Neurosurgery,* 1954, *11,* 268–276.

Lee-Teng, E., & Sherman, S. M. Memory consolidation of one-trial learning in chicks. *Proceedings of the National Academy of Sciences,* 1966, *56,* 926–931.

Leiman, A. L., & Christian, C. N. Electrophysiological analyses of learning and memory. In J. A. Deutsch (Ed.), *The physiological basis of memory.* New York: Academic Press, 1973, 125–165.

Leonard, D. J., & Zavala, A. Electroconvulsive shock, retroactive amnesia, and the single-shock method. *Science,* 1964, *146,* 1073–1074.

Lesse, H. Rhinencephalic electrophysiological activity during "emotional behavior" in cats. *Psychiatry Research Reports,* 1960, *12,* 332–333.

Lettvin, J. Y., Maturana, H. R., McCulloch, W. S., & Pitts, W. H. What the frog's eye tells the frog's brain. *Proceedings of the Institute of Radio Engineers,* 1959, *47,* 1940–1951.

Levison, P. K., & Flynn, J. P. The objects attacked by cats during stimulation of the hypothalamus. *Animal Behavior,* 1965, *13,* 217–220.

Lewis, D. J., & Maher, B. A. Neural consolidation and electroconvulsive shock. *Psychological Review,* 1965, *72,* 225–239.

Lewis, D. J., Miller, R. R., & Misanin, J. R. Control of retrograde amnesia. *Journal of Comparative and Physiological Psychology,* 1968, *66,* 48–52.

Lickey, M. E., & Fox, S. S. Localization and habituation of sensory evoked DC responses in cat cortex. *Experimental Neurology,* 1966, *15,* 437–454.

Lilly, J. C. Learning motivated by subcortical stimulation. In E. R. Ramey & D. S. O'Doherty (Eds.), *Electrical studies on the unanesthetized brain.* New York: Hoeber, 1960.

Lindsley, D. B. Attention, consciousness, sleep and wakefulness. In J. Field (Ed.), *Handbook of physiology; Section I: Neurophysiology,* (Vol. 3). Washington, D.C.: American Physiological Society, 1960, 1553–1593.

Lindsley, D. B., Bowden, J., & Magoun, H. W. Effect upon EEG of acute injury to the brain stem activating system. *Electroencephalography and Clinical Neurophysiology,* 1949, *1,* 475–486.

Lints, C. E., & Harvey, J. A. Altered sensitivity to foot shock and decreased brain content of serotonin following brain lesions in the rat. *Journal of Comparative and Physiological Psychology,* 1969, *67,* 23–31.

Lonowski, D. J., Levitt, R. A., & Larson, S. D. Effects of cholinergic brain injections on mouse killing or carrying by rats. *Physiological Psychology,* 1973, *1,* 341–345.

Loomis, A. L., Harvey, E. N., & Hobart, G. A. Potential rhythms of the cerebral cortex during sleep. *Science,* 1935, *81,* 597–598.

Loomis, A. L., Harvey, E. N., & Hobart, G. A. Cerebral states during sleep as studied by human brain potentials. *Journal of Experimental Psychology,* 1937, *21,* 127–144.

Lorens, S. A. Effects of lesions in the central nervous system on lateral hypothalamic self-stimulation in the rat. *Journal of Comparative and Physiological Psychology,* 1966, *62,* 256–262.

Lovely, R. H. Hormonal dissociation of limbic lesion effects on shuttle box avoidance in rats. *Journal of Comparative and Physiological Psychology,* 1975, *89,* 224–230.

Lubar, J. F. Effect of medial cortical lesions on the avoidance behavior of the cat. *Journal of Comparative and Physiological Psychology,* 1964, *58,* 38–46.

Lubar, J. F., Boyce, B. A., & Schaefer, C. F. Etiology of polydipsia and polyuria in rats with septal lesions. *Physiology and Behavior,* 1968, *3,* 289–292.

Lubar, J. F., Brener, J. M., Deagle, J. H., Numan, R., & Clemens, W. J. Effect of septal lesions on detection threshold and unconditioned response to shock. *Physiology and Behavior,* 1970, *5,* 459–463.

Lubar, J. F., Hermann, T. F., Moore, D. R., & Shouse, M. N. Effects of septal and frontal ablations on species-typical behavior in the rat. *Journal of Comparative and Physiological Psychology,* 1973, *83,* 260–270.

Lubar, J. F., & Perachio, A. A. One-way and two-way learning and transfer of an active avoidance response in normal and cingulectomized cats. *Journal of Comparative and Physiological Psychology,* 1965, *60,* 46–52.

Lubar, J. F., Perachio, A. A., & Kavanagh, A. J. Deficits in active avoidance behavior following lesions of the lateral and posterolateral gyrus of the cat. *Journal of Comparative and Physiological Psychology,* 1966, *62,* 263–269.

Luce, G. G. *Research on sleep and dreams.* Bethesda, Md.: National Institute of Mental Health, 1965.

Luttges, M., Johnston, T., Buck, C., Holland, J., & McGaugh, J. L. An examination of "transfer of learning" by nucleic acid. *Science,* 1966, *151,* 834–837.

Luttges, M. W., & McGaugh, J. L. Permanence of retrograde amnesia produced by electroconvulsive shock. *Science,* 1967, *156,* 408–410.

MacDonnell, M. F., & Flynn, J. P. Attack elicited by stimulation of the thalamus of cats. *Science,* 1964, *144,* 1249–1250.

MacDougall, J. M., Van Hoesen, G. W., & Mitchell, J. C. Anatomical organization of septal projections in maintenance of DRL behavior in rats. *Journal of Comparative and Physiological Psychology,* 1969, *68,* 568–575.

MacInnes, J. W., McConkey, E. H., & Schlesinger, K. Changes in brain polyribosomes following an electroconvulsive seizure. *Journal of Neurochemistry,* 1970, *17,* 457–460.

MacNichol, E. F. Three-pigment color vision. *Scientific American,* 1964, *211,* 48–56.

Madsen, M. C., & Kimble, D. P. The maze behavior

316

References

of hippocampectomized ràts under massed and distributed trials. *Psychonomic Science,* 1965, *3,* 193–194.

Madsen, M. C., & Luttges, M. W. Effect of electroconvulsive shock (ECS) on extinction of an approach response. *Psychological Reports,* 1963, *13,* 225–226.

Mah, C. J., & Albert, D. J. Electroconvulsive shock-induced retrograde amnesia: An analysis of the variation in the length of the amnesia gradient. *Behavioral Biology,* 1973, *9,* 517–540.

Mah, C. J., Albert, D. J., & Jamieson, J. L. Memory storage: Evidence that consolidation continues following electroconvulsive shock. *Physiology and Behavior,* 1972, *8,* 283–286.

Malmo, R. B. Interference factors in delayed response in monkeys after removal of frontal lobes. *Journal of Neurophysiology,* 1942, *5,* 295–308.

Malsbury, C. W. Facilitation of male copulatory behavior by electrical stimulation of the medial preoptic area. *Physiology and Behavior,* 1971, *7,* 797–805.

Mark, V. H., & Ervin, F. R. *Violence and the brain.* New York: Harper & Row, 1970.

Marks, W. B., Dobelle, W. H., & MacNichol, E. F. Visual pigments of single primate cones. *Science,* 1964, *143,* 1181–1182.

Marshall, J. F., & Richardson, J. S. Nigrostriatal bundle damage and the lateral hypothalamic syndrome. *Journal of Comparative and Physiological Psychology,* 1974, *87,* 808–830.

Mason, W. A. The effects of social restriction on the behavior of rhesus monkeys. I. Free social behavior. *Journal of Comparative and Physiological Psychology,* 1960, *53,* 582–589.

Masserman, J. H., & Pechtel, C. How brain lesions affect normal and neurotic behavior (an experimental approach). *American Journal of Psychiatry,* 1956, *112,* 865–872.

Maturana, H. R., Lettvin, J. Y., McCulloch, W. S., & Pitts, W. H. Anatomy and physiology of vision in the frog *(Rana pipiens). Journal of General Physiology,* 1960, *43,* 129–175.

Mayer, Ch., & Stumpf, Ch. Die physostigminwirkung auf die hippocampustätigkeit nach septumläsionen. *Naunyn-Schmiedeberg's Arch. Exp. Pathol. Pharmakol.,* 1958, *234,* 490–500.

Mayer, J. Regulation of energy intake and the body weight. The glucostatic theory and the lipostatic hypothesis. *Annals of the New York Academy of Sciences,* 1955, *63,* 15–43.

Mayer, J., & Marshall, N. B. Specificity of gold thioglucose for ventromedial hypothalamic lesions and hyperphagia. *Nature,* 1956, *178,* 1399–1400.

Mayor, S. J. Memory in the Japanese quail: Effects of puromycin and acetoxycyclohexamide. *Science,* 1969, *166,* 1165–1167.

McCleary, R. A. Response-modulation functions of the limbic system: Initiation and suppression. In E. Stellar & J. M. Sprague (Eds.), *Progress in physiological psychology* (Vol. 1). New York: Academic Press, 1966, 209–272.

McConnell, J. V. Memory transfer through cannibalism in planarians. *Journal of Neuropsychiatry,* 1962, *3, Suppl. 1,* 42–48.

McConnell, J. V., & Jacobson, A. L. Learning in invertebrates. In D. A. Dewsbury & D. A. Rethlingshafer (Eds.), *Comparative psychology: A modern survey.* New York: McGraw-Hill, 1973, 429–470.

McConnell, J. V., Jacobson, A. L., & Kimble, D. P. The effects of regeneration upon retention of a conditioned response in the planarian. *Journal of Comparative and Physiological Psychology,* 1959, *52,* 1–5.

McConnell, J. V., & Shelby, J. M. Memory transfer experiments in invertebrates. In G. Ungar (Ed.), *Molecular mechanisms in memory and learning.* New York: Plenum Press, 1970, 71–101.

McGaugh, J. L. Time-dependent processes in memory storage. *Science,* 1966, *153,* 1351–1358.

McGaugh, J. L., & Alpern, H. P. Effects of electroshock on memory: Amnesia without convulsions. *Science,* 1966, *152,* 665–666.

McGaugh, J. L., & Dawson, R. G. Modification of memory storage processes. *Behavioral Science,* 1971, *16,* 45–63.

McGaugh, J. L., & Herz, M. J. *Memory Consolidation.* San Francisco: Albion, 1972.

McGaugh, J. L., Landfield, P. W., & Dawson, R. G. Delayed development of amnesia following electroconvulsive shock: A further examination. Unpublished. Cited in McGaugh, J. L. & Herz, M. J. *Memory Consolidation.* San Francisco: Albion, 1972.

McGaugh, J. L., & Madsen, M. C. Amnesic and punishing effects of electroconvulsive shock. *Science,* 1964, *144,* 182–183.

McGaugh, J. L., Zornetzer, S. F., Gold, P. E., & Landfield, P. W. Modification of memory systems: Some neurobiological aspects. *Quarterly Reviews of Biophysics,* 1972, *5,* 163–186.

Means, L. W., Harrell, T. H., Mayo, E. S., & Alexander, G. B. Effects of dorsomedial thalamic lesions on spontaneous alternation, maze activity and runway performance in the rat. *Physiology and Behavior,* 1974, *12,* 973–979.

Means, L. W., Huntley, D. H., Anderson, H. P., & Harrell, T. H. Deficient acquisition and retention of a visual-tactile discrimination task in rats with medial thalamic lesions. *Behavioral Biology,* 1973, *9,* 435–450.

Means, L. W., Leander, J. D., & Isaacson, R. L. The effects of hippocampectomy on alternation behavior and response to novelty. *Physiology and Behavior,* 1971, *6,* 17–22.

Mendoza, J. E., & Adams, H. E. Does electroconvulsive shock produce retrograde amnesia? *Physiology and Behavior,* 1969, *4,* 307–309.

Mettler, F. A. (Ed.). *Psychosurgical Problems.* New

York: Blakiston, 1952.

Miczek, K. A., & Grossman, S. P. Effects of septal lesions on inter- and intraspecies aggression in rats. *Journal of Comparative and Physiological Psychology*, 1972, *79*, 37–45.

Miczek, K. A., Kelsey, J. E., & Grossman, S. P. Time course of effects of septal lesions on avoidance, response suppression, and reactivity to shock. *Journal of Comparative and Physiological Psychology*, 1972, *79*, 318–327.

Middaugh, L. D., & Lubar, J. F. Interaction of septal lesions and experience on the suppression of punished responses. *Physiology and Behavior*, 1970, *5*, 233–237.

Mihailović, L., Kržalić, L., Petrović, B., & Čupić, D. Disc electrophoretic analysis of soluble brain proteins in the brain of monkeys subjected to visual discrimination. In G. Adam (Ed.), *Biology of memory*. New York: Plenum Press, 1971, 87–92.

Miles, R. C., & Blomquist, A. J. Frontal lesions and behavioral deficits in monkeys. *Journal of Neurophysiology*, 1960, *23*, 471–484.

Miller, A. J. Variations in retrograde amnesia with parameters of electroconvulsive shock and time of testing. *Journal of Comparative and Physiological Psychology*, 1968, *66*, 40–47.

Miller, N. E. Learning and performance motivated by direct stimulation of the brain. In D. E. Sheer (Ed.), *Electrical stimulation of the brain*. Austin: University of Texas Press, 1961, 387–396.

Miller, N. E. Learning of visceral and glandular responses. *Science*, 1969, *163*, 434–445.

Miller, N. E., Bailey, C. J., & Stevenson, J. A. F. Decreased "hunger" but increased food intake resulting from hypothalamic lesions. *Science*, 1950, *112*, 256–259.

Miller, R. R. Effects of environmental complexity on amnesia induced by electroconvulsive shock in rats. *Journal of Comparative and Physiological Psychology*, 1970, *71*, 267–275.

Miller, R. R., Ott, C. A., Berk, A. M., & Springer, A. D. Appetitive memory restoration after electroconvulsive shock in the rat. *Journal of Comparative and Physiological Psychology*, 1974, *87*, 717–723.

Miller, R. R., & Springer, A. D. Induced recovery of memory in rats following electroconvulsive shock. *Physiology and Behavior*, 1972, *8*, 645–651.

Milner, B. Some effects of frontal lobectomy in man. In J. M. Warren & K. Akert (Eds.), *The frontal granular cortex and behavior*. New York: McGraw-Hill, 1964, 313–334.

Milner, B. Amnesia following operation on the temporal lobes. In C. W. M. Whitty & O. L. Zangwill (Eds.), *Amnesia*. London: Butterworths, 1966, 109–133.

Milner, P. M. *Physiological psychology*. New York: Holt, Rinehart and Winston, 1970.

Mirsky, I. A., Rosvold, H. E., & Pribram, K. H.

Effects of cingulectomy on social behavior in monkeys. *Journal of Neurophysiology*, 1957, *20*, 588–601.

Mishkin, M. Visual discrimination performance following partial ablations of the temporal lobe. II. Ventral surfaces vs. hippocampus. *Journal of Comparative and Physiological Psychology*, 1954, *47*, 187–193.

Mishkin, M. Perseveration of central sets after frontal lesions in monkeys. In J. M. Warren & K. Akert (Eds.), *The frontal granular cortex and behavior*. New York: McGraw-Hill, 1964, 219–241.

Mishkin, M., & Pribram, K. H. Visual discrimination performance following partial ablation of the temporal lobe. I. Ventral vs. lateral. *Journal of Comparative and Physiological Psychology*, 1954, *47*, 14–20.

Mishkin, M., Vest, B., Waxler, M., & Rosvold, H. E. A reexamination of the effects of frontal lesions on object alternation. *Neuropsychologia*, 1969, *7*, 357–364.

Møllgard, K., Diamond, M. C., Bennett, E. L., Rosenzweig, M. R., & Lindner, B. Quantitative synaptic changes with differential experience in rat brain. *International Journal of Neuroscience*, 1971, *2*, 113–128.

Moncrieff, R. W. What is odor? A new theory. *Essential Oils Review*, 1949, *54*, 453–454.

Moniz, E. *Tentatives Opératoires dans le Traitement de Certaines Psychoses*. Paris: Masson, 1936.

Monné, L. Functioning of the cytoplasm. In F. F. Nord (Ed.), *Advances in enzymology* (vol. 8). New York: Interscience, 1948, 1–69.

Montgomery, M. F. The role of the salivary glands in the thirst mechanism. *American Journal of Physiology*, 1931, *96*, 221–227.

Moore, R. Y. Effects on some rhinencephalic lesions on retention of conditioned avoidance behavior in cats. *Journal of Comparative and Physiological Psychology*, 1964, *53*, 540–548.

Morden, B., Mitchell, G., & Dement, W. C. Selective REM sleep deprivation and compensation phenomena in the rat. *Brain Research*, 1967, *5*, 339–349.

Morgan, C. T., & Fields, P. E. The effect of variable preliminary feeding upon the rat's speed of locomotion. *Journal of Comparative and Physiological Psychology*, 1938, *26*, 331–348.

Morgane, P. J. Electrophysiological studies of feeding and satiety centers in the rat. *American Journal of Physiology*, 1961, *201*, 838–844.

Morris, G. O., & Singer, M. T. Sleep deprivation. *Archives of General Psychiatry*, 1961, *5*, 453.

Moruzzi, G., & Magoun, H. W. Brain stem reticular formation and activation of the EEG. *Electroencephalography and Clinical Neurophysiology*, 1949, *1*, 455–473.

Moss, D. E. *Puromycin and memory*. Unpublished doctoral dissertation, Colorado State University, 1973.

Mountcastle, V. B. Pain and temperature sensibilities. In V. B. Mountcastle (Ed.), *Medical physiology* (Vol. 2, 12th ed.). St. Louis: Mosby, 1968, 1424–1464.

Müller, G. E., & Pilzecker, A. Experimentelle Bieträge zur Lehre vom Gedächtniss. *Zeitschrift für Psychologie und Physiologie der Sinnesorgane, Erganzungsband,* 1900, *1,* 1–288.

Müller, J. *Handbuch der Physiologie des Menschen für Vorlesungen* (Vol. 2). Coblenz, 1838.

Murray, E. J. *Sleep, dreams, and arousal.* New York: Appleton-Century-Crofts, 1965.

Myers, R. D. Chemical mechanisms in the hypothalamus mediating eating and drinking in the monkey. *Annals of the New York Academy of Sciences,* 1969, *157,* 918–933.

Myers, R. D. *Methods in Psychobiology* (Vol. 1). New York: Academic Press, 1971.

Myers, R. D. *Handbook of drug and chemical stimulation of the brain: Behavioral, pharmacological and physiological aspects.* New York: Van Nostrand Reinhold, 1974.

Myers, R. D., & Sharpe, L. G. Chemical evaluation of ingestive and other hypothalamic regulatory mechanisms. *Physiology and Behavior,* 1968, *3,* 987–995.

Nakajima, S. Biochemical disruption of memory: A re-examination. In W. B. Essman & S. Nakajima (Eds.), *Current biochemical approaches to learning and memory.* Flushing, New York: Spectrum, 1973, 133–146.

Neff, W. D. Neural mechanisms of auditory discrimination. In W. A. Rosenblith (Ed.), *Sensory communication.* New York: Wiley, 1961, 259–278.

Neff, W. D., & Diamond, I. T. The neural basis of auditory discrimination. In H. F. Harlow & C. N. Woolsey (Eds.), *Biological and biochemical bases of behavior.* Madison: University of Wisconsin Press, 1958, 101–126.

Niki, H. The effects of hippocampal ablation on the behavior in the rat. *Japanese Psychological Research,* 1962, *4,* 139–153.

Niki, H. The effects of hippocampal ablation on the inhibitory control of operant behavior in the rat. *Japanese Psychological Research,* 1965, *7,* 126–137.

Niki, H. Response perseveration following the hippocampal ablation in the rat. *Japanese Psychological Research,* 1966, *8,* 1–9.

Nonneman, A. J., & Isaacson, R. L. Task dependent recovery after early brain damage. *Behavioral Biology,* 1973, *8,* 143–172.

Numan, M. Medial preoptic area and maternal behavior in the female rat. *Journal of Comparative and Physiological Psychology,* 1974, *87,* 746–759.

Nurnberger, J. I. Direct enumeration of cells of the brain. In W. F. Windle (Ed.), *Biology of neuroglia.* Springfield: Charles C Thomas, 1958, 193–202.

Olds, J. Physiological mechanisms of reward. In M. R. Jones (Ed.), *Nebraska Symposium on Motivation* (Vol. 3). Lincoln: University of Nebraska Press, 1955, 73–138.

Olds, J. Pleasure centers in the brain. *Scientific American,* 1956, *195,* 105–116.

Olds, J. Self-stimulation of the brain. *Science,* 1958, *127,* 315–324. (a)

Olds, J. Satiation effects in self-stimulation of the brain. *Journal of Comparative and Physiological Psychology,* 1958, *51,* 675–678. (b)

Olds, J. Differentiation of reward systems in the brain by self-stimulation techniques. In E. R. Ramey & D. S. O'Doherty (Eds.), *Electrical studies on the unanesthetized brain.* New York: Hoeber, 1960, 17–51.

Olds, J. Operant conditioning of single unit responses. *Proceedings of the XXIII International Congress of Physiological Science,* Tokyo, 1965, *4,* 372–380.

Olds, J. The limbic system and behavioral reinforcement. In W. R. Adey & T. Tokizane (Eds.). *Progress in brain research: Structure and function of the limbic system* (Vol. 27). Amsterdam: Elsevier, 1967.

Olds, J. The central nervous system and the reinforcement of behavior. *American Psychologist,* 1969, *24,* 114–132.

Olds, J., & Hirano, T. Conditioned responses of hippocampal and other neurons. *Electroencephalography and Clinical Neurophysiology,* 1969, *26,* 159–166.

Olds, J., & Milner, P. Positive reinforcement produced by electrical stimulation of septal area and other regions of the rat brain. *Journal of Comparative and Physiological Psychology,* 1954, *47,* 419–427.

Olds, J., Mink, W. D., & Best, P. J. Single unit patterns during anticipatory behavior. *Electroencephalography and Clinical Neurophysiology,* 1969, *26,* 144–158.

Olds, J., & Olds, M. E. Interference and learning in paleocortical systems. In J. F. Delafresnaye (Ed.), *Brain mechanisms in learning.* Oxford: Blackwell, 1961, 153–188.

Olds, J., & Olds, M. E. Drives, rewards, and the brain. In T. M. Newcombe (Ed.), *New directions in psychology* (Vol. 2). New York: Holt, Rinehart and Winston, 1965, 327–410.

Olds, M. E., & Olds, J. Approach-avoidance analysis of rat diencephalon. *Journal of Comparative Neurology,* 1963, *120,* 259–295.

Olton, D. S. Discrimination reversal performance after hippocampal lesions: An enduring failure of reinforcement and non-reinforcement to direct behavior. *Physiology and Behavior,* 1972, *9,* 353–356.

Olton, D. S., & Isaacson, R. L. Hippocampal lesions and active avoidance. *Physiology and Behavior,* 1968, *3,* 719–724.

Orbach, J. "Functions" of striate cortex and the

problems of mass action. *Psychological Bulletin,* 1959, *56,* 271–292.

Orbach, J., Milner, B., & Rasmussen, T. Learning and retention in monkeys after amygdalahippocampal resection. *Archives of Neurology,* 1960, *3,* 230–251.

Oshima, K., Gorbman, A., & Shimada, H. Memory-blocking agents: Effects on olfactory discrimination in homing salmon. *Science,* 1969, *165,* 86–88.

Ottoson, D. Analysis of the electrical activity of the olfactory epithelium. *Acta Physiologica Scandinavica,* 1956, *35, Suppl. 122,* 1–82.

Pagano, R. R., Bush, D. F., Martin, G., & Hunt, E. B. Duration of retrograde amnesia as a function of electroconvulsive shock intensity. *Physiology and Behavior,* 1969, *4,* 19–21.

Panksepp, J. Aggression elicited by electrical stimulation of the hypothalamus in albino rats. *Physiology and Behavior,* 1971, *6,* 321–329.

Paolino, R. M., & Hine, B. EEG seizure anomalies following supramaximal intensities of cortical stimulation. *Journal of Comparative and Physiological Psychology,* 1973, *2,* 285–293.

Paolino, R. M., & Levy, H. M. Amnesia produced by spreading depression and ECS: Evidence for time-dependent memory trace localization. *Science,* 1971, *172,* 746–749.

Paolino, R. M., Quartermain, D., & Levy, H. M. Effect of electroconvulsive shock duration on the gradient of retrograde amnesia. *Physiology and Behavior,* 1969, *4,* 147–149.

Papesdorf, J., & Woodruff, M. Effects of bilateral hippocampectomy on the rabbit's acquisition of shuttle-box and passive avoidance responses. *Journal of Comparative and Physiological Psychology,* 1970, *73,* 486–489.

Papez, J. W. A proposed mechanism of emotion. *Archives of Neurology and Psychiatry,* 1937, *38,* 725–743.

Paup, D. C., Coniglio, L. P., & Clemens, L. G. Masculinization of the female golden hamster by neonatal treatment with androgen or estrogen. *Hormones and Behavior,* 1972, *3,* 123–131.

Paup, D. C., Coniglio, L. P., & Clemens, L. G. Hormonal determinants in the development of masculine and feminine behavior in the female hamster. *Behavioral Biology,* 1974, *10,* 353–363.

Pavlov, I. *Conditioned reflexes: An investigation of the physiological activity of the cerebral cortex.* New York: Oxford University Press, 1927.

Paxinos, G., & Bindra, D. Hypothalamic knife cuts: Effects on eating, drinking, irritability, aggression and copulation in the male rat. *Journal of Comparative and Physiological Psychology,* 1972, *79,* 219–229.

Paxinos, G., & Bindra, D. Hypothalamic and midbrain pathways involved in eating, drinking, irritability, aggression, and copulation in rats. *Journal of Comparative and Physiological Psychology,* 1973, *82,* 1–14.

Peeke, H. V. S., McCoy, F., & Herz, M. J. Drive consummatory response effects on memory consolidation for appetitive learning in mice. *Communications in Behavioral Biology,* 1969, *4,* 49–53.

Peck, J. W., & Novin, D. Evidence that osmoreceptors mediating drinking in rabbits are in the lateral preoptic area. *Journal of Comparative and Physiological Psychology,* 1971, *74,* 134–147.

Peele, T. L. *The neuroanatomical basis for clinical neurology.* New York: McGraw-Hill, 1954.

Pellegrino, L. J. Amygdaloid lesions and behavioral inhibition in the rat. *Journal of Comparative and Physiological Psychology,* 1968, *65,* 483–491.

Pellegrino, L. J., & Clapp, D. R. Limbic lesions and externally cued DRL performance. *Physiology and Behavior,* 1971, *7,* 863–868.

Pellegrino, L. J., & Cushman, A. J. *A stereotaxic atlas of the rat brain.* New York: Appleton-Century-Crofts, 1967.

Penfield, W. Speech, perception and the uncommitted cortex. *Pontifasiae Academiae Scientarum, Scripta varia,* 1965, *30,* 319–347.

Penfield, W., & Milner, B. Memory deficits produced by bilateral lesions in the hippocampal zone. *Archives of Neurology and Psychiatry,* 1958, *79,* 475–497.

Penfield, W., & Perot, P. The brain's record of auditory and visual experiences—a final summary and discussion. *Brain,* 1963, *86,* 595–696.

Penfield, W., & Rasmussen, T. *The cerebral cortex of man.* New York: Macmillan, 1950.

Perachio, A. A., & Lubar, J. F. Striate cortex ablation and deficits in conditioned avoidance response. *Physiology and Behavior,* 1970, *5,* 729–733.

Peretz, E. The effects of lesions of the anterior cingulate cortex on the behavior of the rat. *Journal of Comparative and Physiological Psychology,* 1960, *53,* 540–548.

Peretz, E. Extinction of a food-reinforced response in hippocampectomized cats. *Journal of Comparative and Physiological Psychology,* 1965, *60,* 182–185.

Petsche, H., Stumpf, Ch., & Gogolak, G. The significance of the rabbit's septum as a relay station between the midbrain and the hippocampus. I. The control of hippocampus arousal activity by the septum cells. *Electroencephalography and Clinical Neurophysiology,* 1962, *14,* 202–211.

Phillips, A. G., & Lieblich, I. Developmental and hormonal aspects of hyperemotionality produced by septal lesions in male rats. *Physiology and Behavior,* 1972, *9,* 237–242.

Phillips, A. G., & Mogenson, G. J. Self-stimulation of the olfactory bulb. *Physiology and Behavior,* 1969, *4,* 195–197.

Phillips, M. I., & Olds, J. Unit activity: Motivation-dependent responses from midbrain neurons. *Science,* 1969, *165,* 1269–1271.

Phoenix, C. H., Goy, R. W., Gerall, A. A., & Young, W. C. Organizing action of prenatally administered testosterone proprionate on the tissues mediating mating behavior in the female guinea pig. *Endocrinology,* 1959, *65,* 369–382.

Pinsker, H., Kupfermann, I., Castellucci, V., & Kandel, E. Habituation and dishabituation of the gill-withdrawal reflex in *Aplysia. Science,* 1970, *167,* 1740–1742.

Pirch, J. H. Temporary improvement in shuttle-box performance after repeated electroconvulsive shock treatment. *Physiology and Behavior,* 1969, *4,* 517–521.

Polyak, S. *The vertebrate visual system.* Chicago: University of Chicago Press, 1957 (edited by H. Klüver).

Porter, J. H., Allen, J. D., & Arazie, R. Reinforcement frequency and body weight as determinants of motivated performance in hypothalamic hyperphagic rats. *Physiology and Behavior,* 1974, *13,* 627–632.

Pribram, K. H. Some physical and pharmacological factors affecting delayed response performance of baboons following frontal lobotomy. *Journal of Neurophysiology,* 1950, *13,* 373–382.

Pribram, K. H., & Fulton, J. F. An experimental critique of the effects of anterior cingulate ablations in monkey. *Brain,* 1954, *77,* 34–44.

Pribram, K. H., & Weiskrantz, L. A comparison of the effects of medial and lateral cerebral resections on conditioned avoidance behavior of monkeys. *Journal of Comparative and Physiological Psychology,* 1957, *50,* 74–80.

Quartermain, D., McEwen, B. S., & Azmitia, E. C., Jr. Amnesia produced by electroconvulsive shock or cyclohexamide: Conditions for recovery. *Science,* 1970, *169,* 683–686.

Quartermain, D., McEwen, B. S., & Azmitia, E. C., Jr. Recovery of memory following amnesia in the rat and mouse. *Journal of Comparative and Physiological Psychology,* 1972, *79,* 360–370.

Quartermain, D., Paolino, R. M., & Miller, N. E. A brief temporal gradient of retrograde amnesia independent of situational change. *Science,* 1965, *149,* 1116–1118.

Raab, D. H., & Ades, H. W. Cortical and midbrain mediation of a conditioned discrimination of acoustical intensities. *American Journal of Psychology,* 1946, *59,* 59–83.

Rabe, A., & Haddad, R. K. Acquisition of two-way shuttlebox avoidance after selective hippocampal lesions. *Physiology and Behavior,* 1969, *4,* 319–323.

Rabin, B. M. Independence of food intake and obesity following ventromedial hypothalamic lesions in the rat. *Physiology and Behavior,* 1974, *13,* 769–772.

Racine, R. J., & Kimble, D. P. Hippocampal lesions and delayed alternation in the rat. *Psychonomic Science,* 1965, *3,* 285–286.

Raisman, G., & Field, P. M. Sexual dimorphism in the neuropil of the preoptic area of the rat and its dependence on neonatal androgen. *Brain Research,* 1973, *54,* 1–29.

Ranck, J. B., Jr. Studies on single neurons in dorsal hippocampal formation and septum in unrestrained rats. I. Behavioral correlates and firing repertoires. *Experimental Neurology,* 1973, *41,* 461–555. (a)

Ranck, J. B., Jr. A movable microelectrode for recording from single neurons in unrestrained rats. In M. I. Phillips (Ed.), *Brain unit activity during behavior.* Iowa City: University of Iowa Press, 1973, 76–79. (b)

Ransom, B. R., & Goldring, S. Ionic determinants of membrane potential of cells presumed to be glia in cerebral cortex of cats. *Journal of Neurophysiology,* 1973, *36,* 855–868. (a)

Ransom, B. R., & Goldring, S. Slow depolarization in cells presumed to be glia in cerebral cortex of cat. *Journal of Neurophysiology,* 1973, *36,* 869–878. (b)

Ransom, B. R., & Goldring, S. Slow hyperpolarization in cells presumed to be glia in cerebral cortex of cat. *Journal of Neurophysiology,* 1973, *36,* 879–892. (c)

Ranson, S. W. The hypothalamus: Its significance for visceral innervation and emotional expression. The Weir Mitchell Oration, *Transactions and Studies of the College of Physicians of Philadelphia,* Series IV, 1934, *2,* 222–242.

Ranson, S. W. Somnolence caused by hypothalamic lesions in the monkey. *Archives of Neurology and Psychiatry,* 1939, *41,* 1–23.

Raphelson, A. C., Isaacson, R. L., & Douglas, R. J. The effect of limbic damage on the retention and performance of a runway response. *Neuropsychologia,* 1966, *4,* 253–264.

Rappoport, D. A., & Daginawala, H. F. Changes in nuclear RNA of brain induced by olfaction in catfish. *Journal of Neurochemistry,* 1968, *15,* 991–1006.

Ray, O. S., & Barrett, R. J. Disruptive effects of electroconvulsive shock as a function of current level and mode of delivery. *Journal of Comparative and Physiological Psychology,* 1969, *67,* 110–116.

Ray, O. S., & Bivens, L. W. Reinforcement magnitude as a determinant of performance decrement after electroconvulsive shock. *Science,* 1968, *160,* 330–332.

Ray, O. S., Hine, B., & Bivens, L. W. Stability of self-stimulation responding during long test sessions. *Physiology and Behavior,* 1968, *3,* 161–165.

Rechtschaffen, A., & Kales, A. *A manual of standardized terminology, techniques, and scoring system for sleep stages of human subjects.* Bethesda, Md.: National Institutes of Health, 1968.

Reinis, S. The formation of conditioned reflexes in

rats after the parenteral administration of brain homogenate. *Activitas Nervosa Superior,* 1965, *7,* 167–168.

Rickert, E. J., & Bennett, T. L. Performance of hippocampectomized rats on discontinuous negatively correlated reward. *Behavioral Biology,* 1972, *7,* 375–382.

Rickert, E. J., Bennett, T. L., Anderson, G. J., Corbett, J., & Smith, L. Differential performance of hippocampally ablated rats on non-discriminated and discriminated DRL schedules. *Behavioral Biology,* 1973, *8,* 597–609.

Roberts, R. B., Flexner, J. B., & Flexner, L. B. Some evidence for the involvement of adrenergic sites in the memory trace. *Proceedings of the National Academy of Sciences,* 1970, *66,* 310–313.

Roberts, W. W. Both rewarding and punishing effects from stimulation of posterior hypothalamus of cat with same electrode at same intensity. *Journal of Comparative and Physiological Psychology,* 1958, *51,* 400–407. (a)

Roberts, W. W. Rapid escape learning without avoidance learning motivated by hypothalamic stimulation in cats. *Journal of Comparative and Physiological Psychology,* 1958, *51,* 391–399. (b)

Roberts, W. W., Dember, W. N., & Brodwick, M. Alternation and exploration in rats with hippocampal lesions. *Journal of Comparative and Physiological Psychology,* 1962, *55,* 695–700.

Roberts, W. W., Steinberg, M. L., & Means, L. W. Hypothalamic mechanisms for sexual, aggressive, and other motivational behaviors in the opossum, *Didilphis Virginiana. Journal of Comparative and Physiological Psychology,* 1967, *64,* 1–15.

Roeder, F., Orthner, H., & Müller, D. The stereotaxic treatment of pedophilic homosexuality and other sexual deviations. In E. Hitchcock, L. Laitenen, & K. Vaernet (Eds.), *Psychosurgery.* Springfield, Ill.: Charles C Thomas, 1972, 87–111.

Roffwarg, H. P., Muzio, J. N., & Dement, W. C. Ontogenetic development of the human sleep-dream cycle. *Science,* 1966, *152,* 604–619.

Rose, J. E. Organization of frequency sensitive neurons in the cochlear nuclear complex of the cat. In G. L. Rasmussen & W. F. Windle (Eds.), *Neural mechanisms of the auditory and vestibular systems.* Springfield, Ill.: Charles C Thomas, 1960, 116–136.

Rose, J. E., Greenwood, D. D., Goldberg, J. M., & Hind, J. E. Some discharge characteristics of single neurons in the inferior colliculus of the cat. I. Tonotopic organization, relation of spike counts to tone intensity, and firing patterns of single elements. *Journal of Neurophysiology,* 1963, *26,* 294–320.

Rosenzweig, M. R. Effects of environment on development of brain and behavior. In E. Tobach, L. R. Aronson, & E. Shaw (Eds.), *The*

biopsychology of development. New York: Academic Press, 1971, 303–342.

Rosenzweig, M. R., & Bennett, E. L. Cerebral changes in rats exposed individually to an enriched environment. *Journal of Comparative and Physiological Psychology,* 1972, *80,* 304–313.

Rosenzweig, M. R., Bennett, E. L., & Diamond, M. C. Chemical and anatomical plasticity of brain: Replications and extensions, 1970. In J. Gaito (Ed.), *Macromolecules and behavior* (2nd ed.). New York: Appleton-Century-Crofts, 1972, 205–278.

Ross, J. *Neurological findings after prolonged sleep deprivation.* Paper presented to the Association for the Psychophysiological Study of Sleep, 1964.

Rosvold, H. E., & Szwarcbart, M. K. Neural structures involved in delayed-response performance. In J. M. Warren & K. Akert (Eds.), *The frontal granular cortex and behavior.* New York: McGraw-Hill, 1964, 1–15.

Routtenberg, A. Forebrain pathways of reward in *Rattus Norvegicus. Journal of Comparative and Physiological Psychology,* 1971, *75,* 269–276.

Routtenberg, A. Intracranial chemical injection and behavior: A critical review. *Behavioral Biology,* 1972, *7,* 601–641.

Routtenberg, A., & Olds, J. Stimulation of dorsal midbrain during septal and hypothalamic self-stimulation. *Journal of Comparative and Physiological Psychology,* 1966, *62,* 250–255.

Rowland, V. Cortical steady potential (direct current potential) in reinforcement and learning. In E. Stellar & J. M. Sprague (Eds.), *Progress in physiological psychology* (Vol. 2). New York: Academic Press, 1968, 1–77.

Rowland, V., & Anderson, R. Brain steady potential shifts. In E. Stellar & J. M. Sprague (Eds.), *Progress in physiological psychology* (Vol. 4). New York: Academic Press, 1971, 37–51.

Rowland, V., Bradley, H., School, P., & Deutschman, D. Cortical steady potential shifts in conditioning. *Conditional Reflex,* 1967, *2,* 3–22.

Rutherford, W. A. A new theory of hearing. *Journal of Anatomy and Physiology,* 1886, *21,* 166–168.

Saavedra, M. A., Pinto-Hamuy, T., & Oberti, C. Auditory avoidance behavior after extensive and restrictive neocortical lesions in the rat. *Journal of Comparative and Physiological Psychology,* 1965, *60,* 41–45.

Sampson, H. Psychological effects of deprivation of dreaming sleep. *Journal of Nervous and Mental Disease,* 1966, *143,* 305–317.

Sassin, J. F., Parker, D. C., Mace, J. W., Gotlin, R. W., Johnson, L. C., & Rossman, L. G. Human growth hormone release: Relation to slow-wave sleep and sleep-waking cycles. *Science,* 1969, *165,* 513–515.

Sawyer, C. H. Triggering of the pituitary by the central nervous system. In T. H. Bullock (Ed.),

Physiological triggers. Washington, D. C.: American Physiological Society, 1957, 164–174.

Sawyer, C. H. Reproductive behavior. In J. Field (Ed.), *Handbook of Physiology; Section I: Neurophysiology* (Vol. 2). Washington, D. C.: American Physiological Society, 1960, 1225–1240.

Sawyer, C. H., & Robison, B. Separate hypothalamic areas controlling pituitary gonadotrophic function and mating behavior in female cats and rabbits. *Journal of Clinical Endocrinology,* 1956, *16,* 914.

Schiller, P. H., & Chorover, S. L. Short-term amnesic effects of electroconvulsive shock in a one-trial maze learning paradigm. *Neuropsychologia,* 1967, *5,* 155–163.

Schiltz, K. A., Thompson, C. I., Harlow, H. F., Mohr, D. J., & Blomquist, A. J. Learning in monkeys after combined lesions in frontal and anterior temporal lobes. *Journal of Comparative and Physiological Psychology,* 1973, *83,* 271–277.

Schmaltz, L. W., & Isaacson, R. L. The effects of preliminary training conditions upon DRL performance in the hippocampectomized rat. *Physiology and Behavior,* 1966, *1,* 175–182.

Schneider, A. M. Spreading depression: A behavioral analysis. In J. A. Deutsch (Ed.), *The physiological basis of memory.* New York: Academic Press, 1973, 269–304.

Schneider, A. M., Kapp, B., Aron, C., & Jarvik, M. E. Retroactive effects of transcorneal and transpinnate ECS on step-through latencies of mice and rats. *Journal of Comparative and Physiological Psychology,* 1969, *69,* 506–509.

Schneider, R. A. The sense of smell in man—its physiological basis. *New England Journal of Medicine,* 1967, *277,* 299–303.

Schreiner, L. H., & Kling, A. Behavioral changes following rhinencephalic injury in cat. *Journal of Neurophysiology,* 1953, *16,* 643–659.

Schreiner, L. H., Rioch, D., Pechtel, C., & Masserman, J. Behavioral changes following thalamic injury in cat. *Journal of Neurophysiology,* 1953, *16,* 234–246.

Schwartzbaum, J. S., & Donovick, P. J. Discrimination reversal and spatial alternation associated with septal and caudate dysfunction in rats. *Journal of Comparative and Physiological Psychology,* 1968, *65,* 83–92.

Schwartzbaum, J. S., Green, R. H., Beatty, W. W., & Thompson, J. B. Acquisition of avoidance behavior following septal lesions in the rat. *Journal of Comparative and Physiological Psychology,* 1967, *63,* 95–104.

Schwartzbaum, J. S., Kellicutt, M. H., Spieth, T. M., & Thompson, J. B. Effect of septal lesions in rats on response inhibition associated with food-reinforced behavior. *Journal of Comparative and Physiological Psychology,* 1964, *58,* 217–224.

Sclafani, A. Neural pathways involved in the ventromedial hypothalamic lesion syndrome in the rat. *Journal of Comparative and Physiological Psychology,* 1971, *77,* 70–96.

Sclafani, A., Berner, C. N., & Maul, G. Feeding and drinking pathways between medial and lateral hypothalamus in the rat. *Journal of Comparative and Physiological Psychology,* 1973, *85,* 29–51.

Sclafani, A., & Kluge, L. Food motivation and body weight levels in hypothalamic hyperphagic rats: A dual lipostat model of hunger and appetite. *Journal of Comparative and Physiological Psychology,* 1974, *86,* 28–46.

Scoville, W. B. The limbic lobe in man. *Journal of Neurosurgery,* 1954, *11,* 64–66.

Scoville, W. B. Late results of orbital undercutting: Report of 76 patients undergoing quantitative selective lobotomies. *Proceedings of the Royal Society of Medicine,* 1960, *53,* 721–728.

Scoville, W. B., & Milner, B. Loss of recent memory after bilateral hippocampal lesions. *Journal of Neurology, Neurosurgery and Psychiatry,* 1957, *20,* 11–21.

Segal, M., Disterhoft, J., & Olds, J. Hippocampal unit activity during aversive and appetitive conditioning. *Science,* 1972, *175,* 792–794.

Segal, M., & Olds, J. The behavior of units in the hippocampal circuit of the rat during learning. *Journal of Neurophysiology,* 1972, *35,* 680–690.

Segal, M., & Olds, J. Activity of units in the hippocampal circuit of the rat during differential classical conditioning. *Journal of Comparative and Physiological Psychology,* 1973, *82,* 195–204.

Seward, J. P., Uyeda, A. A., & Olds, J. Resistance to extinction following cranial self-stimulation. *Journal of Comparative and Physiological Psychology,* 1959, *52,* 294–299.

Sheafor, P. J., & Rowland, V. Dissociation of cortical steady potential shifts from mass action potentials in cats awaiting food rewards. *Physiological Psychology,* 1974, *2,* 471–480.

Sheer, D. E. (Ed.). *Electrical stimulation of the brain.* Austin: University of Texas Press, 1961.

Sheer, D. E. Electrophysiological correlates of memory consolidation. In G. Ungar (Ed.), *Molecular mechanisms in learning and memory.* New York: Plenum Press, 1970, 177–211.

Siegel, A., Bandler, R. J., Jr., & Flynn, J. P. Thalamic sites and pathways related to elicited attack. *Brain, Behavior, and Evolution,* 1972, *6,* 542–555.

Siegel, A., & Chabora, J. Effects of electrical stimulation of the cingulate gyrus upon attack behavior elicited from the hypothalamus in the cat. *Brain Research,* 1971, *32,* 169–177.

Siegel, A., Edinger, H., & Lowenthal, H. Effects of electrical stimulation of the medial aspect of the prefrontal cortex upon attack behavior in cats. *Brain Research,* 1974, *66,* 467–479.

Siegel, A., & Flynn, J. P. Differential effects of electrical stimulation and lesions of the hippocampus and adjacent regions upon attack behavior in cats. *Brain Research,* 1968, *7,* 252–267.

Siegel, A., & Skog, D. Effects of electrical stimulation of the septum upon attack behavior elicited from the hypothalamus in the cat. *Brain Research,* 1970, *23,* 371–380.

Singer, G., & Montgomery, R. B. Functional relationship of lateral hypothalamus and amygdala in control of drinking. *Physiology and Behavior,* 1969, *4,* 505–507.

Singer, J. J. Hypothalamic control of male and female sexual behavior in the female rat. *Journal of Comparative and Physiological Psychology,* 1968, *66,* 738–742.

Singh, D. Comparison of behavioral deficits caused by lesions in septal and ventromedial hypothalamic areas of female rats. *Journal of Comparative and Physiological Psychology,* 1973, *84,* 370–379.

Singh, D., & Avery, D. D. *Physiological techniques in behavioral research.* Monterey, Calif.: Brooks/Cole, 1975.

Skinner, J. E. *Neuroscience: A laboratory manual.* Philadelphia: W. B. Saunders, 1971.

Slangen, J. L., & Miller, N. E. Pharmacological tests for the function of hypothalamic norepinephrine in eating behavior. *Physiology and Behavior,* 1969, *4,* 543–552.

Smith, D. E., King, M. B., & Hoebel, B. G. Lateral hypothalamic control of killing: Evidence for a cholinoceptive mechanism. *Science,* 1970, *167,* 900–901.

Smith, L. T. The interanimal transfer model: A review. *Psychological Bulletin,* 1974, *81,* 1078–1095.

Smith, O. A. Stimulation of lateral and medial hypothalamus and food intake in the rat. *Anatomical Record,* 1956, *124,* 363–364.

Smith, W. K. The results of ablation of the cingular region of the cerebral cortex. *Federation Proceedings,* 1944, *3,* 42–43.

Snyder, D. R., & Isaacson, R. L. Effects of large and small bilateral hippocampal lesions on two types of passive-avoidance responses. *Psychological Reports,* 1965, *16,* 1277–1290.

Sodetz, F. J., Matalka, E. S., & Bunnell, B. N. Septal ablation and the social behavior of the golden hamster. *Psychonomic Science,* 1967, *7,* 189–190.

Spevack, A. A., & Suboski, M. D. Retrograde effects of electroconvulsive shock on learned responses. *Psychological Bulletin,* 1969, *72,* 66–76.

Spiegel, E. A., Miller, H. R., & Oppenheimer, M. J. Forebrain and rage reactions. *Journal of Neurophysiology,* 1940, *3,* 538–547.

Spiegel, T. A., Hostetter, G., & Thomas, G. J. Effects of bilateral lesions in the hippocampus on acquisition of two-maze problems. *Psychonomic Science,* 1966, *6,* 205–206.

Springer, A. D., Schoel, W. M., Klinger, P. D., & Agranoff, B. W. Anterograde and retrograde effects of electroconvulsive shock and puromycin on memory formation in the goldfish. *Behavioral Biology,* 1975, *13,* 467–481.

Spurzheim, G. *Powers and organs of the mind,* 1834.

Squire, L. R., & Barondes, S. H. Anisomycin, like other inhibitors of cerebral protein synthesis, impairs "long-term" memory of a discrimination task. *Brain Research,* 1974, *66,* 301–308.

Squire, L. R., & Davis, H. P. Cerebral protein synthesis inhibition and discrimination training: Effects of extent and duration of inhibition. *Behavioral Biology,* 1975, *13,* 49–57.

Steggerda, F. R. Observations on the water intake in an adult man with dysfunctioning salivary glands. *American Journal of Physiology,* 1941, *131,* 517–521.

Stein, D. G., & Kimble, D. P. Effects of hippocampal lesions and posttrial strychnine administration on maze behavior in the rat. *Journal of Comparative and Physiological Psychology,* 1966, *62,* 243–249.

Stein, D. G., & Kirkby, R. J. The effects of training on passive avoidance: A reply to Isaacson, Olton, Bauer, and Swart. *Psychonomic Science,* 1967, *7,* 7–8.

Stevens, C. F. *Neurophysiology: A primer.* New York: Wiley, 1966.

Stevenson, J. A. F. Mechanisms in the control of food and water intake. *Annals of the New York Academy of Sciences,* 1969, *157,* 1069–1083.

Stewart, W. W. Comments on the chemistry of scotophobin. *Nature,* 1972, *238,* 202.

Stokman, C. L. J., & Glusman, M. Suppression of hypothalamically produced flight responses by punishment. *Physiology and Behavior,* 1969, *4,* 523–525.

Stokman, C. L. J., & Glusman, M. Amygdaloid modulation of hypothalamic flight in cats. *Journal of Comparative and Physiological Psychology,* 1970, *71,* 365–375.

Stricker, E. M. Extracellular fluid volume and thirst. *American Journal of Physiology,* 1966, *211,* 232–238.

Stricker, E. M., & Jalowiec, J. E. Restoration of intravascular fluid volume following acute hypovolemia in rats. *American Journal of Physiology,* 1970, *218,* 191–196.

Stricker, E. M., & Wolf, G. Blood volume and tonicity in relation to sodium appetite. *Journal of Comparative and Physiological Psychology,* 1966, *62,* 275–279.

Stricker, E. M., & Wolf, G. Behavioral control of intravascular fluid volume: Thirst and sodium appetite. *Annals of the New York Academy of Sciences,* 1969, *157,* 553–568.

Strominger, N. L. Localization of sound in space

after unilateral and bilateral ablation of auditory cortex. *Experimental Neurology,* 1969, *25,* 521–533.

Stumpf, W. E. Estradiol-concentrating neurons: Topography in the hypothalamus by dry mount autoradiography. *Science,* 1968, *162,* 1001–1003.

Stunkard, A. J., Van Itallie, T. B., & Reis, B. B. The mechanism of satiety: Effect of glucagon on gastric hunger contractions in man. *Proceedings of the Society of Experimental Biology and Medicine,* 1955, *89,* 258–261.

Sundsten, J. W. Alterations in water intake and core temperature in baboons during hypothalamic thermal stimulation. *Annals of the New York Academy of Sciences,* 1969, *157,* 1018–1029.

Swanson, H. H., & Crossley, D. A. Sexual behavior in the golden hamster and its modification by neonatal administration of testosterone propionate. In M. Hamburgh & E. J. W. Berrington (Eds.), *Proceedings of the International Conference on Hormones in Development.* New York: Appleton-Century-Crofts, 1971, 677–687.

Teitelbaum, H. A comparison of effects of orbitofrontal and hippocampal lesions upon discrimination learning and reversal in the cat. *Experimental Neurology,* 1964, *9,* 452–462.

Teitelbaum, H., & Milner, P. Activity changes following partial hippocampal lesions in rats. *Journal of Comparative and Physiological Psychology,* 1963, *56,* 284–289.

Teitelbaum, P. Sensory control of hypothalamic hyperphagia. *Journal of Comparative and Physiological Psychology,* 1955, *48,* 156–163.

Teitelbaum, P. Random and food-directed activity in hyperphagic and normal rats. *Journal of Comparative and Physiological Psychology,* 1957, *50,* 486–490.

Teitelbaum, P. Disturbances in feeding and drinking behavior after hypothalamic lesions. In M. R. Jones (Ed.), *Nebraska Symposium on Motivation: 1961.* Lincoln: University of Nebraska Press, 1961, 39–65.

Teitelbaum, P. Appetite. *Proceedings of the American Philosophical Society,* 1964, *108,* 464–472.

Teitelbaum, P., & Epstein, A. N. The lateral hypothalamic syndrome: Recovery of feeding and drinking after lateral hypothalamic lesions. *Psychological Review,* 1962, *69,* 74–90.

Teitelbaum, P., & Stellar, E. Recovery from the failure to eat produced by hypothalamic lesions. *Science,* 1954, *120,* 894–895.

Thomas, C. N., & Gerall, A. A. Effect of hour of operation on feminization of neonatally castrated male rats. *Psychonomic Science,* 1969, *16,* 19–20.

Thomas, G. J. Maze retention by rats with hippocampal lesions and with fornicotomies. *Journal of Comparative and Physiological Psychology,* 1971, *75,* 41–49.

Thomas, G. J., Frey, W. J., Slotnik, B. M., & Kriekhaus, E. E. Behavioral effects of mammillothalamic tractotomy in cats. *Journal of Neurophysiology,* 1963, *26,* 857–876.

Thomas, G. J., Hostetter, G., & Barker, D. J. Behavioral functions of the limbic system. In E. Stellar & J. M. Sprague (Eds.), *Progress in physiological psychology,* (Vol. 2). New York: Academic Press, 1968, 230–311.

Thomas, G. J., & Otis, L. S. Effects of rhinencephalic lesions on conditioning of avoidance responses in the rat. *Journal of Comparative and Physiological Psychology,* 1958, *51,* 130–134.

Thomas, G. J., & Slotnik, B. M. Effects of lesions in the cingulum on maze learning and avoidance conditioning in the rat. *Journal of Comparative and Physiological Psychology,* 1962, *55,* 1085–1091.

Thomas, G. J., & Slotnik, B. M. Impairment of avoidance responding by lesions in cingulate cortex in rats depends on food drive. *Journal of Comparative and Physiological Psychology,* 1963, *56,* 959–964.

Thompson, J. B., & Schwartzbaum, J. S. Discrimination behavior and conditioned suppression (CER) following localized lesions in the amygdala and putamen. *Psychological Reports,* 1964, *15,* Mon. Suppl. 4-V15, 587–606.

Thompson, R. The effects of degree of learning and problem difficulty on perseveration. *Journal of Experimental Psychology,* 1958, *55,* 496–500.

Thompson, R. Localization of the "visual memory system" in the white rat. *Journal of Comparative and Physiological Psychology,* 1969, *69*(4:2), 1–29.

Thompson, R. Localization of the "maze memory system" in the white rat. *Physiological Psychology,* 1974, *2,* 1–17.

Thompson, R., & Langer, S. K. Deficits in position reversal learning following lesions of the limbic system. *Journal of Comparative and Physiological Psychology,* 1963, *56,* 987–995.

Thompson, R., Lesse, H., & Rich, I. Pretectal lesions in rats and cats. *Journal of Comparative Neurology,* 1963, *121,* 161–171.

Thompson, R., & Massopust, L. C. The effect of subcortical lesions on retention of a brightness discrimination in rats. *Journal of Comparative and Physiological Psychology,* 1960, *53,* 488–496.

Thompson, R., & McConnell, J. V. Classical conditioning in the planarian, *Dugesia dorotocephala. Journal of Comparative and Physiological Psychology,* 1955, *48,* 65–68.

Thompson, R. F., & Spencer, W. A. Habituation: A model phenomenon for the study of neuronal substrates of behavior. *Psychological Review,* 1966, *73,* 16–43.

Thompson, R. K. R., & Webster, D. M. C. D. Delayed extinction and drive level effects: Septal self-stimulation compared with natural reward. *Physiology and Behavior,* 1974, *12,* 907–912.

Tigner, J. C. The effects of dorsomedial thalamic lesions on learning, reversal and alternation behavior in the rat. *Physiology and Behavior,* 1974, *12,* 13–17.

Trafton, C. L. Effects of lesions in the septal area and cingulate cortical areas on conditioned suppression of activity and avoidance behavior in rats. *Journal of Comparative and Physiological Psychology,* 1967, *68,* 191–197.

Trafton, C. L., Fibley, R. A., & Johnson, R. W. Avoidance behavior in rats as a function of the size and location of anterior cingulate cortex lesions. *Psychonomic Science,* 1969, *14,* 100–102.

Travis, R. P., Jr., Hooten, T. F., & Sparks, D. L. Single unit activity related to behavior motivated by food reward. *Physiology and Behavior,* 1968, *3,* 309–318.

Travis, R. P., Jr., & Sparks, D. L. Changes in unit activity during stimuli associated with food and shock reinforcement. *Physiology and Behavior,* 1967, *2,* 171–177.

Travis, R. P., Jr., Sparks, D. L., & Hooten, T. F. Single unit response related to sequences of food motivated behavior. *Brain Research,* 1968, *7,* 455–458.

Truax, T., & Thompson, R. Role of the hippocampus in performance of easy and difficult discrimination tasks. *Journal of Comparative and Physiological Psychology,* 1969, *67,* 228–234.

Truex, R. C., & Carpenter, M. B. *Strong and Elwyn's human neuroanatomy* (5th ed.). Baltimore: Williams & Wilkins, 1964.

Tsang, Y. C. The function of the visual areas of the cortex of the rat in the learning and retention of the maze. *Comparative Psychology Monographs,* 1934, *10,* 1–56.

Tsuchitani, C., & Boudreau, J. C. Single unit analysis of cat superior olive S-segment with tonal stimuli. *Journal of Neurophysiology,* 1966, *29,* 684–697.

Ulrich, R. E., & Azrin, N. H. Reflexive fighting in response to aversive stimulation. *Journal of the Experimental Analysis of Behavior,* 1962, *5,* 511–520.

Ungar, G. Transfer of learned information by brain extracts. *Federation Proceedings,* 1967, *26,* 263.

Ungar, G. Learned fear transferred by a brain peptide. *Federation Proceedings,* 1968, *27,* 223.

Ungar, G. Chemical transfer of passive avoidance. *Federation Proceedings,* 1969, *28,* 647.

Ungar, G. Molecular mechanisms in information processing. *International Review of Neurobiology,* 1970, *13,* 223–253. (a)

Ungar, G. (Ed.), *Molecular mechanisms in memory and learning.* New York: Plenum Press, 1970. (b)

Ungar, G., Desiderio, D. M., & Parr, W. Isolation and synthesis of a specific-behavior-inducing peptide. *Nature,* 1972, *238,* 198–202.

Ungar, G., & Oceguera-Navarro, C. Transfer of habituation by material extracted from brain. *Nature,* 1965, *207,* 301–302.

Ursin, H. The effect of amygdaloid lesions on flight and defense behavior in cats. *Experimental Neurology,* 1965, *11,* 61–79. (a)

Ursin, H. Effect of amygdaloid lesions on avoidance behavior and visual discrimination in cats. *Experimental Neurology,* 1965, *11,* 298–317. (b)

Ursin, H. The cingulate gyrus—a fear zone? *Journal of Comparative and Physiological Psychology,* 1969, *68,* 235–238.

Ursin, H., & Kaada, B. R. Functional localization within the amygdaloid complex in the cat. *Electroencephalography and Clinical Neurophysiology,* 1960, *12,* 1–20.

Ursin, R., Ursin, H., & Olds, J. Self-stimulation of hippocampus in rats, *Journal of Comparative and Physiological Psychology,* 1966, *61,* 353–359.

Valatx, J. L., Jouvet, D., & Jouvet, M. Evolution electroencephalographique des differents estats de sommeil chez le chaton. *Electroencephalography and Clinical Neurophysiology,* 1964, *17,* 218–233.

Valenstein, E. S. The anatomical locus of reinforcement. In E. Stellar & J. M. Sprague (Eds.), *Progress in physiological psychology* (Vol. 1.) New York: Academic Press, 1966, 149–190.

Valenstein, E. S. *Brain control.* New York: Wiley, 1973.

Valenstein, E. S., & Campbell, J. F. Medial forebrain bundle-lateral hypothalamic area and reinforcing brain stimulation. *American Journal of Physiology,* 1966, *210,* 270–274.

Valenstein, E. S., Cox, V. C., & Kakolewski, J. W. Polydipsia elicited by the synergistic action of a saccharin and glucose solution. *Science,* 1967, *157,* 552–554.

Valenstein, E. S., Riss, W., & Young, W. C. Experiential and genetic factors in the organization of sexual behavior in male guinea pigs. *Journal of Comparative and Physiological Psychology,* 1955, *48,* 397–403.

Valenstein, E. S., & Valenstein, T. On the interaction of positive and negative reinforcing neural systems. *Science,* 1964, *145,* 1456–1458.

Vanderwolf, C. H. Improved shuttle-box performance following electroconvulsive shock. *Journal of Comparative and Physiological Psychology,* 1963, *56,* 983–986.

Vanderwolf, C. H. Limbic-diencephalic mechanisms of voluntary movement. *Psychological Review,* 1971, *78,* 83–113.

Vanderwolf, C. H., Kramis, R., Gillespie, L. A., & Bland, B. H. Hippocampal rhythmic slow activity and neocortical low voltage fast activity: Relations to behavior. In R. L. Isaacson & K. H. Pribram (Eds.), *The Hippocampus* (Vol. 2):

Neurophysiology and behavior. New York: Plenum Press, 1975, 101–128.

Van Deventer, J. M., & Ratner, S. C. Variables affecting the frequency of response of planaria to light. *Journal of Comparative and Physiological Psychology,* 1964, *57,* 407–411.

Van Dis, H., & Larsson, K. Induction of sexual arousal in the castrated male rat by intracranial stimulation. *Physiology and Behavior,* 1971, *6,* 85–86.

Vaughn, E., & Fisher, A. E. Male sexual behavior induced by intracranial electrical stimulation. *Science,* 1962, *137,* 758–760.

Verney, E. B. The antidiuretic hormone and the factors which determine its release. *Proceedings of the Royal Society,* 1947, *B135,* 25–106.

Victor, M., & Yakovlev, P. S. S. Korsakoff's psychic disorder. *Neurology,* 1955, *5,* 394–407.

Volkmar, F. R., & Greenough, W. T. Rearing complexity affects branching of dendrites in the visual cortex of the rat. *Science,* 1972, *176,* 1445–1447.

Wade, M. The effect of sedatives upon delayed response in monkeys following removal of the prefrontal lobes. *Journal of Neurophysiology,* 1947, *10,* 57–61.

Walter, W. G. The location of cerebral tumours by electroencephalography. *Lancet,* 1936, *2,* 305–308.

Walter, W. G. Slow potential waves in the human brain associated with expectancy, attention and decision. *Archiv für die Psychiatrie und Zeitschrift für die gesamte Neurologie,* 1964, *206,* 309–322.

Wampler, R. S. Increased motivation in rats with ventromedial hypothalamic lesions. *Journal of Comparative and Physiological Psychology,* 1973, *84,* 275–285.

Ward, A. A., Jr. The cingular gyrus: Area 24. *Journal of Neurophysiology,* 1948, *11,* 13–23.

Ward, I. L. Female sexual behavior in male rats treated prenatally with anti-androgen. *Physiology and Behavior,* 1972, *8,* 53–56.

Ward, I. L., & Renz, F. J. Consequences of perinatal hormone manipulation on the adult sexual behavior of female rats. *Journal of Comparative and Physiological Psychology,* 1972, *78,* 349–355.

Warren, J. M. The behavior of carnivores and primates with lesions in the prefrontal cortex. In J. M. Warren & K. Akert (Eds.), *The frontal granular cortex and behavior.* New York: McGraw-Hill, 1964, 168–191.

Warren, J. M., Coutant, L. W., & Cornwell, P. R. Cortical lesions and response inhibition in cats. *Neuropsychologia,* 1969, *7,* 245–257.

Warren, J. M., Warren, H. B., & Akert, K. Learning by cats with lesions in the prestriate cortex. *Journal of Comparative and Physiological Psychology,* 1961, *54,* 629–632.

Warrington, E. K., & Weiskrantz, L. An analysis of short-term and long-term memory defects in man. In J. A. Deutsch (Ed.), *The physiological basis of memory.* New York: Academic Press, 1973, 365–395.

Wasman, M., & Flynn, J. P. Directed attack elicited from hypothalamus. *Archives of Neurology,* 1962, *6,* 220–227.

Webb, W. B. Some effects of prolonged sleep deprivation on the hooded rat. *Journal of Comparative and Physiological Psychology,* 1962, *55,* 791–793.

Webb, W. B., & Agnew, H. W., Jr. Sleep: Effects of a restricted regime. *Science,* 1965, *150,* 1745–1747.

Webb, W. B., & Agnew, H. W., Jr. Stage 4 sleep: Influence of time course variables. *Science,* 1971, *174,* 1354–1356.

Webster, D. B., & Voneida, R. J. Learning deficits following hippocampal lesions in split-brain cats. *Experimental Neurology,* 1964, *10,* 170-182.

Weddell, G., & Verrillo, R. T. Common sensibility. In M. Critchley, J. L. O'Leary, & B. Jennett (Eds.), *Scientific foundations of neurology.* Philadelphia: Davis, 1972, 117–125.

Weiskrantz, L. Neurological studies and animal behavior. *British Medical Bulletin,* 1964, *20,* 49–53.

Weiskrantz, L., Mihailović, L., & Gross, C. G. Effects of stimulation of frontal cortex and hippocampus on behavior. *Brain,* 1962, *85,* 487–504.

Weiskrantz, L., & Mishkin, M. Effects of temporal and frontal cortical lesions on auditory discrimination in monkey. *Brain,* 1958, *81,* 406–414.

Weiss, C. S., & Hertzler, D. R. Facilitation of two-way avoidance of the guinea pig following intrahippocampal injections of procaine hydrochloride. *Physiological Psychology,* 1973, *1,* 305–307.

Wernicke, C. *Der Aphasische Symptomenkomplex.* Breslau: Cohn and Weigart, 1874.

Wetzel, M. C. Self-stimulation aftereffects and runway performance in the rat. *Journal of Comparative and Physiological Psychology,* 1963, *56,* 673–678.

Wever, E. G. *Theory of hearing.* New York: Wiley, 1949.

Wever, E. G. Development of traveling-wave theories. *Journal of the Acoustical Society of America,* 1962, *34,* 1319–1324.

Whalen, R. E., & Edwards, D. A. Hormonal determinants of the development of masculine and feminine behavior in male and female rats. *Anatomical Record,* 1967, *157,* 173–180.

Whalen, R. E., Edwards, D. A., Luttge, W. G., & Robertson, R. T. Early androgen treatment and male sexual behavior in female rats. *Physiology and Behavior,* 1969, *4,* 33–39.

Wheatley, M. D. The hypothalamus and affective

behavior in cats. *Archives of Neurology and Psychiatry,* 1944, *52,* 296–316.

White, N. M., & Fisher, A. E. Relationship between amygdala and hypothalamus in the control of eating behavior. *Physiology and Behavior,* 1969, *4,* 199–205.

Whitty, C. M. W., Duffield, J. E., Tow, P. W., & Cairns, H. Anterior cingulectomy in the treatment of mental disease. *Lancet,* 1952, *1,* 475–481.

Williams, D. R., & Teitelbaum, P. Some observations on the starvation resulting from lateral hypothalamic lesions. *Journal of Comparative and Physiological Psychology,* 1959, *52,* 458–465.

Williams, R. L., Karacan, I., & Hursch, C. J. *Electroencephalography (EEG) of human sleep: Clinical applications.* New York: Wiley, 1974.

Wilson, M. Effects of circumscribed cortical lesions upon somaesthetic and visual discrimination in the monkey. *Journal of Comparative and Physiological Psychology,* 1957, *50,* 630–635.

Winocur, G., & Mills, J. A. Hippocampus and septum in response inhibition. *Journal of Comparative and Physiological Psychology,* 1969, *67,* 352–357.

Winocur, G., & Mills, J. A. Transfer between related and unrelated problems following hippocampal lesions in rats. *Journal of Comparative and Physiological Psychology,* 1970, *73,* 162–169.

Winson, J. The theta mode of hippocampal function. In R. L. Isaacson & K. H. Pribram (Eds.), *The Hippocampus* (Vol.2): *Neurophysiology and behavior.* New York: Plenum Press, 1975, 169–183.

Wisenfeld, Z. Steady potential correlates of T-maze learning in the rat. Unpublished master's thesis, Case Western Reserve University, 1969.

Wood, C. D. Behavioral changes following discrete lesions of temporal lobe structures. *Neurology,* 1958, *8,* 215–220.

Woody, C., Vassilevsky, N. N., & Engle, J. Conditioned eye blink: Unit activity at coronal-precruciate cortex of the cat. *Journal of Neurophysiology,* 1970, *33,* 851–864.

Woolsey, C. N. Patterns of sensory representation in the cerebral cortex. *Federation Proceedings,* 1947, *6,* 437–441.

Wurtz, R. H., & Olds, J. Amygdaloid stimulation and operant reinforcement in the rat. *Journal of Comparative and Physiological Psychology,* 1963, *56,* 941–949.

Zelman, A., Kabat, L., Jacobson, R., & McConnell, J. V. Transfer of training through injection of "conditioned" RNA into untrained planarians. *Worm Runner's Digest,* 1963, *5,* 14–21.

Zigmond, R. E., & McEwen, B. S. Selective retention of oestradiol by cell nuclei in specific brain regions of the ovarectomized rat. *Journal of Neurochemistry,* 1970, *17,* 889–899.

Zinkin, S., & Miller, A. J. Recovery of memory after amnesia induced by electroconvulsive shock. *Science,* 1967, *155,* 102–104.

Zornetzer, S. F., & McGaugh, J. L. Retrograde amnesia and brain seizures in mice. *Physiology and Behavior,* 1971, *7,* 401–408. (a)

Zornetzer, S. F., & McGaugh, J. L. Retrograde amnesia and brain seizures in mice: A further analysis. *Physiology and Behavior, 1971, 7,* 841–845. (b)

Zucker, I. Effect of lesions of the septal-limbic area on the behavior of cats. *Journal of Comparative and Physiological Psychology,* 1965, *60,* 344–352.

Author Index

Subject Index